Aquatic Fitness Professional Manual

Seventh Edition

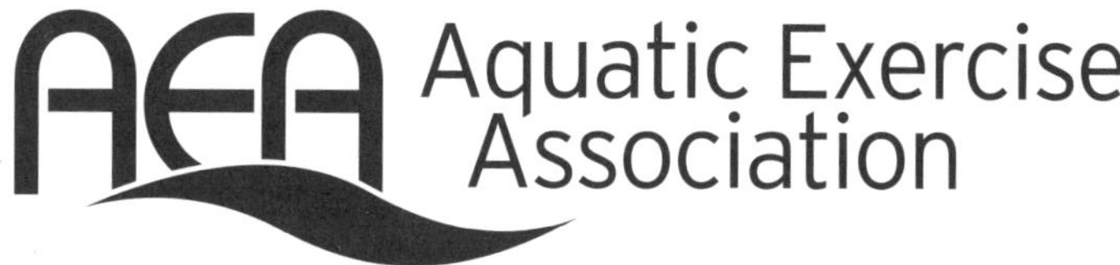

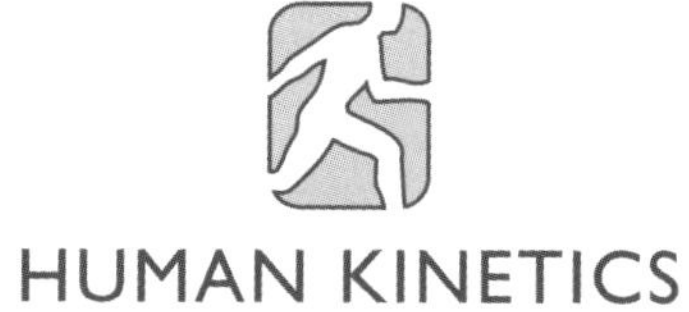

HUMAN KINETICS

Library of Congress Cataloging-in-Publication Data

Names: Aquatic Exercise Association.
Title: Aquatic Fitness Professional Manual / Aquatic Exercise Association.
Description: Seventh Edition. | Champaign, Illinois : Human Kinetics, [2018]
| Includes bibliographical references and index.
Identifiers: LCCN 2017027380 (print) | LCCN 2017011661 (ebook) | ISBN
9781492558460 (ebook) | ISBN 9781492533740 (print)
Subjects: LCSH: Aquatic exercises.
Classification: LCC GV838.53.E94 (print) | LCC GV838.53.E94 A68 2018 (ebook)
| DDC 613.7/16--dc23
LC record available at https://lccn.loc.gov/2017027380

ISBN: 978-1-4925-3374-0 (print)

The web addresses cited in this text were current as of June 2017, unless otherwise noted.

Acquisitions Editor: Michelle Maloney; **Developmental Editor:** Anne Hall; **Managing Editor:** Ann C. Gindes; **Copyeditor:** Joy Hoppenot; **Indexer:** Nan N. Badgett; **Permissions Manager:** Martha Gullo; **Graphic Designers:** Denise Lowry and Angela Snyder; **Cover Designer:** Keri Evans; **Photograph (cover):** © Aquatic Exercise Association; **Photographs (interior):** © Aquatic Exercise Association, unless otherwise noted; **Photo Asset Manager:** Laura Fitch; **Visual Production Assistant:** Joyce Brumfield; **Photo Production Manager:** Jason Allen; **Senior Art Manager:** Kelly Hendren; **Illustrations:** © Human Kinetics, unless otherwise noted; **Printer:** Versa Press

Printed in the United States of America 10 9 8 7 6 5 4 3 2

The paper in this book is certified under a sustainable forestry program.

Human Kinetics
P.O. Box 5076
Champaign, IL 61825-5076
Website: www.HumanKinetics.com

In the United States, email info@hkusa.com or call 800-747-4457.
In Canada, email info@hkcanada.com.
In the United Kingdom/Europe, email hk@hkeurope.com.

For information about Human Kinetics' coverage in other areas of the world, please visit our website: **www.HumanKinetics.com**

E6852

Contents

AEA Mission Statement and Purpose

Our Mission

The Aquatic Exercise Association (AEA) is a nonprofit organization committed to the advancement of aquatic fitness, health and wellness worldwide.

Our Purpose

AEA is committed to increasing awareness, education, and networking opportunities to benefit professionals as well as the general public. With AEA, achieving healthy lifestyles through aquatic fitness is a global team effort.

AEA desires to embrace cultural diversity in our industry to assure that individuals worldwide can enjoy and employ the benefits of aquatic fitness program regardless of age, ability, goals, or interests.

Purpose of Certification

The aquatic fitness professional certification was developed to increase public health, safety, and confidence in aquatic fitness programming led by certified professionals.

The aquatic fitness professional certification is designed to test a standard level of theoretical and practical competence and skill for aquatic fitness professionals to assure the highest level of programming and implementation to a wide range of participants.

The aquatic fitness professional certification offers certified professionals confidence and security through superior standards and current research implementation.

Acknowledgments

The Aquatic Exercise Association (AEA) acknowledges that education is a continuous process. Additionally, knowledge must be shared for it to expand and develop. Fitness is a dynamic field that is ever-changing, and thus requires an open mind and a willingness to continue learning.

This manual is dedicated to aquatic fitness professionals in every country who continue to share their time, talent, and passion to achieve the common goal of global health and quality of life through aquatic exercise.

AEA thanks everyone who has supported aquatic fitness, especially those who have been instrumental in making this educational manual possible.

Introduction

Welcome to the field of aquatic fitness—a vast array of programming options to enhance health and well-being for all ages and abilities. Although water exercise can encompass a wide variety of activities, this manual specifically targets vertical exercise in both shallow and deep water.

Exciting trends continue to emerge in the fitness industry, and aquatic fitness is at the forefront with reduced-impact yet challenging options for group exercise, small-group fitness, and personal training. The properties of water further enhance the benefits of many popular fitness formats, such as cycling, equipment-specific training, circuits, intervals (including HIIT), boot camp training, martial arts, yoga, Pilates, muscle conditioning, walking and jogging, functional fitness, and programs specific for various chronic conditions. Aquatic fitness no longer targets just the senior population. Safe and effective programs can be found for all age groups, including infants, children, teens, young adults, and, of course, the baby boomers.

This manual provides an excellent resource for fitness professionals and students seeking knowledge in aquatic fitness applications, education, and training. AEA sincerely hopes that the following pages inspire you to review, learn, and update those skills necessary to share the benefits of aquatic fitness with others effectively. As an association comprised of aquatic fitness professionals, therapists, personal trainers, athletic trainers, coaches, facility directors and managers, and aquatic fitness participants – may we all work together in the pursuit of a healthier global community.

Part I

Foundations of Fitness and Exercise

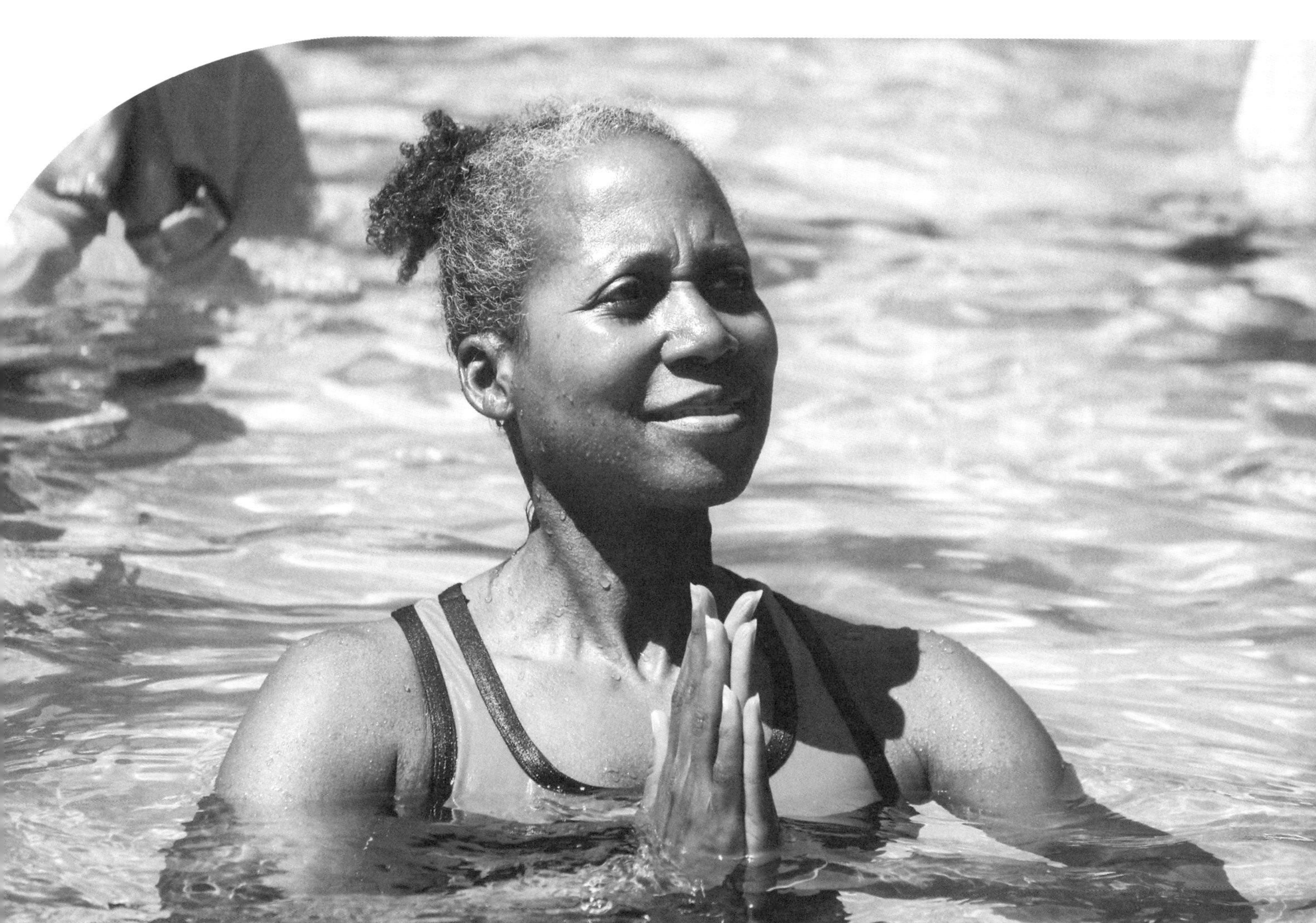

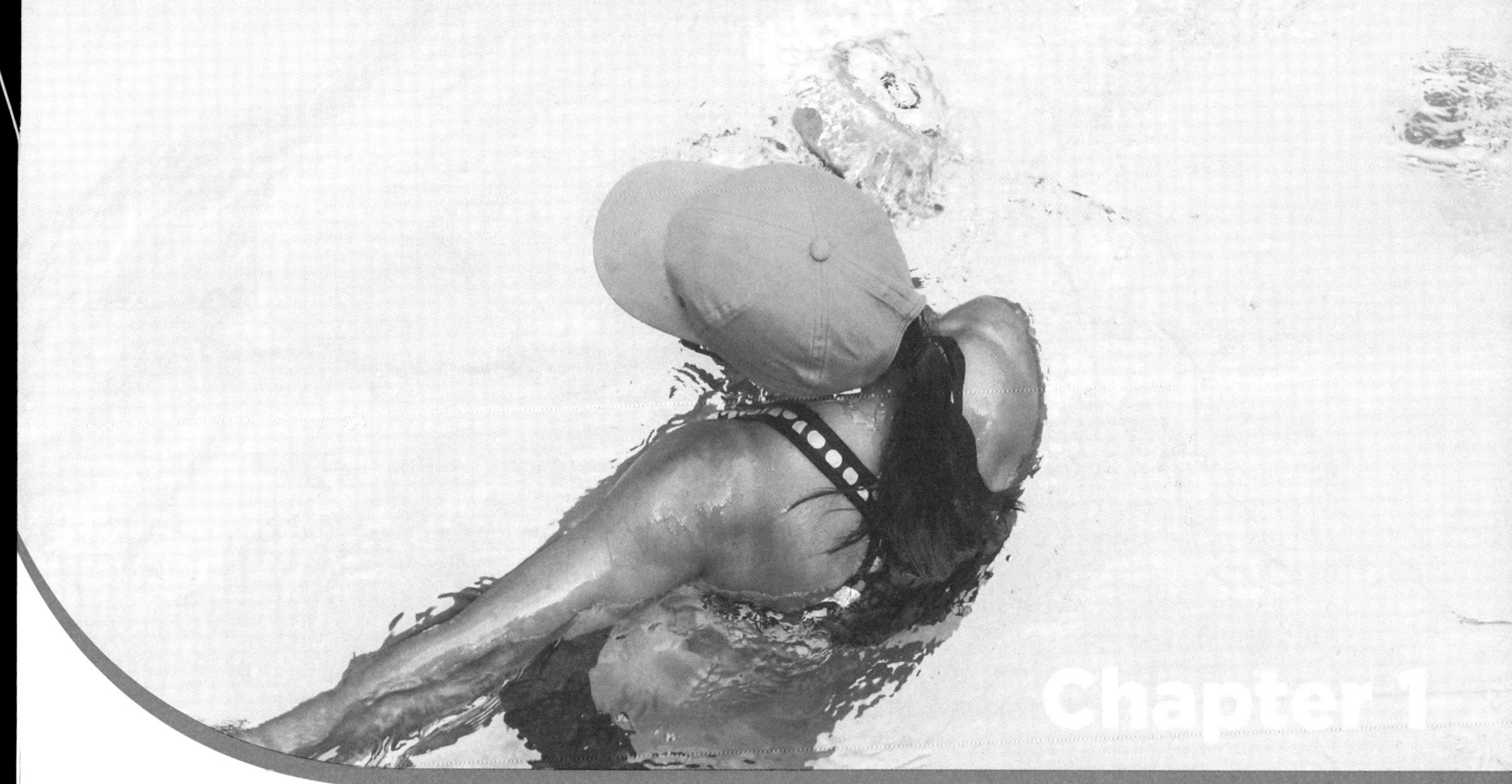

Physical Fitness

Introduction

This chapter highlights the components of physical fitness. Physical fitness describes physical activity with a purpose: the desire to maintain or improve functional capacity or a predetermined fitness level. Guidelines are outlined for the recommended quantity and quality of exercise for developing and maintaining overall fitness in healthy adults. The benefits of regular exercise and moderate-intensity physical activity are discussed as well as their effect on overall health and prevention of chronic disease.

Key Chapter Concepts

- Understand the differences between physical activity, exercise, and physical fitness.
- Define the major health-related components of physical fitness.
- Understand the 2018 American College of Sports Medicine guidelines regarding frequency, intensity, time, type, volume, and progression (FITT-VP) of exercise.
- Understand common methods for monitoring exercise intensity, including rating of perceived exertion and the application of the Kruel Aquatic Heart Rate Deduction.
- Explain the differences between continuous, interval, and circuit training formats.
- Recognize the physiological and psychological benefits of regular exercise as well as the specific benefits associated with aquatic-based exercise.

Physical Activity, Exercise, and Physical Fitness

The **American College of Sports Medicine (ACSM)** defines **physical activity** as movements of the body created by skeletal muscle contractions that result in a substantial increase of energy expenditure compared to resting levels. **Exercise** is a type of physical activity consisting of repetitive movement that is planned and structured to maintain or improve one or more fitness components. **Physical fitness** is a specific set of health-related and skill-related traits associated with the ability to perform physical activity.

Lack of physical activity is considered the fourth leading risk factor for global mortality (6% of deaths) following high blood pressure, the use of tobacco, and elevated blood **glucose** levels (WHO 2009). The U.S. Department of Health and Human Services' 2008 *Physical Activity Guidelines for Americans* describe the major research findings on the health benefits of physical activity:

- Regular physical activity reduces the risk of many adverse health outcomes.
- Some physical activity is better than none.
- For most health outcomes, additional benefits occur as the amount of physical activity increases through higher intensity, greater frequency, or longer duration.
- Most health benefits occur with at least 150 minutes (2 hours and 30 minutes) a week of moderate intensity physical activity, such as brisk walking. Additional benefits occur with more physical activity.
- Both aerobic (endurance) and muscle-strengthening (resistance) physical activities are beneficial.
- Health benefits occur for children and adolescents, young and middle-aged adults, older adults, and those in every studied racial and ethnic group.
- The health benefits of physical activity occur for people with disabilities.
- The benefits of physical activity far outweigh the possibility of adverse outcomes.

According to the Centers for Disease Control and Prevention (CDC), only about one in five American adults are meeting these physical activity guidelines (CDC 2014). However, evidence shows a relationship between increased physical activity and decreased risk for premature death, **stroke**, **hypertension**, type 2 diabetes, falls, and some types of **cancer**, as well as improvements in cognitive function, depression, and functional health (ACSM 2018). Organizations such as the American Cancer Society (ACS), American Heart Association (AHA), and National Heart, Lung, and Blood Institute (NHLBI) also support the importance of physical activity.

Health-Related Components of Physical Fitness

When designing a program to improve physical fitness and health, consider including aerobic, resistance, **flexibility**, and neuromotor exercise training (ACSM 2018). The ACSM exercise guidelines are the recommended targets based on scientific evidence that will provide benefits to most people. Some participants may not be able to include all of the components at the recommended levels.

Major health-related components of physical fitness:

- Cardiorespiratory endurance
- Muscular strength
- Muscular endurance
- Flexibility
- Body composition
- Neuromotor exercise

A fitness instructor must understand all the components that affect a person's fitness level and must be able to design a program that promotes or enhances all components.

Cardiorespiratory Endurance

Cardiorespiratory endurance is defined as the capacity of the cardiovascular and respiratory systems to deliver oxygen to the working muscles for sustained periods of energy production. **Cardiorespiratory fitness** describes the body's physical capacity to supply fuel and eliminate waste in order to perform large muscle movement over a prolonged period of time.. Cardiorespiratory fitness is often termed **aerobic fitness**.

Muscular Strength

Muscular strength is defined as the maximum force that can be exerted by a muscle or muscle group against a resistance in a single effort, referred to as **one-repetition maximum** (one-rep max or 1RM). Added resistance is needed for training for muscular strength; generally, this is achieved by adding equipment. In the water, resistance is influenced by the amount of **buoyancy**, **drag**, or weight being moved as well as the velocity or speed at which the movement is performed.

Training for strength involves greater resistance with fewer repetitions. Although no optimal number of sets and repetitions has been found to elicit maximal strength gains, the accepted range indicated by research for land-based exercise appears to be somewhere between two and five sets of 2 to 10 repetitions at an all-out effort (Fleck and Kraemer 2003). Aquatic resistance training has been found to elicit strength improvements in both genders and various age groups (Pöyhönen et al. 2002; Tsourlou et al. 2006; Colado et al. 2009).

Muscle **hypertrophy** is the term used to describe an increase in the size or girth of muscle tissue. Muscle **atrophy** is the term used to describe the loss or wasting of muscle tissue through lack of use or disease. Both hypertrophy and atrophy can be addressed through proper training unless an underlying clinical condition exists. Muscular hypertrophy can be enhanced and atrophy can be slowed or halted.

Muscular Endurance

Muscular endurance is defined as the capacity of a muscle to exert force repeatedly or to hold a fixed or static contraction over time. Muscular endurance is assessed by measuring the length of time the muscle can hold a contraction or by counting the number of contractions performed in a given length of time.

Once again, there is no optimal number of sets and repetitions for building muscular endurance. As with strength gains, training programs should be individualized and varied to achieve the best results. When focusing on endurance gains, multiple repetitions are usually recommended in sets of 12 to 20 repetitions or more (Van Roden and Gladwin 2002; Coburn and Malek 2012). These sets differ in intensity from the all-out effort in strength training because the goal is to gradually fatigue the muscle over the course of multiple repetitions.

Using the resistance of the water is an excellent way to promote and maintain muscular endurance. Resistance can be progressively increased by applying more force against the water's resistance, increasing the surface area or lever length, or by adding equipment.

> Although it is possible to train specifically for muscular strength or endurance, these two components of fitness are not independent of each other.

Flexibility

Flexibility is defined as the ability of limbs to move at the joints through a complete **range of motion (ROM)**. Flexibility is important in the reduction of the risk of injury as well as for general body mobility. A decrease in flexibility can lead to impaired movement and an inability to perform **activities of daily living (ADLs)**. Loss of flexibility occurs as a natural part of the aging process or as the result of sedentary lifestyles, trauma, injury, or surgery. In order to maintain flexibility, the joints must be taken through their full range of motion on a regular basis.

Immediately following an exercise program is the best time to stretch to maintain and improve flexibility because the muscles are warm and pliable and filled with oxygenated blood. Stretching after exercise is critical for every type of exercise program, including aquatic fitness programs. It is also imperative to stretch correctly.

Ballistic stretching uses momentum of the body part to create the stretch. This type of stretching is generally not recommended for a general fitness class, but may have applications to individuals who engage in activities that require ballistic movements. Ballistic stretching activates the **muscle spindles**, specialized receptors in the muscle that monitor muscle length change and the speed of length change. Muscle spindles stimulate a muscle contraction to prevent overstretching, which might damage the muscle fibers; this is referred to as the **stretch reflex**. Ballistic stretching can oppose the desired effect of stretching by tightening rather than lengthening the muscle.

Static stretching involves slowly stretching to the point of tightness or mild discomfort and holding the elongated position for a period of time. Static stretching is the preferred method for enhancing flexibility for the general population. When performed properly, static stretching does not activate the stretch reflex; therefore, muscles relax and lengthen. Although generally recommended as a safe and effective option, intense static stretching has been shown to reduce maximum force production for up to one hour after the static stretch (Evetovich, Nauman, Conley, and Todd 2003; Young and Behm 2003). Thus, static stretching prior to training or competition might hinder athletic performance in activities that require maximum power, although it would remain acceptable after exercise.

Rhythmic or dynamic stretching involves moving body parts through the full range of motion in a slow, controlled manner. Instead of stopping and holding a static stretch, you may pause briefly in an extended or stretched position before continuing through the full range of motion. For example, a slow front kick with a pause in front will help to lengthen the gluteal and hamstring muscles. Each individual must recognize and respect the normal range of motion and not overstretch to avoid activating the stretch reflex. Rhythmic stretching is generally preferred over static stretching prior to the main segment of the workout. In the pool, adequate heat can be generated during rhythmic stretching to keep participants comfortable and maintain warmth in muscle tissue during the warm-up stage of the workout.

Body Composition

Body composition is defined as the body's relative percentage of fat as compared to lean tissue (bones, muscles, and organs). It is desirable to build and maintain a reasonable level of lean muscle tissue. Adequate levels of muscle tissue increase stamina and strength and boost metabolism. Having too high a relative percentage of fat increases your risk of heart disease, cancer, and other metabolic diseases. Storing excess subcutaneous fat can also impair physical performance and inhibit quality of life.

The aquatic environment can help develop both a favorable body composition and overall physical fitness. Aerobic exercise in the aquatic environment promotes fat loss while working against the three-dimensional resistance of the water builds lean tissue or muscle mass (Colado et al. 2009, Kieres and Plowman 1991, Kravitz and Mayo 1997).

Neuromotor Exercise or Functional Fitness Training

Neuromotor exercise, also referred to as functional fitness training, might include activities to target skill-related components of agility, balance, and coordination; gait training; proprioceptive exercises; and multifaceted activities such as Tai Chi. Though it is comprised of many of the skill-related components of fitness (see next section), neuromotor exercise is different in its goal and how that goal is trained. The primary goal is function, or the ability to perform normal, everyday tasks. The purpose is to allow the body to adapt to daily scenarios that involve movement diversity while having to think through the movement strategy, provide a movement focus, or adjust the movement due to an external stimulus. Various targeted skills are trained simultaneously (instead of targeting one specific skill at a time) to provide more complex activities that challenge physical ability and mental agility at the same time.

Neuromotor exercises have been shown to reduce the risk of falls as well as the fear of falling among older adults. Although the effectiveness of neuromotor exercise training for younger and middle-aged adults has not been established through research, there is probable benefit, especially for individuals who participate in specific activities and sports that require balance, agility, and other motor skills (ACSM 2014). Tai Chi, Ai Chi, Pilates, and yoga are programming options that focus on neuromuscular skills. Incorporating more complex activities of daily living into existing workout routines may also benefit these fitness parameters. (See chapter 11 for more information on Tai Chi, Ai Chi, Pilates and yoga.)

The aquatic environment can offer a comfortable and safe environment for neuromotor exercises, as the risk for falls is lessened while the body is immersed in the water due to buoyancy and reduced gravity (Douris, et al. 2003; Arnold and Faulkner, 2010; Arnold, et al. 2008; Avelar, et al. 2010).

Skill-Related Components of Physical Fitness

In addition to the major health-related components of physical fitness, there are also several **skill-related components of fitness**. These include agility, balance, coordination, power, reaction time, and speed (Sova 2000, The President's Council on Physical Fitness and Sports 2000).

Agility is the ability to change body positioning in space rapidly, quickly, and accurately. **Balance** is the maintenance of equilibrium while stationary (static balance) or moving (dynamic balance). **Coordination** integrates the senses (such as hearing and vision) with movements of the body to smoothly and accurately perform motor tasks. **Power**, a function of strength and speed is the ability to transfer energy into force at a quick rate. The amount of time elapsed between stimulation and acting on the stimulus is **reaction time**, and **speed** is the rate at which a movement or activity can be performed.

Athletes train for these skill-related components primarily to enhance performance in their sport; yet the same components are also important aspects of everyday life. Many of these components are included within an aquatic fitness class, during transitions, in tempo changes, with one-footed moves and so on, and are developed and improved through practice and repetition.

Guidelines for Exercise

Lifestyle diseases have become prevalent in many developed countries due to the population becoming more sedentary and physically inactive, adopting poor eating habits, and being exposed to more environmental hazards. Since the 1940s, long-term or epidemiological research has been conducted in the United States in order to discover which lifestyle factors increase or decrease the risk of various diseases. These types of studies continue to be conducted today. One of the most famous epidemiological studies is the Framingham Study, in which several generations of families in the town of Framingham, Massachusetts, have been studied to monitor risk factors for disease—cardiovascular disease, in particular. A sedentary lifestyle, or physical inactivity, was determined to elevate risk for cardiovascular disease and cancer as well as contribute to elevating risk for many other diseases.

Following the Framingham study, studies were conducted in which researchers collected metabolic and other data to determine the amount and type of exercise necessary to significantly lower risk of disease. The ACSM 2018 recommendations on the quantity and quality of exercise for adults, consistent with the recommendations found in the 2008 Physical Activity Guidelines for Americans (US Department of Health and Human Services), indicate the need for adults to engage in at least 150 minutes of moderate-intensity exercise each week. ACSM points out that it is also important to monitor how much time the individual is sedentary during the day, such as watching television or sitting at a desk.

The 10th edition of ACSM's Guidelines for Exercise Testing and Prescription (2018) designed as a primary resource for professionals that conduct exercise testing and design exercise programs. These guidelines will assist health and fitness professionals in exercise programming through recommendations for the quantity and quality of training needed to develop and maintain cardiorespiratory endurance, muscular strength and endurance, flexibility, and neuromotor exercise in the healthy adult. These recommendations include frequency, intensity, time, and type of exercise as well as recommendations for exercise volume and progression – referred to as the FITT-VP principle.

Frequency

Frequency is how often you exercise or train.

- **Cardiorespiratory Endurance.** Moderate-intensity cardiovascular exercise at least five days a week, or vigorous-intensity training at least three days per week, or a weekly combination of three to five days a week blending moderate and vigorous activities.
- **Muscular Strength and Endurance.** Two to three days per week for each major muscle group. Additionally, at least 48 hours should separate the training sessions for each muscle group to allow adequate recovery and muscle development.
- **Flexibility.** At least two to three days per week is recommended, with the greatest benefits seen with daily stretching. Stretching is most effective when muscles are warm.
- **Neuromotor Exercise.** At least two to three days per week is recommended.

Intensity

Intensity is how hard you exercise.

- **Cardiorespiratory Endurance.** Moderate or vigorous-intensity exercise is recommended for most adults, although deconditioned individuals may benefit from light to moderate intensity exercise.
- **Muscular Strength and Endurance.** Intensity of training will vary based upon the individual's experience with resistance training, age, ability levels and overall goals (endurance, strength or power). For strength gains, two to four sets of 8-12 repetitions (resistance equivalent to 60-80% 1RM) are recommended for most adults. A single set of 10-15 repetitions (resistance equivalent to 40-50% 1RM) is recommended for strength improvements in deconditioned and older adults who are beginning an exercise program. For endurance training, two or more sets of 15-25 repetitions with an intensity that should not exceed resistance equivalent to 50% 1RM are recommended.
- **Flexibility.** Stretching exercises should be performed to the point of mild discomfort within the individual's range of motion. This is generally perceived as the point of tightness.
- **Neuromotor Exercise.** An effective intensity has not been determined.

Time

Time refers to duration, or how long you exercise.

- **Cardiorespiratory Endurance.** Accumulate 30-60 minutes per day of moderate intensity exercise to accumulate a weekly total of at least 150 minutes, or 20-60 minutes per day of vigorous intensity exercise to accumulate a weekly total of at least 75 minutes, or a combination of moderate and vigorous exercise to achieve the recommended target volumes of exercise. Recommended durations can be achieved through one continuous session or bouts of exercise (10 minutes or more) throughout the day. Individuals unable to perform the recommended duration of exercise may still benefit from a shorter duration.
- **Muscular Strength and Endurance.** No specific length of time for training has been determined for optimum effectiveness.
- **Flexibility.** Hold static stretches 10-30 seconds for most adults; 30-60 seconds may be more beneficial for older adults. Perform each stretch 2-4 times to achieve approximately 60 seconds per joint. Note, in the pool both static and dynamic stretches may be used based upon environmental concerns.
- **Neuromotor Exercise.** 20-30 minutes or more per week is currently suggested.

Type

Type describes the mode of exercise being performed.

- **Cardiorespiratory Endurance.** Rhythmic activities that use large muscle groups and can be maintained continuously (aerobic). Aerobic activities are varied and aquatic options include swimming, deep-water running, many shallow-water exercise programs (e.g., kickboxing, martial arts, and aquatic dance formats), aquatic cycling, and walking (shallow water and underwater treadmills). Selected activities should reflect the individual's interests and goals, and be chosen to accommodate the level of fitness and skill.
- **Muscular Strength and Endurance.** All adults should participate in a resistance-training program that includes a combination of multi-joint exercises (involving more than one muscle group) and single-joint exercises. Various types of resistance equipment can be used; aquatic options include drag, buoyancy, weighted, and rubberized (bands, loops and tubing). Aquatic equipment is discussed in more detail in chapter 4 and appendix C.
- **Flexibility.** A series of flexibility exercises targeting the major muscles using a variety of techniques is suggested to improve joint ROM. Environmental considerations of the pool, in particular water and air temperatures, can influence the choice of stretching techniques used.
- **Neuromotor Exercise.** Specific exercises that involve balance, agility, coordination, gait training, or proprioception skills provide neuromotor exercises. Examples include multifaceted activities such as Tai Chi and yoga.

Volume

The **volume** of exercise is based on the total amount of exercise achieved during one week. The volume for cardiovascular and flexibility exercise is the recommended duration or time listed above. The volume for muscular strength and endurance exercises is the sets and reps listed above. According to ACSM, the volume for neuromotor exercise has not yet been determined.

Progression

Progression refers to the rate of advancement of exercise and is dependent upon the individual's health, fitness level, training responses and exercise goals. Progression can be achieved by increasing frequency, intensity, time and type of exercise. The recommended progression for cardiovascular exercise is to gradually adjust the duration, frequency or intensity without increasing the risk of injury or interfering with exercise adherence. The recommended progression for muscular strength and endurance is to gradually increase the intensity, the repetitions or the frequency of training. According to ACSM, the progression for flexibility and neuromotor exercises has not yet been determined.

Monitoring Intensity

Fitness instructors should understand the various ways in which exercise intensity can be measured, although you might only utilize one or two methods during your classes.

Maximal oxygen uptake ($\dot{V}O_2max$) refers to the amount of oxygen an individual can use during maximal exercise. Maximal oxygen uptake is measured in a clinical setting, using specialized equipment to collect and measure the volume and oxygen concentration on inhaled and exhaled air. Oxygen consumption follows linearly with exercise intensity (as intensity increases, oxygen consumption increases) up to the point where oxygen consumption plateaus; this point marks $\dot{V}O_2max$. Using a percentage of $\dot{V}O_2max$ to measure intensity is not practical for use in an exercise class but is important for understanding research as well as basic fitness information.

More common ways to measure intensity of aerobic exercise use a percentage of a person's **maximal heart rate (HRmax)** or **heart rate reserve (HRR).** A person's maximal heart rate is determined the same way a $\dot{V}O_2max$ is determined. To test this, a person runs on a treadmill with a heart monitor until exhaustion; this is the point where maximal exercise heart rate is reached. Because measuring maximal heart rate in this manner is not practical in fitness classes, we use an estimated maximal heart rate instead. There are several commonly used equations for estimating maximal heart rate, including the "220 minus age" formula, which is generally accepted as a reasonably accurate estimate of maximal heart rate. Recommendations for aerobic training include 30 to 60 minutes of moderate intensity (40-59% HRR or 64-76% of HRmax) five days per week, or 20 to 30 minutes of vigorous exercise (60-89% HRR or 77-95% HRmax) three days per week.

A more accurate way to measure intensity is the heart rate reserve method, also known as **Karvonen's formula**. Karvonen's formula personalizes heart rate measurement by factoring the individual's **resting heart rate** into the equation. A true resting heart rate (HRrest) is determined by taking an average of three 60-second heart rate measurements; each measurement is taken prior to rising from bed on three separate days. Note that this is most accurate when waking naturally instead of via an alarm, as the alarm can increase heart rate.

$$(220 - \text{age} - \text{HRrest}) \times \text{Recommended Percentage} + \text{HRrest} = \text{Desired Intensity}$$

Many factors can affect the training heart rate, including stress, caffeine, medication, general health, and environmental factors. Additionally, research indicates that the exercise heart rate during aquatic exercise is reduced compared to the heart rate observed during exercise of the same intensity on land (Heithold and Glass, 2002; Alberton, et al. 2009). This aquatic suppression of heart rate is influenced by water temperature, reduced gravity, compression, partial pressure, and reduction of body mass (table 1.1). Similarly, it is recommended that a 6-second count be used for monitoring heart rate during aquatic exercise. Informal data collected indicates that a 10-second heart rate might not be as accurate because of the cooling factor of the water in addition to the inherent effects of immersion (mentioned above), which lowers the exercise heart rate more quickly.

Research indicates that a standard percent or a standard number of beats per minute may not be as accurate as a personalized deduction in determining aquatic heart rate calculations. Several studies comparing physiological responses for land and water that included hundreds of people concluded that two heart rate measures (in the water and out of the water) are needed to determine an individual's aquatic deduction (Coertjens et al. 2000; Kruel et al. 2002). The **Kruel Aquatic Heart Rate Deduction** is the differ-

Table 1.1 Factors Influencing Aquatic Exercise Heart Rates

Temperature	Water cools the body more efficiently than air. This cooling effect will reduce the effect of thermic stress (heat) resulting in a lowered heart rate response. In other words, since the aquatic environment allows the body to cool more efficiently, the heart is not working as hard to eliminate the excess heat produced during exercise.
Gravity	Water reduces the effect of gravity on the body. Blood flows from below the heart back up to the heart with less effort, resulting in a lowered heart rate.
Compression	The water is thought to act like a compressor on all body systems, including the vascular system, causing a smaller venous load to the heart than equivalent land exercise. In other words, the heart has to work less to return blood from the limbs back to the heart.
Partial pressure	A gas enters a liquid more readily under pressure. The gas would be oxygen and the liquid blood. It is believed more efficient gas transfer might occur because of water pressure. This improved gas exchange results in a reduced need to increase blood flow and heart rate leading to a reduced workload of the heart.
Reduced body mass	Research indicates that a reduction in body mass (you weigh less in the water) might at least be partially responsible for lower aquatic heart rates.

ence between land-based heart rate and heart rate measured while immersed in the water (see protocol below). This deduction is then included when using the Karvonen formula for determining target heart rate.

The following example shows how to implement the Kruel Aquatic Heart Rate Deduction with the Karvonen formula to determine an individual's target aquatic heart rate. The equation is based upon a 50-year-old individual with a resting heart rate of 70 who wants to train at 65% of heart rate reserve and who has found his or her aquatic deduction to be 8. See appendix E for more information on the Kruel Aquatic Heart Rate Deduction, including a worksheet to assist with calculations.

Stand on deck for 3 minutes to get Deck Heart Rate: Result = 76 beats per minute (BPM)

Stand in chest depth water for 3 minutes to get Water Heart Rate: Result = 68 BPM

76 (Deck Heart Rate) – 68 (Water Heart Rate) = 8

220 – 50 (age) = 170

170 – 70 (resting heart rate) = 100 (heart rate reserve)

100 – 8 (aquatic deduction) = 92

92 × 0.65 (intensity level) = 59.8 (round number to 60)

60 + 70 (resting heart rate) = 130 BPM

Many fitness professionals, both land and water instructors, utilize **rating of perceived exertion (RPE)** to have participants determine exercise intensity. Rating of perceived exertion is a subjective method of assessing

Protocol for Determining the Kruel Aquatic Heart Rate Deduction

Determine a one-minute heart rate after standing out of the pool for three minutes and a one-minute heart rate after standing in the water (at armpit depth) for three minutes. The **aquatic heart rate deduction** is determined by subtracting the heart rate standing in the water from the heart rate standing out of the water. Environmental conditions, medication, caffeine, and excessive movement when entering the pool can affect heart rate response. Care should be taken to minimize these factors.

effort, strain, discomfort, or fatigue experienced during exercise (Noble and Robertson, 1996). Participants are advised to increase their respiration rate, break a sweat (depending on water temperature), and feel as if they are working "somewhat hard" to "hard" (between 7 and 8) according to the scale of perceived exertion (see table 1.2). The Aquatic Exercise Intensity Scale was developed to take into consideration the unique aspects of training in the water, and it includes an RPE scale (0-10), an aquatic heart rate reference, and a standard description of exertion plus an added description to help individuals assess intensity levels better. In this manual, future references to measurements on the RPE scale are based upon the Aquatic Exercise Intensity Scale (see table 1.2).

Perceived exertion is a viable way to measure **intensity** without the influence of additional

Table 1.2 Aquatic Exercise Intensity Scale

Rating & % Aquatic HR	Description (Standard)	Added Description
0-1	Nothing at all (lying down)	Relaxing on the couch or lying in your bed are two examples of this range.
2	Extremely little	You are not breathing hard; your heart rate is low or near resting, and you could sing a song.
3	Very easy	You are not breathing hard, but you feel a slight increase in heart rate; you can speak in complete paragraphs without becoming short of breath.
4 **~ 40% Aq HR**	Easy	This may feel like light housework or an easy walk on flat terrain. You can still speak in full sentences without an issue and you feel like you could do this all day without any problems.
5 **~ 50% Aq HR**	Somewhat easy	You feel like you could exercise for hours. Your heart and breathing rates are slightly increased, but it is still easy for you to speak in full sentences and carry on a conversation.
6 **~ 60% Aq HR**	Moderate (could do this for a long time)	Your heart and breathing rates are starting to increase noticably. You are sweating. Your body is telling you that you are starting to go beyond your normal activity level, and your muscles feel like they are working. This is still a level you could maintain for a while before having to stop. You may compare this to a brisk walk or to walking up a slight incline. You can say four to five words before having to take a breath.
7 **~ 70% Aq HR**	Somewhat hard (starting to feel it)	Your heart rate, your breathing pattern, and your muscles are telling you that you are working hard. You have to breathe through your mouth; nose breathing isn't enough to give you the oxygen you need. You can say only four to five words before you need to take a breath. You are past the point of feeling like you could do the exercise all day.
8 **~ 80% Aq HR**	Hard (making an effort to keep up)	Your heart is pounding, you are breathing hard, and you would rather breathe than talk. You can say two to three words before you have to take a breath. Your muscles start to feel warm from the inside out (that is lactate trying to tell you that you need more oxygen). This intensity is uncomfortable and it cannot be maintained for a long time.
9 **~ 90% Aq HR**	Very hard	Forget talking; at this intensity, you may be able to belt out one word at a time, but you don't want to because breathing is your goal. You shouldn't be able to do this intensity for long and your body is telling you to stop. Your muscles are screaming for oxygen; therefore, your breathing and your heart rate are rapid. This intensity is reserved for shorter intervals and you are so glad that there is a time limit. Your body is saying "No more."
10 **100% Aq HR**	Maximum effort (can't go any further)	All you can think about is how hard you are working and how much you would like to stop. Picture trying to get away from a man-eating shark that is swimming after you; that is how hard you are working right now!

factors that can affect heart rate measurements, such as medications or environmental conditions. With healthy middle-aged and elderly adults, research indicates that rating of perceived exertion (RPE) is not affected by aging and can be a useful tool for monitoring exercise intensity, especially when used in conjunction with heart rate monitoring (Groslambert and Mahon 2006). Because so many factors affect resting and exercise heart rate in the water, it is prudent to use both aquatic adjusted heart rate (Kruel Aquatic Heart Rate Deduction) and perceived exertion.

Another subjective intensity measurement is the **talk test**. It is believed that participants are working above their aerobic threshold—that is, at too high of an intensity for aerobic exercise—if they cannot talk while exercising. This method proves useful for some exercise settings and with certain populations.

Monitoring intensity of resistance training is also important for achieving safe and effective training results. The ACSM (2018) guidelines recommend that adults perform two to four sets of an exercise for each muscle group. A rest period of two to three minutes between sets helps to improve muscular fitness. Deconditioned participants and older adults who are beginning an exercise program should train with a resistance that would allow them to reach muscular fatigue with one set of 10-15 reps, or the equivalent of 40-50% 1RM.

Aerobic Formats

Several aerobic conditioning formats are commonly used for group exercise classes as well as for individual training sessions, including continuous, interval, and circuit training. All three types of training can be used to add variety to your aquatic fitness classes.

Continuous training resembles a bell curve. After warming up, participants maintain a relatively constant level of training within the targeted training zone for a designated length of time (figure 1.1). During this time, minimal fluctuation in intensity occurs. Here is an example of continuous training: Warm up for 10 to 15 minutes, beginning with water walking and gradually increasing effort to jogging or running. Bring heart rate or RPE up to desired training intensity and maintain that for 15 to 30 minutes by performing exercises such as running, jumping jacks, and cross-country skis. The cross-country ski exercise, performed in shallow or deep water, involves the legs moving forward and backward in opposition (i.e., the motion used in cross-country skiing; see appendix A). Conclude the session with a 10- to 15-minute cool-down by slowing down the movements and highlighting range of motion for reducing heart rate and respiration rate.

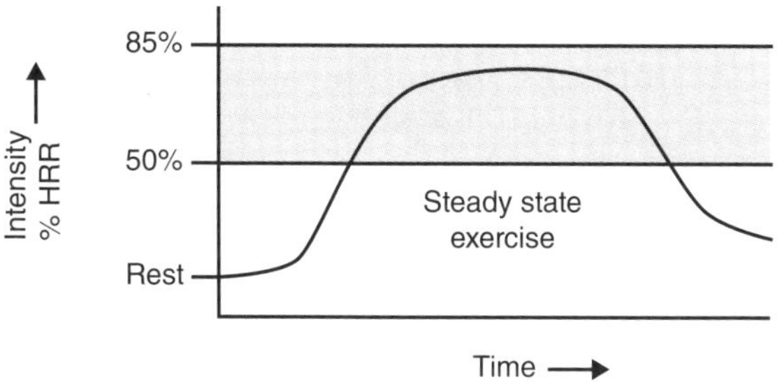

Figure 1.1 Continuous training.

Interval training consists of harder bouts of exercise interspersed with easier bouts, also called work and **recovery** cycles. The goal of most interval programs is to maintain easy and hard intervals within the recommended training zone (figure 1.2). Some interval programs include exercise bouts below the minimum training threshold to train deconditioned participants or beginner exercisers who cannot tolerate continuous training within the training threshold. **High-intensity interval training (HIIT)** is another interval format that includes short periods of very intense anaerobic training. Generally not recommended for beginning exercisers or deconditioned participants, HIIT has become popular in the aquatic setting. An example of an interval class may

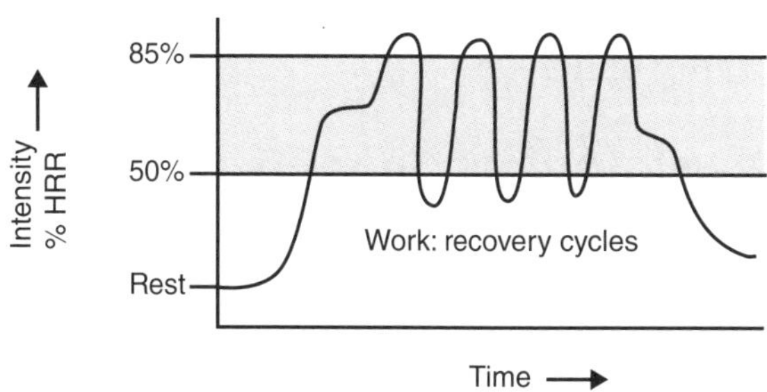

Figure 1.2 Interval training.

look something like this: Warm up for 10 to 15 minutes, including movements that participants will be performing during their intervals. Use intervals of 1 minute of hard to very hard work (80% or greater HRR or 8-9 on the RPE scale), such as fast sprints, followed by 1 minute of active recovery (below 50% HRR or under 5 on the RPE scale), such as walking with a long stride. Repeat these intervals 8 to 10 times with different exercises. Conclude the class with a cool-down appropriate to the training.

Circuit training is often conducted in a station format that uses equipment, but there are many ways to design this type of class or training session. Circuit training may be designed to elicit a cardiorespiratory response; alternate aerobic work with resistance training, neuromotor exercises, or skill-related activities; or focus on muscle conditioning (see chapter 11).

Incorporate different methods of training to add variety, increase motivation, and ensure continued **progression** for your participants. An entire class does not have to be dedicated to one method of training. For example, you may choose to add 10 minutes of interval training during the cardio portion or plan a circuit format for the resistance-training segment of class.

Benefits of Regular Exercise

Increasing functional capacity or physical fitness results in several **physiological** and **psychological** benefits. Many of these benefits have been confirmed through research. Some benefits, such as the psychological benefits, are harder to isolate and confirm. Safe and effective physical training can improve physical appearance, health, and quality of life.

Physiological Benefits of Regular Exercise

Many people initiate an exercise program to improve their physical appearance. Regular fitness training can improve physical appearance, and is instrumental in achieving and maintaining a healthy weight and body composition. People who continue to exercise on a regular basis often do so because of how it makes them feel, which is the result of physical and chemical changes that occur in the body. Because of these physical and chemical changes, exercise reduces risk for cardiovascular disease, cancer, and many other diseases.

Regular aerobic exercise increases the functional capacity of the respiratory and cardiovascular systems. The respiratory system becomes more efficient by increasing the volume of air inhaled and exhaled with each breath. Intercostal (breathing) muscles become more fit and the ability of the lungs to hold air increases. The heart becomes stronger with use, increasing its ability to eject more blood with each beat **(stroke volume)**. This increased stroke volume improves the heart's ability to supply blood to the body. Due to these adaptations, a fit person generally has a lower resting heart rate. Regular exercise also strengthens the walls of the blood vessels, promotes the development of capillary beds, and provides a better blood supply to the body. The body's ability to extract oxygen from blood increases as well, elevating cardiorespiratory endurance levels.

Exercise is also beneficial for the muscular and skeletal systems. Regular exercise strengthens the skeletal system and increases bone density. Because muscles and tendons attach to the bones, adding **overload** to the muscles can strengthen bone and connective tissue and help reduce risk of osteoperosis. Repetitive use of the muscles in aerobic training combined with resistance training actually increases the girth and density of muscle tissue (Merideth-Jones et al 2009). When proper flexibility training is included, the skeletal muscles become not only stronger but also more flexible. Strong, flexible muscles protect **joints** from injury and enable the body to move and function with ease.

The efficiency of the endocrine system, nervous system, and lymphatic system also improves with regular exercise. The endocrine system becomes more efficient at regulating hormones and the lymphatic system becomes more efficient at protecting the body from disease. Motor pathways are developed and enhanced, allowing the nervous system to better regulate the quality of movement and other nervous functions. Metabolic functions improve, favorably altering blood lipid levels and metabolism, making it easier to lose **fat** and improve body composition.

Many organs, such as the liver, intestines, and kidneys, benefit from regular exercise as well. Regular exercise enhances blood flow, fluid transfer, and oxygenation in the body. The body's functional capacity drops 5 to 10 percent per decade between the ages of 20 to 70 years. Muscle tissue and flexibility are also lost in the aging process. Regular exercise promotes the maintenance of functional capacity, muscle tissue, and flexibility at any age. The health benefits of exercise are truly staggering. Our bodies evolved as active machines, made to move. Physical inactivity and lack of use can have detrimental health effects. Regular physical activity protects the body from injury and disease.

> "The Human Body is the only machine that breaks down when you don't use it."
> –Thomas Cureton (Kautz, 108 1966)

Psychological and Cognitive Benefits of Regular Exercise

Exercise can influence psychological function and is often recommended to reduce depression and anxiety. Regular exercisers report reduced stress and tension, improved sleep habits, increased energy, increased productivity, improved self-esteem and an increased sense of self control. Exercise has been related to improvements in mental health through the improvement in self-esteem and cognitive function, and by reducing depression, anxiety and negative mood (Callaghan 2004). Psychological benefits as well as the psychology related to exercise are discussed in chapter 5.

A survey of older adults showed that brain health was the second most important component to maintaining a healthy lifestyle after heart health (AARP 2014). Research has shown the cognitive benefits of aerobic exercise (Neeper 1995). Additional research has shown improvements in cognitive function as a result of participating in a resistance training (Nagamatsu et al. 2012). Participation in programs that include exercise, cognitive training, dietary guidance and social interaction have been proven to improve overall cognitive performance (Kivipelto et al. 2013).

Specific Benefits of Aquatic Exercise

This manual focuses on exercise specific to the aquatic environment that is performed in a vertical position (as opposed to swimming). Research has shown positive benefits in many areas of health and fitness relating directly to aquatic exercise including the following (Yazigi 2014):

- Cardiorespiratory endurance (Wilber et al 1996; Bushman et al. 1997; Frangolias et al. 1997; Burns and Lauder 2001)
- Muscular strength (Bravo et al. 1997; Suomi and Koceja 2000; Suomi and Collier 2003; Gusi et al. 2006)
- Flexibility (Templeton, Booth, and O'Kelly 1996; Driver et al. 2004; Wang et al. 2007)
- Body composition (Colado et al. 2009; Volaklis, Spassis, and Tokmakidis 2007; Tsourlou et al. 2006)
- Balance (Gusi et al. 2006; Devereux, Robertson, and Briffa 2005; Noh et al. 2008; Tomas-Carus et al. 2007; Cancela Carral and Ayan Perez 2007; Lee 2006)
- Functional capacity (Templeton et al. 1996; Driver et al. 2006)
- Musculoskeletal conditions (Bacon et al. 1991; Ay and Yurtkuran 2005)
- Psychological considerations (Wantanabe et al. 2000)
- Quality of life (Hinman, Heywood, and Day 2007)

Summary

A fitness professional should understand the differences between physical activity, exercise, and physical fitness as well as recognize the health benefits of each. Programs should be developed to achieve specific fitness goals as well as to increase activity levels that target healthy lifestyle changes.

Regular exercise programs need to include the major components of physical fitness. It is essential to target cardiorespiratory endurance, muscular strength and endurance, flexibility, neuromotor abilities, and body composition. Developing all of the components promotes overall fitness and good health.

Following the ACSM (2018) guidelines for frequency, intensity, time, type, volume, and progression of exercise provides optimal benefits and functional capacity. These guidelines apply to cardiorespiratory endurance, muscular strength and endurance, flexibility, and neuromotor exercise. These guidelines ensure an effective exercise program for increasing physical fitness and reducing risk of chronic disease.

Aerobic conditioning could include continuous, interval, and circuit training formats. Providing variety in class structure enhances motivation and continued progression of training.

Regular exercise provides physiological, psychological, and cognitive health benefits.

Review Questions

1. ________________________ is defined as the maximum force that can be exerted by a muscle or muscle group against a resistance.
2. What type of stretching activates the muscle spindles, specialized receptors in the muscle that monitor muscle length change and the speed of muscle length change?
3. Name the six skill-related components of fitness.
4. What is the difference between maximal heart rate and heart rate reserve?
5. How does compression lower your heart rate in the water?
6. What is the ACSM's (2018) recommended frequency for resistance training?
7. Define body composition.
8. List five benefits of regular exercise.
9. When calculating exercise intensity, a popular method is the Karvonen Formula, which is also known as the _________.
   a. heart rate minimum method
   b. heart rate reserve method
   c. maximal heart rate method
   d. rating of perceived exertion

10. _______________is a subjective method of assessing effort, strain, discomfort, and fatigue experienced during exercise.

See appendix D for answers to review questions.

References and Resources

Alberton, C.L., M.P. Tartaruga, S.S. Pinto, E.L. Cadore, E.M. Da Silva, and L.F.M. Kruel. 2009. Cardiorespiratory responses to stationary running at different cadences in water and on land. *Journal of Sports Medicine and Physical Fitness* 49(2):142.

American College of Sports Medicine. 2018. *Guidelines for exercise testing and prescription.* 10th edition. Baltimore: Lippincott, Williams & Wilkins.

American College of Sports Medicine. 2014. *Guidelines for exercise testing and prescription.* 9th edition. Baltimore: Lippincott, Williams & Wilkins.

American Council on Exercise. 2000. *Group fitness instructor manual.* San Diego: Author.

———. 2003. *Personal trainer manual.* 3rd edition. San Diego: Author.

Arnold, C.M., A.J. Busch, C.L. Schachter, E.L. Harrison, and W.P. Olszynski. 2008. A randomized clinical trial of aquatic versus land exercise to improve balance, function, and quality of life in older women with osteoporosis. *Physiotherapy Canada* 60(4):296-306.

Arnold, C.M., and R.A. Faulkner. 2010. The effect of aquatic exercise and education on lowering fall risk in older adults with hip osteoarthritis. *Journal of Aging and Physical Activity* 18(3):245-260.

Avelar, N.C.P., C. Alessandra, M.A. Bastone, M.A. Alcântara, and W.F. Gomes. 2010. Effectiveness of aquatic and non-aquatic lower limb muscle endurance training in the static and dynamic balance of elderly people. *Brazilian Journal of Physical Therapy* 14(3):229-236.

Ay, A., and M. Yurtkuran. 2005. Influence of aquatic and weight-bearing exercises on quantitative ultrasound variables in postmenopausal women. *American Journal of Physical Medicine & Rehabilitation* 84(1):52-61.

Bacon, M.C., C. Nicholson, H. Binder, and P.H. White. 1991. Juvenile rheumatoid arthritis. Aquatic exercise and lower-extremity function. *Arthritis Care & Research* 4(2):102-105.

Bravo, G., P. Gauthier, P.M. Roy, H. Payette, and P. Gaulin. 1997. A weight-bearing, water-based exercise program for osteopenic women: Its impact on bone, functional fitness, and well-being. *Archives of Physical Medicine and Rehabilitation* 78(12):1375-1380.

Burns, A.S., and T.D. Lauder. 2001. Deep water running: An effective non-weightbearing exercise for the maintenance of land-based running performance. *Military Medicine* 166(3):253-258.

Bushman, B.A., M.G. Flynn, F.F. Andres, C.P. Lambert, M.S. Taylor, and W.A. Braun. 1997. Effect of 4 wk of deep water run training on running performance. *Medicine & Science in Sports & Exercise* 29(5):694-699.

Callaghan P. 2004. Exercise: a neglected intervention in mental health care? *J Psychiatr Ment Health Nurs.* 11:476–483.

Cancela Carral, J.M., and C. Ayan Perez. 2007. Effects of high-intensity combined training on women over 65. *Gerontology* 53(6):340-346.

Coburn, J.W., and M.H. Malek. 2012. *NSCA's essentials of personal training.* 2nd edition. Champaign, IL. Human Kinetics.

Coertjens, M., A.B.C Dias, R.C Silva, A.C.B. Rangel, L.A.P. Turtle., and L.F.M. Kruel. 2000. Determination of bradycardia during vertical immersion in the liquid medium. XII Scientific Initiation Hall, Federal University of Rio Grande do Sul, Porto Alegre, Rio Grande do Sul 341.

Centers for Disease Control and Prevention. n.d. FastStats: Leading causes of death. www.cdc.gov/nchs/fastats/leading-causes-of-death.htm.

Centers for Disease Control and Prevention. 2014. Facts about Physical Activity. www.cdc.gov/physicalactivity/data/facts.htm.

Colado, J.C., V. Tella, N.T. Triplett, and L.M. Gonzalez. 2009. Effects of a short-term aquatic resistance program on strength and body composition in fit young men. *Journal of Strength and Conditioning Research* 23(2):549-559.

David, P. and V. Gelfeld. 2014. Brain Health Research Study. AARP Research www.aarp.

org/research/topics/health/info-2015/staying-sharper-study.html.

Devereux, K., D. Robertson, and N.K. Briffa. 2005. Effects of a water-based program on women 65 years and over: A randomised controlled trial. *Australian Journal of Physiotherapy* 51(2):102-108.

Douris, P., V. Southard, C. Varga, W. Schauss, C. Gennaro, and A. Reiss. 2003. The effect of land and aquatic exercise on balance scores in older adults. *Journal of Geriatric Physical Therapy* 26(1):3-6.

Driver, S., J. O'Connor, C. Lox, and K. Rees. 2004. Evaluation of an aquatics programme on fitness parameters of individuals with a brain injury. *Brain Injury* 18(9):847-859.

Driver, S., K. Rees, J. O'Connor, and C. Lox. 2006. Aquatics, health-promoting self-care behaviours and adults with brain injuries. *Brain Injury* 20(2):133-141.

Evetovich, T.K., N.J. Nauman, D.S. Conley, and J.B. Todd. 2003. Effect of static stretching of the biceps brachii on torque, electromyography, and mechanomyography during concentric isokinetic muscle actions. *Journal of Strength and Conditioning Research* 17(3):484-488.

Fleck, S., and W. Kraemer. 2003. *Designing resistance training programs.* 3rd edition. Champaign, IL: Human Kinetics.

Frangolias, D.D., J.E. Taunton, E.C. Rhodes, J.P. McConkey, and M. Moon. 1997. Maintenance of aerobic capacity during recovery from right foot Jones fracture: A case report. *Clinical Journal of Sports Medicine* 7(1):54-57; discussion 57-58.

Graef, Fabiane Inês, and Luiz Fernando Martins Kruel. 2006. Heart rate and perceived exertion at aquatic environment: differences in relation to land environment and applications for exercise prescription-a review. *Revista Brasileira de Medicina do Esporte*. 12(4):221-228.

Groslambert, A., and A.D. Mahon. 2006. Perceived exertion: Influence of age and cognitive development. *Sports Medicine* 36(11):911-928.

Gusi, N., P. Tomas-Carus, A. Hakkinen, K. Hakkinen, and A. Ortega-Alonso. 2006. Exercise in waist-high warm water decreases pain and improves health-related quality of life and strength in the lower extremities in women with fibromyalgia. *Arthritis & Rheumatology* 55(1):66-73.

Haff, G.G., and N.T. Triplett. 2015. *Essentials of strength training and conditioning.* 4th edition. Champaign, IL: Human Kinetics.

Heithold, K., and S.C. Glass. 2002. Variations in heart rate and perception of effort during land and water aerobics in older women. *Medicine & Science in Sports & Exercise* 34(5):S74.

Hinman, R.S., S.E. Heywood, and A.R. Day. 2007. Aquatic physical therapy for hip and knee osteoarthritis: Results of a single-blind randomized controlled trial. *Physical Therapy* 87(1):32-43.

Kautz, J. 1966. Focus on elementary education. *Physical Educator* 12(3):108.

Kieres, J., and S. Plowman. 1991. Effects of swimming and land exercises versus swimming and water exercises on body composition of college students. *The Journal of Sports Medicine and Physical Fitness*. 31(2):189-195.

Kivipelto, M. et al. 2013. The Finnish geriatric intervention study to prevent cognitive impairment and disability (FINGER): study design and progress. *Alzheimer's & Dementia* 9(6): 657-665.

Kruel, Luiz Fernando Martins, et al. 2009. Effects of hydrostatic weight on heart rate during water immersion. *International Journal of Aquatic Research and Education*. 3(2):8.

Lee, H.Y. 2006. Comparison of effects among Tai-Chi exercise, aquatic exercise, and a self-help program for patients with knee osteoarthritis. *Taehan Kanho Hakhoe Chi* 36(3):571-580.

Meredith-Jones, K., M. Legge, and L.M. Jones. 2009. Circuit-based deep water running improves cardiovascular fitness, strength and abdominal obesity in older, overweight women. *Med Sport* 13(1):5-12.

Nagamatsu, L. S. et al. 2012. Resistance training promotes cognitive and functional brain plasticity in seniors with probable mild cognitive impairment. *Archives of Internal Medicine* 172(8):666-668.

Neeper, S.A., F. Goauctemez-Pinilla, J. Choi, and C. Cotman. 1995. Exercise and brain neurotrophins. *Nature* 373(6510):19.

Noble, B.J., and R.J. Robertson. 1996. *Perceived exertion.* Champaign, IL: Human Kinetics.

Noh, D.K., J.Y. Lim, H.I. Shin, and N.J. Paik. 2008. The effect of aquatic therapy on postural balance and muscle strength in stroke survivors—a randomized controlled pilot trial. *Clinical Rehabilitation* 22(10-11):966-976.

Pöyhönen, T., S. Sipilä, K.L. Keskinen, A. Hautala, J. Savolainen, and E. Mälkiä. 2002. Effects of aquatic resistance training on neuromuscular performance in healthy women. *Medicine & Science in Sports & Exercise* 34(12):2103-2109.

The President's Council on Physical Fitness and Sports. *Definitions—Health, fitness, and physical activity*. Washington, D.C.: The President's Council on Physical Fitness and Sports. www.webharvest.gov/peth04/20041023064714/http://fitness.gov/digest_mar2000.htm.

Sova, R. 2000. *Aquatics: The complete reference guide for aquatic fitness professionals*. 2nd edition. Pt. Washington, WI: DSL.

Suomi, R., and D. Collier. 2003. Effects of arthritis exercise programs on functional fitness and perceived activities of daily living measures in older adults with arthritis. *Archives of Physical Medicine and Rehabilitation* 84(11):1589-1594.

Suomi, R., and D.M. Koceja. 2000. Postural sway characteristics in women with lower extremity arthritis before and after an aquatic exercise intervention. *Archives of Physical Medicine and Rehabilitation* 81(6):780-785.

Templeton, M.S., D.L. Booth, and W.D. O'Kelly. 1996. Effects of aquatic therapy on joint flexibility and functional ability in subjects with rheumatic disease. *Journal of Orthopaedic & Sports Physical Therapy* 23(6):376-381.

Tomas-Carus, P., A. Hakkinen, N. Gusi, A. Leal, K. Hakkinen, and A. Ortega-Alonso. 2007. Aquatic training and detraining on fitness and quality of life in fibromyalgia. *Medicine & Science in Sports & Exercise* 39(7):1044-1050.

Tsourlou, T., A. Benik, K. Dipla, A. Zafeiridis, and S. Kellis. 2006. The effects of a twenty-four-week aquatic training program on muscular strength performance in healthy elderly women. *Journal of Strength and Conditioning Research* 20(4):811-818.

U.S. Centers for Disease Control and Prevention and ACSM. 1993. Summary statement: Workshop on physical activity and public health sports medicine bulletin 28:4. Washington, D.C.: President's Council on Physical Fitness.

Van Roden, J., and L. Gladwin. 2002. *Fitness theory & practice*. 4th edition. Sherman Oaks, CA: Aerobic & Fitness Association of America.

Volaklis, K.A., A.T. Spassis, and S.P. Tokmakidis. 2007. Land versus water exercise in patients with coronary artery disease: Effects on body composition, blood lipids, and physical fitness. *American Heart Journal* 154(3):560.e1-560.e6

Wang, T.J., B. Belza, E. Thompson, J.D. Whitney, and K. Bennett. 2007. Effects of aquatic exercise on flexibility, strength and aerobic fitness in adults with osteoarthritis of the hip or knee. *Journal of Advanced Nursing* 57(2):141-152.

Watanabe, E., N. Takeshima, A. Okada, and K. Inomata. 2000. Comparison of water- and land-based exercise in the reduction of state anxiety among older adults. *Perception and Motor Skills* 91(1):97-104.

Wilber, R.L., R.J. Moffatt, B.E. Scott, D.T. Lee, and N.A. Cucuzzo. 1996. Influence of water run training on the maintenance of aerobic performance. *Medicine & Science in Sports & Exercise* 28(8):1056-1062.

World Health Organization. 2009. *Global health risks: Mortality and burden of disease attributable to selected major risks*. Geneva: Author.

Yázigi, F. 2014. *Knee osteoarthritis and obesity: effectiveness of PICO aquatic exercise program on symptoms, physical fitness and quality of life*. PhD thesis, University of Lisbon, Portugal. Retrieved from http://hdl.handle.net/10400.5/7449

Young, W.B., and D.G. Behm. 2003. Effects of running, static stretching and practice jumps on explosive force production and jumping performance. *Journal of Sports Medicine & Physical Fitness* 43(1):21-27.

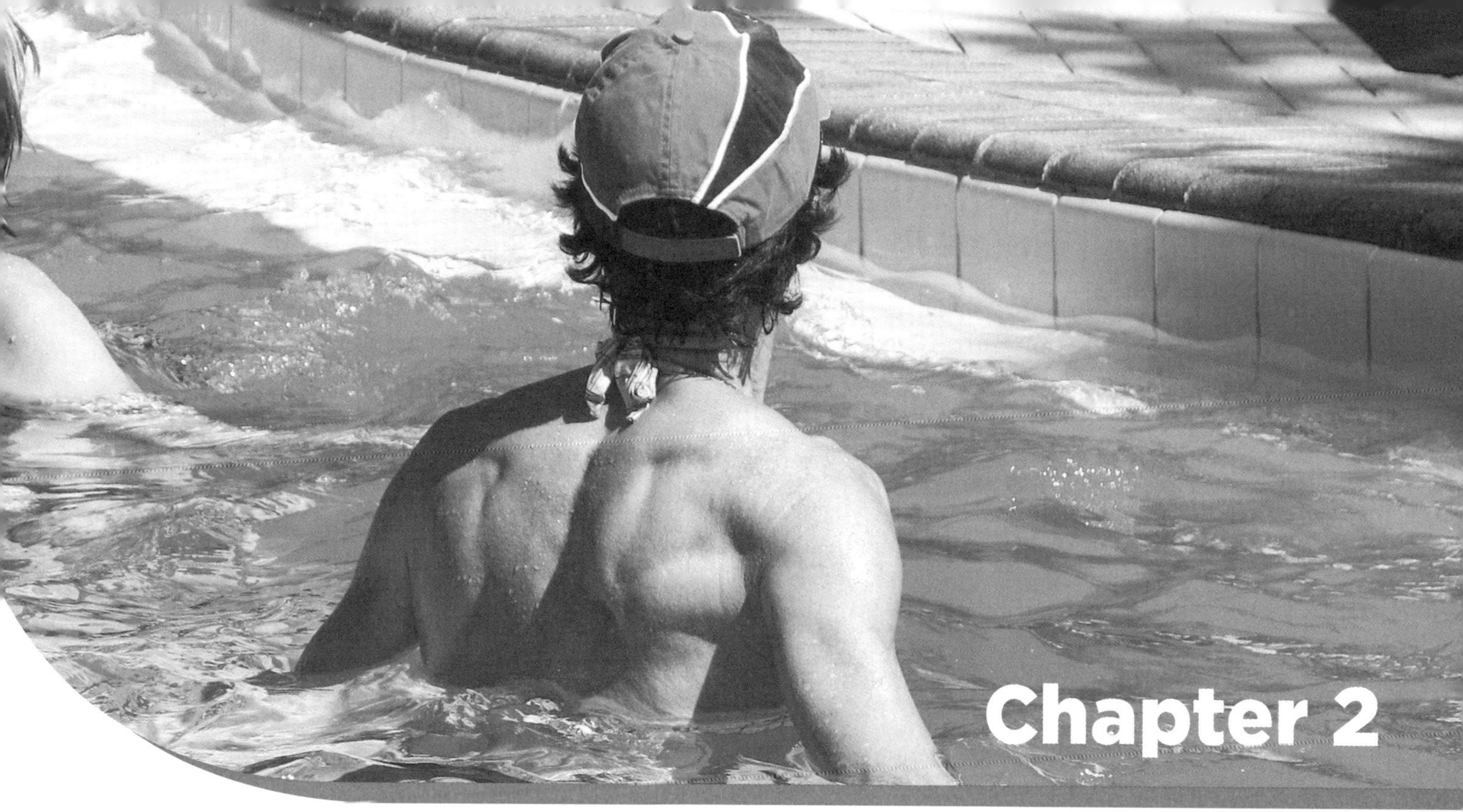

Exercise Anatomy

Introduction

Chapter 2 presents an overview of the organization of the human body, with an in-depth look at the five systems of the body most closely related to exercise: the skeletal, muscular, nervous, respiratory, and cardiovascular systems. It shows how these five systems work together to create movements involved in exercise.

Key Chapter Concepts

- Recognize the structural organization of the human body.
- Understand the five systems of the body that are most pertinent to fitness instructors.
- Explain how bones grow, including the influence of exercise and nutrition.
- Differentiate between the axial skeleton and the appendicular skeleton.
- Define the four principle characteristics of muscle tissue.
- Describe how muscles are arranged in the human body.
- Identify and locate the major muscles, including the joints moved.
- Describe how the nervous system works with the muscular system to create movement.
- Explain how oxygen and carbon dioxide are exchanged within the respiratory system.
- Describe the role of the cardiovascular system during exercise.
- Explain the flow of blood through the body.

Structural Organization of the Human Body

Think of your body as consisting of several levels of structural organization. Each level is more and more complex than the previous level, and is associated with other levels in several ways.

The first level, called the **chemical level**, consists of all the chemical substances found in the body that are essential for maintaining life. The next level is called the **cellular level**, which consists of the basic structural and functional unit of the body called the *cell*. The body is composed of various types of cells, including muscle cells, blood cells, and adipose or fat cells. Cells are grouped together based on their function and structure to form tissues. Tissues make up the next level of structural organization, called the **tissue level**. The body is composed of various types of tissues, including muscle tissue, nervous tissue, and connective tissue. Various types of tissues are combined based on their function to make organs. Organs comprise an even higher level of organization, called the **organ level**. Examples include the heart, liver, stomach, and brain.

The next level of organization is called the **system level**. A system is several organs grouped together to perform a particular function such as digestion, hormone secretion, or supplying the body with blood and oxygen. All of the systems of the body work together to make up a functional living human. We will focus on the systems that work together to create movements associated with exercise.

Systems of the Human Body

The human body is divided into 11 systems that work together in several ways to allow humans to function as a whole person. One example of systems working together that is of interest to fitness instructors is how the skeletal, muscular, and nervous systems work together to create movements, specifically exercise.

The 11 systems of the body are organized as follows:

- **Cardiovascular system:** includes the heart, the blood vessels, and the blood.
- **Digestive system:** includes the digestive tract—a series of organs joined in a long tube—and other organs involved in digestion, including the liver, gallbladder, and pancreas.
- **Endocrine system:** includes all the glands that produce hormones. The endocrine system and the hormones it produces play an important role in regulating many exercise processes.
- **Integumentary system:** includes the skin and all the structures derived from the skin (e.g., hair, nails).
- **Lymphatic system:** includes lymph, lymph nodes, lymph vessels, and lymph glands. The lymphatic system is part of the immune system and works to protect the body against diseases.
- **Muscular system:** includes all the skeletal muscles, visceral muscles, cardiac muscle, tendons, and ligaments.
- **Nervous system:** includes the brain, spinal cord, nerves, and sensory organs (eyes and ears).
- **Reproductive system:** includes organs that produce, store, and transport reproductive cells.
- **Respiratory system:** includes the lungs and the various passageways that lead into and out of the lungs.
- **Skeletal system:** includes all the bones of the body, the cartilage associated with the bones, and the joints.
- **Urinary system:** includes organs that produce, collect, and eliminate urine.

The systems of particular interest to fitness instructors are the skeletal, muscular, nervous, cardiovascular, and respiratory systems. This chapter presents a basic understanding of the function and role that these five systems play in the process of movement and exercise.

Skeletal System

The skeletal system provides our bodies with support, protection, and structure. The rib cage and scapulae protect vital organs like the lungs, kidneys, and liver. The skull surrounds and houses the brain. The muscles attach to the bones to provide the shape and support of the body while delivering the leverage needed for movement. Bones also manufacture red blood cells and store **minerals**.

The human skeleton consists of 206 bones. It is divided into two parts: the **axial skeleton** and the **appendicular skeleton**. The axial skeleton consists of the bones found around the axis (the imaginary midline of the body) and includes the skull, vertebral column, sternum, and ribs. The appendicular skeleton refers to the bones associated with the appendages and includes the bones in the arms, shoulders, legs, and hips.

This section focuses on the major bones in the body associated with movements and exercise: sternum, vertebral column, ribs, clavicle, scapulae, humerus, ulna, radius, phalanges (hands and feet), skull, carpals, metacarpals, patella, calcaneus, pelvic girdle, femur, tibia, fibula, tarsals, and metatarsals (figure 2.1).

The **vertebral column** is made up of 26 bones called **vertebrae** (figure 2.2). The vertebrae are divided into five sections. The portion of the vertebral column found in the neck is called the **cervical spine**. It contains seven small vertebrae. The part of the vertebral column found behind the rib cage is called the **thoracic** spine. It consists of 12 midsized vertebrae. The lower back area of the vertebral column is called the

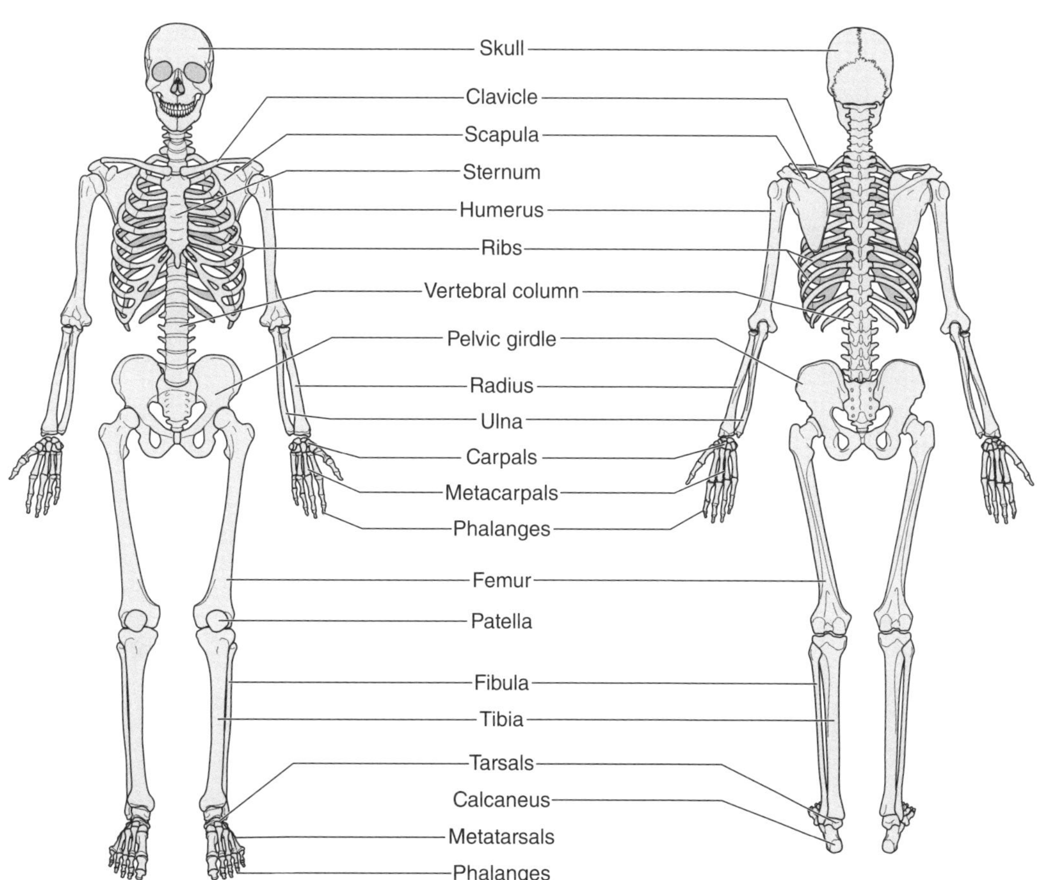

Figure 2.1 The human skeleton.

lumbar spine. It consists of five large vertebrae. Below the lumbar spine is the **sacrum**, which is one bone made up of five fused sacral vertebrae. The **coccyx**, or tailbone, is made up of four vertebrae fused into one or two bones. A fibrocartilaginous tissue called an **intervertebral disc** is found between each vertebra. This tissue can be injured through trauma or overuse, especially in the weight-bearing lumbar area or in the delicate cervical area of the spine. Disc problems are not as common in the thoracic area because of the support and stability the ribs provide the vertebral column.

An **articulation**, or joint, is the point of contact between bones or between cartilage and bone. **Cartilage** is a dense connective tissue that is able to withstand considerable force. It provides a smooth surface between two bones and acts as a shock absorber for movements in the joint. Joints are classified as immovable, slightly movable, or freely movable, and are discussed in greater depth in chapter 4. The amount of movement possible at a joint depends on the way in which the bones fit together, the tightness of the tissue that surrounds the joints, and the position of the ligaments, muscles, and tendons. **Ligaments** are dense connective tissue that attach bone to bone at movable joints. They help make the joint more stable and protect it from dislocation. **Tendons** connect the muscles to the bones. They are discussed in more detail in the section on the muscular system.

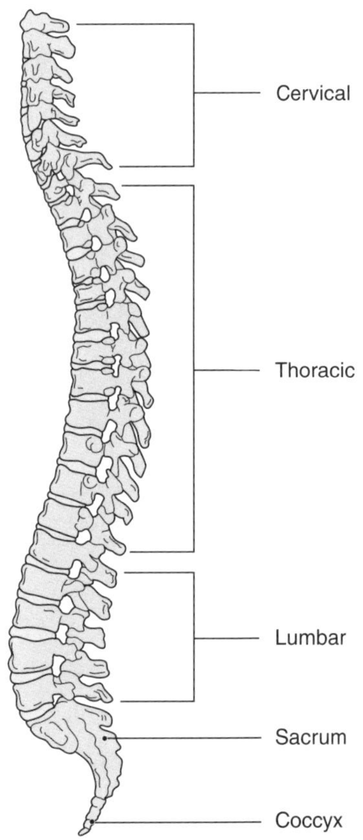

Figure 2.2 The vertebral column.

Structural Composition of Bone

A bone is made of many parts, with the proportions of each part depending on the size and shape of the bone (figure 2.3). The rigid part of the bone is made of spongy and compact bone. The spongy bone is less dense, and contains spaces so blood vessels and other nutrients can be supplied to the bone. The compact part of the bone contains few spaces and provides protection and strength. The **periosteum** is a dense, white fibrous sheath that covers the surface of the bone. This is where muscles and tendons attach to the bone. The **medullary cavity** is the space in the center of the bone filled with bone marrow. Bone marrow is where blood cells are produced. The **endosteum** is the layer of

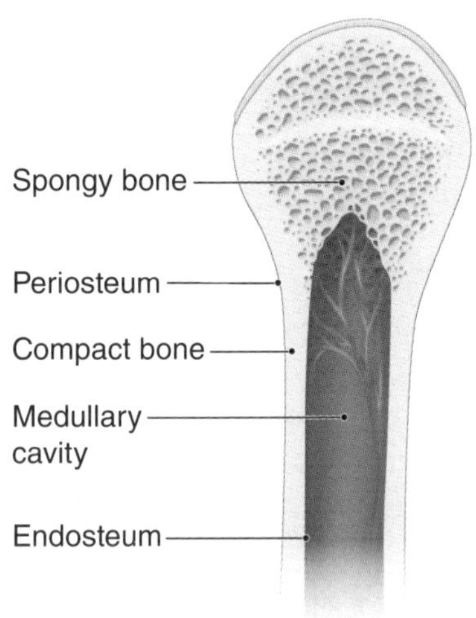

Figure 2.3 Parts of a bone.

old bone cells that line the medullary cavity. These cells are reabsorbed as part of the growth process to prevent the bones from becoming too thick.

How Bones Grow

New bone formation occurs when **osteoblasts** (bone formation cells) manufacture **proteins** or collagen molecules in response to mechanical loading or stress on the bone, such as resistance training or weight-bearing exercises. These molecules are layered on the outer surface of the periosteum. The process is called **ossification**. **Osteoclasts** remove old bone from the endosteum (inner surface), leaving the new, stronger bone tissue. Long bones, such as the bones in your arms and legs, have cartilaginous growth plates located at either end called **epiphyseal plates**. Initially, these plates are not completely hardened, allowing for growth to occur in the bone. These fragile growth plates can be damaged in growing children or teens, affecting bone development. The epiphyseal plates harden as a person matures. Bone growth stops between the ages of 21 and 25.

The structures in bones are continually layering new bone and removing old bone. In fact, most of the bone making up the adult skeleton is replaced every 10 years (Office of the Surgeon General 2004). Exercise, adequate rest, and nutrition promote healthy bone tissue development and reduce the risk of bone disease such as osteoporosis.

Muscular System

The human body has more than 600 muscles. The muscular system works with other systems to create movement and to maintain posture. It also assists with the proper function of many of the other systems of the body, such as the circulatory and digestive systems. The muscular system is composed of visceral, cardiac, and skeletal muscles. **Visceral muscle** is the smooth involuntary muscle found in the walls of organs such as the intestines and esophagus. **Cardiac muscle** is found in the heart. **Skeletal muscle** is the striated voluntary muscle that attaches to the bones and works with the skeletal system to create movement. Most movements require the skeletal and muscular systems to work together, so those two systems are referred to as the musculoskeletal system.

Characteristics of Muscle Tissue

All muscle tissue possesses four principle characteristics:

- **Excitability** allows the muscle to receive and respond to stimuli. A stimulus is some kind of change that occurs in the muscle itself or a change that occurs in the external environment of the muscle tissue. This change must be strong enough to initiate a nerve impulse. This relationship between the nervous system and the muscular system is referred to as the neuromuscular system.
- **Contractility** is simply the ability of muscle tissue to shorten or contract when it is stimulated.
- **Extensibility** is the ability of a muscle to stretch. The ability of muscles to contract (shorten) and extend (lengthen) is what allows movement to occur in the body.
- **Elasticity** allows the muscle to return to its original shape (somewhat like a rubber band) so it can contract or extend again to repeat the same movement or cause a different movement.

Muscle Structure and Arrangement

Structurally, muscles are bands of fibers anchored firmly to bones by **tendons**. Tendons are made of very strong, fibrous connective tissue. They connect the **fascia**, the covering on the muscles, to the periosteum, the fibrous membrane covering the bones. Most muscles have at least two tendons, each one attaching to a different bone. One of these attachments is stationary or immobile, and is referred to as the muscle's **origin**. The other attachment is more mobile, and is called the muscle's **insertion**.

The muscles in the human musculoskeletal system are primarily organized in pairs throughout the body. These muscle pairs tend to be arranged around the same joint on opposite sides (figure 2.4), allowing movement to occur in more than one direction. Muscle pairs have a relationship that allows one muscle to relax or stretch while the other muscle is shortening or contracting. The muscle that is actively contracting is referred to as the **agonist**, or prime mover. To remember the term, think of this contracting muscle as having the agony of doing the work. The other muscle of the muscle pair must relax or stretch so that the agonist can contract. This relaxed or stretched muscle is referred to as the **antagonist**. The agonist and antagonist in a muscle pair work together to contract and relax on either side of a joint so movement can occur in different directions and at various angles. A contraction in both muscles at the same time would prevent movement at that joint and is referred to as **stabilizing** the joint.

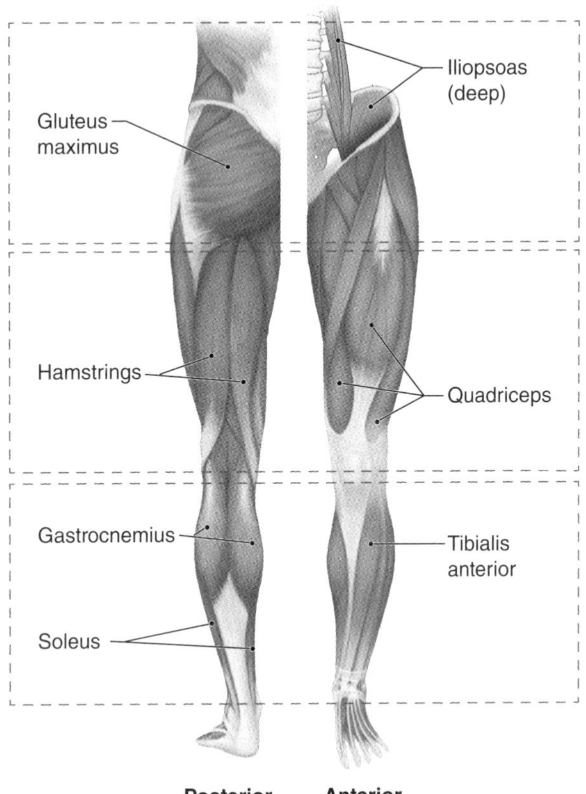

Figure 2.4 Muscle pairs in the lower body.

The biceps and triceps in the upper arm are one example of a muscle pair. The biceps muscle is in the front of the upper arm. It crosses the elbow joint and attaches into the forearm. A contraction of the biceps muscle bends the elbow, raising the forearm toward the upper arm. The triceps muscle, located on the back of the upper arm, also crosses the elbow and attaches into the forearm. The triceps muscle must relax and stretch for the bicep to bend the elbow. Likewise, a contraction of the triceps muscle straightens the arm. The biceps must relax or stretch to allow the arm to straighten. The arrangement of these paired muscle groups throughout the body allows us to perform a variety of movements.

Some other common muscle pairs affecting gross movements include the following:

- Anterior deltoid and posterior deltoid—front and back of the shoulder joint
- Rectus abdominis and erector spinae—front and back of the lumbar spine
- Iliopsoas and gluteus maximus—front and back of the hip joint
- Hip abductors and adductors—inside and outside of the hip joint
- Quadriceps and hamstrings—front and back of the hip joint and the knee joint
- Tibialis anterior and the gastrocnemius together with the soleus—front and back of the ankle joint

Fitness instructors should pay close attention to muscle pairs when designing exercise programs. This is discussed in more detail in chapter 3.

Major Muscle Groups

Fitness instructors should have a general understanding of the basic muscle groups and their involvement in movement in order to design and implement effective exercise programs. You must be aware of which muscles are responsible for which movements with every exercise or move in your choreography. This chapter will show you the location of the major muscle groups and the joints that they move. See figure 2.5 for a full view of the major superficial muscles in the body. See table 2.1 for the names of the major muscle groups, their location in the body, and the joints moved by each muscle group.

Muscles of the Upper Torso and Extremities

Several muscle groups are involved in movement in the upper torso, but here we focus on only the major muscle groups: the sternocleidomastoid, pectoralis major, trapezius, latissimus dorsi, deltoids, biceps brachii, triceps brachii, wrist flexors, and wrist extensors.

Sternocleidomastoid (ster-no-kli-do-MAS-toid) The sternocleidomastoid is located in the front of the neck. This muscle attaches from the sternum and clavicle up to the jaw area and moves the cervical or neck area intervertebral spine joints (figure 2.6).

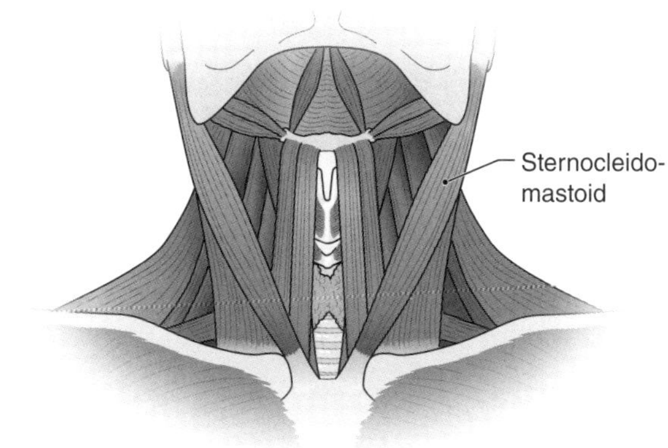

Figure 2.6 Sternocleidomastoid.

Pectoralis major (pek-tor-A-lis) The pectoralis major muscle is located in the chest. It originates at the sternum, clavicle, and ribs and attaches into the upper arm. The primary joint moved is the shoulder joint. The pectoralis major also moves the sternoclavicular joint, where the sternum and the clavicle meet (see figure 2.7).

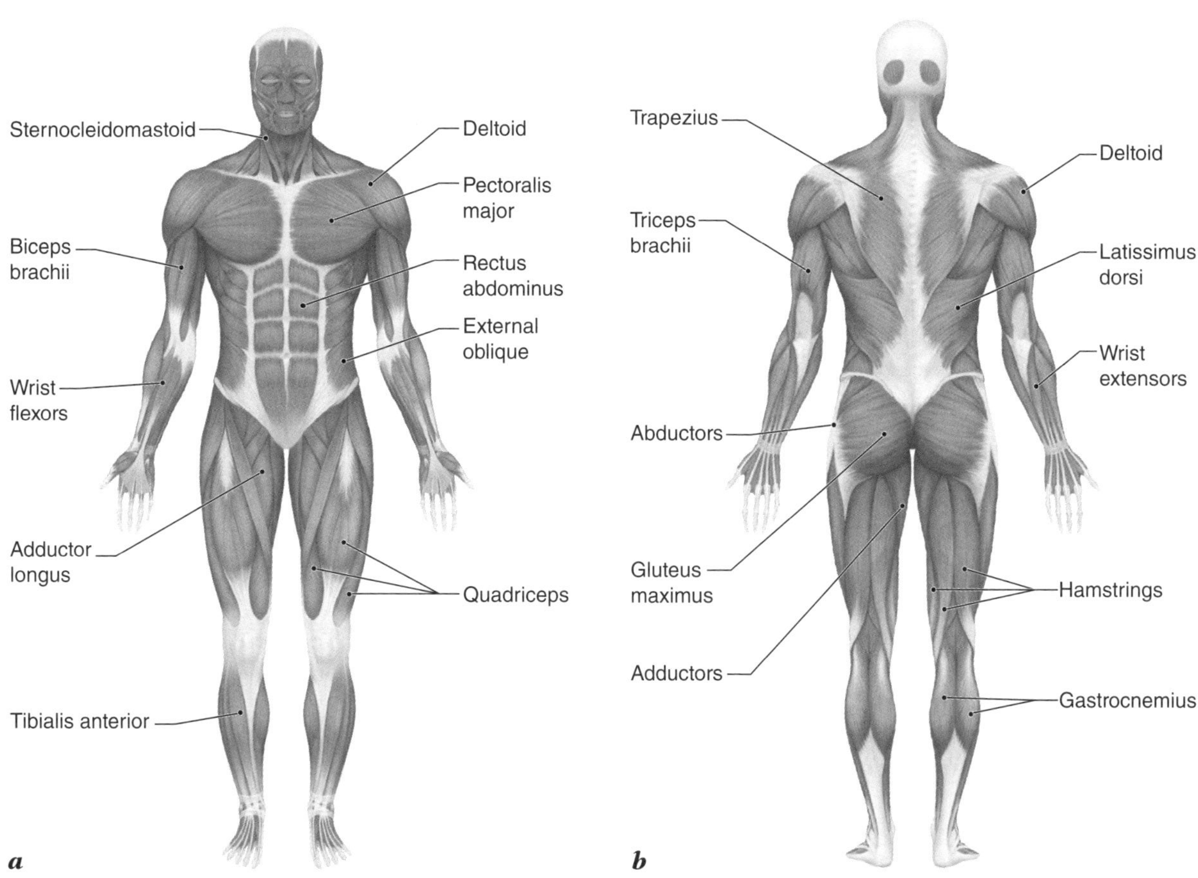

Figure 2.5 *(a)* Anterior and *(b)* posterior views of muscles in the body.

Table 2.1 Major Muscles of the Body

Name of muscle	Location in anatomical position	Joints moved
Sternocleidomastoid	Front of the neck	Cervical spine
Pectoralis major	Chest	Shoulder Sternoclavicular
Trapezius • Upper • Middle • Lower	Upper back and neck	Scapulae Sternoclavicular Cervical spine
Latissimus dorsi	Middle and low back	Shoulder
Deltoid • Anterior • Medial • Posterior	Cap of shoulder	Shoulder
Biceps brachii	Front of upper arm	Elbow Shoulder Radioulnar
Triceps brachii	Back of upper arm	Elbow Shoulder
Wrist flexors	Front of the forearm	Wrist Phalanges
Wrist extensors	Back of the forearm	Wrist Phalanges
Erector spinae	Back, along spine	Intervertebral joints of spine
Quadratus lumborum	Low back	Lumbar spine
Rectus abdominis	Abdomen	Lumbar spine
Internal and external obliques	Abdomen	Lumbar spine
Transversus abdominis	Abdomen	Abdominal compression Lumbar stabilization
Iliopsoas (psoas major and minor, iliacus)	Front of hip	Hip
Gluteus maximus	Back of hip	Hip
Hip abductors (gluteus medius and minimus)	Outer thigh	Hip
Hip adductors	Inner thigh	Hip
Quadriceps femoris (rectus femoris, vastus medialis, vastus intermedius, vastus lateralis)	Front of thigh	Hip (rectus femoris) Knee
Hamstrings (biceps femoris, semimembranosus, semitendinosus)	Back of thigh	Hip Knee
Gastrocnemius	Back of lower leg	Ankle Knee
Soleus	Back of lower leg	Ankle
Tibialis anterior	Front of lower leg	Ankle

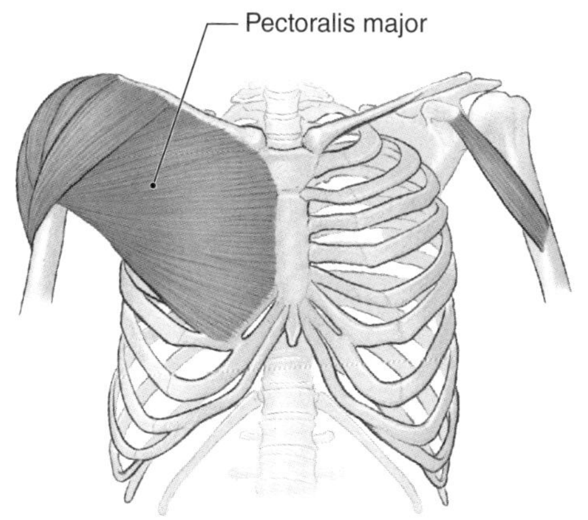

Figure 2.7 Pectoralis major.

Trapezius (tra-PE-ze-us) The trapezius is a large diamond-shaped muscle located in the upper back and the back of the neck. The muscle is divided into three parts based on the direction of the fibers and the movements for which each section is responsible. The fibers in the upper trapezius run at an angle from the spine up the neck to the head and out toward the scapulae (shoulder blades). The middle trapezius fibers run horizontally from the spine across the upper back to the scapulae. The lower trapezius fibers run at an angle from the spine up and out toward the scapulae. The trapezius muscle does not cross the shoulder joint or attach to the humerus (upper arm); therefore, it is not responsible for movements at the shoulder joint. The trapezius moves the scapulae and the sternoclavicular joint. The upper trapezius extends the neck (figure 2.8).

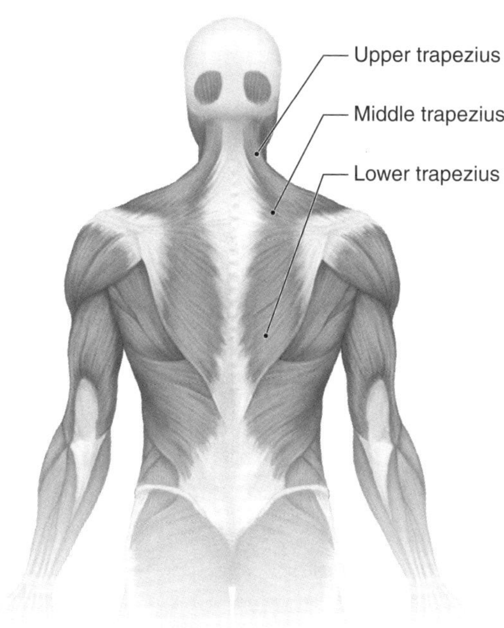

Figure 2.8 Trapezius.

Latissimus dorsi (la-TIS-i-mus DOR-si) The latissimus dorsi muscle is located in the middle and lower back. It is a large, flat muscle that attaches to the pelvic bone and the vertebral column. It runs up and out either side of the lower back to attach to the humerus. The primary joint this muscle moves is the shoulder (figure 2.9).

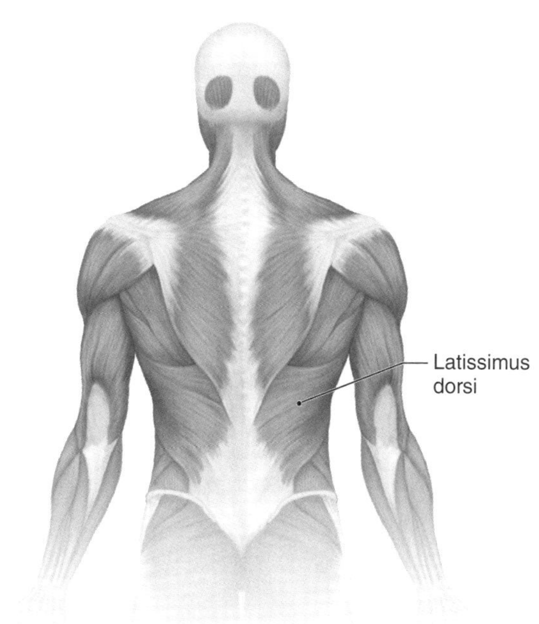

Figure 2.9 Latissimus dorsi.

Deltoid (DEL-toyd) The deltoid is the muscle that caps the shoulder. This muscle is divided into the anterior (front), medial (middle), and posterior (back) muscle fibers. This allows the muscle to be involved in three different movements. The deltoid muscle runs over the top of the shoulder and attaches into the humerus. This muscle moves the shoulder joint (figure 2.10).

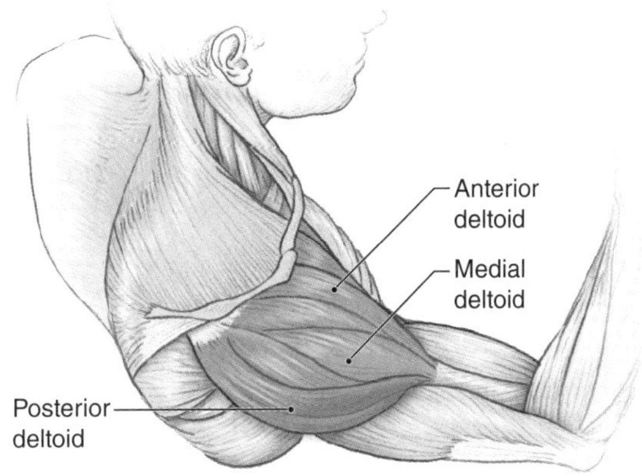

Figure 2.10 Deltoid.

Biceps brachii (BI-ceps BRA-ke-i) The biceps brachii muscle is located on the front of the upper arm. It crosses three joints. The muscle is so named (bi-ceps) because it has two origins on the scapula. The muscle fibers come together to form one attachment on the forearm. The biceps is the prime mover in the elbow joint, but also moves the shoulder and radioulnar joints (figure 2.11).

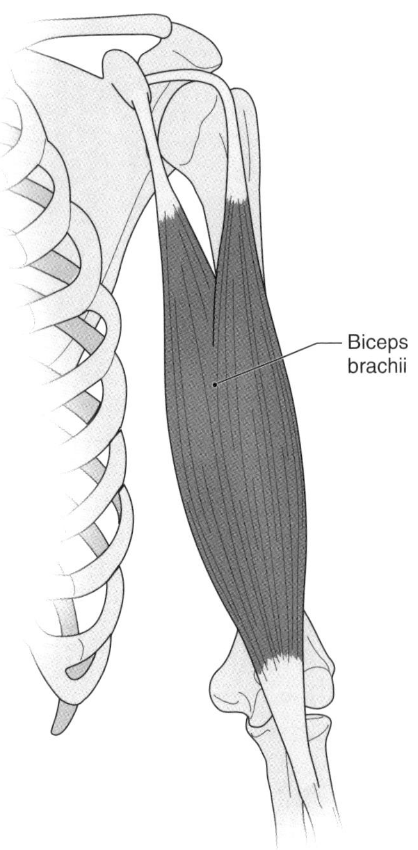

Figure 2.11 Biceps brachii.

Triceps brachii (TRI-ceps BRA-ke-i) The triceps brachii muscle is located in the back of the upper arm. This muscle is so named (tri-ceps) because it has three origins in the shoulder. The muscle fibers come together to form one attachment on the forearm. The triceps is the prime mover in the elbow joint, but also moves the shoulder joint (figure 2.12).

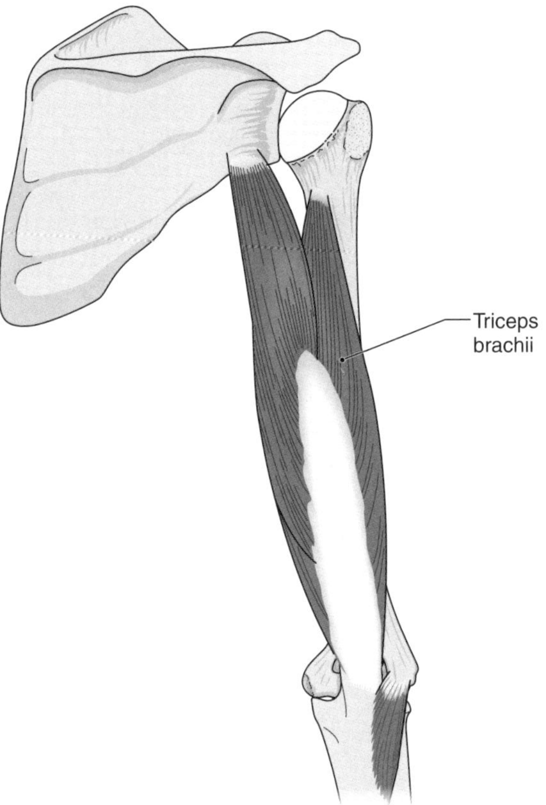

Figure 2.12 Triceps brachii.

Wrist flexors The wrist flexors are a group of muscles located in the front of the forearm. They move the wrist and fingers (phalanges). Their arrangement and attachment from the arm into the hand allow flexion of the wrist as well as movement in the hand and the thumb (figure 2.13).

Wrist extensors The wrist extensors are a group of muscles located in the back of the forearm that work in opposition to the wrist flexors. They also move the wrist and fingers (phalanges). Their attachment from the arm into the hand allows extension of the wrist and movement in the hand and thumb (figure 2.14).

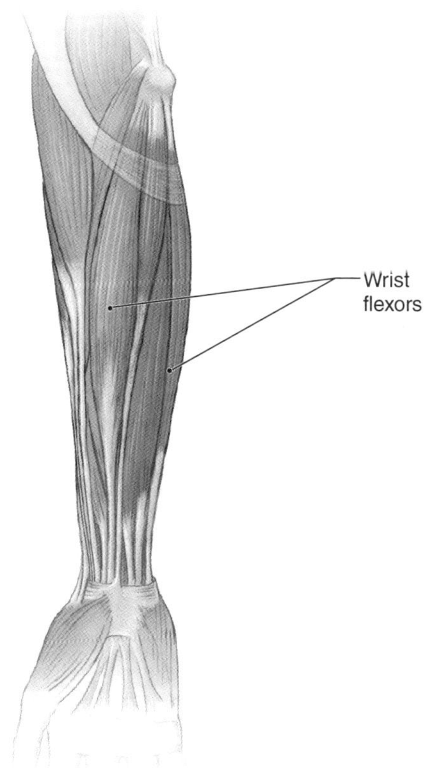

Figure 2.13 Wrist flexors.

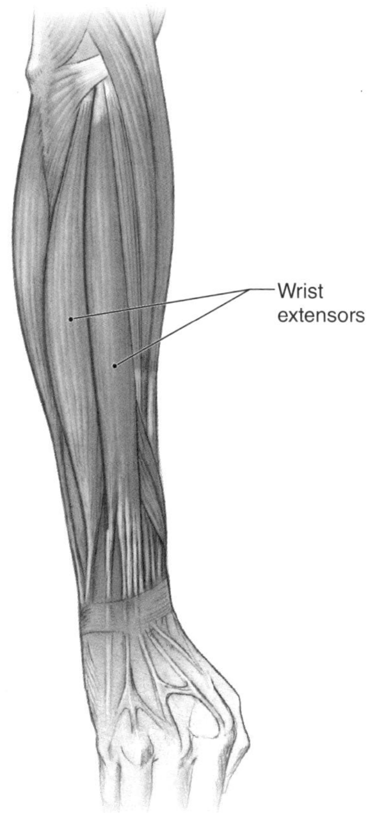

Figure 2.14 Wrist extensors.

Muscles of the Torso

Major muscles in the midsection of the body include the erector spinae, quadratus lumborum, rectus abdominis, internal and external obliques, and the transversus abdominis. These muscles provide support and stability for the lumbar or weight-bearing area of the vertebral column. Adequate strength and flexibility in these muscles enhance postural alignment, improve functional mobility and reduce risk of lower-back problems.

Erector spinae (e-REK-tor SPI-ne) The erector spinae muscles are located in the back, running along the entire length of the vertebral column. This muscle group is a large mass of tissue that splits and attaches in an overlapping fashion to the vertebrae. The erector spinae move the intervertebral spine joints (figure 2.15).

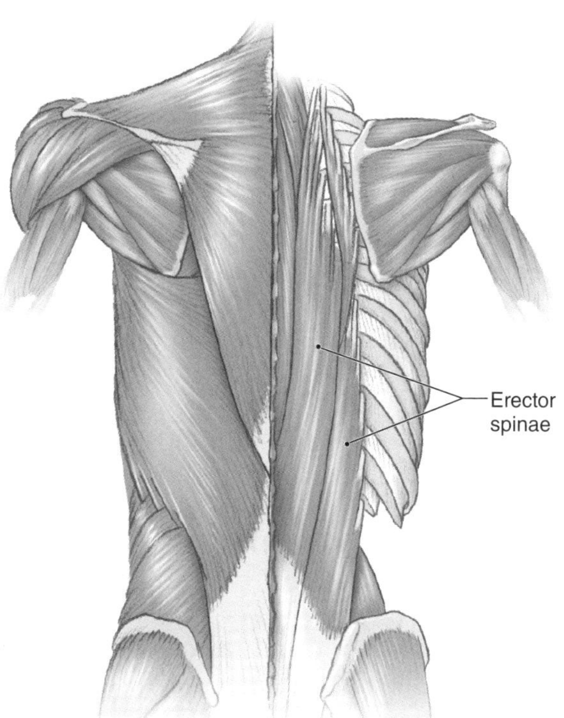

Figure 2.15 Erector spinae.

Quadratus lumborum (kwod-RA-tus lum-BOR-um) The quadratus lumborum muscle is located in the lower back. It attaches from the pelvic bone up into the ribs and lumbar vertebrae. The fibers run at a slight angle and can flex the spine laterally

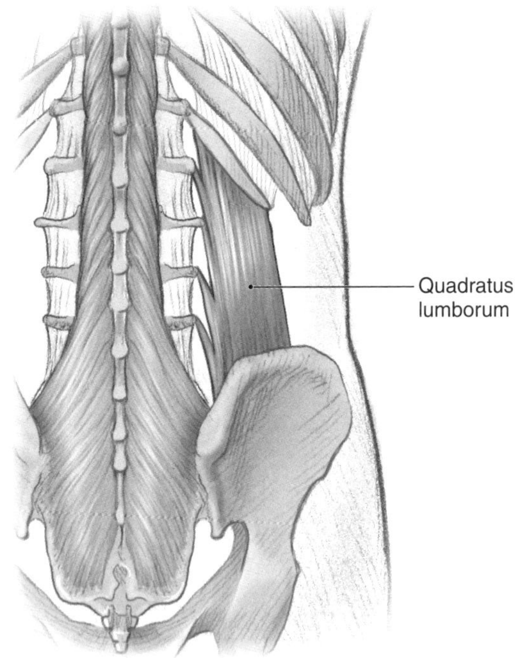

Figure 2.16 Quadratus lumborum.

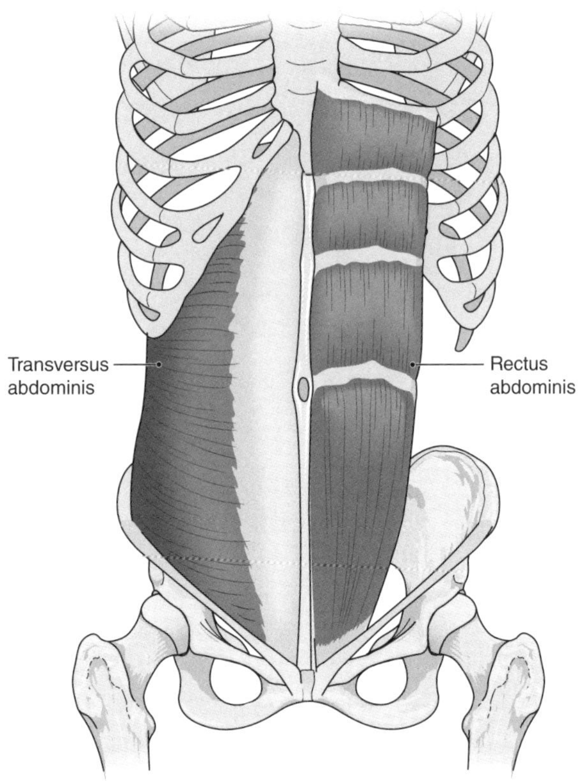

Figure 2.17 Transversus abdominis and rectus abdominis.

(bending sideways) if only one side is contracted. These muscles help with supporting the lower back when both sides contract simultaneously (figure 2.16).

Rectus abdominis (REK-tus ab-DOM-in-is) This long, flat muscle runs from the pubic bone in the abdomen up into the sternum and ribs. Many people believe that exercises such as leg lifts, bicycles, or lifting your legs while hanging from a noodle in the pool actively work the rectus abdominis muscle. However, these exercises involve movement at the hip joint and so do not actively involve the rectus abdominis because it does not cross the hip joint. The rectus abdominis muscle is contracted to stabilize the pelvis and protect the lower back when lifting the legs and moving from the hip. It is not actively doing the work. The rectus abdominis moves the intervertebral joints of the lumbar spine (figure 2.17).

Transversus abdominis (tranz-VER-sus ab-DOM-in-is) The fibers of the transversus abdominis run horizontally across the front of the abdominal cavity. Contraction of this muscle compresses the abdomen and stabilizes the lumbar spine and pelvis. Instructors often cue participants to tighten their abdominal muscles by "pulling their belly button into their spine." The purpose of this cue is to engage the transversus abdominis to support and stabilize the torso so that the exercise will be more effective (figure 2.17).

Internal and external obliques (o-BLEK) The term oblique refers to muscle fibers that run diagonal to the midline. The internal obliques are located under the external obliques in an inverted V pattern (figure 2.18). The external obliques are more superficial than the internal obliques. They are arranged in the opposite direction, forming a V pattern (figure 2.19). Both the internal and external oblique muscles wrap around the waist and move the intervertebral joints of the lumbar spine.

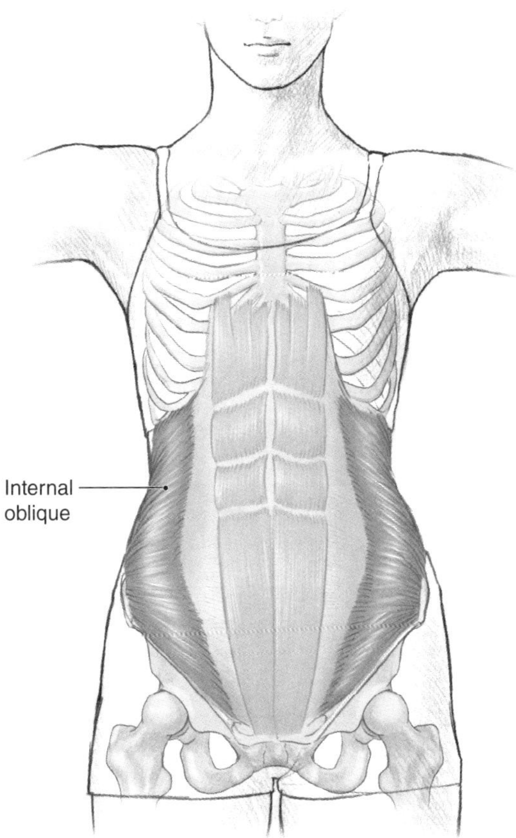

Figure 2.18 Internal oblique.

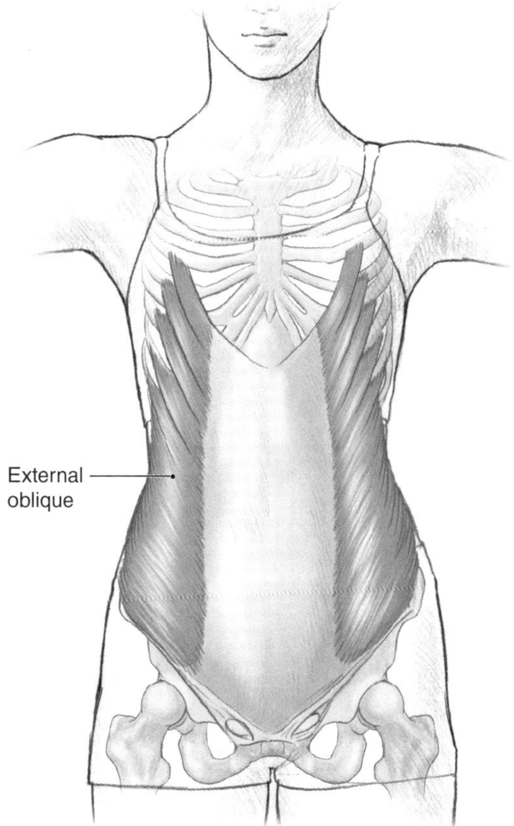

Figure 2.19 External oblique.

Muscles of the Lower Torso and Extremities

Muscles of the lower extremities include all the major muscles in the hips and legs. Some of these muscles are the largest skeletal muscles in the body and are capable of powerful contractions to move the weight of the body. These muscles include the iliopsoas, gluteus maximus, hip abductors and adductors, the quadriceps femoris, hamstrings, gastrocnemius, soleus, and the tibialis anterior.

Iliopsoas (il-e-o-SO-as) The iliopsoas is composed of three muscles: the psoas major, psoas minor, and iliacus. These three muscles are referred to as the hip flexors. They originate on the lumbar vertebrae and pelvis and insert onto the upper leg or femur. They are often confused with the abdominal muscles because they run through the lower abdomen. The iliopsoas actually moves the hip joint and works independently of the abdominal muscles (figure 2.20).

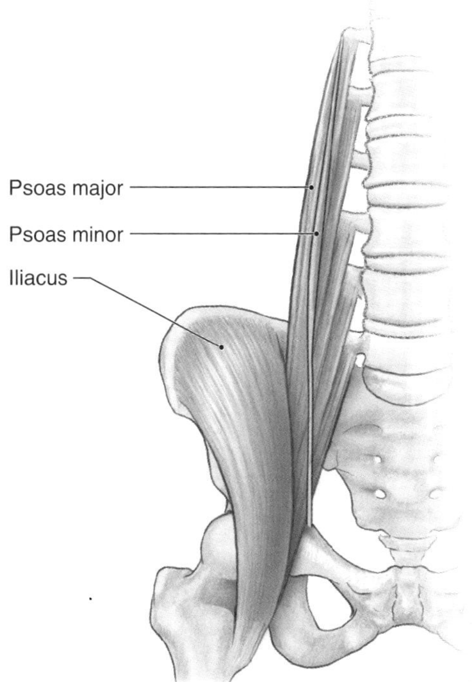

Figure 2.20 Iliopsoas.

Gluteus maximus (GLOO-te-us MAK-si-mus) This muscle is the largest of the three gluteal muscles. It is located in the buttocks. It originates along the lower vertebrae and along the pelvis and inserts onto the femur. The gluteus maximus moves the hip joint (figure 2.21).

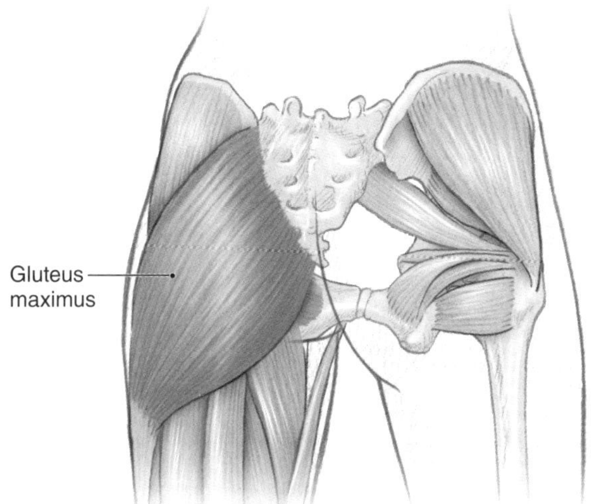

Figure 2.21 Gluteus maximus.

Hip abductors These muscles are located in the outer thigh and are named after the movement they initiate (**abduction**). The hip abductors include the gluteus medius and gluteus minimus. They originate along the back crest of the pelvis and attach onto the femur. The hip abductors move the hip joint (figure 2.22).

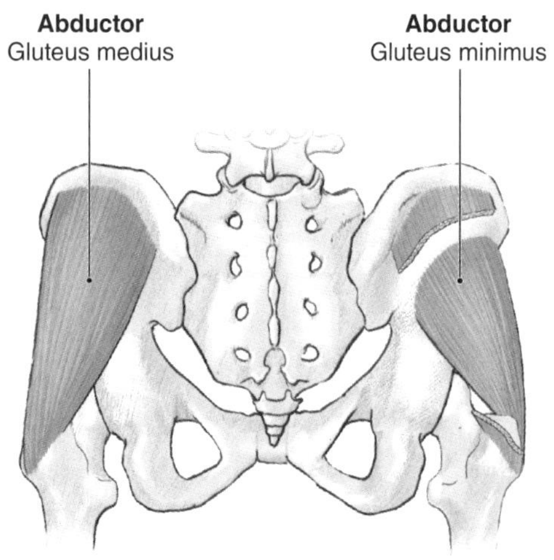

Figure 2.22 Gluteus medius and gluteus minimus.

Hip adductors The hip adductors work in opposition to the hip abductors. They are named after the movement they initiate (hip **adduction**). This muscle group is made up of five small muscles located on the inside of the thigh. They originate on the lower center part of the pelvis, called the *pubis*, and insert onto the femur. The hip adductors move the hip joint (figure 2.23).

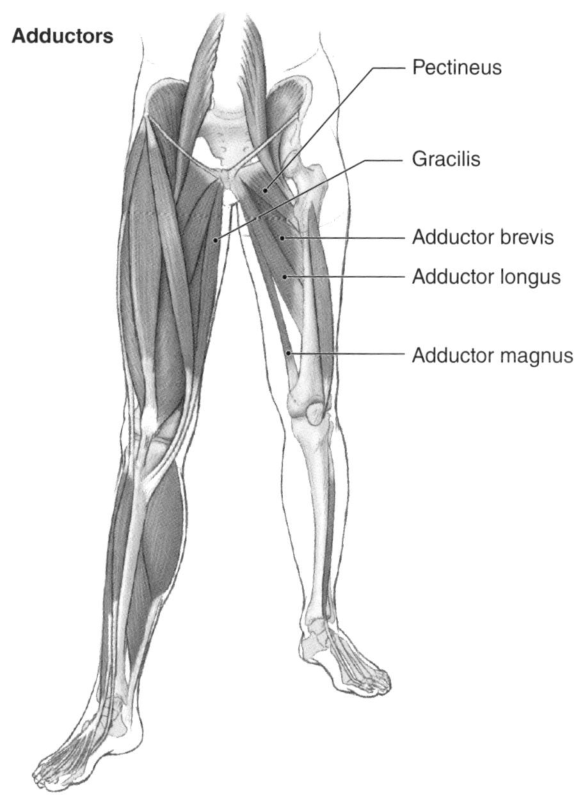

Figure 2.23 Hip adductors.

Quadriceps femoris (KWOD-ri-ceps FEM-or-is) The quadriceps femoris is located in the front of the thigh. The quadriceps femoris muscle group has four parts. The rectus femoris (fibers running parallel to the midline of the femur) is a large, long muscle that originates above the hip. It is the only part of the quadriceps group that moves the hip. The three vastus muscles—the vastus lateralis, vastus intermedius, and vastus medialis—originate on the femur. All four parts of the quadriceps muscle cross the knee joint and insert onto the lower leg. The quadriceps femoris muscle group moves the knee joint (figure 2.24).

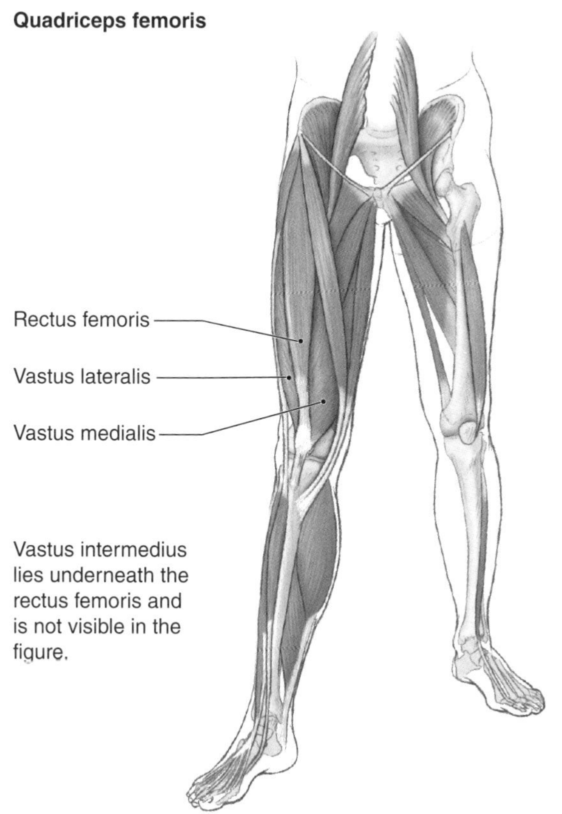

Figure 2.24 Quadriceps femoris.

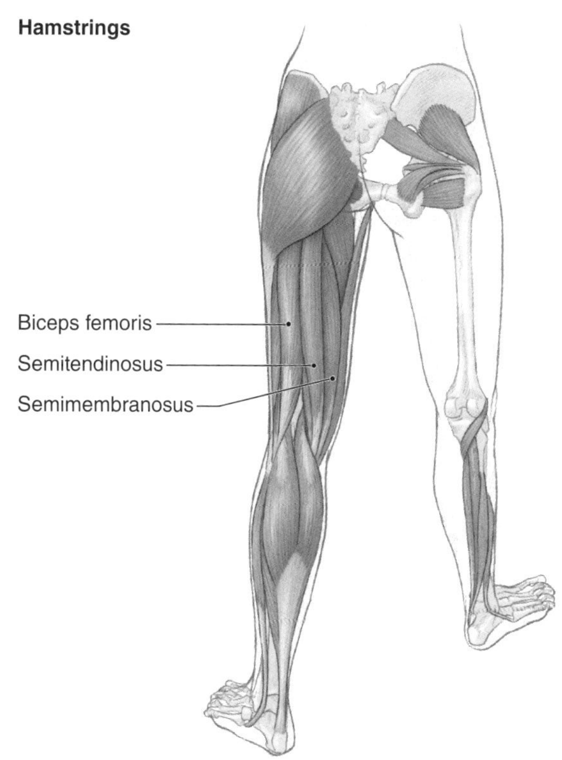

Figure 2.25 Hamstrings.

Hamstrings The hamstrings, composed of three muscles, are located in the back of the thigh. The biceps femoris has two origins. One part originates above the hip and one originates on the femur. The semimembranosus and the semitendinosus originate above the hip, and all three insert onto the lower leg. The hamstrings muscles move the hip and knee joints (figure 2.25).

Gastrocnemius (gas-trok-NE-me-us) The gastrocnemius muscle is the large muscle located in the calf. The gastrocnemius originates at the very lower end of the femur and the back of the knee and inserts onto the underside of the heel by way of the large Achilles tendon. The gastrocnemius crosses the knee; therefore, it is involved in movements at the knee, but its primary role is moving the ankle joint (figure 2.26).

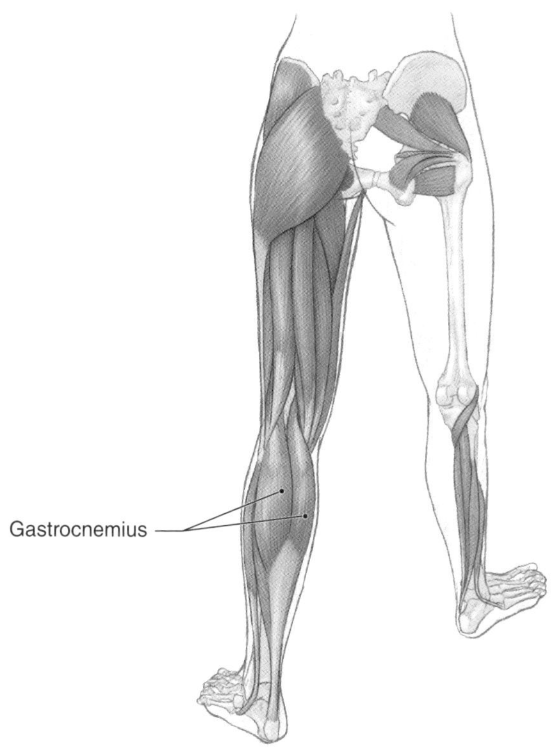

Figure 2.26 Gastrocnemius.

Soleus (SO-le-us) The soleus is located directly under the gastrocnemius in the calf. The soleus muscle originates near the

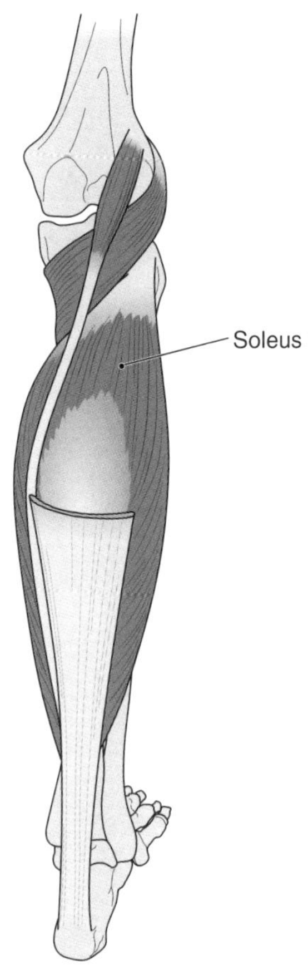

Figure 2.27 Soleus.

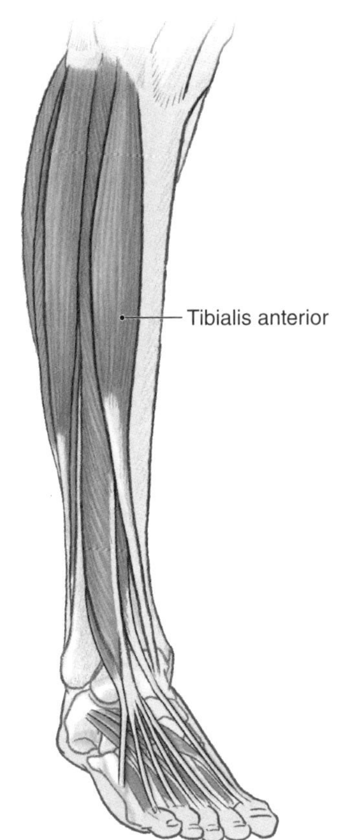

Figure 2.28 Tibialis anterior.

gastrocnemius on the tibia and fibula (lower leg) and inserts onto the underside of the heel by way of the large Achilles tendon. The soleus works with the gastrocnemius to move the ankle joint (figure 2.27).

Tibialis anterior (tib-e-A-lis) The tibialis anterior is located in front of the tibia bone, or in the shin. It originates on the front of the lower leg and inserts onto the top of the foot. The tibialis anterior moves the ankle joint (figure 2.28).

Nervous System

The nervous system is composed of the brain, spinal cord, nerves, and the sense organs. It serves as the control center and communication network within the body (figure 2.29). The split-second reactions determined by the nervous system and carried out by nerve impulses are instrumental in keeping the body functioning efficiently.

The nervous system has three primary functions. First, internal and external changes are sensed by a variety of sense organs and tissues. Next, the nervous system interprets these changes. Last, it responds to these interpretations through muscular contractions or glandular secretions. During water exercise, for example, the nervous system senses that the body is moving against greater resistance than normal. It then recognizes that more force is needed to move against the water and signals the muscles to work harder. A general understanding of how the nervous system is organized is particularly important when creating exercise modifications for people who are experiencing discomfort or limitations with movement due to a musculoskeletal injury or a chronic condition affecting the nervous system.

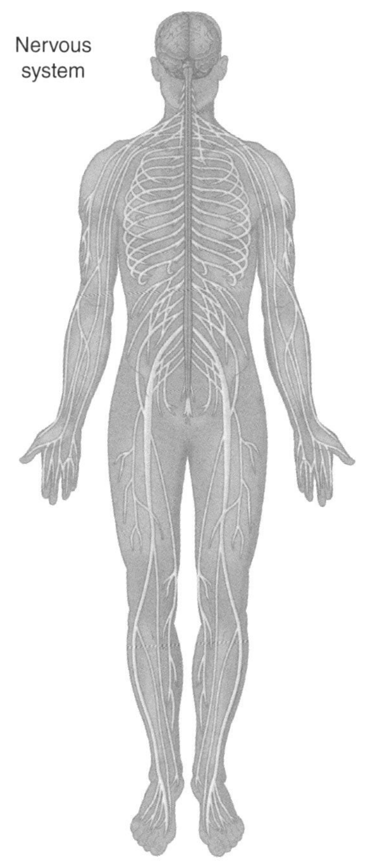

Figure 2.29 The nervous system.

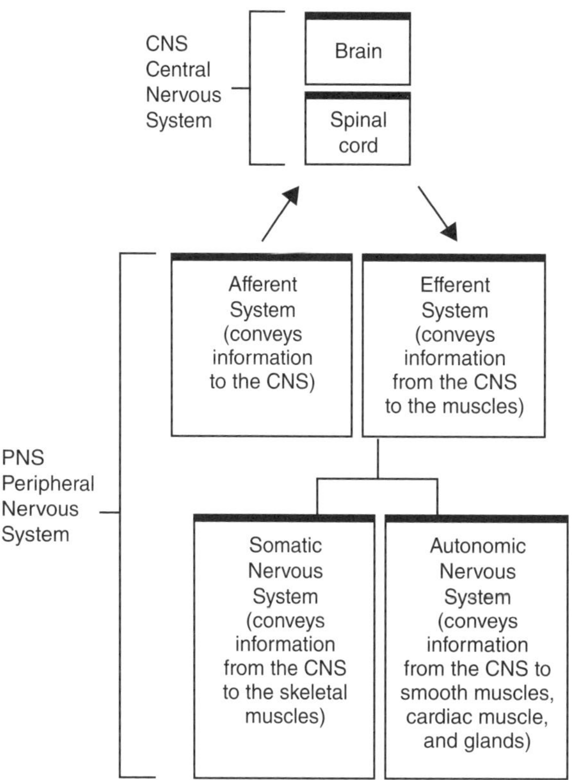

Figure 2.30 Divisions of the nervous system.

Organization of the Nervous System

The brain and spinal cord are the primary structures in the nervous system. They are classified as the **central nervous system** (CNS). The various nerve processes that branch off from the spinal cord and brain constitute the **peripheral nervous system** (PNS). The peripheral nervous system connects the brain and spinal cord with receptors, muscles, and glands.

The peripheral nervous system can be broken down into the **afferent** and **efferent nervous systems** (figure 2.30). The afferent system conveys information from sensors in the periphery of the body to the central nervous system via **neurons**, or nerve cells. This system conveys incoming information about position and tone from the muscles to the central nervous system. This information might include how much force will be needed to complete the movement or exercise.

The efferent neurons, also known as **motor neurons**, relay outgoing information from the central nervous system to the muscle cells. This information might include how many muscle fibers are needed to perform a certain exercise. The efferent system is further divided into the **somatic** and **autonomic nervous systems**.

The autonomic system consists of efferent neurons that transmit impulses to involuntary muscles and glands such as the heart and the muscles involved in respiration. The somatic system consists of efferent neurons that transmit messages or impulses to voluntary skeletal muscle. The somatic nervous system is important to fitness instructors in that it represents the link between the mind and the muscles to control movements. A single motor neuron in the brain may stimulate several neurons in the spinal cord, which in turn stimulate several fibers in a muscle.

Thus, a single impulse from the brain will result in the contraction of multiple muscle fibers.

During water exercise, the afferent nervous system sends sensory information to the brain about the resistance met as the body moves through the water. The brain recognizes that greater force is needed to create movement in the water. The somatic branches of the efferent nervous system carry messages to the skeletal muscles, signaling the agonist muscles to contract with the amount of force necessary to move against the resistance of the water. The somatic nervous system will also signal the antagonist muscles to relax or stretch to allow the movements to occur. The neuromuscular system will continue to send signals to the brain as exercises change; the brain will interpret the signals and respond to the signals with the appropriate muscle contractions as long as the body continues to exercise.

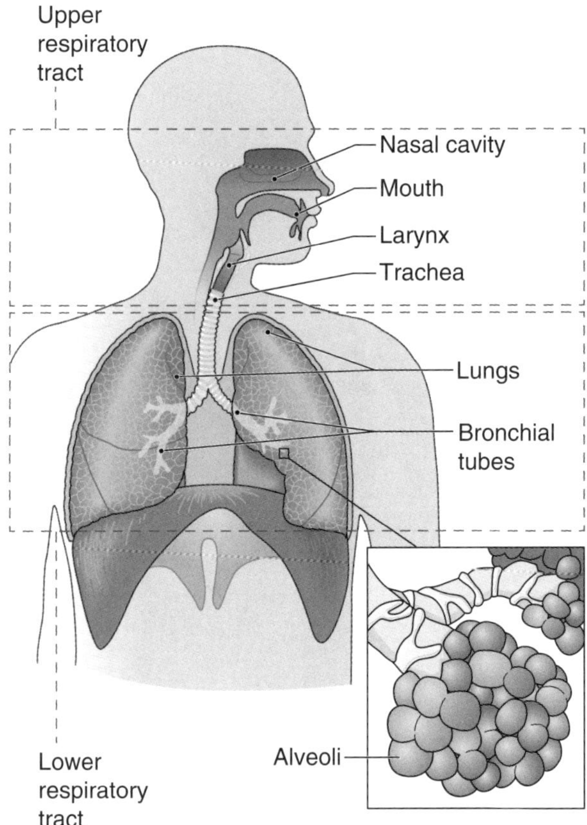

Figure 2.31 Respiratory system.

Respiratory System

The respiratory system is made up of the lungs and a series of passageways leading into and out of the lungs. The respiratory system is important in exercise because it functions to supply oxygen from the air we breathe to the body. Oxygen is critical in the production of energy used for muscular contractions during exercise. The respiratory system is also responsible for eliminating carbon dioxide, a by-product of energy production, through exhalation.

Organization of the Respiratory System

The respiratory system is divided into upper and lower respiratory tracts (figure 2.31). The upper respiratory tract consists of the parts located outside the chest cavity, including the mouth, nose, and nasal cavities as well as the upper **trachea** (the tube that connects the nasal passages to the lungs). The lower respiratory tract consists of the lower trachea and the lungs, which include the bronchial tubes and alveoli.

Oxygen Flow in the Respiratory System

Air enters and leaves the respiratory system through the nose and mouth. The nose is composed of bone and cartilage covered by skin. It contains tiny hairs that block dust and other pollutants from entering the body. Inhaled air travels through the nasal cavity, the larynx (voice box), and into the upper trachea. The trachea is 4 to 5 inches (10-12 cm) long and contains several C-shaped cartilaginous segments that hold it open. The air continues traveling in the trachea as it splits into the right and left primary **bronchi**. These two bronchi enter the lungs and continue to split and branch into smaller and smaller **bronchial tubes**. The smallest bronchial tubes connect to small balloon-like air sacs in the lungs, known as the **alveoli**.

In the alveoli, oxygen and carbon dioxide are exchanged through the vascular system. The alveoli are surrounded by a rich supply of pulmonary capillaries (very small blood vessels). Oxygen crosses into the pulmonary capillaries from the alveoli to be transported by the bloodstream to the heart and eventually pumped to the rest of the body. Carbon dioxide is carried from the heart and then to the lungs via the bloodstream. Carbon dioxide crosses from the blood into the alveoli, where it is exhaled through the respiratory tract.

Inhalation and exhalation are involuntary responses controlled primarily by the autonomic nervous system. Involuntary nerve impulses to the diaphragm and the intercostal muscles cause them to contract, assisting with inhalation. The **diaphragm** moves downward, and the intercostal muscles, which are located between the ribs, contract to expand the rib cage. This expansion of the chest cavity creates pressure that causes the lungs to expand and fill with air. When the pressure in the lungs and outside of the lungs is equal, a normal inhalation is completed. A more forceful contraction of the diaphragm and intercostal muscles further expands the lungs, allowing for an even deeper breath.

Exhalation is a much simpler process. When the nerve impulses are decreased, the diaphragm and intercostal muscles relax. The chest cavity becomes smaller and compresses the lungs and alveoli tissue, forcing air out through the respiratory tract.

Breathing correctly during exercise is critical to the efficiency of the circulatory and respiratory system as well as the delivery of oxygen to the body. Holding one's breath during the exertion phase of an exercise creates an unequal pressure in the chest, causing blood pressure to drop and decreasing blood flow to the heart. Resuming normal breathing creates a surge in blood to the heart, causing a sharp increase in blood pressure. This is known as the **Valsalva maneuver**, and can create dangerous conditions for people with high blood pressure or **cardiovascular disease**.

Cardiovascular System

The **cardiovascular system** is responsible for many functions in the body. The two that are most important to fitness professionals are the distribution of oxygen and **nutrients** to the cells and the removal of carbon dioxide and waste from the cells.

Organization of the Cardiovascular System

The cardiovascular system includes the heart, the blood vessels, and the blood. The heart is an organ located within the chest cavity that serves as the pump for the system. The blood vessels are a series of tubes that carry blood away from the heart throughout the body and eventually return the blood back to the heart. Blood is the fluid that the heart pumps through the blood vessels to deliver oxygen and nutrients to all parts of the body (figure 2.32).

Heart

Your heart is a hollow, fist-sized muscle found slightly to the left of your sternum in your chest cavity (figure 2.33). It is made up of four chambers—two receiving chambers called atria and two sending, or pumping, chambers called ventricles. A wall or **septum** is found between the right and left sides of the heart. Several membranous folds called **valves** open to allow blood to flow into the heart's chambers and then close to prevent the backflow of blood.

Blood flows in only one direction through the heart. Blood enters the **right atrium** of the heart through two large veins called the **superior vena cava** (carries blood from the upper body) and the **inferior vena cava** (carries blood from the lower body). Blood then flows through a valve into the **right ventricle**. The right ventricle contracts to force blood through the **pulmonary artery** to the cap-

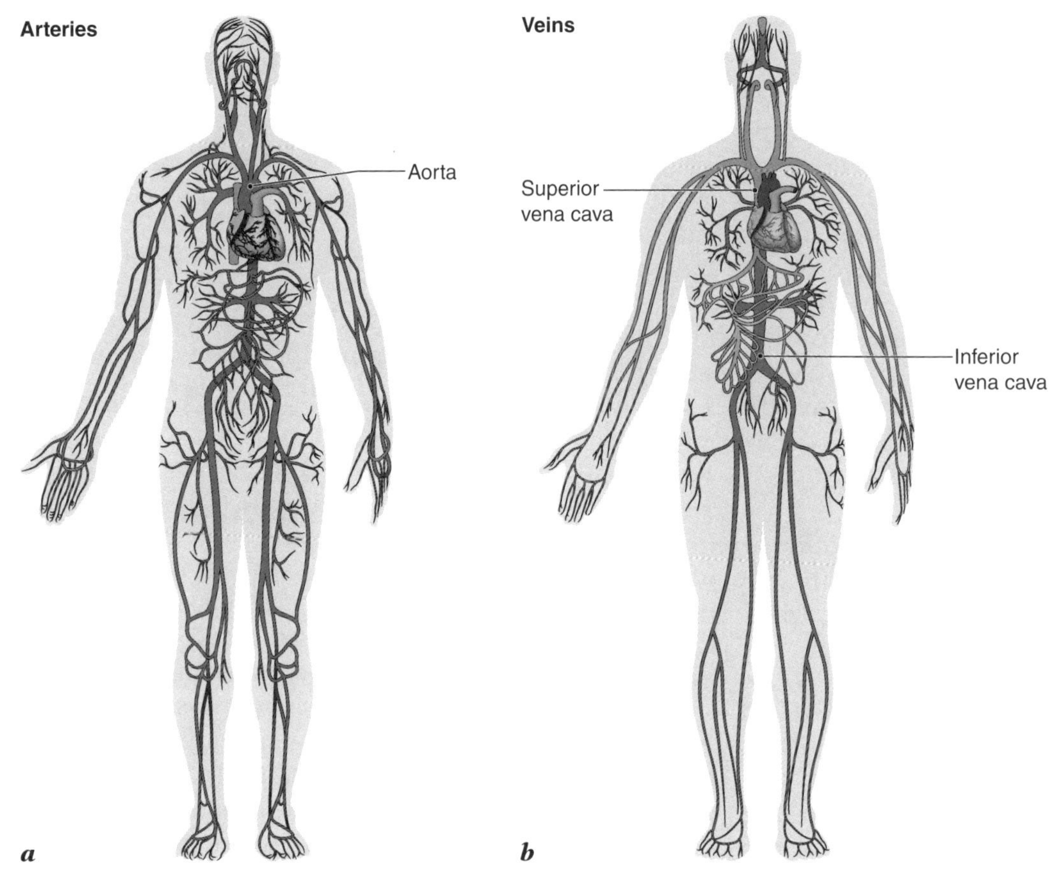

Figure 2.32 *(a)* Arteries and *(b)* veins of the cardiovascular system.

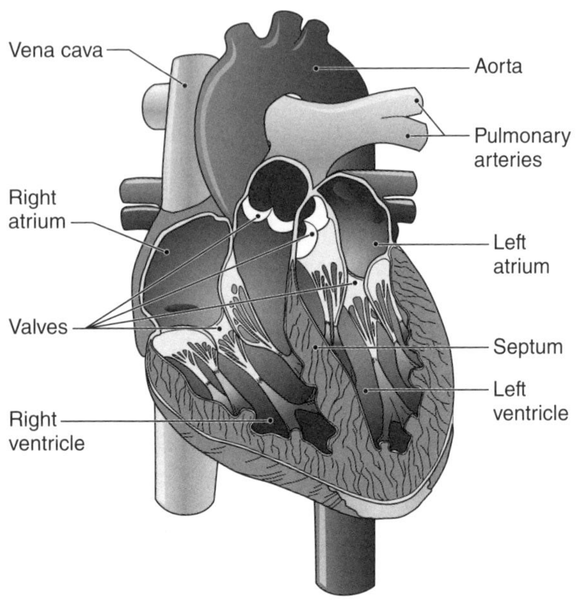

Figure 2.33 The heart.

illaries at the alveoli in the lungs. Here the blood is oxygenated (picks up oxygen) and sent back to the **left atrium** of the heart via the **pulmonary veins**. The blood then travels through a valve into the **left ventricle**, where it is forcefully pumped out of the heart through a large **artery**, called the **aorta**, to the body.

The heart itself is made of cardiac muscle. Therefore, it must be supplied with nutrients and oxygen of its own from the blood. The heart has its own supply of blood vessels called **coronary arteries**. A blockage in one of the coronary arteries restricts the blood flow and limits the amount of oxygen being supplied to the heart. Lack of oxygen to the heart significantly increases the risk of a **heart attack**, which could result in damage to the cardiac muscle tissue. Damage to the heart muscle would make the heart less efficient at pumping blood, oxygen, and nutrients to the body (figure 2.34).

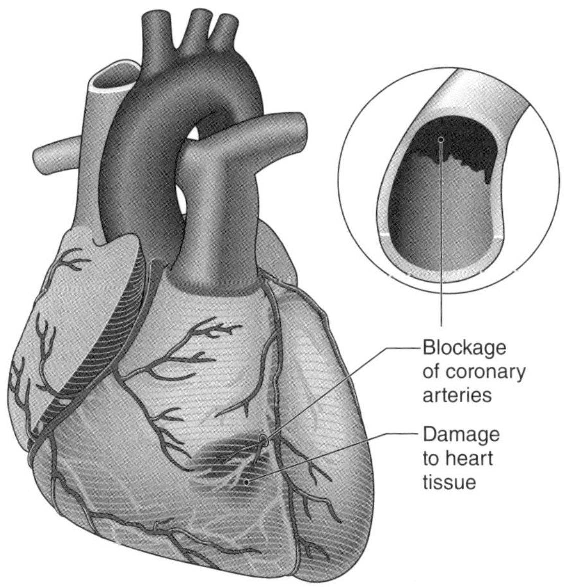

Figure 2.34 Heart attack.

Vessels

Blood vessels are divided into **arteries**, **capillaries**, and **veins**. All arteries, except for the pulmonary arteries, carry oxygenated blood away from the heart to all parts of the body. The aorta, the largest artery, carries blood from the left ventricle of the heart to the rest of the body. The blood continues to travel through smaller and smaller arteries throughout the body until it reaches the smallest branches of arteries, called **arterioles**. Arterioles are located at the capillary beds. Capillaries are where the arteries and veins meet. They have very thin membranes, allowing the exchange of oxygen and nutrients for carbon dioxide and waste products.

After the blood passes through the capillaries, exchanging the oxygen and nutrients for carbon dioxide and waste products, it then passes through the **venules**, which are the smallest branches of the veins. All veins, except for the pulmonary veins, carry deoxygenated blood back through the body to the heart. Blood travels through the venules to larger and larger veins until reaching the inferior and superior vena cava, which are the largest veins that carry blood into the heart. Many veins have valves to assist with venous return (blood flow back to the heart).

The blood vessels are like miles and miles—an estimated 60,000 miles (96,560 km)—of tubes carrying blood in a continuous loop from the heart, through the body, and back to the heart again (Loe and Edwards 2004).

Blood

Humans have between 4 and 6 liters of blood. General functions of the blood include transportation, regulation, and protection. The blood transports nutrients, gases, hormones, and waste products. It helps regulate body temperature and maintain fluid and electrolyte balance. **Red blood cells** contain the protein **hemoglobin**, which is where oxygen is carried in the blood. Iron, an essential component of hemoglobin, bonds with oxygen for transportation to the cells of the body. **White blood cells** protect the body from infectious diseases and provide immunity. **Platelets** are cells that function in several ways to clot blood to prevent blood loss during an injury.

Blood Flow and Oxygenation

The following is a review of the path blood takes to pick up oxygen, deliver it throughout the body, and remove carbon dioxide from the body (figures 2.35).

- Deoxygenated blood enters the right atrium through the inferior and superior venae cavae.
- The right atrium contracts to pump the deoxygenated blood through a valve into the right ventricle.
- The right ventricle contracts to pump deoxygenated blood through the pulmonary artery to the lungs.
- The pulmonary artery branches into smaller and smaller vessels called arterioles at the capillary beds of the lungs.
- At the capillary beds, oxygen and carbon dioxide are exchanged through the alveoli of the lungs.
- The oxygenated blood travels through the venules that branch into larger vessels to form the pulmonary veins.

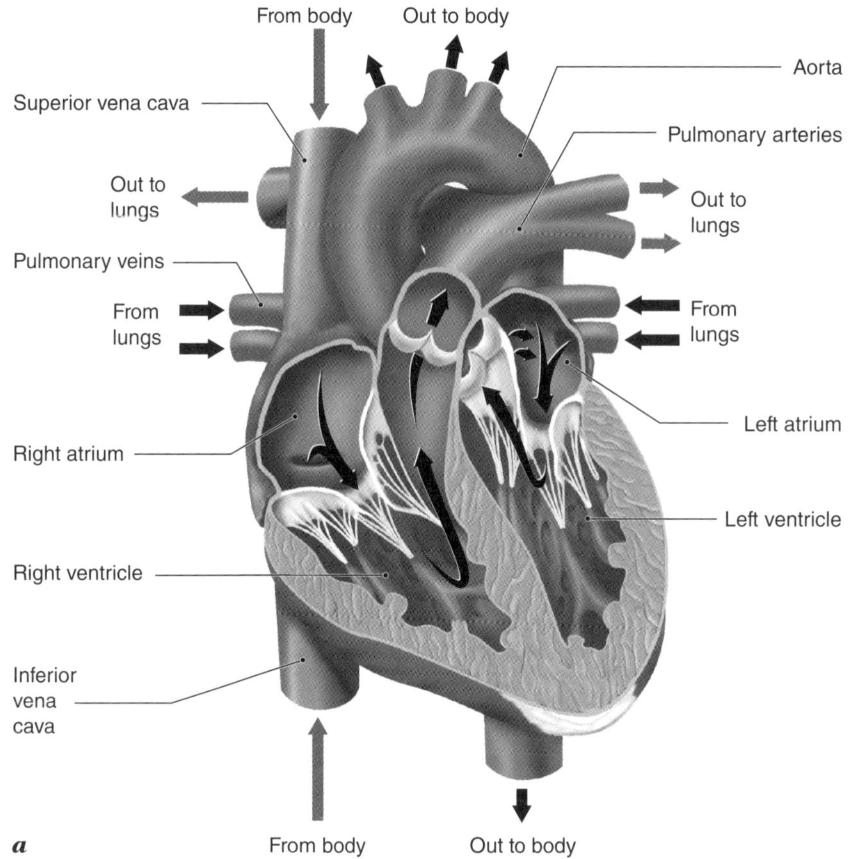

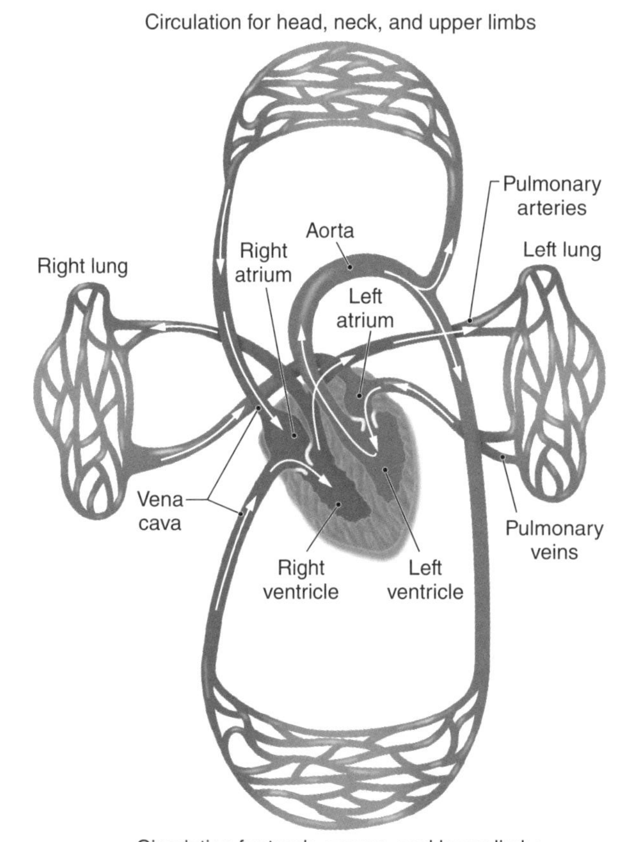

Figure 2.35 Blood flow through heart *(a)* and through the body *(b)*.

- Oxygenated blood enters the left atrium of the heart through the pulmonary veins.
- The left atrium contracts to pump oxygenated blood through a valve into the left ventricle.
- The left ventricle contracts forcefully to pump oxygenated blood through the aorta to the miles of arteries throughout the body.
- Oxygenated blood is carried through the arteries as they branch into smaller and smaller arterioles and finally into capillaries located at the capillary beds in various tissues of the body.
- At the capillary beds, oxygen and nutrients from the blood are exchanged for carbon dioxide and waste products from tissue fluids.
- The blood passes into the venules, which combine with larger and larger veins until reaching the inferior and superior venae cavae.
- The process begins again in an unending cycle that allows for normal function of the body.

When you start to exercise, the body recognizes that more oxygen will be needed to continue the exercise. Messages are sent to the respiratory system to bring in more oxygen through inhalation. Messages are also sent to the cardiovascular system to deliver more oxygen to the working muscle groups by increasing the heart rate to increase blood flow to the muscles. The cardiovascular and respiratory systems also work harder and faster to eliminate carbon dioxide through exhalation. These two systems, referenced together as the **cardiorespiratory system**, will continue to work at a higher rate as long as the body is continuing to exercise or recovering from exercise.

Cardiovascular Terms

Cardiac cycle: Simultaneous contraction of the atria followed by simultaneous contraction of the ventricles. This sequence of events is one heartbeat.

Systole: The active contraction of the heart muscle during the cardiac cycle. Ventricular contraction forces blood into the arteries.

Diastole: Relaxation of the heart muscle during the cardiac cycle.

Blood pressure: The force the blood exerts against the blood vessel walls. Two numbers are obtained (the systolic blood pressure and the diastolic blood pressure) and are normally expressed as a fraction. Systolic blood pressure is the pressure in the blood vessels during an active contraction of the heart muscle during the cardiac cycle (systole). This number is considered normal if it is less than 120. A diastolic blood pressure is the pressure in the vessels when the heart is relaxed during the cardiac cycle (diastole). Normal diastolic pressure is less than 80. A blood pressure of less than 120/80 is considered normal, a blood pressure between 120/80 and 139/89 is referred to as prehypertension, and blood pressure of 140/90 is considered high blood pressure. High blood pressure can weaken the blood vessel walls and increase the risk of cardiovascular disease and strokes.

Heart rate: The number of times the heart beats or completes a cardiac cycle in 1 minute. Heart rate is lower when at rest, and increases as activity level increases.

Stroke volume: The amount of blood pumped by the heart in one beat.

Cardiac output: The volume of blood pumped by the heart in 1 minute. Usually expressed as $CO = SV \times HR$, or cardiac output equals stroke volume times heart rate.

Arrhythmia: An abnormal or **irregular heart rhythm** resulting in an irregular heartbeat.

Tachycardia: An abnormally rapid or high heart rate.

Bradycardia: An abnormally slow or low heart rate.

Atherosclerosis: An abnormal collection of fat and other materials on the walls of arteries that narrow the openings and increase the risk of blockages.

Coronary artery disease: When atherosclerosis affects the arteries of the heart muscle.

Angina: Chest pain caused by lack of oxygen to the heart muscle. Angina is a symptom of heart disease.

Heart murmur: An abnormal or extra heart sound caused by the malfunctioning of a heart valve.

Summary

The 11 systems in the body interact to allow the body to function properly. Five systems (the skeletal, muscular, nervous, respiratory, and cardiovascular systems) allow us to move and sustain prolonged exercise. Each system plays a special role in the initiation and continuation of movements and exercise.

The skeletal system provides the rigid structure for muscles to attach and the leverage necessary for movement to occur. The muscular system provides the force that moves the skeleton. Our muscles attach from bone to bone across joints and have the ability to contract to move the bones. Tendons are fibrous connective tissues that attach muscles to bones, whereas ligaments attach bones to bones and provide stability to the joints. The muscles are primarily organized in pairs arranged on opposite sides of the same joint.

Coordinated, or voluntary, movement of the musculoskeletal system is made possible by the nervous system. The nervous system gives us the mind-to-muscle connection we need to move. Without the nervous system, we would not be able to control the quality or quantity of our muscle contractions.

The respiratory and cardiovascular systems provide the oxygen and nutrients needed for muscles to contract. The cardiovascular and respiratory systems also play a critical role in removing carbon dioxide and wastes from our bodies. We would not be able to sustain muscle contractions during exercise without these two systems.

Review Questions

1. The skeletal system provides our bodies with support, protection, and ______________________.
2. During the cardiac cycle, ________ is the active contraction of the heart muscle and ___________ is the relaxation of the heart muscle.
3. Which characteristic of muscle allows it to shorten and thicken?
4. The ________________________ muscle group flexes the leg at the knee.
5. What is a motor neuron?
6. Describe the Valsalva maneuver.
7. Name the five systems of the body most actively involved in movement and exercise.
8. In a muscle pair, the muscle that is actively contracting is referred to as the ___________, or prime mover.
9. List the three types of muscle tissues in the human body.
10. The process by which bones grow in the body is called ______________________.

See appendix D for answers to review questions.

References and Resources

American Council on Exercise. 2000. *Group fitness instructor manual.* San Diego: Author.

Haff, G.G., and N.T. Triplett. 2015. *Essentials of strength training and conditioning.* 4th edition. Champaign, IL: Human Kinetics.

Gray, H. 1901. *Gray's anatomy.* New York: Crown.

Loe, M.J., and W.D. Edwards. 2004. A light-hearted look at a lion-hearted organ (or, a perspective from three standard deviations beyond the norm). Part 1 (of two parts). *Cardiovascular Pathology* 13(5):282-292.

Office of the Surgeon General (US). 2004. *Bone health and osteoporosis: A report of the Surgeon General.* Rockville, MD: Author.

Riposo, D. 1990. *Fitness concepts: A resource manual for aquatic fitness instructors.* 2nd edition. Pt. Washington, WI: Aquatic Exercise Association.

Scanlon, V., and T. Sanders. 2003. *Essentials of anatomy and physiology.* 4th edition. Philadelphia: Davis.

Thompson, C.W., and R.T. Floyd. 1994. *Manual of structural kinesiology.* 12th edition. St. Louis: Mosby-Year Book.

Tortora, G., and S. Grabowski. 2002. *Principles of anatomy and physiology.* 10th edition. Indianapolis: Wiley.

Van Roden, J., and L. Gladwin. 2002. *Fitness: Theory & practice.* 4th edition. Sherman Oaks, CA: Aerobic & Fitness Association of America.

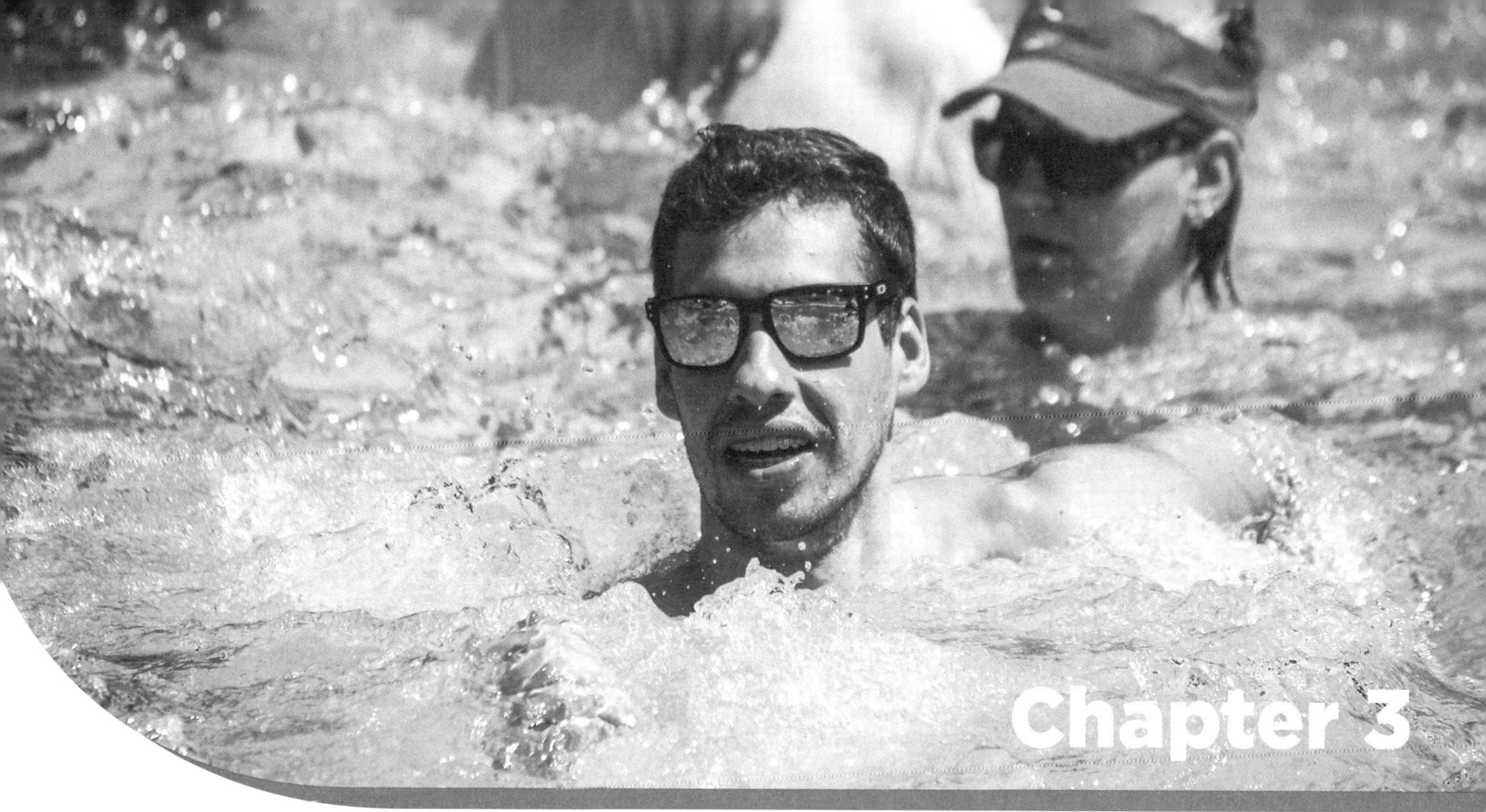

Exercise Physiology

Introduction

This chapter presents a basic explanation of the physiological principles governing the body's acute and chronic response to exercise. Exercise physiology helps to explain why our bodies adapt to different types of training, how we use various energy sources, and why it is important to provide a variety of aquatic programming.

Key Chapter Concepts

- Define the eight physiological principles required for improving fitness.
- Understand the three metabolic systems the body uses to produce ATP and how they work together during exercise.
- Recognize the difference between fast-twitch and slow-twitch muscle fibers.
- Differentiate between isometric, isotonic, and isokinetic muscle actions and contractions.
- Understand the importance of maintaining muscle balance and how muscle balance is promoted in the aquatic environment.
- Understand the acute physiological responses to both aerobic and anaerobic exercise.

Physiological Principles

Basic physiological principles must be applied in exercise programs in order to see advancements in fitness. Understanding these principles helps the fitness professional recognize how the body changes and responds to exercise. Appling these principles helps the fitness professional to offer effective aquatic programming based on the body's response to different exercise stimuli. These exercise principles will allow you to guide your participants in appropriate and effective programing that provides lasting results. They will also help you educate participants on the reasoning behind exercise programming.

Overload

Definition: A greater-than-normal stress or demand placed on a physiological system or organ typically resulting in an increase in strength or function.

This principle explains the method through which you become more fit. **Overload** occurs when a stimulus to the body is greater than that to which the body is accustomed. When the exercise frequency, intensity, or **duration** of the exercise being performed is changed to provide a greater challenge, the body adapts to the increased demand. A **threshold of training**, or a given overload, must be exceeded in order to see improvements in fitness. Overload is something that instructors need to consider in programming; otherwise, participants will not see progress. For instance, if an instructor teaches the same class with the same exercises at the same intensity day after day, participants will experience minimal or no change in their fitness levels. However, if the instructor provides new physiological stimuli in the form of new exercises, varied intensity levels, or added equipment, participants will be more likely to experience gains in their fitness levels.

If you want to increase function or fitness, you must overload the muscle or system where you want to see the change occur. The overload principal must be employed to improve all components of fitness. The water's resistance and the use of aquatic resistance equipment place additional demands on the muscle groups being targeted, resulting in increased muscular endurance, strength, or function. The cardiorespiratory system must be overloaded through exercise frequency, intensity, or duration to achieve increases in cardiorespiratory fitness or function. The overload principle must also be employed to promote gains in flexibility.

Progressive Overload

Definition: A gradual, systematic increase in the stress or demand placed on a physiological system or organ to promote fitness gains while avoiding the risk of chronic fatigue or injury.

The need to modify exercise programming by manipulating the exercise frequency, intensity, duration, or **mode** is important in producing fitness gains. However, if these modifications are too abrupt, adverse results may occur. Improper overload in a fitness program can pose a physiological threat to the body. Doing too much too fast can lead to injury or chronic fatigue. It is safer to progress through graduated levels of additional overload with less risk of injury. For example, an unfit participant needs to participate in several class sessions before adding resistance equipment. This person might also need to take brief rest breaks or reduce the intensity of the exercise when first participating in class. Properly using **progressive overload** increases participant compliance while promoting fitness gains. Progressive overload can be achieved by incrementally increasing intensity, duration, or frequency of exercise. It may also be incorporated by introducing new movement patterns or exercises gradually and at lower intensities. Alterations in rest and recovery should also be considered and progressed over time (rest and recovery are discussed later in the chapter).

Adaptation

Definition: The ability of a body part, system, or organ to adjust to additional stress, or overload, over time by increasing in strength or function.

The human body becomes more fit by adapting to additional demands or overload. If the body repeatedly performs the same type of exercise at the same workload, that particular exercise will become easier to perform. If you want to continue to increase function, you must continue to incrementally, or progressively, overload as the body adapts to each new challenge. **Adaptation** is one of the prizes of a regular exercise program. Instructors should understand and recognize the adaptation that occurs in their group fitness classes. Adaptation should cue the instructor that new exercise stimulus is needed to allow for greater participant fitness gains.

Specificity

Definition: You train only that part of the system or body that is overloaded in the way that it is overloaded.

Physiological adaptation is specific to the system or part of the body that is overloaded. If you lift weights to train the biceps muscles, you will see little or no benefit for the triceps muscles, deltoid muscles, or leg muscles. To see improvements, you must specifically train that muscle, muscle group, or metabolic system within the parameters that you want them to perform. Because of **specificity**, you must perform exercises to train for all of the activities that you wish to be able to complete. This should include all components of fitness as well as task-specific, or functional, training.

Specificity can refer to metabolic systems, neurological patterns, or muscular contractions. Therefore, exercise planning should consider the purpose of each exercise. In other words, training for a marathon would have a far different exercise prescription than training to participate in football. Instructors should consider what muscles, movement patterns, components of fitness, and metabolic systems are used for the exercise goal and mimic these within the exercise class. The most optimal exercise session is one that considers the individual needs of the participants. Though improvements in fitness help you better perform any type of exercise, your body will perform exercises for which you have specifically trained with less effort and greater efficiency.

Variability (Cross-Training)

Definition: The varying of intensity, duration, or mode (cross-training) of exercise sessions to obtain better overall fitness.

Increasing demand on a variety of muscle groups or physiological systems creates more widespread adaptation within the body. **Variability** is necessary because of the law of specificity. Athletes must train specifically to improve skills and performance for a particular sport while including cross-training techniques to assist with general health, reduced injury rate, and **muscle balance**. Conversely, the average adult seeking overall health and fitness should practice a variety of exercise modes, intensities, and durations to challenge the body and develop a more widespread base of overall fitness. The concept of variability or cross-training can easily be incorporated into aquatic fitness classes simply by altering the class variables. Instructors can change the exercises being performed, the intensity to which they are performed, the equipment used, and the duration of the activities.

Reversibility

Definition: The body will gradually revert to pretraining status when exercise is discontinued.

Fitness cannot be stored. When you do not exercise, physiological function or strength will decrease to pretraining levels over time. The old adage, "If you don't use it, you lose it.," rings true with the **reversibility** principle. A reduction in fitness due to discontinuing exercise is commonly called detraining. Fitness losses can happen rapidly once exercise ceases. This is an important educational topic for instructors to share with their participants.

One encouraging point is that our bodies do store muscle or fitness memory. Because of many factors associated with muscle memory, a previously fit person finds it much easier to get back into shape compared to someone who has never exercised. Encourage your participants not to use a two-week layoff as an excuse to abandon exercise completely. Getting started again might be difficult for the first few exercise sessions, but fitness will return quickly.

Recovery

Definition: The body's return to *homeostasis*.

Recovery pertains to two segments of exercise training: (1) recovery during exercise and (2) recovery after an exercise session. Recovery is an integral component of fitness that is necessary for the body to continually adapt. Recovery between exercise bouts, also termed short-term recovery, provides participants rest between intense bouts of exercise. This allows participants to work at a higher intensity level than what would be possible if rest was not incorporated. The recovery time between exercise sessions is known as training recovery, and allows a more complete return to homeostasis at the cellular level. Both types of recovery are important to consider for optimal fitness gains.

Overtraining

Definition: Long-term reductions in performance and overall ability to exercise due to an imbalance in the amount of exercise and amount of recovery.

Overtraining occurs when people take part in extensive amounts of exercise without allowing for recovery. Physical and psychological symptoms that commonly accompany overtraining include a reduction in performance and **coordination**, elevated resting heart rate and blood pressure, loss of appetite, soreness, increased illness or infection, issues with sleep, depression, and reduced self-esteem. Fitness professionals should be aware of these signs and symptoms, not only for their class participants, but also for themselves. Usually, overtraining can be avoided by adhering to the progressive overload principle and incorporating appropriate training recovery between exercise sessions.

Energy Metabolism

The conversion of energy within the human body, or **energy metabolism**, is a fascinating and ongoing process. The body must maintain a continuous energy supply to support all of the necessary functions when working and while at rest. The primary energy supply for our body is derived from the foods that we eat. These foods must be converted to an energy source that our body can easily use. This energy source is known as **adenosine triphosphate**, or ATP. ATP is an immediately available source of energy for our body that is stored in small amounts within our cells. It can also be produced, or synthesized, from fuel that has been stored (fat and **glycogen**). Due to fluctuating energy needs, the body has several pathways to provide the necessary ATP for the work being performed. Aquatic fitness professionals can use their knowledge of these pathways to design and implement workouts that emphasize the different systems. By stressing all of the energy

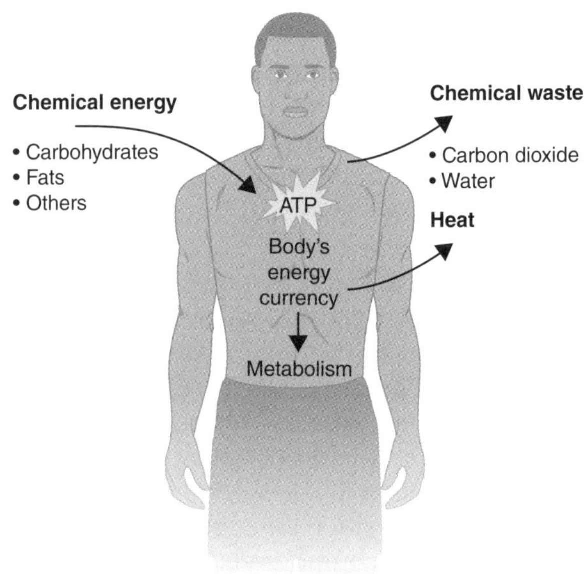

Figure 3.1 Energy conversion chain.

pathways, you can help your participants achieve a greater level of fitness.

Adenosine Triphosphate (ATP)

Adenosine triphosphate, more commonly known as ATP, is the most immediate source of energy for a cell. The amount of ATP stored in the cell is able to provide enough energy for several seconds of maximal, explosive exercise. Then, the stores are depleted. Additional ATP must be supplied for exercise lasting longer than a few seconds. Three systems manufacture energy for the muscle cells. The primary energy system activated depends specifically on the exercise being performed. Active muscle has an immediate source of energy available (the ATP-PC system), a short-term source of energy (the anaerobic glycolysis or glycolytic system), and a long-term source of energy (the aerobic or oxidative system). These three systems work together to meet the ATP demands that the body requires.

ATP-PC System

The **ATP-PC system** supplies the working muscle with an immediate source of energy. Activities with a high-energy demand over a short period of time depend primarily on ATP generated from this system. A rapidly available source of ATP is supplied to the muscles for contractions involving a relatively short series of chemical reactions that does not require oxygen. Because this system does not require oxygen for the synthesis of ATP, it is considered to be **anaerobic** (or without oxygen). The ATP-PC system is the primary source of energy for muscle contractions during the first few seconds of exercise regardless of exercise intensity or duration. This means that going from sitting in a chair to standing up uses the ATP-PC system to initiate that movement. The total amount of ATP energy available from this system is very limited; it would be exhausted after about 10 seconds of maximal exercise.

During their classes, aquatic professionals can incorporate intervals lasting 8 to 10 seconds while providing ample recovery to target the ATP-PC system. As you stress this system, the body will adapt and be able to produce more power, burn more **calories**, and enhance the energy system.

- Intensity: Up to maximal levels of exercise
- Type: Anaerobic
- Duration: 0-10 seconds
- Examples: 10 seconds of sprinting, 5-10 squat jumps, getting up from a chair

Glycolytic System

The **glycolytic system**, or **anaerobic glycolysis**, is the primary source of ATP for intermediate energy or for activities lasting more than a few seconds up to approximately 2 minutes. The glycolytic system uses glycogen or sugar stored in the muscles to create ATP. Like the ATP-PC system, it does not require oxygen. The series of chemical reactions occurring during anaerobic glycolysis results in a by-product known as **lactic acid**. When lactic acid builds up in the muscle and blood, it leads to muscle fatigue and ultimately to muscle failure.

The anaerobic glycolysis system can be enhanced by using intervals with the purpose of either teaching the body to better tolerate the lactic acid buildup in the muscles or developing the body's ability to remove lactic acid more proficiently. To assist in improving the body's tolerance to lactic acid, use intervals that require 30 seconds to 2 minutes of hard work paired with near full recovery. If you want to teach the body to clear, or buffer, lactic acid more proficiently, perform intervals lasting 30 seconds to 2 minutes with less than full recovery so that the lactic acid can accumulate and your body will be forced to adapt.

- Intensity: Up to maximal levels of exercise
- Type: Anaerobic
- Duration: 10 seconds to 2 minutes
- Examples: Sprint repeats, 1 minute of squat jumps, high-intensity running from one end of the pool to the other

Oxidative System

The **oxidative system** produces a substantially greater number of ATP molecules and uses oxygen to generate ATP. It is activated to produce energy for long-duration exercise. This system requires an uninterrupted supply of oxygen in order to continue to produce ATP, but can supply virtually unlimited energy in the presence of oxygen. This aerobic system uses both glycogen (derived from **carbohydrate**) and fatty acids (derived from fat).

Aerobic glycolysis is the breakdown of glycogen in the presence of oxygen. The difference between anaerobic glycolysis, discussed previously, and aerobic glycolysis is that oxygen prevents the accumulation of lactic acid. The lower intensity of the exercise being performed allows the body to meet the oxygen demands, thus making oxygen readily available for use in ATP production and lactic acid buffering. If fatty acids are used for fuel instead of glycogen, more oxygen is needed, but the yield of ATP is substantially higher. Fatty acids are considered to be calorically dense, meaning that fatty acids can provide more energy to the body than any other fuel source. For this reason, fat is the preferred source of fuel for low-intensity exercise. Higher-intensity exercise limits the amount of oxygen that is available, and will require ATP production from anaerobic glycolysis. Glycogen derived from carbohydrate is the preferred source of fuel for higher-intensity exercises.

As with the other metabolic systems, the oxidative system can be trained to become more efficient. Unlike the anaerobic systems, the aerobic systems are not power oriented. The oxidative system is focused on lower-intensity, long-duration exercise. This system can be trained with steady-state continuous exercise, intervals with shorter durations of rest, or varied-intensity continuous exercise. Increasing the intensity of the exercise sessions allows the body to adapt so that the oxidative system will be more efficient during higher intensities of exercise. This means that you train your body to use the oxidative system, both glycogen and fatty acids, more efficiently.

- Intensity: Low to moderate levels of exercise
- Type: Aerobic
- Duration: More than 2 minutes
- Examples: Low- to moderate-intensity running for 30 minutes, 3 minutes of shallow water squats, completing most **activities of daily living (ADLs)** such as bathing and getting dressed and **instrumental activities of daily living (IADLs)**, such as cooking and cleaning.

How These Systems Interact

Although energy systems are activated in response to specific types of exercise or activity, one system does not shut off as another is activated. All systems are being used at all times, but one system will dominate (figure 3.2). For instance, in times of low energy demands or physical inactivity, the oxidative system is the dominant fuel production system. Once the body initiates movement or exercise, the ATP-PC, glycolytic, and oxidative systems are engaged. Because it takes a few seconds for these systems to begin producing ATP, the immediate stores of ATP are used (0-10 seconds). By then, the glycolytic system

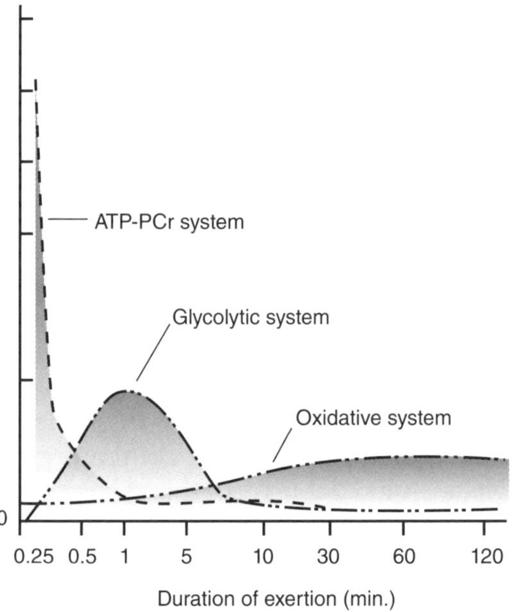

Figure 3.2 How the metabolic systems work together.

is working at full capacity and can continue the ATP production at a high rate for up to 2 minutes. Once the body's anaerobic systems have exhausted their resources, or the intensity of the exercise decreases, the oxidative system, which has been producing ATP this entire time, takes the lead role of supplying the body with the necessary ATP for the work being accomplished. At any point during the exercise session that the body requires more power or a higher level of intensity, the ATP-PC and glycolytic systems will become the dominating systems once more.

Skeletal Muscle Tissue

As with the various energy systems and their specialized functions, skeletal muscle (figure 3.3) is similarly composed of different kinds of fibers, each with unique characteristics. The fiber types and energy systems are interrelated in their function. In other words, some fiber types are made for quick, powerful movements related to the anaerobic energy systems, while others are constructed for long-duration, lower-intensity exercise corresponding to the oxidative energy systems.

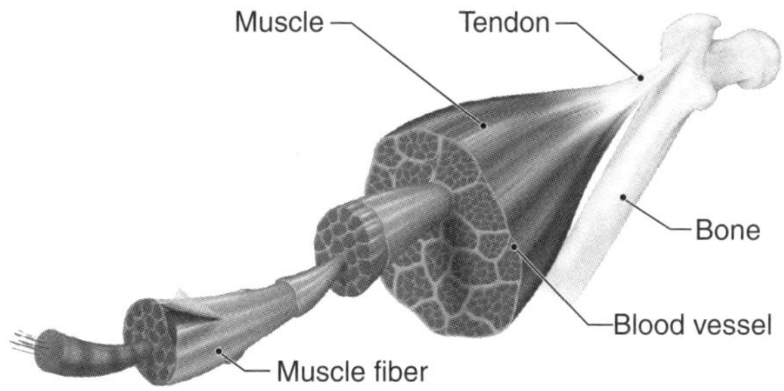

Figure 3.3 Skeletal muscle.

Types of Skeletal Muscle Fibers

The duration of contraction of various muscles depends on their function in the body. Eye movements must be rapid, so the duration of contraction of eye muscles is less than 1/100th of a second. The erector spinae muscle in the back does not depend on rapid movement to function properly, so the duration of contraction for this muscle is about 1/30th of a second. Faster contracting muscles, like the muscles around the eye, are made up primarily of "white muscle," or **fast-twitch (Type II)** muscle fibers. Slower contracting muscles, like those in the erector spinae, are made up primarily of "red muscles," or **slow-twitch (Type I)** muscle fibers.

Slow-twitch muscle fibers are slow to fatigue, and are made for submaximal prolonged exercise. They contain additional oxygen-rich components for more aerobic energy production, and are reddish in color. Slow-twitch fibers are the first recruited. They can sustain repeated contractions for extended periods of time. For this reason, muscle groups that need endurance more than power, such as those involved in posture maintenance, are predominately composed of slow-twitch muscle fibers.

Fast-twitch muscles, on the other hand, are specialized for high-intensity contractions and therefore fatigue more readily. They depend more on anaerobic energy production and are whitish in appearance because they do not store much blood. When the demand for force exceeds that of what the slow-twitch fibers can sustain, the fast-twitch fibers are recruited. Fast-twitch fibers make up the bulk of our skeletal muscles (muscles responsible for movement) and contribute to increasing muscle size. Although muscle groups may be dominated by one muscle fiber type, all muscles are made up of Type I and Type II fibers. This is important to know when understanding how muscles will adapt to movements.

These two types of muscle fibers are classified by the energy systems they use and their ability to contract. It is estimated that 45 percent of muscle fiber type is genetically predetermined in humans; the other primary variables are the environment and its related stimuli (Wilmore and Costill 2001; Simoneau and Bouchard 1995). It is likely that muscle fibers can take on the characteristics of another type in response to aerobic or anaerobic training (Wilson et al. 2012). In other words, it is possible for us to alter our muscle fibers by training our body in a specific way. Most untrained people have an approximate 50/50 muscle composition (fast and slow twitch). However, it is found that long-distance runners have more slow-twitch endurance fibers and sprinters have more fast-twitch anaerobic fibers. This finding could be supported by both genetic and environmental factors (training). Regardless, all skeletal muscles possess both types of fibers, but predominant muscle fiber type in any given skeletal muscle depends on several factors, including the function of the muscle, genetics, and how the muscle has been trained.

Types of Skeletal Muscle Contractions and Actions

Skeletal muscle can generate three types of muscle actions: **isotonic**, **isometric**, and **isokinetic**.

Isotonic contractions occur when muscles shorten and lengthen and movement occurs at the joint. Isotonic contractions cause, as well as control, joint movement. The force generated by the contraction changes with the length of the muscle and the angle of the joint. Isotonic contractions consist of two parts—the shortening, or concentric phase, and the lengthening, or eccentric phase (see figure 3.4). The concentric phase occurs when the muscle is creating tension while shortening or contracting (for example, raising a weight resisted by gravity in a forearm curl). The eccentric phase happens when the weight is lowered while assisted by gravity, or when tension is retained in a muscle as it lengthens. The eccentric part is often referred to as negative work.

Technically, the eccentric phase is considered a muscle action instead of a contraction because the muscle is lengthening instead of shortening, as the term contraction implies (Ostdiek and Bord 1994). However, the terms muscle action and muscle contraction are often used interchangeably, as we will do in this manual.

Concentric and eccentric muscle actions are of particular interest in the aquatic environment. Primarily concentric contractions are used in aquatic exercise because the drag property of the water provides more resistance than gravity or buoyancy. In the water, both muscles of a muscle pair are worked concentrically. This is different than on land (gravity environment), where one muscle is being worked concentrically and eccentrically. For example, when doing an arm curl on land, the bicep contracts concentrically (shortens) to bend the elbow against gravity. The bicep contracts eccentrically (lengthens) to slowly straighten the arm, in the direction of gravity, back to the starting position. Doing an arm curl in the water, the bicep contracts concentrically to bend the elbow against the resistance of the water. The triceps contracts concentrically to straighten the arm against the resistance of the water.

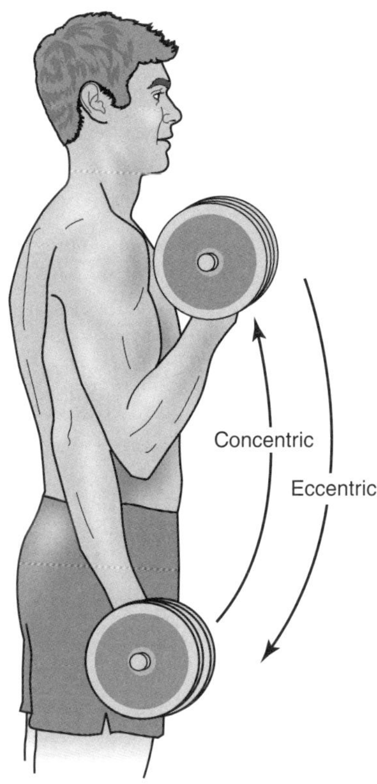

Figure 3.4 Concentric and eccentric phases of the isotonic contraction.

It is a common misconception that eccentric contractions are significantly better at building strength in a muscle. Research indicates that eccentric training results in no greater gains in isometric, eccentric, and concentric strength than normal resistance training with dumbbells (Fleck and Kraemer 2003). Aquatic strength training programs have been shown to improve all aspects of strength for all age groups, including maximal strength and muscular endurance. Research clearly indicates that strength gains can be achieved through appropriate aquatic training programs (Colado et al. 2009; Katsura et al. 2010; Arazi and Asadi 2011). Although muscle contractions done in water are predominately concentric, eccentric muscle actions are achievable. Eccentric actions can be introduced for variety through the use of buoyant, weighted, and rubberized equipment. The influence of equipment on muscle actions in the aquatic environment is discussed more fully in chapter 4.

Isometric muscle actions occur when tension is developed in the muscle without movement at the joint or a change in the muscle length. Isometric literally means equal length. In an isometric action, the tension remains constant because the length of the muscle does not change. Examples of isometric actions are holding a push-up in the down position and trying to move an immovable object, such as pressing against a door frame. Because no movement is involved, this muscle action is often called a static contraction. Isometric muscle actions have the ability to recruit the entire muscle for the contraction, but will only strengthen the muscle or muscle group at the angle where engaged. In other words, if you are isometrically contracting your arm to hold a 90-degree angle at the elbow, then the muscles will get stronger at that angle. Isometric muscle actions were once considered dangerous for people with high blood pressure, but more recent findings support the use of isometric muscle actions to assist with reductions in blood pressure (Cornelissen and Smart 2013; Owen, Wiles, and Swaine 2010). In fact, when compared to dynamic aerobic and dynamic strength training, isometric training resulted in greater reductions in blood pressure.

Isokinetic muscle actions are, in a sense, a combination of isometric and isotonic contractions. Because of this, some consider isokinetic muscle actions to be a technique as opposed to another type of muscle contraction (Thompson and Floyd 2000). An isokinetic muscle action is a dynamic muscle action performed at a constant velocity. Isokinetic actions are not performed in aqua exercise because this type of muscle action requires very specialized, expensive equipment. Isokinetic equipment is primarily used in physical therapy and athletic training facilities.

Muscle Balance

Muscle pairs (discussed in chapter 2) surrounding any given joint need to be reasonably equal in both strength and flexibility to promote optimal mobility and function. Muscular imbalance in strength, flexibility, or both can affect the integrity of the involved joint and increase risk of injury. Many **acute** and **chronic injuries** can be traced to poor joint integrity or stability as a result of muscle imbalance in either strength or flexibility. Muscle balance should be considered for the front and back, left and right sides, and upper and lower parts of the body. For instance, when designing exercises involving the upper leg, perform exercises that work on the front and back of the thigh, inner and outer thigh, and the bottom (near the knee) and top (near the hip) portions of the thigh.

The human body craves symmetry and **balance**. It is very common for a variety of asymmetries (imbalances) to exist throughout the body that can lead to acute or chronic issues. These issues usually arise from activities that we perform frequently, such as movements necessary for our occupation, participation in a sport, or how we move in general. Muscle balance is one of the factors that instructors must pay close attention to when designing classes.

Muscle balance (or imbalance) carries over to all forms of exercise. If you train using only one type of exercise or only one certain type of program, you could be promoting muscle imbalance. For example, biking places emphasis on the quadriceps muscles. Therefore, other types of exercise that emphasize the hamstrings should be combined with a bike training program to maintain equality in strength in the thigh muscles to maintain integrity in the knee joint. Remember that both muscles in a muscle pair should also be stretched during each workout to maintain equality in flexibility.

The aquatic environment enhances muscle balance. The resistance of the water surrounds you when you are exercising and therefore affects every movement in every direction. This provides resistance for both muscles in a muscle pair in both directions of movement unless specific equipment is being used. This topic is covered in more detail in chapter 4.

Acute Responses to Aerobic and Anaerobic Exercise

Prolonged aerobic exercise, such as a water aerobics class, elicits certain physiological responses within the body. When beginning to exercise, an immediate demand is placed on the body for more oxygen. Unfortunately, the body cannot immediately supply increased amounts of oxygen to the working muscle. It takes time to transport the oxygen from the air, through the respiratory system, through the cardiovascular system to the muscle cells. This time of inadequate oxygen supply is referred to as **oxygen deficit**. During this time, ATP is primarily synthesized by the anaerobic systems (ATP-PC and anaerobic glycolysis), resulting in accumulation of lactic acid in the muscle tissue. Eventually, the body is able to supply the oxygen needed for exercise, and oxygen supply meets oxygen demand. This is referred to as **steady-state exercise**.

At the cessation of exercise, oxygen supply exceeds oxygen demand. Your heart rate and respiratory rate do not drop immediately to resting rates; rather, they do so gradually over time to allow the body to account for the time spent in oxygen deficit. This time of excess oxygen supply is referred to as **oxygen debt** or **excess post-exercise oxygen consumption (EPOC)**. During this time, extra oxygen is needed to help return the body back to homeostasis by ridding the body of waste products, such as lactic acid, that were created during exercise (figure 3.5). The duration of EPOC depends on the intensity and duration of the exercise session. The larger the oxygen deficit, the longer it takes for the oxygen debt (EPOC) to be repaid.

In anaerobic or very high-intensity exercise, the body never reaches steady state exercise because oxygen supply never meets oxygen demand (figure 3.6). In this type of exercise, energy stores are depleted and the respiratory system becomes distressed, lactic acid builds up, body temperature rises, and muscles fatigue. Because the body has experienced a greater amount of physiological stress, it will take longer to recover. During this recovery period, the body uses greater amounts of energy to return all of the body's

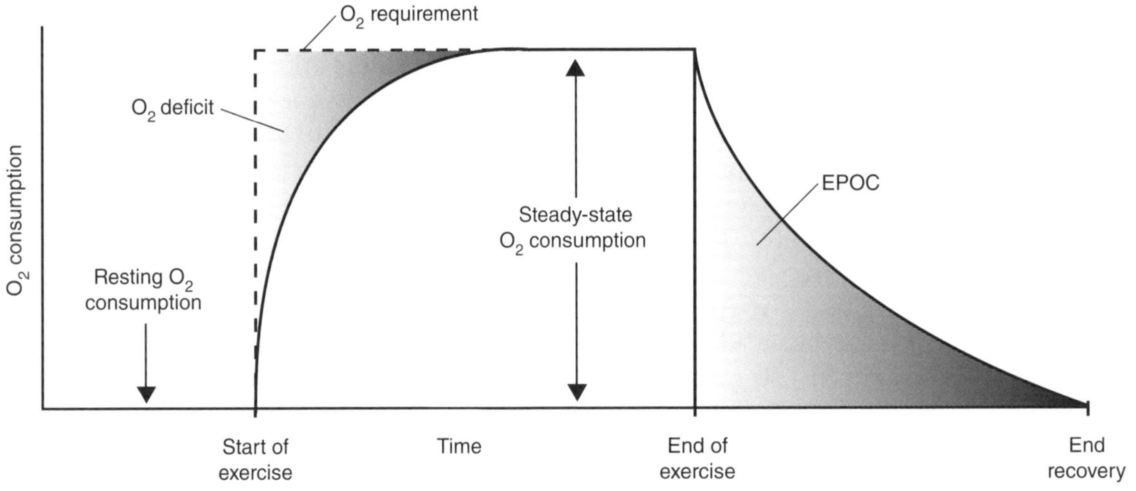

Figure 3.5 Steady-state aerobic exercise.

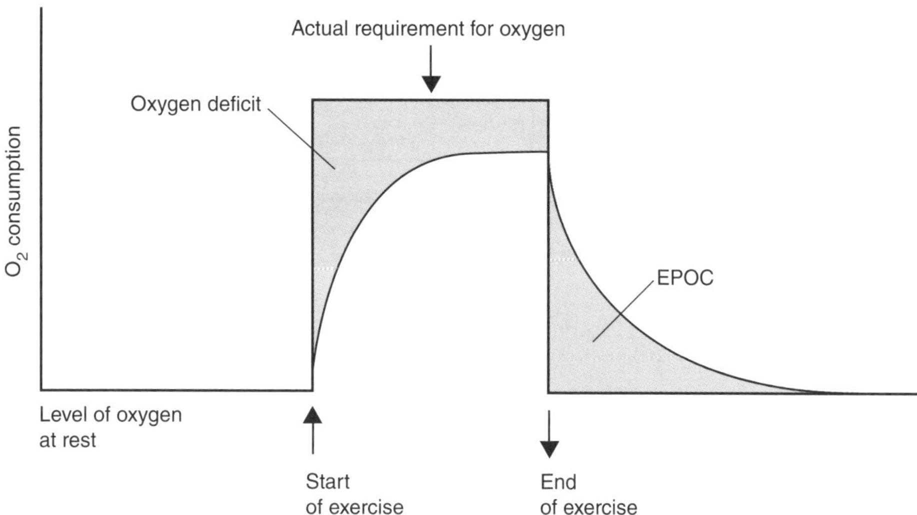

Figure 3.6 Anaerobic exercise.

systems back to homeostatic levels. For this reason, the recovery time following anaerobic exercise is commonly called the afterburn, otherwise known as EPOC, due to the increased caloric expenditure still occurring in the body.

The physiological status of the body during recovery supports the need for properly cooling down and stretching after an exercise session. Continuing dynamic movement while reducing the speed and intensity assists in gradually returning the body back to homeostatic levels. The cardiovascular, respiratory, and muscular systems should be the primary focus during the cool-down. Permitting these systems to gradually return to pre-exercising levels reduces the tendency of blood to pool in the legs, reduces risk of cardiac events after exercise, and decreases the risks of feeling light-headed or dizzy.

Summary

Eight physiological principles govern the body's response to exercise. These principles are overload, progressive overload, adaptation, specificity, variability, reversibility, recovery, and overtraining.

The body uses three energy systems to synthesize ATP for muscle contractions. For immediate energy (up to 10 seconds), the ATP-PC system is primarily used. For intermediate energy (10 seconds to 2 minutes), the glycolytic system (or anaerobic glycolysis) is primarily used. For long-term energy (greater than 2 minutes), the oxidative system supplies most of the ATP needed.

Two basic types of muscle fibers are found in human skeletal muscle: fast-twitch (white) Type II muscle fibers used for intense or explosive exercises and slow-twitch (red) Type I muscle fibers used for moderate-intensity exercise at longer durations.

Three basic types of muscle actions exist: isotonic contractions consisting of concentric and eccentric muscle actions, isometric contractions or actions in which tension is developed without movement, and isokinetic contractions that require specialized equipment.

Responses to aerobic exercise include oxygen deficit, steady state, and EPOC. In anaerobic exercise, the body never achieves steady state. Recovery from exercise is the time when energy stores are replenished and lactic acid and other waste products are removed.

Review Questions

1. ____________________ states that you train only that part of the system or body that is overloaded.
2. Muscle balance should be considered for the front and back, left and right sides, and ________________ parts of the body.
3. Which metabolic system yields the highest amount of ATP for the working muscle?
4. Recovery pertains to two segments of training: recovery _____________ exercise and recovery _______ an exercise session.
5. List five physical and psychological symptoms that commonly accompany overtraining.
6. Which type of muscle tissue is best suited for endurance activities?
7. Concentric and eccentric muscle actions are part of a(n) ____________________ muscle contraction.
8. When initiating exercise, the time of inadequate oxygen supply is called ____________________.
9. A given overload must be exceeded in order to see improvements in fitness. This is referred to as ____________________.
10. Name the three types of muscle actions that skeletal muscle can generate.

See appendix D for answers to review questions.

References and Resources

American Council on Exercise. 2000. *Group fitness instructor manual.* San Diego: Author.

———. 2003. *Personal trainer manual.* 3rd edition. San Diego: Author.

Arazi, H., and A. Asadi. 2011. The effect of aquatic and land plyometric training on strength, sprint, and balance in young basketball players. *Journal of Human Sport and Exercise* 6(1):101-111

Colado, J.C., V. Tella, N.T. Triplett, and L.M. González. 2009. Effects of a short-term aquatic resistance program on strength and body composition in fit young men. *Journal of Strength & Conditioning Research* 23(2):549-559.

Cornelissen, V.A., and N.A. Smart. 2013. Exercise training for blood pressure: A systematic review and meta-analysis. *Journal of the American Heart Association*. 2(1):e004473.

Fleck, S., and W. Kraemer. 2003. *Designing resistance training programs.* 3rd edition. Champaign, IL: Human Kinetics.

Katsura, Y., T. Yoshikawa, S.-Y. Ueda, T. Usui, D. Sotobayashi, H. Nakao, H. Sakamoto, T. Okumoto, and S. Fujimoto. 2010. Effects of aquatic exercise training using water-resistance equipment in elderly. *European Journal of Applied Physiology.* 108(5):957-964.

Ostdiek, V., and D. Bord. 1994. *Inquiry into physics.* 3rd edition. St. Paul: West.

Owen, A., J. Wiles, and I. Swaine. 2010. Effect of isometric exercise on resting blood pressure: A meta analysis. *Journal of Human Hypertension* 24(12):796-800.

Schiaffino, S., and C. Reggiani. 2011. Fiber types in mammalian skeletal muscles. *Physiological Reviews* 91(4):1447-1531.

Simoneau, J.-A., and C. Bouchard. 1995. Genetic determinism of fiber type proportion in human skeletal muscle. *FASEB Journal* 9(11):1091-1095.

Thompson, C., and R. Floyd. 2000. *Manual of structural kinesiology.* 14th edition. New York: McGraw-Hill.

Tortora, G., and S. Grabowski. 2002. *Principles of anatomy and physiology.* 10th edition. Indianapolis: Wiley.

Van Roden, J., and L. Gladwin. 2002. *Fitness: Theory & practice.* 4th edition. Sherman Oaks, CA: Aerobic & Fitness Association of America.

Wilmore, J., and D. Costill. 2001. *Physiology of sport and exercise.* 3rd edition. Champaign, IL: Human Kinetics.

Wilson, J.M., J.P. Loenneke, E. Jo, G.J. Wilson, M.C. Zourdos, and J.-S. Kim. 2012. The effects of endurance, strength, and power training on muscle fiber type shifting. *Journal of Strength & Conditioning Research* 26(6):1724-1729.

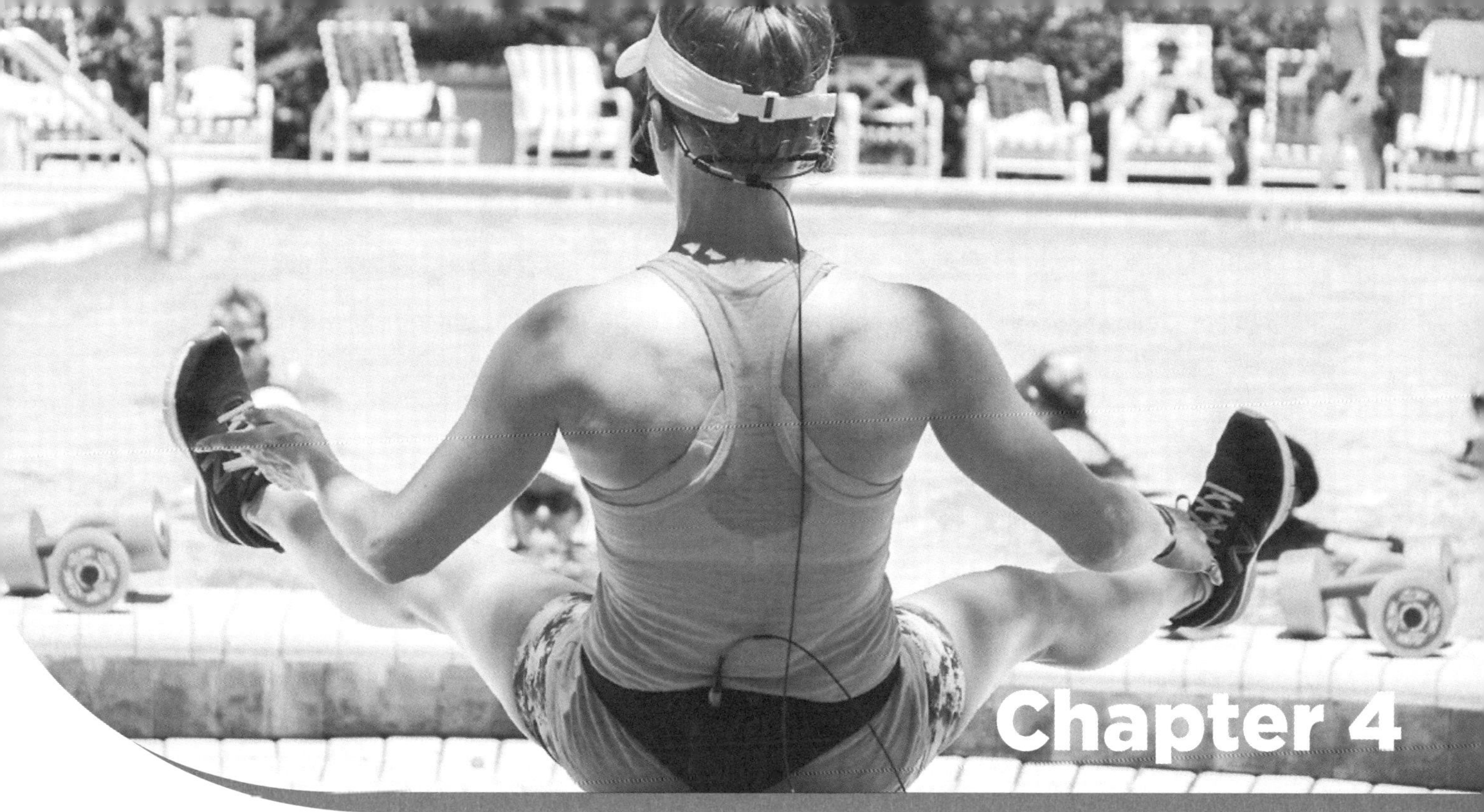

Movement Analysis

Introduction

This chapter covers **kinesiology**, the study of human motion, and **biomechanics**, the area of kinesiology that deals specifically with the analysis of movement. You need to learn both the fundamental concepts of biomechanics and how to analyze all the movements and stabilizing activities that occur during an exercise. The ability to evaluate each movement one joint at a time will help you become aware of exactly what is happening in the body with each exercise. This will allow you to create, sequence, and modify exercises and movements to benefit your participants.

Key Chapter Concepts

- Define and describe anatomical position and understand key anatomical reference terms.
- Describe the difference between center of gravity and center of buoyancy and how each influences posture, alignment, and balance in the water.
- Explain the three planes of movement and the joint actions that occur in each.
- Understand the basic structure of the synovial joints most involved with exercise design and recognize movements that occur at each joint.
- Recognize the interaction between the skeletal and the muscular systems in producing movement.
- Understand how movement in water differs from movement on land and how different types of aquatic equipment influence the muscle actions.

Anatomical Position

The first step in movement analysis is to understand **anatomical position**. All literature about the structure and function of the human body is referenced to the anatomical position, and all movements begin and end in anatomical position. In anatomical position, the body is erect (or lying supine as if erect) with the arms by the sides, palms facing forward, legs together, and feet directed forward (figure 4.1). The joints and body segments are in a neutral position (not flexed, extended, hyperextended, or rotated) except for the forearms, which are supinated (palms facing forward). This is the position of reference for definitions and descriptions of movements.

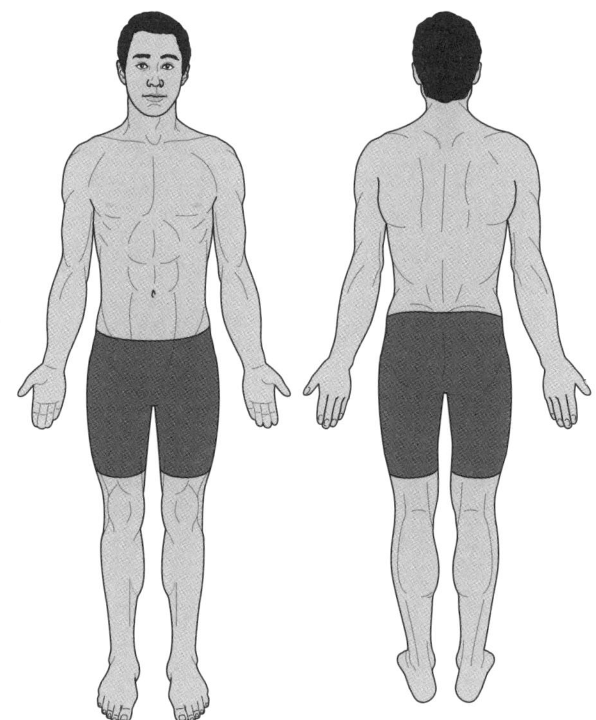

Figure 4.1 Anatomical position.

Anatomical Reference Terms

Several anatomical terms refer to the location and position of parts of the body:

- **Superior**, which means *above*
- **Inferior**, which means *below*
- **Anterior**, which means *in front of*
- **Posterior**, which means *behind*
- **Medial**, which means *toward* the midline of the body
- **Lateral**, which means *away* from the midline of the body

These terms are typically used in exercise when describing the location of one part of the body in relation to another part of the body. For example, the quadriceps muscles, located in the front of the thigh, could be described as being anterior to (in front of) the hamstring muscles, which are located in the back of the thigh. The pectoralis muscle located in the chest would be considered superior to the rectus abdominis muscle located in the abdomen. The adductor muscles located in the inner thigh would be considered medial to the abductor muscles located in the outer thigh. The humerus bone in the upper arm would be considered lateral to the ribs. The tibia bone located in the lower leg would be considered inferior to the femur bone located in the upper leg.

The next two terms describe positioning of the body. The term **supine** refers to the body lying in a face-up position. The term **prone** refers to the body lying in a face-down position. These terms are often used to describe the body's position when starting, performing, or finishing a particular exercise. The next three terms describe a surface of the body independent of its positioning in space. The term **ventral** describes the front surface of the body. The term **dorsal** describes the back surface of the body. Dorsal also refers to the top part of the foot or the instep. **Plantar** refers to the bottom surface or the sole of the foot.

Posture, Alignment, and Balance

Posture, alignment, and balance are interrelated. Posture is determined by alignment, while the ability to balance hinges on both posture and alignment.

Neutral body alignment means that the ankles, knees, hips, and shoulders are even and parallel with the floor. A vertical line should pass just anterior to the ankles, through the center of the knee, hip, and shoulder joints and through the center of the ear (figure 4.2). Maintaining neutral alignment during exercise is very important because it is the safest position for the spine when lifting or exerting force (ACE 1997). The ability to maintain neutral body alignment as well as neutral spinal alignment and balance is important for proper exercise execution as well as injury prevention.

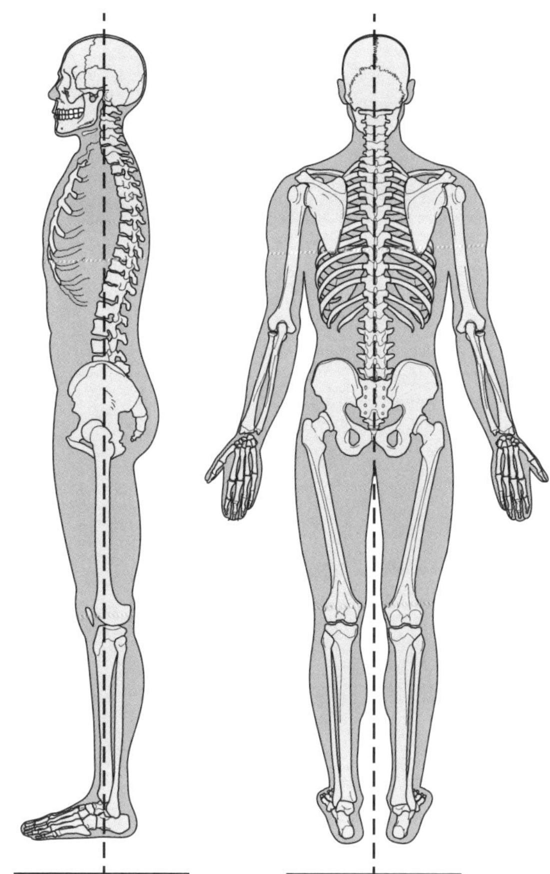

Figure 4.2 Neutral posture.

Neutral spinal alignment is a specific component of neutral body alignment. From a lateral view, the spine has three natural curves—cervical, thoracic, and lumbar (figure 4.3). From a posterior or anterior view, the vertebrae are aligned vertically.

When the spine is in neutral alignment, the pelvis is also neutral, not tilting in any direction (pelvic tilt is discussed later in this chapter).

From a mechanical perspective, maintaining balance involves controlling the position of the body's **center of gravity**. The center of gravity is typically located in the object's geometric center. In the human body, the position of the body parts determines the location of the center of gravity. Each time

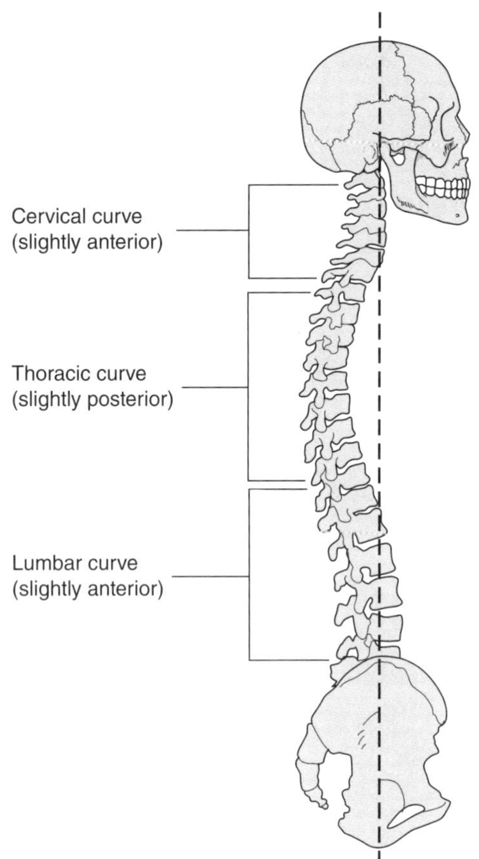

Figure 4.3 Normal curves of the spine.

any part of the body moves, a redistribution of body mass occurs and the center of gravity shifts. Movement of large body parts (e.g., legs) has a greater effect on center of gravity than moving smaller body parts (e.g., arms).

To maintain balance, the body's center of gravity must remain within the base of support. The base of support is the area of the body in contact with the ground; in most cases, this is the feet plus the area between the feet. Keeping the base wide and the body low to the ground helps ensure that the center of gravity stays within the base of support. When you lean in any direction, the center of gravity shifts. If you lean too far, the center of gravity moves outside the base of support, making you more likely to lose your balance. Maintaining neutral alignment will help you keep your center of gravity within your base of support and maintain your balance.

The concepts of center of gravity and balance still apply in the pool, especially in shallow water. You still have a base of support in contact with the pool bottom. As you reach in different directions, your center of gravity moves outside your base of support, causing you to lose your balance. Balance is a key consideration in exercise design. Off-balanced moves can lead to such problems as loss of coordination and compromised alignment. Compromised alignment during exercise may increase risk of injury and decrease ability to perform the exercise. On the other hand, some exercises specifically challenge balance. These exercises should be given careful consideration, proper cueing, and appropriate progression to ensure correct alignment and control.

The deeper the water, the more you have to consider the **center of buoyancy**. Center of buoyancy can be defined as the center of the volume of the body displacing the water or the center of a floating object. Center of buoyancy is usually located in the chest region near the lungs; however, it will vary based on the body composition and lung volume of the participant. The center of buoyancy and center of gravity are in a vertical line, but the distance between them depends on body fat patterns, the amount of air in the lungs, and muscle mass. A person with excess body fat floats easily, while a muscular person sinks. Fat and air have greater water-displacement volume than bone, organs, and muscle. All of these factors influence one's ability to maintain balance and neutral alignment in deeper water.

Aquatic exercise design should encourage awareness of posture, alignment, and balance. Cue the participants to reestablish neutral body alignment frequently, especially between changes of movement patterns and changes of direction. Allowing time for water turbulence to settle by offering a centering activity, such as a bounce or jog between traveling moves, also helps the body remain in alignment.

Planes of Movement

The body is capable of many different movements. Movement occurs in three planes that are based on dimensions in space: forward and backward, up and down, and side to side. The planes are at right angles to each other. The **sagittal plane** is vertical, and extends from front to back, dividing the body into right and left parts. The **frontal plane** is vertical, and extends from side to side, dividing the body into anterior and posterior (front and back) segments. This plane is easy to visualize if you stand in a doorway. The doorway divides the body into front and back. The **transverse plane** is horizontal, and divides the body into upper and lower portions. Think of this plane as a table because transverse movements are similar to moving on a table that encircles the body (figure 4.4).

Understanding the planes of movement will help you address muscle balance when designing exercise programs. For example, if your choreography or workout includes movements in only the sagittal plane, it will fail to target the muscles responsible for lateral movements in the frontal plane. The participants would not have the opportunity to develop the muscle balance needed for safe and effective functional mobility. Knowledge of the planes of movement will also help you to choose exercises that target the appropriate muscle groups without overworking other muscle groups. For example, bringing your arms straight up in front (in the sagittal plane) will use different muscle groups than lifting your arms out to the side (in the frontal plane).

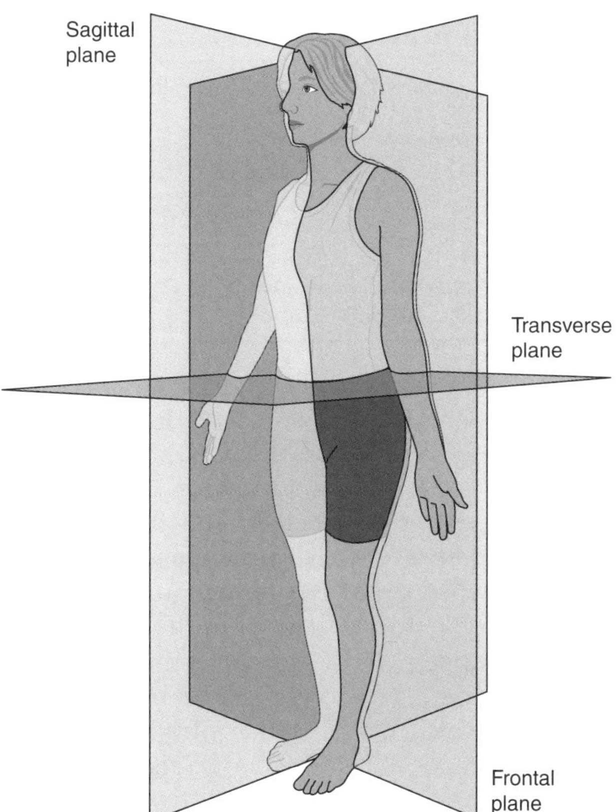

Figure 4.4 The three planes of the body.

The body does not move in a purely linear manner. In fact, most movements are **multiplane movements;** they occur in more than one plane. The fluid nature of water encourages multiplane movements. During exercise, the resistance of the water also stimulates a more efficient overload of movements in the transverse plane than land-based exercises do. Water fitness instructors should take advantage of this when designing choreography and exercise programs by adding purposeful transverse-focused movements.

Joint Actions

The term joint actions identifies movements that the joints are capable of performing. These terms are usually described as opposing movements: **flexion** and **extension**, **abduction** and **adduction**, **medial (internal) rotation** and **lateral (external) rotation**, **elevation** and **depression**, **protraction** and **retraction**, **pronation** and **supination**, and **inversion** and **eversion**. These movements can occur at more than one joint in the body or may be unique to only one joint. Flexion and extension happen in the shoulder, elbow, wrist, spine, hip, and knee, while inversion and eversion happen only in the foot. Three other joint actions that are often used in exercise are hyperextension, circumduction, and tilt. Use table 4.1 and the following text and figures to review the definitions of the fundamental movements.

Flexion and extension can be visually described in reference to anatomical position. Flexion is moving out of anatomical position, whereas extension is returning to anatomical position. Flexion is defined as a decrease in the angle at a joint. Extension is defined as an

Table 4.1 Fundamental Movements From Anatomical Position

Flexion	Decreasing the angle between two bones (e.g., bending the arm at the elbow joint, moving out of anatomical position)
Extension	Increasing the angle between two bones (e.g., straightening the arm at the elbow, returning to anatomical position)
Hyperextension	Continuing extension past neutral position (e.g., moving the head at the neck to look up)
Abduction	Movement away from the body's midline (e.g., raising your leg to the side)
Adduction	Movement toward the body's midline (e.g., returning your leg from a side leg raise)
Medial (internal) rotation	Rotary movement around the long axis of a bone toward the midline of the body (e.g., rotating your arm inward from the shoulder)
Lateral (external) rotation	Rotary movement around the long axis of a bone away from the midline of the body (e.g., rotating the arm outward from the shoulder)
Circumduction	Circular movement of a limb that describes a cone; a combination of flexion, extension, abduction, and adduction (e.g., arm or leg circles)
Elevation	Movement of the shoulder girdle toward the head (e.g., shrugging the shoulders upward)
Depression	Movement of the shoulder girdle toward the feet (e.g., pressing your shoulders downward)
Protraction	Forward movement of the shoulder girdle away from the spine (abduction of the scapula)
Retraction	Backward movement of the shoulder girdle toward the spine (adduction of the scapula)
Pronation	Rotating the forearm medially (turning the palm down or backward)
Supination	Rotating the forearm laterally (turning the palm up or forward)
Plantar flexion	Movement at the ankle where the foot moves away from the body (e.g., pointing the toes)
Dorsiflexion	Movement at the ankle where the top of the foot moves toward the shin
Inversion	Turning the sole of the foot inward (medially)
Eversion	Turning the sole of the foot outward (laterally)
Tilt	Movements of the pelvis (e.g., moving the top of the pelvis forward [anterior pelvic tilt], backward [posterior pelvic tilt], or to the right or left [lateral pelvic tilt])

increase in the angle at a joint. A straight arm is in anatomical or neutral position. When the arm bends at the elbow, flexion is occurring as the angle in the joint decreases. Straightening the arm (increasing the angle in the joint) is extension. Flexion and extension typically occur in the sagittal plane (figure 4.5).

Hyperextension is defined as going beyond anatomical position or neutral position. It typically occurs in the sagittal plane. From anatomical position, with the arm straight down to the side, hyperextension of the shoulder would involve moving the arm backward from the shoulder (figure 4.6). Hyperextension is a functional movement, and slow, controlled hyperextension of some joints is an appropriate joint action for strengthening specific muscle groups. Hyperextension of the hip engages the gluteus maximus and the hamstring muscles. Hyperextension of the shoulder engages several muscles in the posterior shoulder and back. Hyperextension of one joint resulting from movement in another joint is not safe, and could possibly increase the risk of injury to the joint. For example, uncontrolled hyperextension of the spine as a result of hip hyperextension, such as arching the back during a

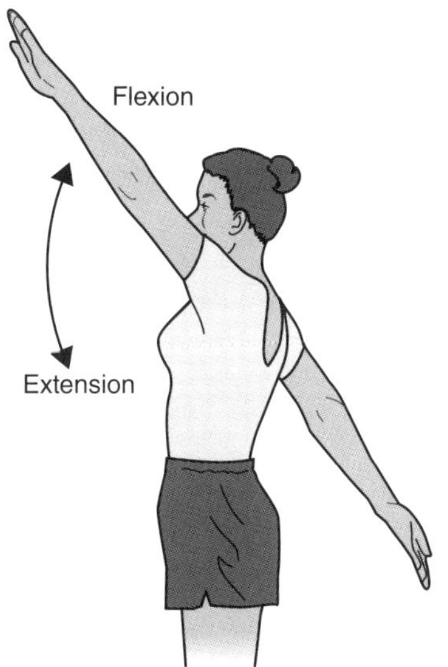

Figure 4.5 Flexion and extension.

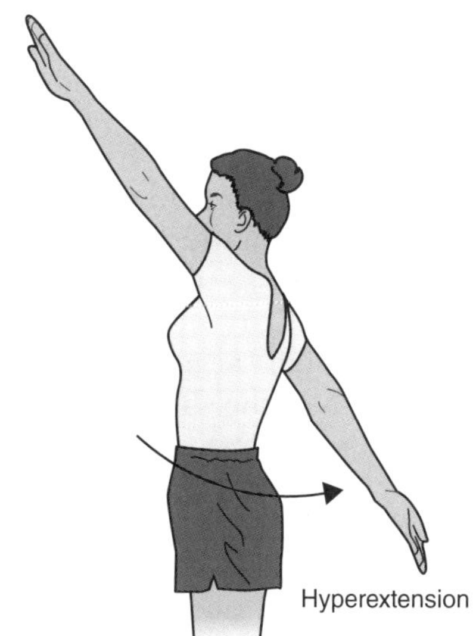

Figure 4.6 Hyperextension.

back kick, might increase the risk of injury to the spine. During the performance of a back kick, both the spine and pelvis should remain in a neutral position. Movement should occur only at the hip joint, not at the lumbar spine.

Abduction and **adduction** refer to movement away from (abduction) and toward (adduction) the midline (center) of the body. Several joints in the body are capable of abduction and adduction, but in exercise design, we tend to focus on abduction and adduction in the hips and shoulders. Jumping jacks, side steps, side leg lifts, and lifting your arms out to the sides are examples of abduction and adduction movements in the frontal plane, or movement to the side (figure 4.7). Abduction and adduction movements also occur in the transverse plane, or parallel to the ground. Transverse (sometimes called "horizontal") abduction and adduction occur at the hip and shoulder. Holding the arms out to the side at shoulder height and bringing the arms together in front of the body (moving toward the midline) involve transverse adduction. Returning the arms from the front of the body to the sides at shoulder height (moving away from the midline) is transverse abduction.

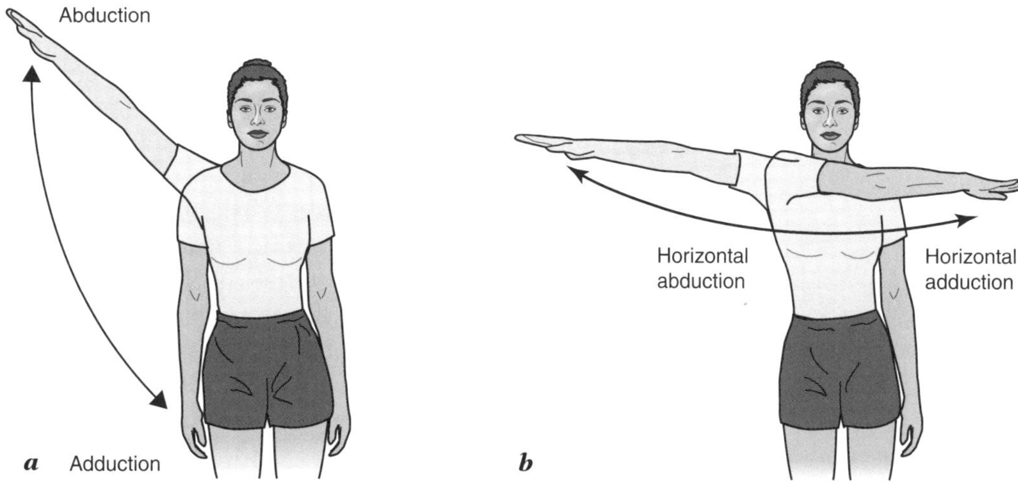

Figure 4.7 Abduction and adduction in the *(a)* frontal plane and the *(b)* transverse plane.

Rotation refers to movement around the longitudinal axis of the limb or spine (figure 4.8). Rotational movements occur in the transverse plane. Twisting to the right or left is an example of spinal rotation. Rotation can also occur in the shoulder and hip. For example, rotation toward the midline is medial (internal) rotation; rotation away from midline is lateral (external) rotation. Turning the arm at the shoulder toward the center of the body is an example of medial rotation. Turning the arm at the shoulder away from the center of the body is an example of lateral rotation. Likewise, turning the leg at the hip toward the center of the body is an example of medial rotation. Turning the leg at the hip away from the center of the body is an example of lateral rotation.

Pronation and **supination** are terms specific to movement of the forearm. Pronation of the forearm is medial rotation (palm down or back), and supination of the forearm is lateral rotation (palm up or forward). It is beneficial to include pronation and supination exercises in your water exercise program to strengthen the forearm muscles (figure 4.9).

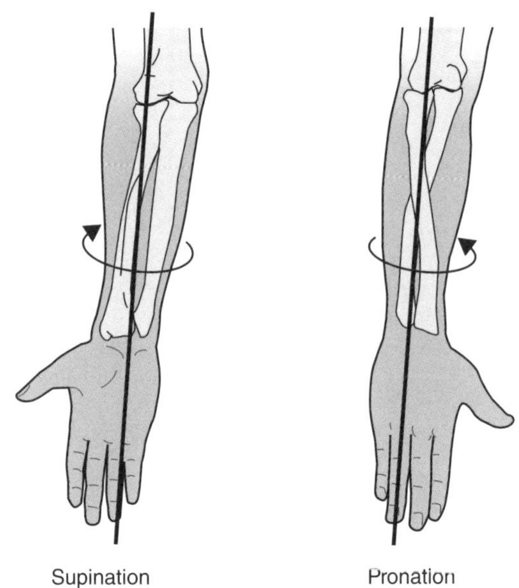

Figure 4.9 Pronation and supination.

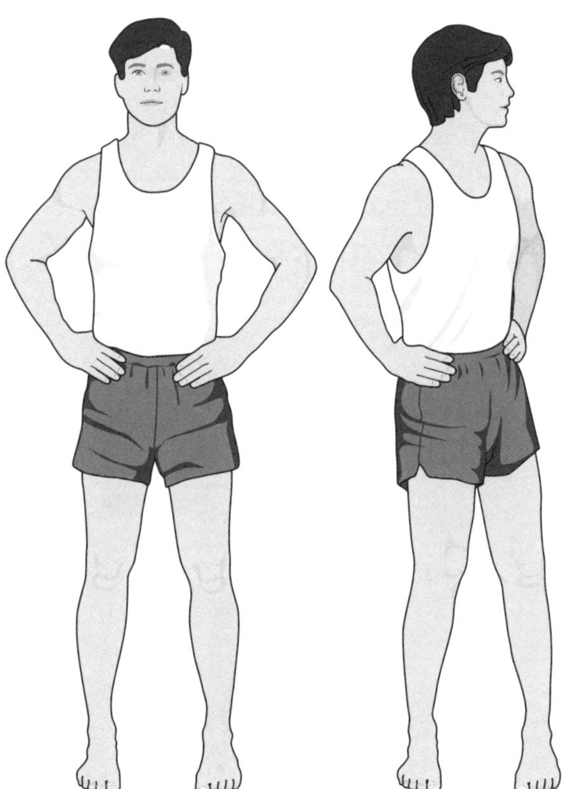

Figure 4.8 Rotation.

Elevation, **depression**, **protraction**, and **retraction** refer to movements occurring in the shoulder girdle (clavicles and scapulae). Elevation is movement of the shoulder girdle upward, as if shrugging your shoulders. Depression is movement of the shoulder girdle down toward the hips. Protraction is movement of the shoulder blades forward, away from the spine (abduction of scapulae). Retraction is movement of the shoulder blades back toward the spine (adduction of scapulae). Sitting at a computer and other repetitive tasks performed in front of the body tend to cause extensive scapular elevation and protraction. Fitness instructors should include exercises to strengthen the muscles that are responsible for scapular depression and retraction to offset this postural imbalance associated with daily activities.

Plantar flexion and **dorsiflexion** are movements at the ankle. Plantar flexion is moving the plantar surface (sole) of the foot away from the body, often referred to as pointing the toes. Dorsiflexion is moving the dorsal surface of the foot (top of foot) toward the shin (figure 4.10).

Inversion and **eversion** are terms specific to movement of the foot. Inversion is turning

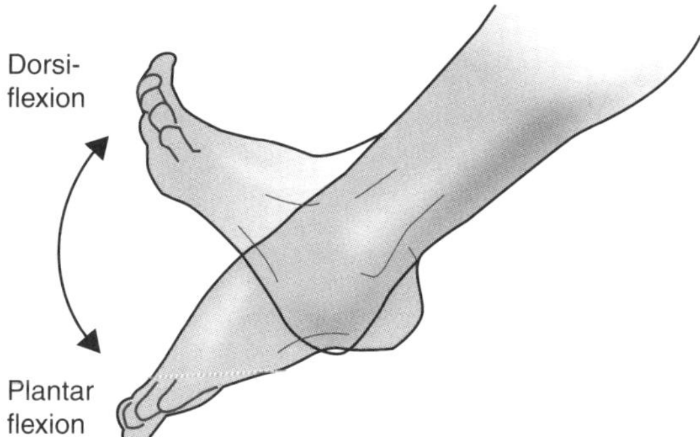

Figure 4.10 Plantar and dorsiflexion.

the sole (bottom) of the foot inward. Eversion is turning the sole of the foot outward (figure 4.11).

Circumduction is movement at a joint in a circular direction. It is a combination of

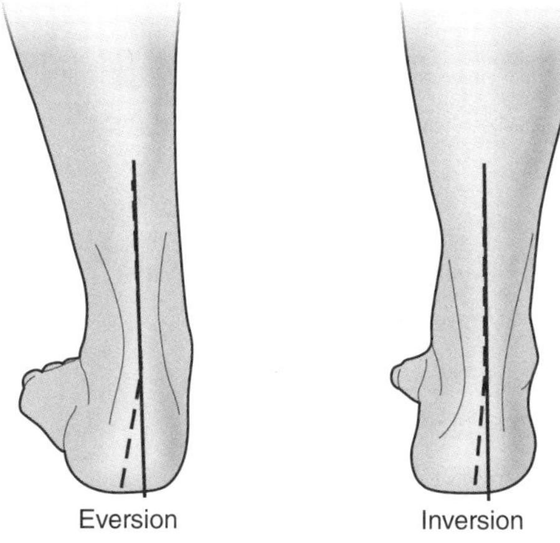

Figure 4.11 Eversion and inversion.

flexion, extension, abduction, and adduction. Common examples of circumduction are arm circles (circumduction at the shoulder) and leg circles (circumduction at the hip) (figure 4.12). Circumduction should be performed both clockwise and counterclockwise to maintain muscle balance.

Tilt describes certain movements of the pelvis. The pelvis is capable of tilting anteriorly, posteriorly, and laterally. The direction of the pelvic tilt is determined from movement of the top part of the pelvis. **Anterior tilt** is when the top part of the pelvis moves forward (figure 4.13). **Posterior tilt** is when the top part moves backward. With **lateral**

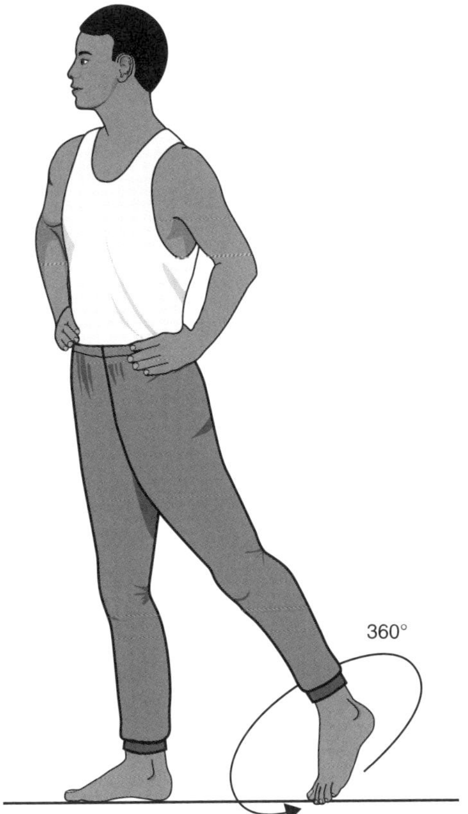

Figure 4.12 Circumduction.

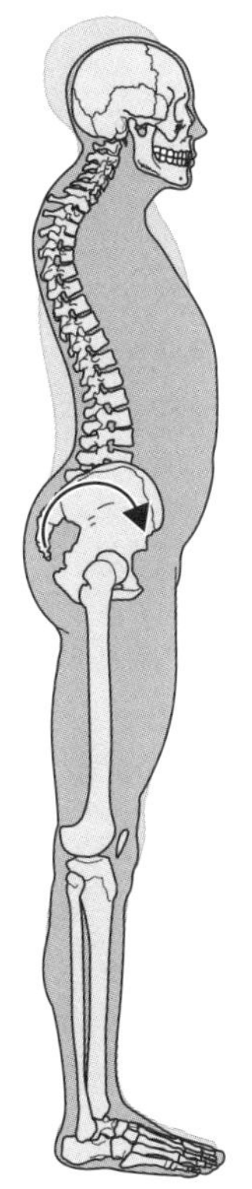

Figure 4.13 Anterior pelvic tilt.

Table 4.2 Muscle Groups and Movements

Name of muscle	Joints moved	Primary movement
Sternocleidomastoid	Cervical spine	Flexion, lateral flexion, and rotation of the neck
Pectoralis major	Shoulder	Flexion and transverse adduction of the arm at the shoulder
Trapezius Upper (U) Middle (M) Lower (L)	Scapula Cervical spine	(U) Scapular elevation and neck extension (M) Scapular retraction (L) Scapular depression
Latissimus dorsi	Shoulder	Extension and adduction of the arm at the shoulder
Deltoid Anterior (A) Medial (M) Posterior (P)	Shoulder	(A) Transverse adduction of the arm at the shoulder (M) Abduction of the arm at the shoulder (P) Transverse abduction of the arm at the shoulder
Biceps brachii	Elbow Shoulder	Flexion of the forearm at the elbow Flexion of the arm at the shoulder
Triceps brachii	Elbow Shoulder	Extension of the forearm at the elbow Extension of the arm at the shoulder
Wrist flexors	Wrist Phalanges	Flexion of the hand at the wrist Flexion of the phalanges
Wrist extensors	Wrist Phalanges	Extension of the hand at the wrist Extension of the phalanges
Erector spinae	Spine	Extension of the trunk along the spine
Quadratus lumborum	Lumbar spine	Lateral flexion of the spine
Rectus abdominis	Lumbar spine	Flexion of the spine
Internal and external obliques	Lumbar spine	Flexion and rotation of the spine
Transversus abdominis	Lumbar spine	Abdominal compression and lumbar stabilization
Iliopsoas (psoas major and minor, iliacus)	Hip	Flexion of the leg at the hip
Gluteus maximus	Hip	Extension of the leg at the hip
Hip abductors (gluteus medius and gluteus minimus)	Hip	Abduction of the leg at the hip
Hip adductors (pectineus, gracilis, adductor brevis, adductor longus and adductor magnus)	Hip	Adduction of the leg at the hip
Quadriceps femoris (rectus femoris, vastus medialis, vastus intermedius, vastus lateralis)	Hip (rectus femoris) Knee	Flexion of the leg at the hip Extension of the lower leg at the knee
Hamstrings (biceps femoris, semimembranosus, semitendinosus)	Hip Knee	Extension of the leg at the hip Flexion of the lower leg at the knee
Gastrocnemius	Ankle	Plantar flexion at the ankle
Soleus	Ankle	Plantar flexion at the ankle
Tibialis anterior	Ankle	Dorsiflexion at the ankle

tilt of the pelvis, the top part of the pelvis moves to the right or left. It is easy to remember pelvic movements by thinking of the pelvis as a bucket of water. When the top of the bucket spills forward, it is an anterior tilt. When the top of the bucket spills backward, it is a posterior tilt. When the bucket spills to either side, it is a lateral tilt.

Refer to table 4.2 for a summary of the joints, joint actions, and the muscles responsible for each movement.

Refer to table 4.3 to see which joint actions occur in each of the three movement planes.

Table 4.3 Movement Planes and Joint Actions

Plane	Description of plane	Joint actions
Frontal	Divides body into front and back parts	Abduction, adduction, and lateral flexion
Sagittal	Divides body into right and left parts	Flexion, extension, and hyperextension
Transverse	Divides body into upper and lower body	Medial and lateral rotation, transverse abduction and adduction

Types of Joints

A basic knowledge of joint structure is another tool that helps instructors make safe, effective exercise choices. Joints are the mechanisms by which bones are held together. An anatomical joint, or articulation, is formed where two bones meet. The type of joint determines the possible range of movement. Sometimes the bones are so close that there is no significant movement, as in an immovable joint. In other joints, the connection is quite loose, allowing tremendous freedom of movement. Joints might provide total stability, stability in one direction with freedom in the other direction, or freedom in all directions.

The amount of movement within a specific joint is limited by several factors, including bony limitations (how the bones articulate) and limitations with ligaments or the connective tissue components of muscle, such as tightness or excessive scar tissue. Movement may also be limited by the attachment of the surrounding muscles.

Three basic categories of joints are based on the movement allowed at the articulation.

Immovable joints—Bones are held together by fibrous connective tissue that forms an interosseous (i.e., connecting or lying between bones) ligament or membrane. These joints generally hold two parts of the body together, such as the bones in the skull (figure 4.14).

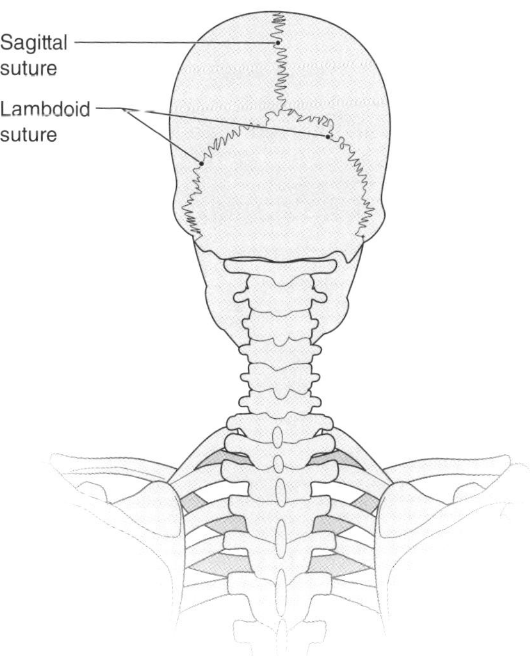

Figure 4.14 Immovable joints.

Slightly movable joints—Bones are held together by strong fibrocartilaginous membranes. The sacroiliac joint (holds the back of the pelvis to the sacrum) and symphysis pubis (holds the front lower part of the pelvis together) are slightly movable joints (figure 4.15).

Freely movable (synovial joints)—Bones are held together by synovial membranes. The joint cavity is filled with synovial fluid that allows movement to occur with minimal friction. Located between bones, ligaments, tendons, and muscles are bursae (sacs filled

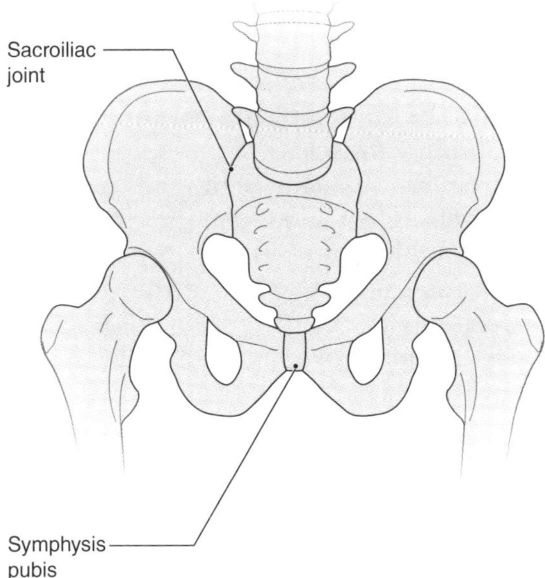

Figure 4.15 Slightly movable joints.

with synovial fluid) that also act as friction reducers for adjacent moving surfaces. Most joints in the body related to exercise are freely movable synovial joints.

Table 4.4 summarizes several types of synovial joints and the joint actions and provides examples in the human body.

The following are descriptions of some of the synovial joints involved in exercise.

Ball and Socket

Examples: Hip joint and shoulder joint

A ball-shaped surface articulates with a cup-shaped surface. Movements can occur in all three planes of movement. Flexion and extension, abduction and adduction, rotation, and circumduction are possible in **ball-and-socket joints** (figure 4.16). The hip joint is the articulation of the pelvis with the head of the femur (figure 4.17). The shoulder joint (glenohumeral joint) is the articulation of the

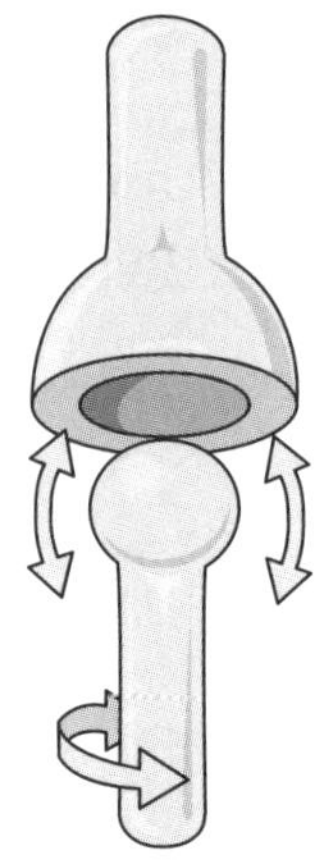

Figure 4.16 Ball and socket joint.

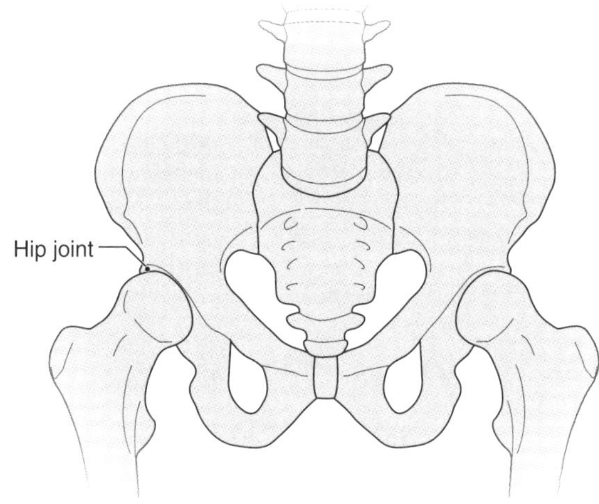

Figure 4.17 Hip joint.

Table 4.4 Classification of Synovial Joints

Articulation	Joint action	Example
Ball and socket	All joint movements	Hip and shoulder
Hinge	Flexion and extension	Elbow, knee, and ankle
Condyloid	All except rotation (bones allow movement in two planes without rotation)	Radiocarpal (wrist)
Saddle	All except rotation	Thumb (first joint)
Plane or gliding	Gliding	Intertarsal (ankle) and intercarpal (wrist)
Pivot	Supination, pronation, and rotation	Radioulnar (forearm)

head of the humerus with the glenoid cavity of the scapula.

Hinge

Examples: Elbow joint, knee joint, and ankle joint

A **hinge joint** involves two articular surfaces that restrict movement, largely to the sagittal plane. Hinge joints usually have strong collateral ligaments that provide reinforcement to the joint (figure 4.18). Flexion and extension are the primary movements.

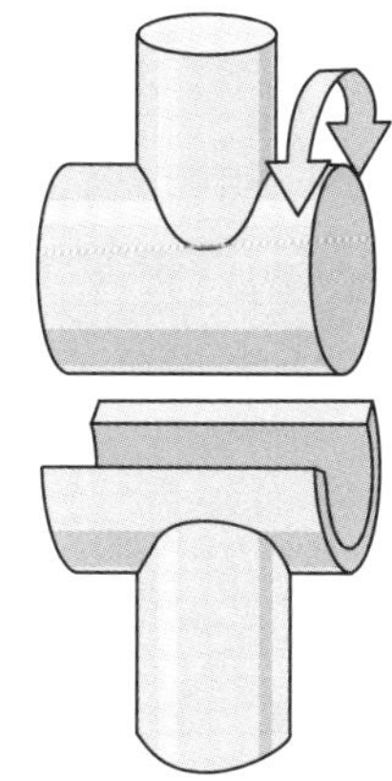

Figure 4.18 Hinge or joint.

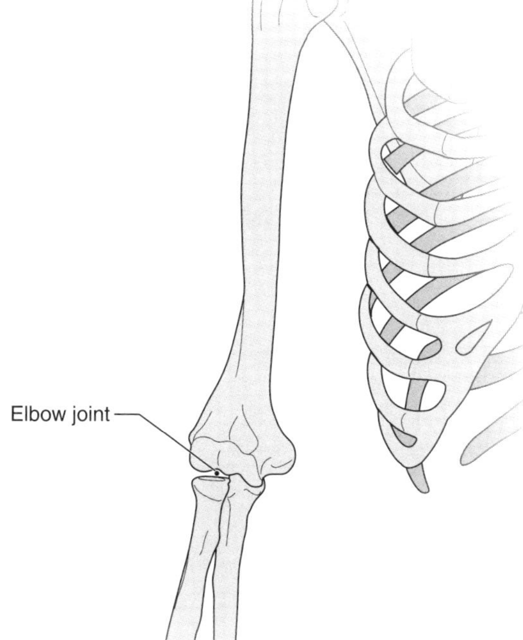

Figure 4.19 Elbow joint.

The elbow joint is the articulation of the humerus with the ulna and radius (figure 4.19). The knee joint is formed by the articulations of the femur, the tibia, and the patella (kneecap) (figure 4.20). The ankle is the articulation of the tibia and fibula with the talus bone in the foot (figure 4.21).

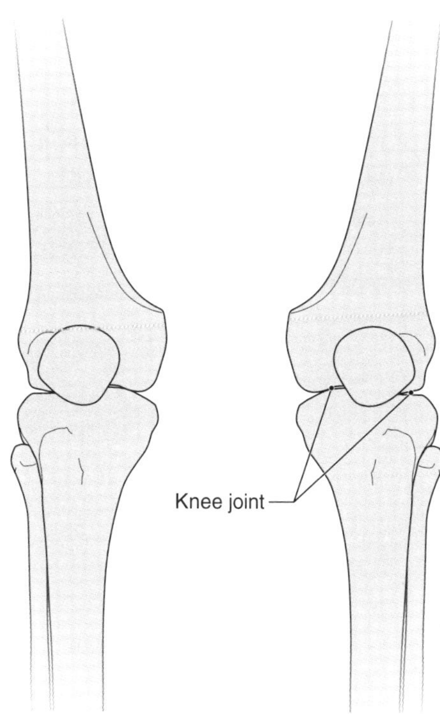

Figure 4.20 Knee joint.

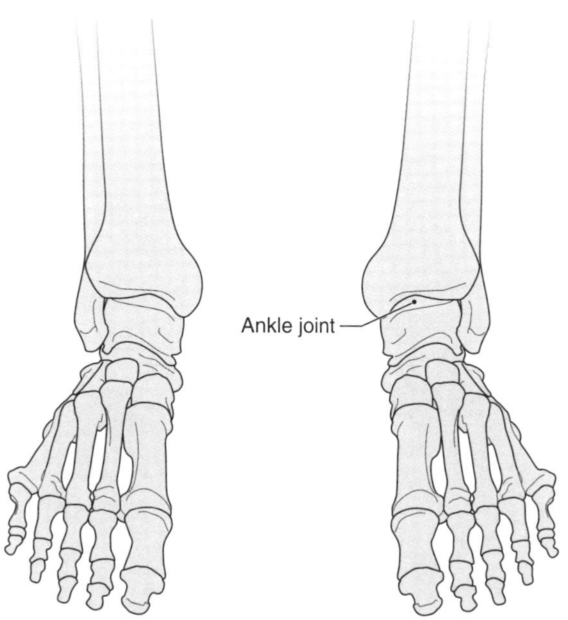

Figure 4.21 Ankle joint.

Condyloid

Example: Wrist joint

A **condyloid joint** is formed by a convex surface placed near a concave surface. This articulation provides movement in two planes (figure 4.22). Wrist extension and flexion occur in the sagittal plane and abduction and adduction occur in the frontal plane (figure 4.23).

Circumduction (wrist circle) is possible by combining the radioulnar joint and the midcarpal joint, but the movement is not as free as a true ball-and-socket joint.

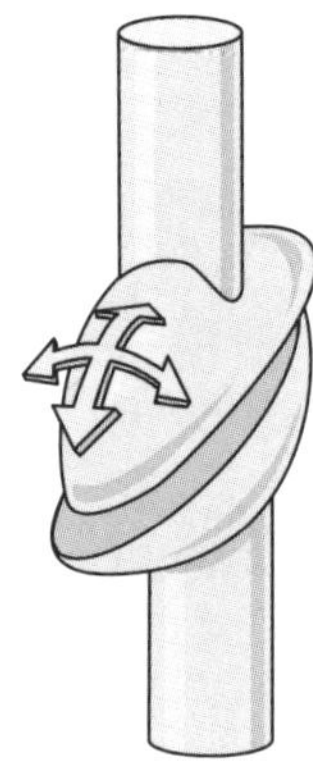

Figure 4.22 Condyloid joint.

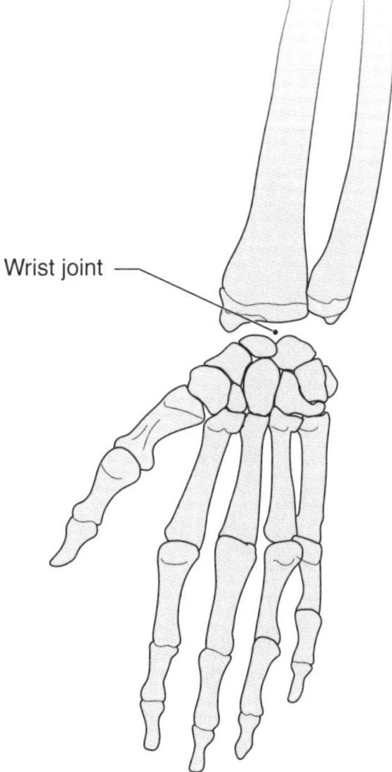

Figure 4.23 Wrist joint.

Saddle

Example: First carpometacarpal joint (thumb)

All movements except rotation are possible at a **saddle joint** (figure 4.24). The thumb joint is formed by the articulation of the trapezium with the first metacarpal (figure 4.25).

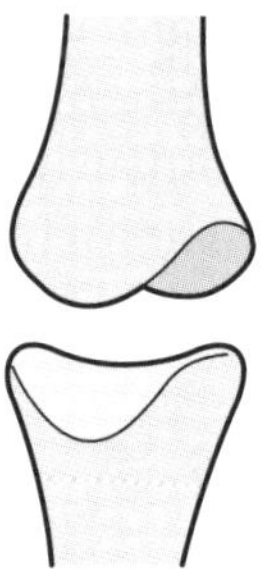

Figure 4.24 Saddle joint.

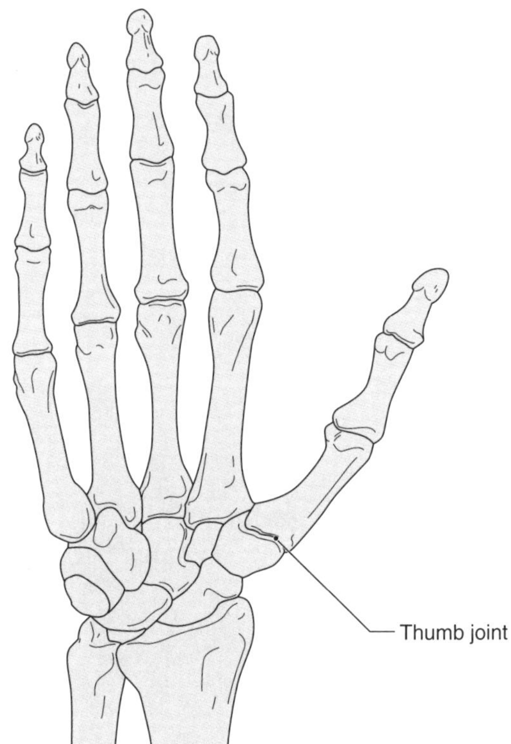

Figure 4.25 Thumb joint.

Plane or Gliding

Example: Intertarsal joints (in the foot) and intercarpal joints (in the wrist)

Gliding (plane) joints are formed by the proximity of two relatively flat surfaces, allowing gliding movements to occur (figure 4.26). An example of an intertarsal joint with gliding action is the subtalar joint, the articulation of the talus and the calcaneus (figure 4.27).

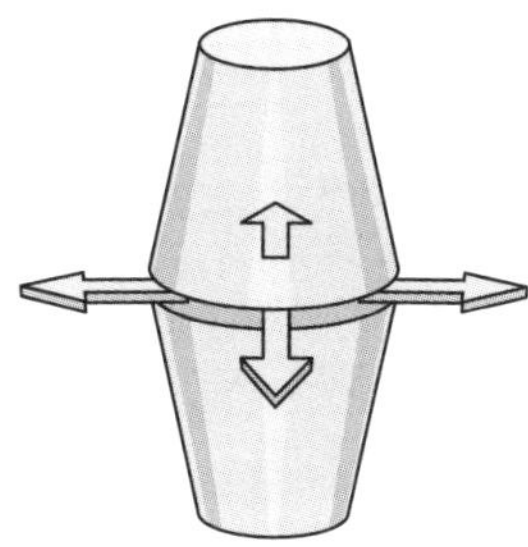

Figure 4.26 Plane or gliding joint.
© LifeART®

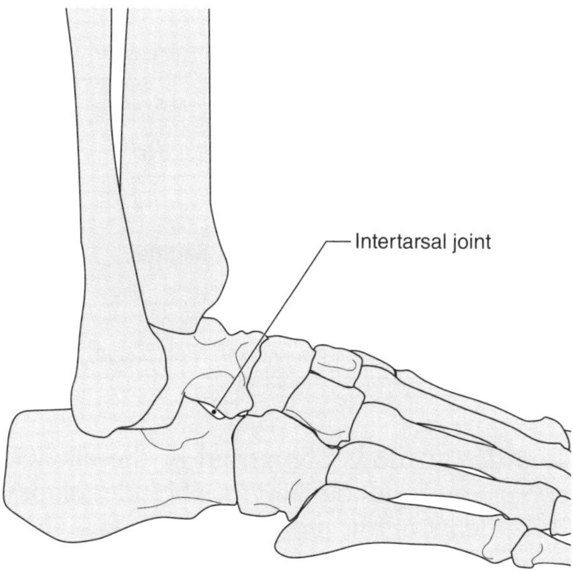

Figure 4.27 Intertarsal joint.

Pivot

Example: Superior radioulnar joint

A **pivot joint** consists of a central bony pivot, a ring of bone and ligament that permits only rotatory movement (figure 4.28). Pronation and supination of the forearm are considered rotation of the radioulnar joint (figure 4.29).

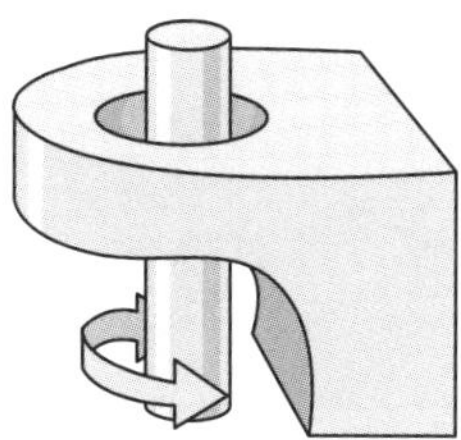

Figure 4.28 Pivot or troichoid joint.
© LifeART®

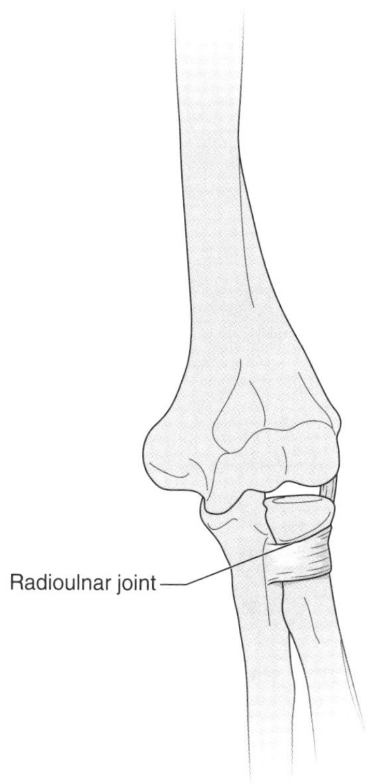

Figure 4.29 Radioulnar joint.

See table 4.5 for summaries of joints, joint actions, and movement planes.

Table 4.5 Joints, Joint Actions, and Planes

Joint	Joint action	Plane
Vertebral column (various types of joints)	Flexion, extension, and hyperextension	Sagittal
	Lateral flexion	Frontal
	Rotation	Transverse
	Circumduction	Multiplanar
Hip (ball and socket)	Flexion, extension, and hyperextension	Sagittal
	Abduction and adduction	Frontal
	Rotation	Transverse
	Circumduction	Multiplanar
	Transverse abduction and adduction	Transverse
Knee (hinge)	Flexion and extension	Sagittal
Ankle (hinge)	Dorsiflexion and plantar flexion	Sagittal
Shoulder (ball and socket)	Flexion, extension, and hyperextension	Sagittal
	Abduction and adduction	Frontal
	Rotation	Transverse
	Circumduction	Multiplanar
	Transverse abduction and adduction	Transverse
Elbow (hinge)	Flexion and extension	Sagittal
Radioulnar (pivot)	Pronation and supination	Transverse
Wrist (condyloid)	Flexion, extension, and hyperextension	Sagittal
	Abduction and adduction	Frontal
	Circumduction (also involves midcarpal joint)	Multiplanar

Joints Most Involved in Exercise Design

The following sections discuss basic structure and movements of the joints most involved with exercise design.

Shoulder Girdle

What we call the shoulder really consists of the shoulder girdle and the shoulder joint. It has a larger range of motion than any other body part. The muscles of the shoulder girdle provide stabilization, allowing the arms and hands to perform fine motor skills. The shoulder girdle is composed of the clavicle (collarbone) and the scapula (shoulder blade). Movements of the shoulder girdle have their pivotal point at the junction of the clavicle and sternum (sternoclavicular joint), but we are more aware of, and concerned with, movements in the scapula. The scapula is attached to the rib cage and vertebral column by muscles and is capable of elevation, depression, protraction, and retraction. Contractions of these muscles produce rotary as well as linear movements. You can help participants maintain adequate strength and range of motion in the shoulder girdle by including exercises for the muscles that move the scapulae. You should also teach participants how to engage these muscles to stabilize the scapulae, since scapular stabilization is necessary for safely and efficiently performing many activities of daily living and maintaining posture.

Shoulder Joint

The shoulder joint (glenohumeral joint) is a ball-and-socket joint where the head of the humerus (ball) attaches into the glenoid cavity of the scapula (socket). The shoulder joint is capable of abduction and adduction, transverse abduction and adduction, rotation, circumduction, and flexion, extension, and hyperextension. Movements of the shoulder joint are independent of movements of the shoulder girdle, and often require shoulder girdle stabilization for efficient performance.

Elbow Joint

The elbow is a hinge joint. Motion in this joint is basically limited to flexion and extension. Movements that flex and extend the elbow, thereby working the biceps and triceps, are often included in exercises that also involve the shoulder. Therefore, you may want to consider including some exercises that isolate the elbow joint in your workouts to specifically target the biceps and triceps. Although pronation and supination of the forearm occur at the radio-ulnar joint rather than at the elbow joint, these movements are often associated with exercises involving the elbow.

Spine and Pelvic Girdle

The individual vertebrae in the spine have only slight movement, but combined, they allow the vertebral column to perform a considerable range of motion. The spine is capable of flexion, circumduction, extension, hyperextension, lateral flexion, and rotation. The muscles affecting the spine should be balanced in strength and flexibility to maintain the normal curves (see figure 4.3). Range of motion in the spine is increased when we add the motion of the pelvis. Motion of the pelvis corresponds to motion of the spine, but occurs in the opposite direction. In other words, as the spine flexes forward, the pelvis tilts backward (posterior pelvic tilt). The opposite occurs for spinal extension (anterior pelvic tilt).

Maintaining or retraining the normal curves of the spine can be a primary focus in exercise programs. A large percentage of the population experiences back problems. Many of these problems are caused or made worse by imbalances in muscular strength and flexibility, or body mechanics. Because we are vertically oriented creatures, these imbalances become exaggerated by the pull of gravity. For example, weak abdominal muscles allow the pelvis to move further forward (greater anterior tilt), causing lumbar hyperextension. Prolonged sitting causes tight hip flexors, again increasing the anterior tilt, forcing the lumbar spine into hyperextension. This increased curve in the lumbar spine can be a contributing factor to lower-back pain. Similarly, an exaggerated posterior pelvic tilt eliminates the normal curve of the lumbar spine, also causing lower-back pain. Abdominal exercises are recommended for correcting an extreme anterior tilt to improve posture and alignment. Strengthening the erector spinae muscles will help control unnatural posterior pelvic tilt. The general exercise recommendations are to stretch the muscles that are tight and strengthen the muscles that are weak to improve or maintain neutral alignment.

We may also see abnormal curvatures of the spine that result in postural deviations. The three most common postural deviations are **scoliosis**, **kyphosis**, and **lordosis** (figure 4.30*a* and *b*) Scoliosis refers to a lateral curvature and rotation of the spine. The shoulders and pelvis appear uneven and the rib cage might be twisted. Kyphosis (rounded shoulders) refers to an exaggerated curve in the thoracic spine. The head is often too far forward, with rounded shoulders and sunken chest. Lordosis is an increased curve in the lumbar spine. Lordosis is often accompanied by an increased anterior pelvic tilt. The abdomen and the buttocks protrude and the arms hang farther back. These conditions might be considered permanent from congenital or disease-related abnormalities; if so, exercise will not correct them. However, if the condition is due to muscle imbalance, flexibility issues, or strength deficits, exercise may reduce or eliminate the condition.

Our aim is to establish, and to continually re-establish, the normal curves of the spine in order to maintain neutral body alignment. When doing any type of exercise, including water exercise, the body should always assume a position as close to neutral alignment as possible before beginning the exercise. Neutral body alignment occurs easily if there is muscular balance. Unfortunately, many of our daily habits put inappropriate stress on our muscles and cause imbalances. Examples include looking down while texting on a cell phone or sitting at the computer for hours. Even in exercise programs, imbalances are seen, especially if the workout includes only hip flexor exercises, such as knee lifts and front kicks, without including exercises that focus on the back of the body. Plan to provide ways to balance muscle strength and flexibility from right to left sides, from front to back, and from the upper body to lower body. You should also balance strength ratios in opposing muscle pairs within the exercise program.

Maintaining neutral spine is particularly relevant with the popularity of flotation devices and other resistance equipment for water exercise. This equipment provides an additional challenge to balance and coordination. If a participant cannot control neutral posture while exercising with equipment, the equipment should not be utilized.

Hip Joint

The hip joint is a ball-and-socket joint, like the shoulder, but the hip joint has greater

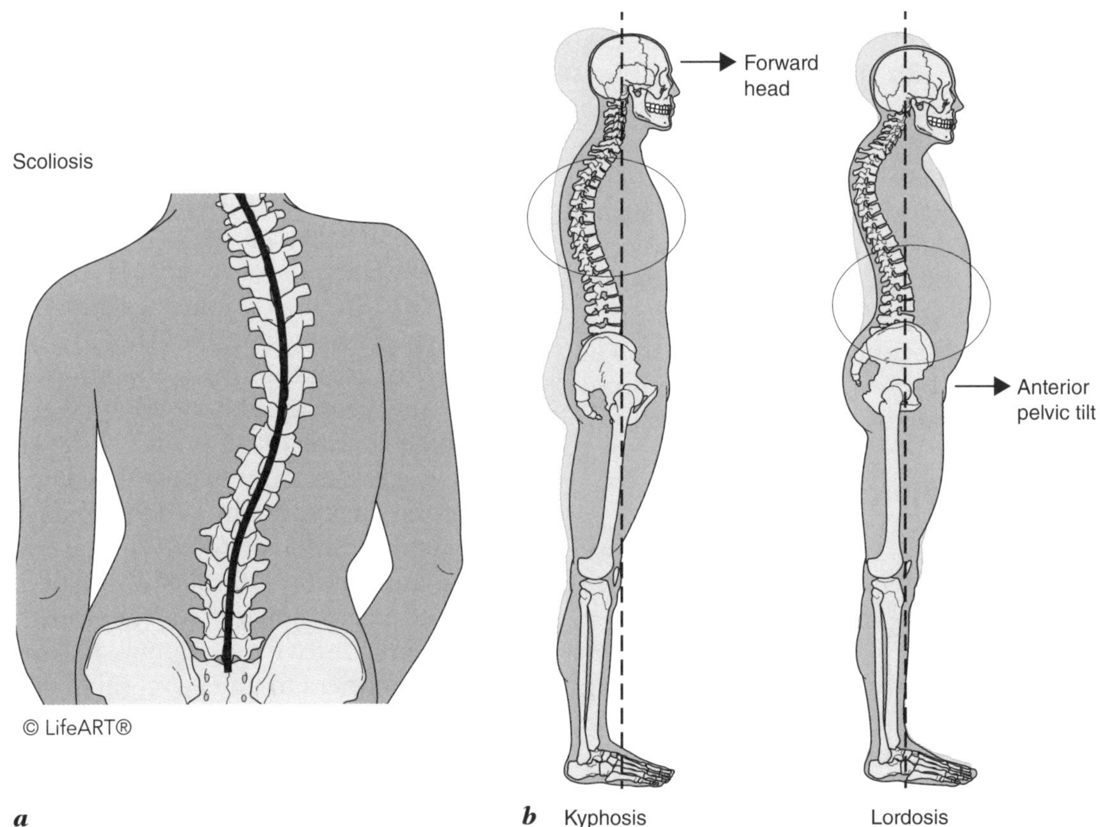

Figure 4.30 Structural deviations of the spine: *(a)* scoliosis, and *(b)* thoracic (kyphosis) and lumbar (lordosis) regions.

stability mainly because of its weight-bearing role. Just as the shoulder joint interacts with the shoulder girdle, the hip joint interacts with the pelvic girdle. Movements at the hip joint include abduction and adduction, transverse abduction and adduction, lateral and medial rotation, circumduction, and flexion, extension, and hyperextension. The important point for instructors to remember is that some of the muscles crossing the hip joint also have attachments on the spine (such as the iliopsoas), so hip movements can affect changes in the lumbar spine. Hip flexion can involve either lifting the leg in front, as with a front kick, or bending forward at the hips.

Knee Joint

The knee is a hinge joint that performs flexion and extension. The main muscles acting on the knee are the quadriceps and hamstrings. The patella bone (kneecap) acts as a pulley to increase the effective strength of the quadriceps by increasing leverage or mechanical advantage. Water exercise, if designed properly, can provide the important muscle balance needed between the quadriceps and the hamstrings.

Interaction Between the Skeletal and Muscular Systems

To understand movement, look at the interaction between the skeletal and muscular systems. Muscular contractions are responsible for movements at each joint. When muscles contract, they pull on the bones to create movement.

The body moves through the use of a system of **levers**. Levers consist of rigid bars that turn around an axis. In the body, the bones represent the rigid bars, called lever arms, and the joints represent the axes, or fulcrum. The axis, or **fulcrum** (F), can be visualized as a pivot point. Two different forces act on the lever: **resistance** (R) and **effort** (E). Resistance can be regarded as a force to overcome, such as a weight in your hand or the resistance of the water when exercising in a pool. Effort is the amount of force needed to create the movement, such as the muscle contractions necessary for lifting a weight or moving through the water.

Three basic types of levers exist: first-class lever, second-class lever, and third-class lever (figure 4.31). The type of lever is based on the arrangement of the fulcrum, the resistance, and the effort. In a first-class lever, the fulcrum is between the effort and the resistance. An example of a first-class lever in the body is the head sitting on top of the cervical vertebrae. The joint between the base of the skull and cervical vertebrae acts as the fulcrum. The effort is represented by the muscle contraction occurring in the upper back and neck to tilt the head backward into hyperextension. The resistance is provided by the weight of the face and jaw area of the head (figure 4.31*a*).

In a second-class lever, the resistance is between the fulcrum and the effort. Rising

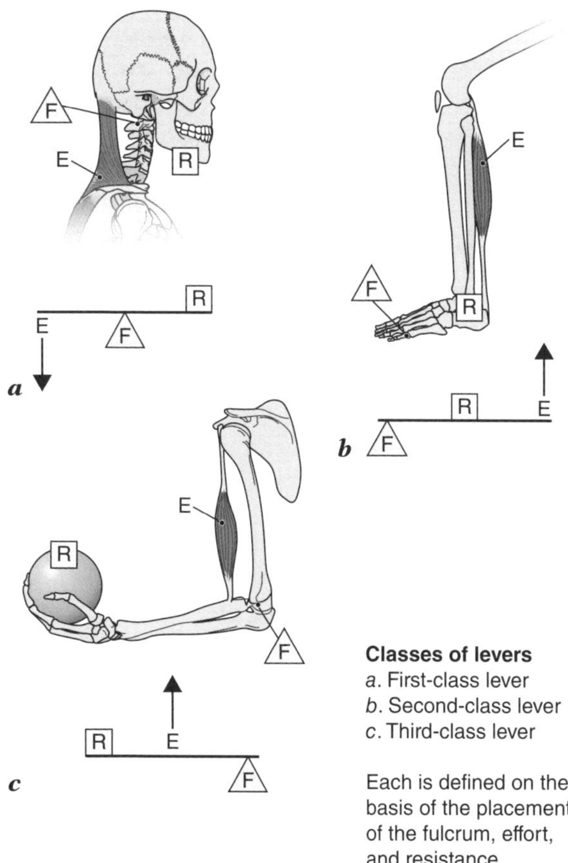

Figure 4.31 Classes of levers.

up onto the toes is an example of using a second-class lever. The weight of the body is the resistance, whereas the fulcrum is the ball of the foot. The effort occurs when the calf muscles contract to lift the heels (figure 4.31*b*).

In a third-class lever, the effort is in between the fulcrum and the resistance. Bending the elbow to do an arm curl is an example of a third-class lever. Here, the weight of the forearm (or the weight held in the hand) is the resistance and the contraction of the biceps muscle (that inserts at the forearm) is the effort. The elbow joint acts as the fulcrum (see figure 4.31*c*). Most of the joints in the body related to exercise are third-class levers, such as the shoulder joint shown in figure 4.32.

Movement also involves a complex and coordinated effort of activation (contraction) of certain muscles **(agonists)**, deactivation (relaxation) of others **(antagonists)**, or a cocontraction of both agonists and antagonists, as with stabilization. Muscles that contract to stabilize (or fixate) a joint or bone so that another body part can exert force against a fixed point are called **synergists**.

Stabilization occurs frequently in the torso. The erector spinae, transversus abdominis, rectus abdominis, internal obliques, and external obliques stabilize the torso, allowing for more efficient movements in the arms and legs. Muscles in the shoulder also stabilize the shoulder and shoulder girdle to allow efficient movements in the upper body. The water is a great place to work on the torso and shoulder stabilizers. The trunk stabilizers are particularly challenged in deep water, where control of the body is totally focused on the dynamic stabilization of the trunk muscles to maintain neutral alignment. Significant improvements are often seen in postural alignment following a consistent deep- or shallow-water exercise program.

Of particular note for exercise instructors are muscle groups that cross more than one joint. Contracting the muscle to create movement at one joint can cause limited motion in the other joint. An example of this is trying to do a back kick (hip extension) with your knee bent (knee flexion). This may be challenging because the hamstring muscle group is responsible for both joint actions.

The length of a muscle may also prevent full range of motion at the joint or joints that the muscle crosses. For example, the hamstring crosses the hip and the knee,

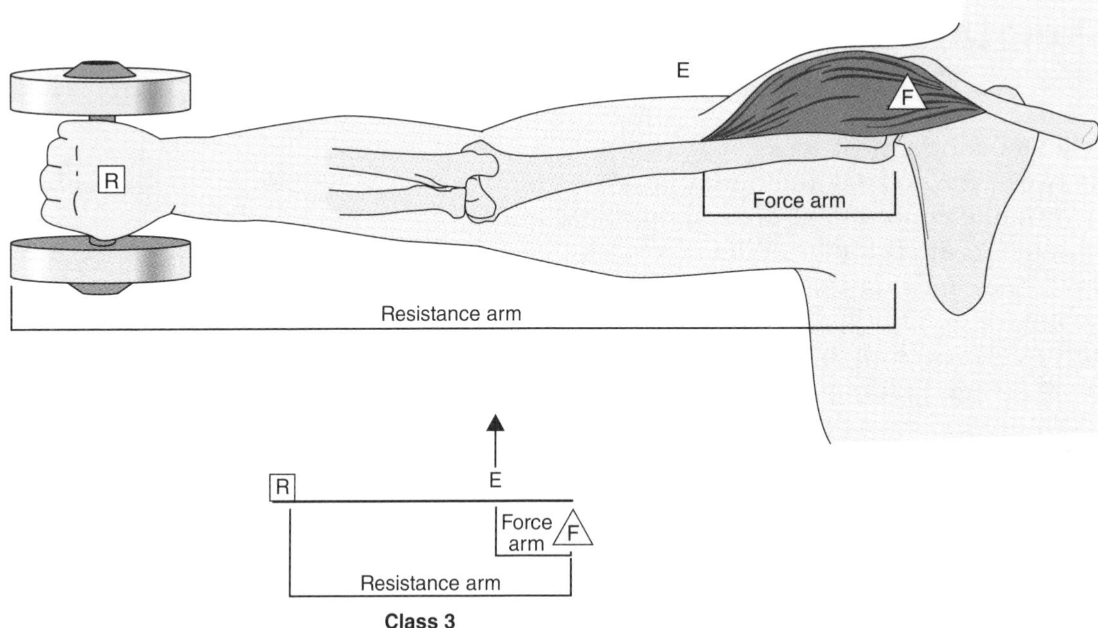

Figure 4.32 The shoulder joint is a third-class lever.

so it is easier to lift your leg in front of you when your knee is bent than when your leg is straight. In other words, you have greater range of motion at the hip when the knee is flexed than when the knee is extended.

Movement and Muscle Actions With Aquatic Exercise

The movements of the body are the same whether you are moving in or out of the water. The difference is that movements on land are affected by gravity, whereas movements in the water are met with resistance in all directions and influenced by the type of equipment being used in the pool.

Pure Movement

Pure movement is muscle action void of gravity, water, or equipment. If you were in outer space, there would be no environmental impact and your movement would be caused by the contraction of the muscles that move that joint; this is pure movement. Table 4.6 shows pure movement of the biceps and triceps muscles shown in figures 4.33 and 4.34. You should understand muscle actions in isolation before trying to understand the effect of various environments and types of equipment on muscle actions.

Table 4.6 Example of Pure Movement: Flexion and Extension of the Arm at the Elbow While Standing Upright

Flexion	Biceps brachii (figure 4.33)	To bend the forearm up or move it out of anatomical position
Extension	Triceps brachii (see figure 4.34)	To lower the forearm down or return it to anatomical position

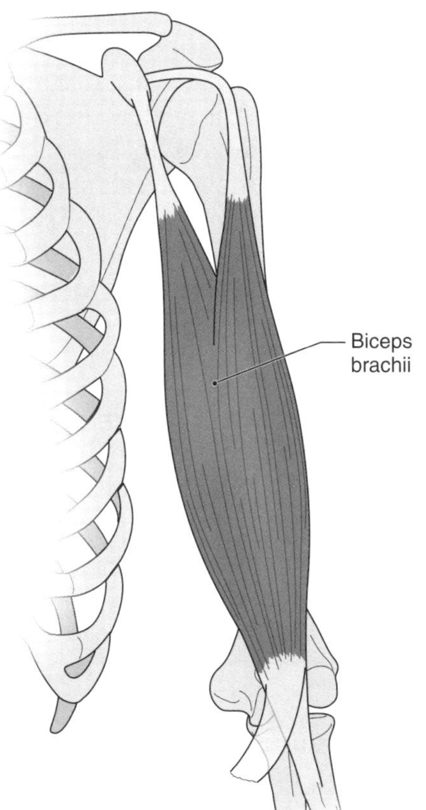

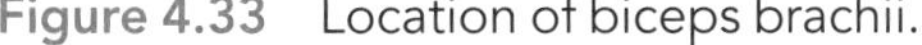

Figure 4.33 Location of biceps brachii.

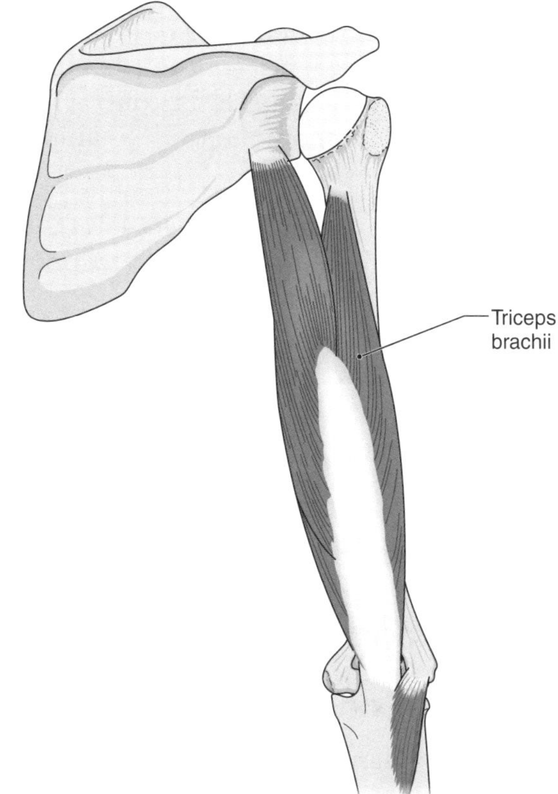

Figure 4.34 Location of triceps brachii.

Resisted and Assisted Movements

Assisted movement refers to any part in the range of motion of an exercise movement that is facilitated by gravity or buoyancy or by the properties of the equipment. The movement is an eccentric muscle action because the muscle is generating tension while lengthening to control the movement. Examples include the following:

- The return movement toward the anchored point when using rubberized resistance equipment (equipment assisted)
- Movement toward the pool bottom when using weighted equipment (gravity assisted)
- Movement toward the surface of the water when using buoyant equipment (**buoyancy assisted**)

Resisted movement refers to any part in the range of motion of an exercise movement that is impeded by the forces of gravity or buoyancy or by the properties of the equipment. The movement is a concentric muscle action because the muscle is contracting and shortening to move the load. Examples include the following:

- Movement that pulls rubberized equipment away from its anchored point (equipment resisted)
- Movement toward the surface of the water, or upward out of the water, when using weighted equipment (gravity resisted)
- Movement toward the pool bottom when using buoyant equipment (**buoyancy resisted**)
- Any submerged movement when using drag equipment (water resisted)

Movement on Land

Movement on land is affected by the pull of gravity. Any movement performed away from the ground is gravity resisted, and requires a concentric muscle action. Any movement performed toward the ground is gravity assisted. Because gravity assists downward movement, lowering a limb or body part toward the ground requires an eccentric muscle action. If you relax the muscle involved, the limb or body part falls downward rather than being moved downward with control. Movements performed on land typically consist of concentric and eccentric muscle actions of the same muscle due to gravitational forces (table 4.7).

Table 4.7 Example of Muscle Action on Land in Gravity: Flexion and Extension of the Arm at the Elbow While Standing Upright

Flexion	Biceps brachii	Concentric muscle action
Extension	Biceps brachii	Eccentric muscle action

Submerged Movement

Submerged movements are affected by the water's buoyancy and viscosity. Submerged movement without equipment will primarily be influenced by drag, which relates to the water's viscosity. The water surrounds you and affects movements in every direction; therefore, every movement in every plane is resisted in the water. Every submerged movement without equipment requires a concentric contraction due to the water's viscosity (table 4.8).

Table 4.8 Example of Muscle Action in Submerged Movement: Flexion and Extension of the Arm at the Elbow While Standing Upright

Flexion	Biceps brachii	Concentric muscle action
Extension	Triceps brachii	Concentric muscle action

Table 4.9 summarizes the muscles involved during pure movement, land movement, and submerged movement in common exercises.

Table 4.9 Summary of Muscle Actions During Pure Movement, Land Movement, and Submerged Movement

Exercise	Pure movement	Land movement	Submerged movement without equipment
Arm curl			
Flexion of the forearm	Biceps brachii	Concentric biceps brachii	Concentric biceps brachii
Extension of the forearm	Triceps brachii	Eccentric biceps brachii	Concentric triceps brachii
Leg curl			
Flexion of the lower leg	Hamstrings	Concentric hamstrings	Concentric hamstrings
Extension of the lower leg	Quadriceps	Eccentric hamstrings	Concentric quadriceps
Lateral arm raise			
Abduction of the arm	Deltoid	Concentric deltoid	Concentric deltoid
Adduction of the arm	Latissimus dorsi	Eccentric deltoid	Concentric latissimus dorsi
Lateral leg lift			
Abduction of the leg	Abductors	Concentric abductors	Concentric abductors
Adduction of the leg	Adductors	Eccentric adductors	Concentric adductors
Horizontal arm sweep			
Transverse adduction	Pectoralis and anterior deltoid	Primarily isometric deltoids to hold the arm up at shoulder height	Concentric pectoralis and anterior deltoid
Transverse abduction	Posterior deltoid	Primarily isometric deltoids to hold the arm up at shoulder height	Concentric posterior deltoid
Front arm raise			
Flexion of the arm	Anterior deltoid/pectoralis/biceps brachii	Concentric anterior deltoid/pectoralis/biceps brachii	Concentric anterior deltoid/pectoralis/biceps brachii
Extension of the arm	Posterior deltoid/latissimus dorsi/triceps	Eccentric anterior deltoid/pectoralis/biceps brachii	Concentric posterior deltoid/latissimus dorsi/triceps
Straight-leg front lift			
Flexion of the leg	Iliopsoas/rectus femoris	Concentric iliopsoas/rectus femoris	Concentric iliopsoas/rectus femoris
Extension of the leg	Gluteus maximus/hamstrings	Eccentric iliopsoas/rectus femoris	Concentric gluteus maximus/hamstrings

Influence of Aquatic Equipment

The type of equipment—buoyant, weighted, drag, or rubberized—affects muscle actions and exercise outcomes in aquatic exercise.

Buoyant Equipment

Buoyant equipment is specific to the aquatic environment. This equipment is made of a material such as foam or something like rubber or plastic that can be filled with air so that it floats on the surface of the water.

Any movement toward the bottom of the pool goes against the object's tendency to float or to be supported by the water's buoyancy. Movement toward the pool bottom is buoyancy resisted and is usually a concentric muscle action. Any movement toward the surface of the water is buoyancy assisted and is usually an eccentric muscle action (table 4.10).

Table 4.10 Example of Muscle Action in the Water With Buoyant Equipment: Flexion and Extension of the Arm at the Elbow While Standing Upright

Flexion	Triceps brachii	Eccentric muscle action assisted by buoyancy
Extension	Triceps brachii	Concentric muscle action resisted by buoyancy

Weighted Equipment

Muscle action for weighted resistance in the water is very similar to actions done on land. Weighted equipment sinks in the water, and is influenced by the force of gravity. Although the effects of gravity are reduced in the water, as long as the weighted resistance is denser than water (it sinks), it will be affected by gravity. Any movement performed upward against gravity is gravity resisted, and usually creates a concentric muscle action. Any movement performed downward is assisted by gravity, and usually creates an eccentric muscle action (table 4.11). When compared, buoyed and weighted muscle actions are the opposite of each other.

Table 4.11 Example of Muscle Action in the Water With Weighted Equipment: Flexion and Extension of the Arm at the Elbow While Standing Upright

Flexion	Biceps brachii	Concentric muscle action resisted by gravity
Extension	Biceps brachii	Eccentric muscle action assisted by gravity

Weighted and buoyed equipment complement each other well in programming. For example, it is difficult to work the medial deltoids, hip abductors, iliopsoas, and erector spinae with buoyant equipment in the water unless you assume some awkward positions or risk injuring the lower back. Most movements for these muscle groups are buoyancy assisted, so they work primarily as antagonists. Using weighted equipment engages these muscles as agonists or prime movers. On the other hand, it is difficult to work the hip adductors, latissimus dorsi, and rectus abdominis while standing in the water with weights. These muscle groups are prime movers with buoyant equipment, but are antagonists with weighted equipment. Once again, you must understand the effects of each type of equipment and carefully plan your resistance programming in the water if you are going to use equipment. Weighted equipment should be carefully supervised and monitored if used at all in deep water.

Drag Equipment

Drag equipment addresses muscle balance more simply than the use of weighted or buoyant resistance. Introducing drag equipment simply increases the drag forces of the water. Muscle actions with drag equipment are the same as the muscle actions for movements in the water without equipment; however, the resistive force has been magnified. You are using primarily concentric contractions in all directions of movement (figure 4.12). Drag equipment usually increases the surface area or turbulence to create additional resistance for muscle action. Drag

Table 4.12 Example of Muscle Action in the Water With Drag Equipment: Flexion and Extension of the Arm at the Elbow While Standing Upright

Flexion	Biceps brachii	Concentric muscle action resisted by water
Extension	Triceps brachii	Concentric muscle action resisted by water

equipment can be cumbersome, and may actually reduce the potential for full range of motion due to the increased surface area. Body positioning may need to be adjusted to accommodate the equipment. Regardless of these disadvantages, drag equipment is often preferred by fitness professionals and participants alike. The movement and resistive forces feel most consistent with natural movement in the water.

Table 4.13 compares the muscle actions involved in common exercises based on the type of equipment utilized (buoyant, weighted, or drag).

Rubberized Equipment

Rubberized equipment is composed of bands, loops, or tubes in various configurations. The muscle action created by rubberized equipment is virtually the same regardless of the environment. Any muscle action away from the anchored point is resisted and concentric. Any muscle action toward the anchored point is assisted and eccentric. The position of the anchor point determines the muscle group being worked. In the example given in table 4.14, if you anchor or hold the band lower than the elbow, you work the biceps concentrically and eccentrically. If you anchor the band higher than the elbow, you work the triceps eccentrically and concentrically.

Table 4.15 compares the muscle actions involved in common exercises with rubberized equipment based on the location of the anchor point.

As you can see, your choice of equipment offers a very specific outcome on muscle actions in aquatic fitness. Table 4.16 summarizes muscle action for a standing arm curl. This table combines information from the previous tables in this chapter to help you better see the entire picture of muscle action. Notice that the same movement—flexion and extension at the elbow—results in different muscle involvement and actions depending on the environment and type of equipment. Although it might take time to completely understand muscle actions and equipment use in the water, it is necessary for you to learn this information so you can understand the result of each movement and the benefit of each exercise you include in your program.

Table 4.13 Muscle Actions for Common Exercises Using Buoyant, Weighted, and Drag Equipment

Exercise	Buoyant equipment	Weighted equipment	Drag equipment
Arm curl			
Flexion of the forearm	Eccentric triceps brachii	Concentric biceps brachii	Concentric biceps brachii
Extension of the forearm	Concentric triceps brachii	Eccentric biceps brachii	Concentric triceps brachii
Leg curl			
Flexion of the lower leg	Eccentric quadriceps	Concentric hamstrings	Concentric hamstrings
Extension of the lower leg	Concentric quadriceps	Eccentric hamstrings	Concentric quadriceps
Lateral arm raise			
Abduction of the arm	Eccentric latissimus dorsi	Concentric deltoids	Concentric deltoids
Adduction of the arm	Concentric latissimus dorsi	Eccentric deltoids	Concentric latissimus dorsi
Lateral leg lift			
Abduction of the leg	Eccentric adductors	Concentric abductors	Concentric abductors
Adduction of the leg	Concentric adductors	Eccentric abductors	Concentric adductors
Horizontal arm sweep			
Transverse adduction	Primarily isometric latissimus dorsi/lower trapezius to hold the buoyancy underwater. Concentric pectoralis/anterior deltoid from the drag resistance.	Primarily isometric deltoids to hold the arm up at shoulder height. Concentric pectoralis/anterior deltoid from the drag resistance.	Concentric pectoralis/anterior deltoid
Transverse abduction	Primarily isometric latissimus dorsi/lower trapezius to hold the buoyancy under water. Concentric posterior deltoid from the drag resistance.	Primarily isometric deltoids to hold the arm up at shoulder height. Concentric posterior deltoids from the drag resistance.	Concentric posterior deltoids
Front arm raise			
Flexion of the arm	Eccentric posterior deltoid/latissimus dorsi/triceps	Concentric anterior deltoid/pectoralis/biceps brachii	Concentric anterior deltoid/pectoralis/biceps brachii
Extension of the arm	Concentric posterior deltoid/latissimus dorsi/triceps	Eccentric anterior deltoid/pectoralis/biceps brachii	Concentric posterior deltoid/latissimus dorsi/triceps
Straight-leg front lift			
Flexion of the leg	Eccentric gluteus maximus/hamstrings	Concentric iliopsoas/rectus femoris	Concentric iliopsoas/rectus femoris
Extension of the leg	Concentric gluteus maximus/hamstrings	Eccentric iliopsoas/rectus femoris	Concentric gluteus maximus/hamstrings

Table 4.14 Example of Muscle Action in the Water With Rubberized Equipment: Flexion and Extension of the Arm at the Elbow While Standing Upright

Anchored low, below the elbow		
Flexion	Biceps brachii	Concentric muscle action resisted away from the anchored point
Extension	Biceps brachii	Eccentric muscle action assisted toward the anchored point
Anchored high, above the elbow		
Flexion	Triceps brachii	Eccentric muscle action assisted toward the anchored point
Extension	Triceps brachii	Concentric muscle action resisted away from the anchored point

Table 4.15 Muscle Actions for Common Exercises Using Rubberized Equipment

Exercise and movement	Anchor	Anchor
Arm curl	**High**	**Low**
Flexion of the forearm	Eccentric triceps brachii	Concentric biceps brachii
Extension of the forearm	Concentric triceps brachii	Eccentric biceps brachii
Leg curl	**Front**	**Back**
Flexion of the lower leg	Concentric hamstrings	Eccentric quadriceps
Extension of the lower leg	Eccentric hamstrings	Concentric quadriceps
Lateral arm raise	**High**	**Low**
Abduction of the arm	Eccentric latissimus dorsi	Concentric deltoid
Adduction of the arm	Concentric latissimus dorsi	Eccentric deltoid
Lateral leg lift	**Medial**	**Lateral**
Abduction of the leg	Concentric abductor	Eccentric adductor
Adduction of the leg	Eccentric abductor	Concentric adductor
Horizontal arm sweep	**Front**	**Back**
Transverse adduction	Eccentric posterior deltoid	Concentric pectoralis/anterior deltoid
Transverse abduction	Concentric posterior deltoid	Eccentric pectoralis/anterior deltoid
Front arm raise	**Front**	**Back**
Flexion of the arm	Eccentric posterior deltoid/latissimus dorsi/triceps	Concentric anterior deltoid/pectoralis/biceps brachii
Extension of the arm	Concentric posterior deltoid/latissimus dorsi/triceps	Eccentric anterior deltoid/pectoralis/biceps brachii
Straight-leg front lift	**Front**	**Back**
Flexion of the leg	Eccentric gluteus maximus/hamstrings	Concentric iliopsoas/rectus femoris
Extension of the leg	Concentric gluteus maximus/hamstrings	Eccentric iliopsoas/rectus femoris

Table 4.16 Muscle Actions for a Standing Arm Curl

Environment and equipment	Muscle	Muscle action	Resisted or assisted
	Pure movement		
Flexion	Biceps brachii		
Extension	Triceps brachii		
	Land, no equipment		
Flexion	Biceps brachii	Concentric	Gravity resisted
Extension	Biceps brachii	Eccentric	Gravity assisted
	Submerged, no equipment		
Flexion	Biceps brachii	Concentric	Water resisted
Extension	Triceps brachii	Concentric	Water resisted
	Buoyant equipment		
Flexion	Triceps brachii	Eccentric	Buoyancy assisted
Extension	Triceps brachii	Concentric	Buoyancy resisted
	Weighted equipment		
Flexion	Biceps brachii	Concentric	Gravity resisted
Extension	Biceps brachii	Eccentric	Gravity assisted
	Drag equipment		
Flexion	Biceps brachii	Concentric	Water resisted
Extension	Triceps brachii	Concentric	Water resisted
	Rubberized equipment Anchored low		
Flexion	Biceps brachii	Concentric	Equipment resisted
Extension	Biceps brachii	Eccentric	Equipment assisted
	Rubberized equipment Anchored high		
Flexion	Triceps brachii	Eccentric	Equipment assisted
Extension	Triceps brachii	Concentric	Equipment resisted

Summary

A basic understanding of movement analysis is necessary for creating safe and effective programming. This includes understanding anatomical position and reference terms. A clear understanding of the purpose of each exercise will allow you to increase the benefits of the program.

Posture and alignment are necessary for the effective performance of exercises and injury prevention. Proper posture and alignment should be taught and promoted in any aquatic exercise program. Include movement in all three planes—frontal, sagittal, and transverse—in order to achieve muscle balance and functional mobility.

Joint actions related to exercise include abduction and adduction, medial and lateral rotation, circumduction, tilt, supination and pronation, inversion and eversion, elevation and depression, retraction and protraction, and flexion, extension, and hyperextension. These joint actions are referenced in relation to anatomical position.

Several types of joints exist in the human body. Movement at any joint is determined by the type of joint, bones surrounding the joint, and the muscles and associated soft tissue involved in the movement. You should know the muscles associated with each joint, the type of joint, and safe movement options at each joint.

The skeletal and muscular systems work together as a system of levers to create movement. Most movements related to exercise result from third-class levers and involve a complex and coordinated effort of activation, deactivation, or cocontraction of muscles.

Although the movements of the body are the same, movements on land are affected by gravity, whereas movements in the water are met with resistance in all directions. Adding equipment to submerged movement influences the muscle actions and exercise outcomes.

Review Questions

1. __________________ is moving away from the midline of the body.
2. Flexion and extension are performed primarily in the __________________ plane.
3. In a third-class lever, the __________________ is between the __________________ and __________________.
4. What type of joint is the elbow?
5. Name the three natural curves in the spine.
6. The deeper the water in which you are exercising, the more you have to consider the center of ____________.
7. List and define at least six terms used to identify joint actions.
8. Define anatomical position.

9. ________________ refers to any part in the range of motion of an exercise movement that is facilitated by the forces of gravity or buoyancy or by the properties of the equipment.

10. Movement toward the pool bottom with buoyant equipment is buoyancy resisted and is usually a ________________muscle action.

See appendix D for answers to review questions.

References and Resources

American College of Sports Medicine. 2013. *Guidelines for exercise testing and prescription.* 9th edition. Baltimore: Lippincott, Williams & Wilkins.

American Council on Exercise. 1997. *Personal training manual.* San Diego: American Council on Exercise.

———. 2000. *Group fitness instructor manual.* San Diego: American Council on Exercise.

April, E. 1984. *Anatomy (National Medical Series).* Indianapolis: Wiley.

Burke, R. 1993. *Kinesiology and applied anatomy: The science of human movement.* 7th edition. Philadelphia: Lea & Febiger.

Clarkson, H. 2000. *Musculoskeletal assessment: Joint range of motion and manual muscle strength.* 2nd edition. Baltimore: Lippincott, Williams & Wilkins.

Heyward, V. 2014. *Advanced fitness assessment & exercise prescription.* 7th edition. Champaign, IL: Human Kinetics.

Kendall, F., E. McCreary, P. Provance, M. McIntyre, and W. Romani. 2005. *Muscles: Testing and function with posture and pain.* 5th edition. Baltimore: Lippincott, Williams & Wilkins.

Kreighbaum, E., and M. Barthels. 1995. *Biomechanics: A qualitative approach for studying human movement.* 4th edition. San Francisco: Cummings.

Riposo, D. 1990. *Fitness concepts: A resource manual for aquatic fitness instructors.* 2nd edition. Pt. Washington, WI: Aquatic Exercise Association.

Sweigard, L. 1974. *Human movement potential: Its ideokinetic facilitation.* New York: Harper and Row.

Thompson, C., and R. Floyd. 2000. *Manual of structural kinesiology.* 14th edition. New York: McGraw-Hill.

Todd, M. 1980. *The thinking body: A study of the balancing forces of dynamic man.* Highstown, NJ: Princeton Book.

Tortora, G., and S. Grabowski. 2002. *Principles of anatomy and physiology.* 10th edition. Indianapolis: Wiley.

Van Roden, J., and L. Gladwin. 2002. *Fitness theory & practice.* 4th edition. Sherman Oaks, CA: Aerobic & Fitness Association of America.

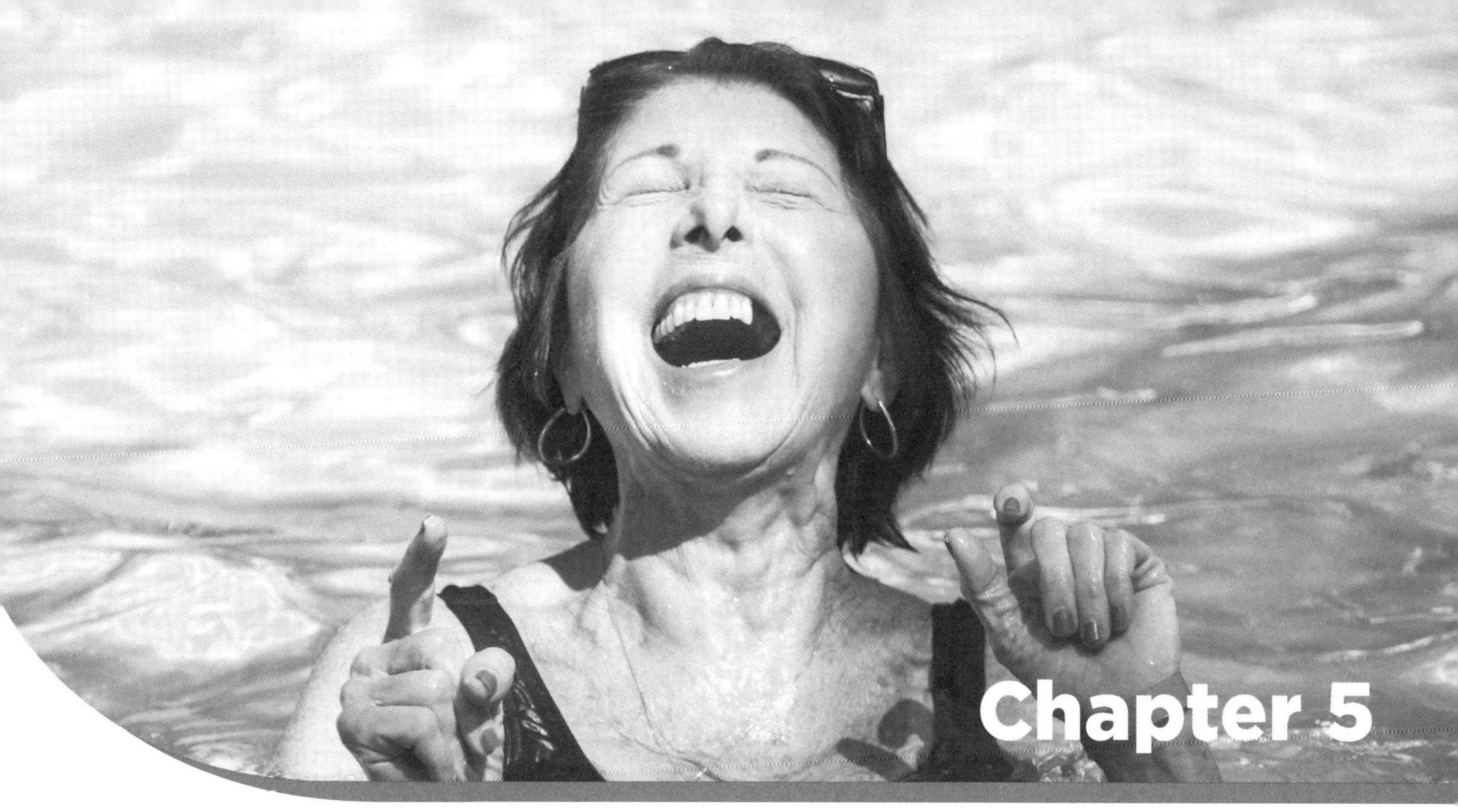

Exercise Motivation and Behavior

Introduction

One of the most rewarding aspects of working in the aquatic fitness industry is helping participants integrate regular exercise into their lives with the goal of improved health. We all love to share our passion for active living, and many times this enthusiasm rubs off and helps our participants overcome barriers, injuries, and other challenges to reach their goals. Yet, as you have surely experienced, some of the biggest frustrations—a lack of participant motivation and inconsistent adherence—often emerge within each program or class. How can we reduce these frustrations and reach the maximum number of participants with our efforts? The purpose of this chapter is to share several reasons why participants struggle to maintain regular exercise and to provide a set of specific practices that aquatic fitness professionals can integrate into their work.

Key Chapter Concepts

- Understand the three key principles regarding the complexity of behavior change for exercise participants.
- Explain and apply the three strategies for motivating exercise participants for sustained change.
- Define the terms of autonomy, competence, and relatedness as they relate to the theory of self-determination.
- Understand the process of motivational interviewing to assist participants with motivation and exercise adherence.
- Explore two case scenarios that give insight into providing exercise motivation for a group setting and assisting participants through exercise barriers.

Foundations of Behavior Change

Why is it so hard to change? Thousands of articles and books have been written about exercise motivation and behavior. Countless theories address participant attitudes, knowledge, intentions, and behavior with the goal of understanding how to help others change. A few core principles from this exhaustive list of research may more clearly guide your understanding of the complexity of change relating to **exercise behavior.**

Principle 1: It takes more than goals and willpower to change.

When working with new participants (who often seem highly motivated), one of the biggest mistakes you can make is assuming that their initial motivation and attitude will be sustained long term. As humans living in an achievement-oriented society, we place value on setting ambitious outcome goals and appearing motivated (i.e., "talking the talk") at the beginning of any new effort. We love to create New Year's resolutions, set goals for a wedding or an anniversary, or try out a new exercise regimen.

The research in this area is quite clear, however. Although initial outcome goals can provide short-term motivation for initiating a behavior, they rarely last more than a few weeks or months without being connected to a meaningful piece of a person's identity or life priorities (Kimiecik 2002). We also know that it takes approximately six months of sustained efforts to turn a new habit into one that will be maintained (Prochaska and DiClemente 1992), which can extend longer than some aquatic classes or programs. Thus, a corollary here is that starting exercise is easy, but sticking with it is not.

A typical mistake participants make in the early phase of their efforts is to overestimate their own willpower, take on an exercise routine they are not ready to sustain, and underestimate the potential influence of any personal or situational barriers that might emerge. Many new exercisers embody this "go big or go home" mentality. Unfortunately, this lands most participants back home far too soon. Those who are successful plan effectively, use support, and integrate their new routine into their weekly schedule.

Successful regular exercisers often report that the reasons that motivate them to maintain their exercise habit are not the same reasons that motivated them to start. Thus, one of the roles aquatic fitness professionals can fill is to help participants take advantage of their initial motivation to start strong and use this to prepare them for the transition in motivation that may be necessary should they either reach their goal or come to the conclusion that their initial goal is no longer relevant. Knowing that there is more to creating a successful exercise routine than willpower can help normalize the struggle that many participants will go through. Finally, helping participants plan (i.e., schedule exercise sessions into their week like a medical appointment) and self-monitor (i.e., record their exercise on a daily basis) can help them stick with exercise, since new exercisers often underuse these tools.

Principle 2: There are multiple levels of influence on motivation.

We interact with our participants in a limited context, typically before, during, and after a planned exercise session. We observe their attitude, mood, and behavior in this setting and then learn something about their overall personality and life story. But we need to move beyond participants' attitudes and experiences to understand the context in which they are trying to apply exercise.

The best fitness professionals go beyond the exercise prescription and provide lifestyle coaching to help participants connect their fitness pursuits to other pieces of their lives that hold greater meaning. We cannot expect that all participants will share the same level of passion for fitness and active living that we do. To explore the context in which they are living, consider learning more about the micro- and mesoenvironmental factors that might be influencing their exercise attitudes and behavior (Stokols 1996).

At the microenvironmental level, you can ask questions about their work schedule, social commitments, and their friends and family members. You might find it helpful to ask about specific supports (e.g., workout partner, flexible work schedule) as well as hindrances and social sabotage (e.g., family and social obligations). At the next level, it is useful to ask about their home neighborhood, safe walking routes near home and work, and access to home exercise equipment. Knowing this specific contextual information will allow you to customize your suggestions for adherence to class and provide input on any home exercise program that might be relevant. If the overall goal is long-term adherence to exercise, then we need to understand these environmental variables so the plan fits with the rest of their lives.

Principle 3: Finding meaning in exercise and being healthy are important.

It is easy to assume that everyone who shows up to an aquatic session or class is a motivated participant who values their health. At that moment, yes, they have made a choice to be with you, but that choice may be different in the future if they don't find a way to incorporate exercise among their other priorities. This process is especially important for participants who do not identify strongly with being a healthy or active person.

For nearly all of us in the fitness industry, being active is a large part of our identity; thus, our choices to exercise regularly confirm that piece of our identity, and those choices are made easily (Kimiecik 2002). For new exercise participants, much of the exercise adoption process can feel quite unnatural, from the physical sensations (e.g., breathing hard, sweating, lack of endurance or strength) to the psychosocial experiences (e.g., poor body image, perceived pain). With repeated exposure and the right level of reinforcement, participants can learn to tolerate these sensations and then excel in exercise settings. Their bodies adapt to the physical challenges in a few weeks, and they can begin to experience positive mood and energy benefits within a few days. When participants tune into these welcome changes and shift their focus away from outcome goals, such as the number on the scale or inches around their waist, they can start to develop a stronger identity as an active person.

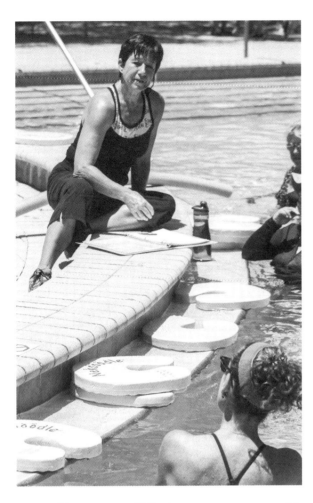

A good instructor will find a way to connect with participants who may be unsure of their progress and help them feel more comfortable with the experience.

This is one area where the aquatic class setting can match novice exercisers particularly well because they are likely to experience less of the negative physical sensations. Support is also built in from the fitness professional and their peers. Research across a variety of exercise settings indicates that substantial psychological benefits exist for moderate amounts of physical activity, including reduced depression and anxiety and improved energy (Lox, Martin-Ginis, and Petruzzello 2014). It is common for lifelong exercisers to report that these psychological benefits are the reasons they continue to exercise on a daily basis compared to the physical fitness or weight management benefits. Thus, it is our job to help participants find meaning in an activity by making them aware of the many psychosocial benefits of it, helping them build an identity as an active participant, and teaching them how being a healthier version of themselves will have a positive influence on their lives outside the water in their roles as a parent, employee, or colleague. Yet the bridge from awareness of the benefits of exercise to being a regular exerciser is still full of challenges. The fact is that we all struggle to incorporate exercise into our busy lives; it just so happens that some of us have more practice doing this, and therefore we have more tools in our toolbox for sustaining this habit. Transferring these tools to our participants is the focus of the next section.

Motivating Participants for Sustained Change

As an aquatic fitness professional, you will spend countless hours working toward your certification and then designing a quality program or class session for your participants. By applying your training knowledge, you can design workouts and programs to maximize participant fitness and enjoyment. You can also apply sound theory to create a group environment that maximizes participant motivation. The following strategies are drawn from experience working with numerous people and are supported by several research theories and techniques from individual and group counseling. The overall approach focuses on building choice, support, and competence into your instructional style while also developing individual interviewing skills so that your interactions outside of the water will be more structured.

Strategy 1: Create a task-focused, growth-oriented climate.

This strategy involves both a macro-level philosophy, focused on helping participants improve their own skills and fitness, and micro-level techniques for modifying your instructions and activities to build and sustain participant motivation. On the macro level, a **growth mind-set** involves getting your participants to focus on their own effort and improvement and to shift attention away from comparing their abilities with others. This idea comes from Carol Dweck (2006), who examined work from various researchers in achievement motivation. Dweck (2006) showed the importance of a task-oriented approach to learning. This orientation embraces the use of specific feedback and the value of failure (i.e., struggling) as useful information in the learning process. Experiences, feedback, and even failure can teach us how to become better and more adherent exercisers. Most certainly, you will have participants of a wide range of abilities, shapes, and sizes under your care, and this approach will help you reach all of them where they need to be reached.

The theory of self-determination provides a set of more specific strategies for building health behavior motivation. This line of research suggests that if participants can meet their needs for **autonomy** (i.e., freedom of choice), **competence** (i.e., confidence in their skills, improvement), and **relatedness** (i.e., meaningful connections to others) through exercise, then they will experience stronger and more sustained motivation (Ryan et al. 2008). An example of a strategy that promotes both autonomy and competence would be to provide exercise modifications that allow participants to choose an easier, less strenuous option and a more difficult and intense option for each phase of a class or training session. It is also useful to give an outline of what to expect for the class in terms of exercises and intensities (e.g., four circuits of four exercises, each done for 30 seconds, and each circuit will be completed two times). This outline allows your participants to choose (autonomy) how hard they can push themselves based on what is coming up and to gauge their own progress through the workout (competence). As the class progresses, you may want to ask them to notice if a specific circuit or set was less difficult for them so they can be aware of their increasing fitness and skill (competence).

Additional strategies could involve allowing participants some autonomy in the order of a workout, or choosing or demonstrating the next exercise in a combination. The group context of an aquatic class naturally promotes relatedness within the class session, and you could extend these relationships outside of class to encourage choosing workout partners, ride sharing, and so on. For competence, you can have participants demonstrate specific exercises when they are learning, give them specific form-related feedback and encouragement, and then engage them in class leadership as they gain experience. Encouraging participants to make notes of improvements in their ability to perform exercises or daily activities can also help build competence.

Strategy 2: Use a motivational interviewing approach for individual encounters.

This builds on strategy 1 well because it allows you to extend the group climate into individual conversations that naturally happen in your fitness center, in the locker room, or on the pool deck. **Motivational interviewing** is a set of counseling questions and techniques that helps participants who are unmotivated or ambivalent to change (Rollnick, Miller, and Butler 2008). The tone of this approach is empathetic and encouraging, and puts you in a position of a partner, not an expert. Thus, you spend less time telling them what they need to do and more time helping them explore what they want to do.

This approach will help your participants feel supported. The interactions will force them to develop their own reasons for change, as opposed to being convinced by you. Participants won't care how much you know until they know how much you care. Here are a few examples of the types of questions that can lead to fruitful conversations with your participants:

- What have you noticed about . . . ? (e.g., your changes in fitness, your mood or energy levels after class, your level of comfort in class)
- Of all the options we talked about for home exercise plans, what makes the most sense to you?

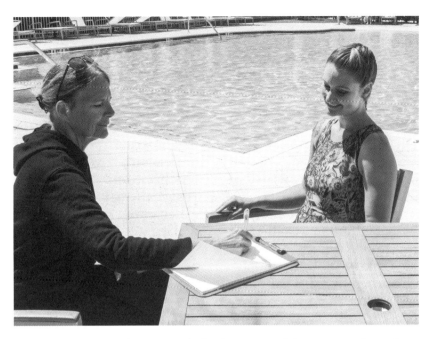

One-on-one interviews can help keep participants motivated to achieve their goals through personalized support.

- How might things be different if you . . . ? (e.g., worked a bit harder in class, came more often, exercised more on your own)
- In what way would an exercise partner affect your motivation?

These kinds of questions lead participants to explore their own ambivalence and to produce their own solutions. The tone and wording of the questions is important, too, because they send implied messages that *you* are supportive, but *they* have the authority to choose from among the options and make the final decision. To gain more experience in this useful technique, seek out workshops or additional training in motivational interviewing that might be offered in your local area or at regional or national conferences.

Strategy 3: Before they drop out, help participants identify and proactively address barriers to their exercise goals.

This final tip focuses specifically on the personal and situational barriers that regularly emerge in participants' lives. The big difference in those participants who stick with exercise long term and those who drop out is not the presence of barriers (we all have them) but instead the use of self-regulation strategies to prevent relapse. We often frame this discussion in terms of having a Plan A and a backup plan for your exercise each day.

A week or two into your program or class, ask your participants, "What are some of the barriers you are experiencing related to getting to your exercise session or completing your exercise?" For each barrier, brainstorm a prevention plan that includes the specific contextual information related to when, where, and how that barrier occurs. When speaking one on one with a participant (before or after class, or even outside the class setting), listen carefully—the details matter. For example, if the participant is having a problem with attendance at the early morning class due to hitting the snooze button too many times, first discuss plans for making the morning process easier (e.g., preparing the night before with clothes for work and exercise, food for the day, and so on). Begin these plans with strategies they already use on the days they do make it to class, and then add in cues in their environment to help them

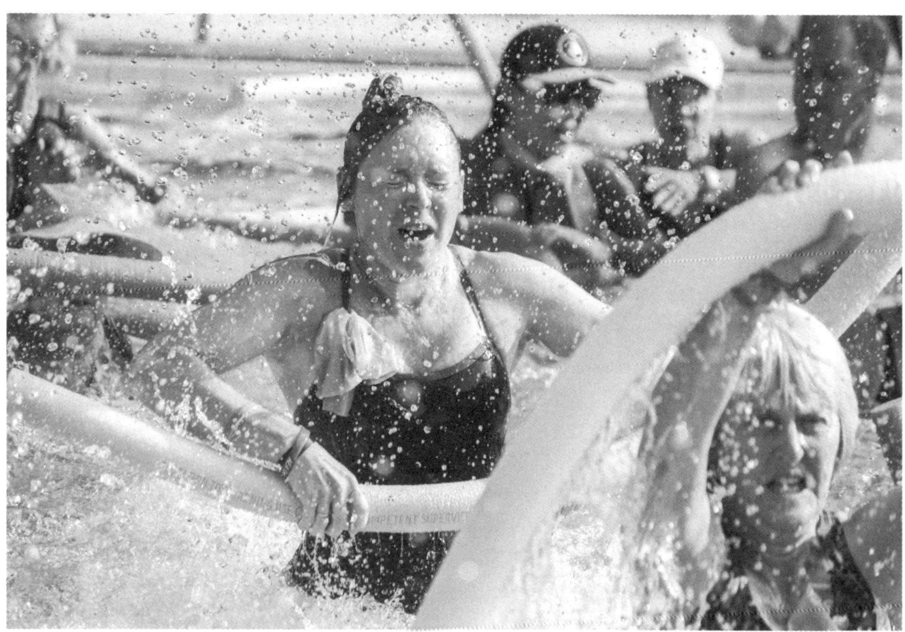

One barrier to exercise is boredom. Keeping participants entertained while exercising will improve class attendance.

make the decision easier (e.g., reminder notes on the mirror or their phone's home screen, swimsuit by the front door). Next, talk with them about backup plans if they miss class and remind them that they can still make up their exercise in another way. This conversation naturally leads to the development of appropriate home-based exercise plans and will allow you to integrate micro- and mesoenvironmental questions, too.

The primary idea here is recognizing that we cannot prevent all barriers. So, when participants do encounter difficulty, we want them to have a specific plan so they feel more confident in their ability to manage that barrier. This discussion strategy can also work well within the class setting, allowing you the opportunity to address common barriers and solutions during the warm-up or cool-down or as part of your daily education and inspiration, if that is something you include in your program. By providing ideas for staying motivated and allowing interaction within the class, you can build camaraderie and a feeling of inclusion. It can be encouraging for participants to realize that they are not alone in the struggle to keep the exercise commitment.

Case Scenarios

Instructors can incorporate these ideas to create a motivating and empowering group fitness environment in many different ways. Case 1 presents a few examples about how to integrate these ideas, but use your creativity to come up with additional ways to honor your participants' need for autonomy, competence, and relatedness. The more these needs become part of your class environment, the happier your participants will be and the more likely they will be to come back and to recommend your class to others!

Case 2 is one example of how we can incorporate some principles of motivational interviewing to help participants better understand their motivation and barriers to exercising. Participants are usually unaware of all challenges that need to be overcome and, as a result, blame themselves for not making exercise happen. You are in a great position to provide support to participants who are struggling by asking them questions that help explore their environment so they can develop an effective plan for increasing their activity and reaching their goals.

Case 1: Create a group fitness environment that builds motivation.

In this first case, we present some strategies for building a motivational group fitness environment by incorporating the ideas presented in this chapter. Specifically, we focus on how to build autonomy, competence, and relatedness into your class. Teacher dialogue is presented on the left and connections to the theoretical basis for it is on the right.

Fitness Leader Dialogue and Analysis for Building Motivation

Fitness leader dialogue	Analysis
"Welcome to class. It's great to see so many of you made the commitment to be here today! I have a fun workout planned. We will start with our warm-up and then we will work through 4 different circuits before finishing with our cool-down."	• Acknowledging the commitment it took to come to class gets participants thinking about what steps they took to be there and why coming to class is meaningful to them. • Giving a plan for the day gives them a sense of control over what is coming so they can then choose (autonomy) how intensely to push and monitor their progress through the workout (competence).
"Let me run through our first circuit. We have 4 exercises that we will do for 45 seconds each. I will demonstrate each exercise briefly with one modification to add some difficulty for those of you who want to challenge yourselves today. Then we will run through the circuit 2 times."	• Giving options helps participants choose (autonomy) what they feel comfortable doing. We won't want our participants to feel like they failed if they can't complete an exercise (lack of competence), so it's better to structure the workout so that people can step up to a higher difficulty rather than step down. If participants choose to step up the difficulty, they will have the opportunity to experience progress and accomplishment, making them more likely to come back to your class.
"Steve, great job on your level III cross-country skis! You are getting a great range of motion today."	• Knowing participant names is huge (relatedness), since it allows you to give specific feedback to each person about their progress (competence).
"Great job today! You brought excellent energy to those exercises. Give yourself some kudos!"	• Acknowledging the energy or effort helps participants focus on their identity as someone who works hard and puts good energy into what they commit to rather than on being a good or perfect exerciser. • Reinforcing effort and attendance also builds the growth mind-set in your class, because no matter their health, shape, or size, they can show up and work hard!
"While we cool down, chat with your neighbor about what steps you took to be here today and how it feels now to have done that."	• Reflecting on what got them to class helps solidify the positive habits they already have. Reflecting on how it feels when they make a commitment to themselves will help connect exercise with their own personal values that underlie coming to class. • Having them share with their neighbors allows them to build connections (relatedness), which will build motivation. In addition, having a structure for each class that includes a specific time for socializing can help cut down on unwanted talking during the workout portion of the class.

Case 2: Help a participant work through barriers to exercise.

This second case study focuses on a one-on-one conversation with a participant who is feeling down about their progress because of a struggle to make it to class on a regular basis.

Fitness Leader Dialogue and Analysis for Helping a Participant

Dialogue	Analysis
Aquatic fitness professional (AFP): "Hey, Nancy—you brought great energy to class today!"	
Nancy: "Well, I'd better have good energy since this is the only class I've made it to this week. I always start the week with great plans for exercising more but can never seem to follow through. I just don't know what I am doing wrong!"	• She starts attributing blame to herself. In doing so, she prevents any exploration of why she might be struggling to make it to class more often. • Resist jumping right into problem-solving mode; first, help explore her situation.
AFP: "That's frustrating, but finding time to exercise isn't easy. What steps did you take to make it happen today?"	• Honor her feelings and normalize the struggle of trying to fit exercise into her schedule. Then shift the focus to helping her explore.
Nancy: "Hmm . . . well, last night I looked up the schedule for classes because I saw I had time this morning and then I just made sure to get up with enough time to make it."	
AFP: "Nice work! So, you planned ahead by looking up the schedule for classes and comparing that with your schedule, and then you made a commitment to yourself to get up early enough to make it. And what happens on days you don't make it to class?"	• This starts to shift the focus from blaming herself to looking at her schedule and exploring how exercise can fit.
Nancy: "Well, usually I just forget and then all of sudden the class is about to start and I am in the middle of something."	• Understanding the situations around when she does or doesn't exercise will help her develop an effective plan for making exercise a regular routine.
AFP: "It takes a lot of effort and planning to make exercise happen."	• Normalize the struggle!
Nancy: "Yeah, I guess so. I just thought it would happen, like if you are motivated to exercise, you'd just be able to make it work."	• This is typical. We all tend to think it should be easy and then beat ourselves up when it's not. It takes more than willpower to make new habits! And beating yourself up regularly is no fun. Eventually, people just quit.
AFP: "That'd be nice! So, what are 1 or 2 steps you could take next week to make it to one more class than you did this week?"	• Let her come up with some ideas. Yes, we know planning is important, but let her come up with her own ideas about how this will work for her.

Planning for Success

Advance planning may help you prepare participants for a successful exercise experience. The following five questions can help participants recognize their reasons for participating in exercise, expectations they hold about the program, personal goals, and possible barriers. Appendix E offers a similar set of questions in a worksheet format, which works well as a homework assignment for your class. Answering these questions opens doors for participants to communicate with you individually and also offers you the opportunity to address the topics during class, which helps to develop relatedness within the group.

1. What is the main reason you are joining this exercise program?
2. What are your personal expectations for participating in this exercise program? What do you hope to get out of the exercise program?
3. What are your personal fitness goals?
4. Why are these goals important to you?
5. Has anything held you back from trying to achieve these goals in the past?

Summary

Three basic core principles form the foundation for helping participants achieve changes to exercise behavior.

1. It takes more than goals and willpower to change.
2. There are multiple levels of influence on motivation.
3. It is important to find meaning in exercise and being healthy.

Although the physiological benefits of exercise are obviously important, you must help participants recognize the psychosocial benefits as well. This allows people to build an identity as active participants and helps them understand how improved health has a positive influence on their entire life.

Aquatic fitness professionals have strategies to help motivate participants for sustained change. The overall approach focuses on building choice, support, and confidence into your instructional style while also developing individual interviewing skills so that your interactions outside of class will have a greater effect. Create a task-focused, growth-oriented climate in your classes and sessions. Use motivational interviewing for individual encounters. Help participants identify and proactively address exercise barriers—before they drop out.

The theory of self-determination provides a set of more specific strategies for building health behavior motivation. This line of research suggests that if participants can meet their needs for autonomy (i.e., freedom of choice), competence (i.e., confidence in their skills, improvement), and relatedness (i.e., meaningful connections to others) through exercise, then they will experience stronger and more sustained motivation.

Review Questions

1. What are three key principles of exercise behavior change?
2. It takes approximately _____________ of sustained efforts to turn a new habit into one that will be maintained.
3. Helping participants plan and self-monitor can help them stick with exercise, since new exercisers often underuse these tools.
   a. True
   b. False
4. With the initiation of an exercise program, the body adapts to the physical challenges in a few weeks; participants can expect to see positive mood and energy benefits within ___________.
   a. a few minutes
   b. a few days
   c. a few weeks
   d. a few months
5. How can you use the psychosocial benefits of exercise to help your participants sustain their motivation long term?
6. What are the three strategies for motivating participants for sustained change?
7. The idea of a growth mind-set means to get your participants to focus on __________________ rather than on their ability, especially as compared to others.
8. What are the three needs within self-determination theory that guide motivation?
9. Asking participants to make notes of their improvements with exercise and daily activities can help build __________________.
   a. Competence
   b. Autonomy
   c. Relatedness
   d. All of these
10. __________________________ is a set of counseling questions and techniques that helps participants who are unmotivated or ambivalent to change.

See appendix D for answers to review questions.

References and Resources

Dweck, C.S. 2006. *Mindset: The new psychology of success.* New York: Random House.

Kimiecik, J.C. 2002. *The intrinsic exerciser: Discovering the joy of exercise.* Boston: Houghton Mifflin Harcourt.

Lox, C.L., K.A. Martin Ginis, and S.J. Petruzzello. 2014. *The psychology of exercise.* Scottsdale, AZ: Holcomb Hathaway.

Prochaska, J.O., and C.C. DiClemente, 1992. The transtheoretical approach. In *Handbook of psychotherapy integration*, edited by J.C. Norcross and M.R. Goldfried, 300-334. New York: Basic Books.

Rollnick, S., W.R. Miller, and C.C. Butler. 2008. *Motivational interviewing in health care: Helping patients change health behavior.* New York: Guildford Press.

Ryan, R.M. and E.L. Deci. 2008. A self-determination theory approach to psychotherapy: The motivational basis for effective change. *Canadian Psychology/Psychologie Canadienne.* 49(3): 186.

Stokols, D. 1996. Translating social ecological theory into guidelines for community health promotion. *American Journal of Health Promotion* 10(4):282-298.

Zizzi, S., and K. Gilchrist. 2014. A theory-based model for health performance consultations. In *Becoming a sport, exercise, and performance psychology professional: International perspectives*, edited by G. Cremedes and L. Tashman, 102-110. New York: Taylor & Francis.

Zizzi, S., and V. Shannon. 2013. The ethical practice of exercise psychology. In *Ethics in sport and exercise psychology*, edited by J. Watson and E. Etzel, 77-87. Morgantown, WV: FIT Information Technology.

Part II

The Aquatic Environment

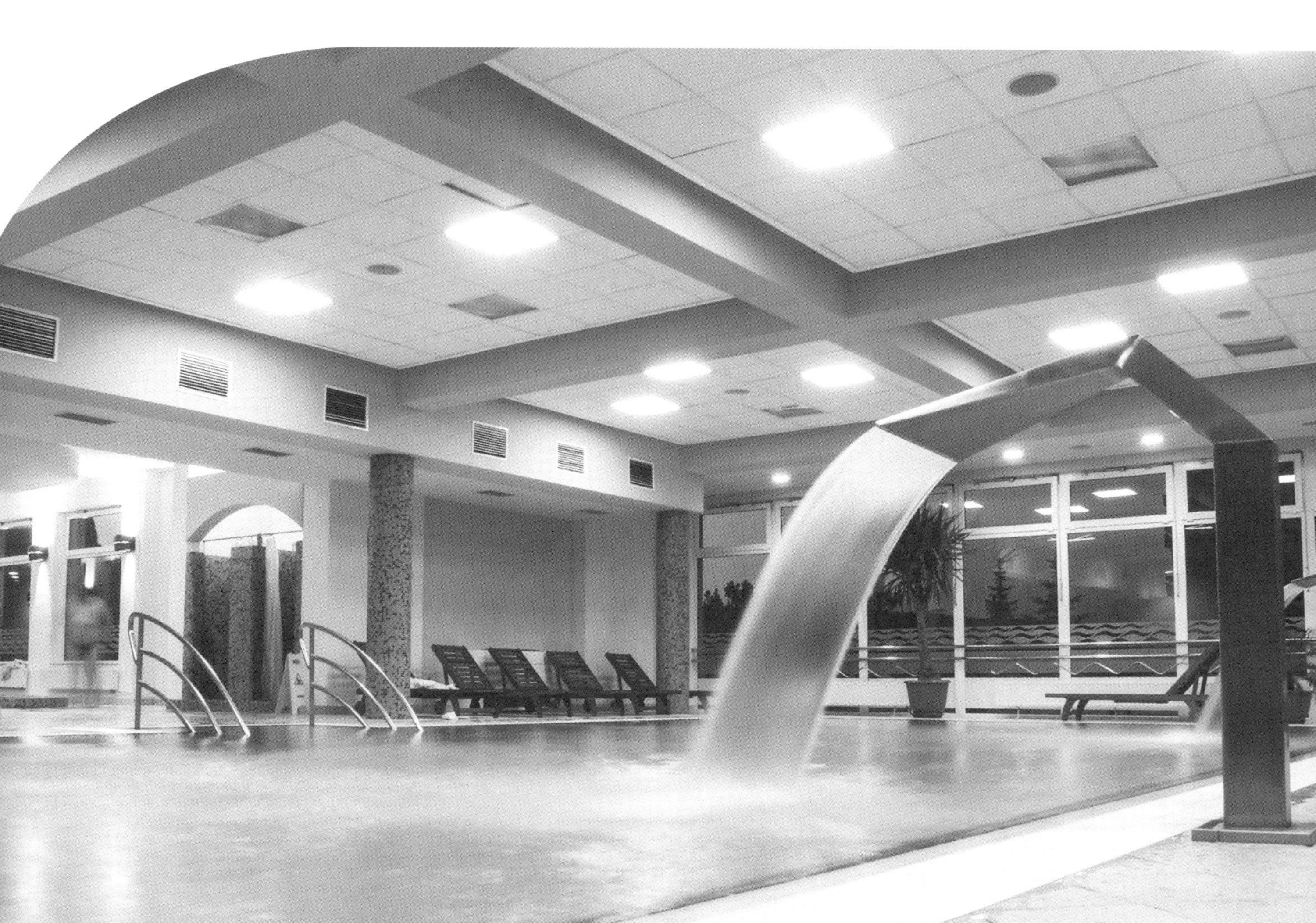

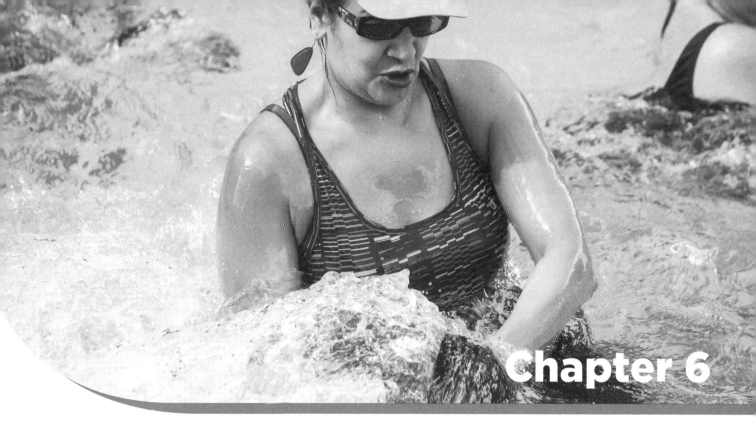

Physical Laws as Applied to the Aquatic Environment

Introduction

In this chapter, we provide information needed to gain a clear understanding of how the water works or, more correctly stated, how to work the water. Your body reacts to movement in the water differently than to movement on land. On land, gravity is the primary force affecting movement. The water provides a unique environment where the level of exertion is a function of the properties and principles of water as well as the physical laws of motion. Increasing your knowledge of the principles that govern water exercise allows you to maximize the benefits of your programs and keep participants coming back.

Key Chapter Concepts

- Recognize the physiological benefits of water immersion and how these are influenced by individual differences of participants, environmental concerns, and programming.
- Explain how buoyancy affects individual participants differently and how this property of water can influence outcomes of vertical water exercise.
- Understand how water's resistance is influenced by viscosity and differentiate between streamlined and turbulent flow.
- Define drag, hydrostatic pressure, and surface tension and explain how each influences aquatic exercise.
- Understand Newton's laws of motion (inertia, acceleration, and action and reaction) as they relate to aquatic exercise program design.
- Recognize how to apply the principles of levers, frontal resistance, and speed of movement to alter aquatic exercise intensity.

One of the most helpful lessons for a beginning aquatic fitness professional is how to put together programming that uses the water to its fullest potential. Instructors who try to simply drop their land-based program into the pool quickly discover that things just do not work the same way in water. Ineffective use of the aquatic environment is a common mistake made by those who do not have a solid understanding of how the water affects submerged movement. An effective aquatic fitness professional knows how to make the most of the fluctuating aquatic environment and to manipulate the unique properties of water to provide a practical workout for a wide range of clientele.

In this chapter, we define and explain Newton's laws of motion, the properties of viscosity and buoyancy, the physiology of immersion, and the use of levers, frontal resistance, and hand positions for manipulating the intensity of an aquatic workout. In addition, we discuss practical applications for each principle in relation to an aquatic fitness workout. These laws and principles can be employed to increase the effectiveness of any water exercise programing, including shallow-water aerobics, water walking, deep-water exercise, aquatic dance formats, one-on-one aquatic training, water therapy, sport-specific training, and even the use of equipment in the aquatic environment.

Motion

Humans are capable of running, jumping, hopping, dancing, walking, bending, twisting, and moving in many other ways. Our bodies were designed to be active, moving machines. Motion for the human machine takes the form of physical activity or exercise, and is essential to normal functioning and health.

Exercise professionals study motion in the human body to determine safe, effective, and efficient ways to move the entire body or its parts. Safe movement might save the body from an injury, chronic disease, or wear over time. Effective means that the movement is accomplishing its desired intention. That intention might be to increase cardiorespiratory endurance, flexibility, or muscular strength and endurance, or it might be functional, such as to maneuver a grocery cart through a crowded store. Efficient movement is the best and quickest way—or the least costly way, from a movement perspective—to achieve your desired intention. During water exercise, motion of the body or its parts is affected by the water's viscosity and buoyancy and somewhat by gravity.

Research studies on movement in water support that muscle activity in water changes with direction, speed, water current, and even the participant's age (Masumoto and Mercer 2008; Pinto et al. 2011; Torres-Ronda and del Alcázar 2014). Additionally, muscle activity changes from land to water, and range of motion at the joints has been shown to increase in water when compared to land (Masumoto and Mercer 2008). These alterations should be considered when designing aquatic programming for clients.

Water Immersion

Water exercise is a powerful tool that can be used to improve every parameter of fitness while making exercise attainable and fun for all populations. What is so interesting is that even before we begin to exercise, the aquatic environment starts affecting our bodies. Just being immersed in water can directly affect physiological, psychological, and emotional outcomes (Cole and Becker 2004).

A wide base of research supports the idea that immersion has a vast array of effects on many systems within the body. Physiological responses to water immersion include the following:

- Alterations in circulation, blood volume, and the heart
- Reduction in both resting and exercise heart rates (reduced cardiac workload)
- Changes in thermal regulation and body core temperature, with heat dissipation primarily through conduction and convection
- Influence on renal (kidney) output due to an increased production of urine and an increase in blood fluid
- Hydrostatic pressure influence on surface (skin) and internal body organs
- Reduction in hydrostatic weight, with reduced stress on joints
- Decompression of the spine in deep water
- Reduced swelling in the extremities, especially the legs and ankles
- Anatomical and physiological benefits in prenatal participants
- Effects on oxygen transport and oxygen consumption
- Musculoskeletal adjustments to movement in a more viscous environment, including an increase in muscular effort and rating of perceived exertion
- Biomechanical changes in movement patterns (concentric versus eccentric muscle actions)
- Changes in pulmonary function, pulmonary blood distribution, and added load to the respiratory muscles
- Facilitation of recovery from exercises performed in the water and on land

Immersion offers many beneficial outcomes during exercise. Your participants may experience less stress on the heart and vessels during exercise, reduced joint pain, or reduced blood pressure. Participants may recover faster from exercise sessions. Healing may occur at a more rapid rate due to the influx of blood flow to the muscles and tissues. The respiratory muscles may become stronger and more efficient. Immersion will affect people differently depending on their age, gender, physical condition, and body composition. Additionally, the extent to which a participant will experience these effects depends on a variety of environmental factors and programming options, including the following:

- Water temperature
- Water depth or depth of immersion
- Dunking (temporary submersion of the head and face)
- Intensity of exercise (rest, submaximal exercise, or maximal exercise)

All of these factors should be taken into consideration when designing programming that will meet the needs of your participants while maximizing the positive effects of the water.

Essential Properties of Water

The physical properties of water make aquatic exercise extremely unique. Due to these fundamental properties, aquatic exercise professionals must understand the principles of the physics of water and how to use them to change, challenge, and adapt exercises in order to meet everyone's needs (Torres-Ronda and del Alcázar 2014).

Buoyancy

According to **Archimedes' principle**, the loss of weight of a submerged body equals the weight of the fluid displaced by the body. In other words, the amount of buoyancy a body will experience is reflected by the amount of water that it displaces.

Archimedes' principle describes the buoyant property of water. When standing in water, you are subjected to two opposing forces: the downward vertical force of gravity and the upward vertical force of **buoyancy**. Both size and **density** (density = mass/volume) influence whether you sink or float. Have you ever heard the adage that muscle weighs more than fat? In reality, muscle is more dense than fat. This is the basic premise of why muscular people sink and people with more adipose tissue float. A compact, denser body (a small muscular person) displaces a relatively small amount of water, so the weight of the body is more than the weight of the water displaced; therefore, the person sinks. A person with excess body fat displaces a larger amount of water because fat is less compact than muscle (i.e., fat has more volume). Since the weight of the body is less than the weight of the water displaced, the person will float (figure 6.1). Most people are buoyant to varying degrees, depending on their body size, density, lung capacity, and percentage of fat. Only a small percentage of the population is considered to be true sinkers.

The concept of floating and sinking is important because it will help you determine the best water depth for your participants. The deeper clients go in the water, the more water they will displace, resulting in a greater buoyant effect. Participants who tend to float when immersed to the shoulders may find it difficult to keep their feet in contact with the pool bottom, which may compromise alignment. In some situations, you will want to take advantage of buoyancy, for example, with participants who must limit weight-bearing exercise.

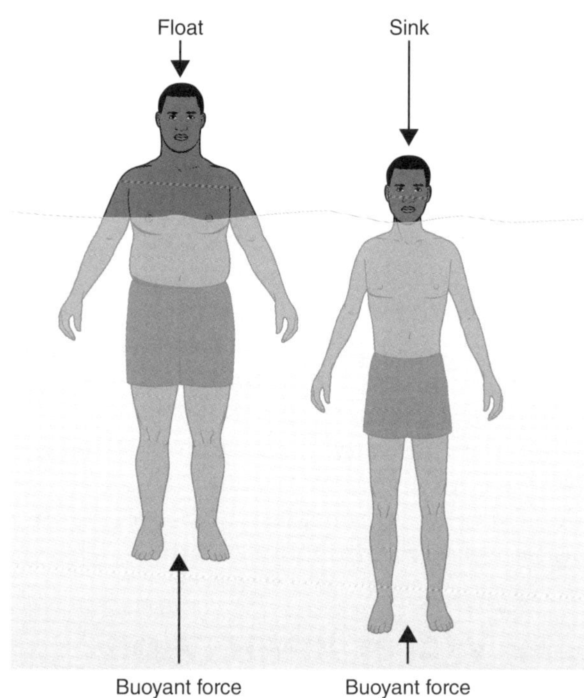

Figure 6.1 Variations in buoyancy due to body size and body composition.

Buoyancy provides many benefits for water exercisers. It decreases the effects of gravity and reduces weight bearing or compression of joints. Many people who cannot exercise on land, where they must bear their full weight, can exercise comfortably and vigorously in the water. As stated previously, buoyancy depends on the depth of immersion because being immersed in deeper water displaces more water. A body immersed to the neck bears approximately 10 percent of its body weight. A body immersed to the chest bears approximately 25 to 35 percent and a body immersed to the waist bears about 50 percent of its body weight. These percentages are general, and vary with body composition and gender.

Increases in **kinesthetic awareness** (the body's abilities to coordinate motion and awareness of where the body is in time and space) and muscular stabilization are required as the depth of immersion increases. Most people can exercise comfortably at mid-chest depth because they still experience enough body weight (effect of gravity) to control their movements. For shallow-water programs, movement speed and control are hindered when immersed past armpit depth.

If the **center of gravity** (typically in the hip and waist area) and the **center of buoyancy** (typically in the chest area) are vertically aligned, the body is relatively stable in the water (figure 6.2). If center of gravity and center of buoyancy are not vertically aligned, the body will roll or turn until balance is achieved. A great example of this is when you tuck into a ball and try to float in a prone position. The body will rotate and roll until the center of buoyancy and center of gravity are aligned. The center of buoyancy and center of gravity are dynamic, meaning that they change with movement. Therefore, plan transitions and traveling movements in the water that will keep the body in alignment or provide participants with opportunities to realign the body between movements. Carefully cue specific training to challenge balance and provide options to reduce the risk of injury.

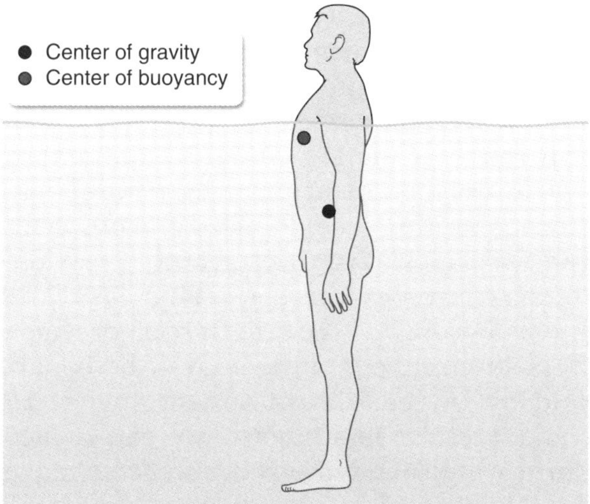

Figure 6.2 Center of gravity versus center of buoyancy.

When suspended in the water, as with deep-water exercise, your body turns around your center of buoyancy. Although the center of gravity is not as important a consideration when the body is suspended, proper alignment of the body remains important. In vertical suspended exercise, proper body alignment increases the effectiveness of the workout and reduces risk of injury. A more vertical alignment also increases the surface area of the body and therefore increases effort and intensity, resulting in a greater number of calories burned. Additionally, the use of buoyancy equipment for support, flotation, or resistance permits for a greater ability to maintain alignment and the potential to elicit greater overload on working muscles.

As discussed in chapter 4, movement of a buoyant object toward the pool bottom is buoyancy resisted and movement toward the surface of the pool is buoyancy assisted. Any movement floating on the surface of the water or movements parallel to the pool bottom while suspended below the surface are considered to be **buoyancy supported**. When moving the body in the water without equipment, you tend to work more against the water's resistance as opposed to its buoyancy. When buoyancy equipment is added, buoyancy and gravity become more involved, affecting muscle use and contractions.

Viscosity

Viscosity refers to the friction between molecules of a liquid or gas, causing the molecules to adhere to each other **(cohesion)** and, in water, to a submerged body **(adhesion)**. Water is more viscous than air, just as molasses is more viscous than water. Viscosity increases as temperature decreases, as is evident with frozen water. Air, water, and molasses are more viscous when cold; however, a change in water viscosity is not noticeable in the small temperature fluctuations we experience in water exercise.

This friction between molecules is what causes resistance to motion. Because water is more viscous than air, water provides more resistance to motion than air. A combination of the surface area of an object and its speed determines the resistance to the motion caused by the fluid viscosity (drag). In other words, the size, shape, and speed of the object determine how much drag resistance will be experienced. During exercise, additional resistance increases the intensity of the movement and thus requires greater muscular effort. Greater energy expenditure causes higher caloric expenditure.

Water resistance can be altered in many ways. **Streamlined flow** is continuous, steady movement of a fluid (figure 6.3). The rate of movement at any fixed point remains constant. A swimmer attempts to streamline the body by reducing frontal surface area and creating smooth, efficient stroke mechanics to minimize friction or resistance while traveling through the water. A streamlined swimmer can go farther faster and with less energy expenditure.

In vertical water exercise, using movements where the water continues to move in a single direction is an illustration of streamlined flow. An example of this would be when all class participants are walking in a straight line, following one another in a circular pattern around the pool. The water is moving in a streamlined position, making the movement easier to perform.

One purpose of vertical water exercise is to increase energy expenditure. Creating additional drag and impedance with turbulent flow can increase resistance (figure 6.4). **Turbulent flow** is irregular movement of a fluid with the rate of movement varying at any fixed point. This type of movement is less efficient. It creates rotary movements called **eddies** and increases the water's resistance (figure 6.5). Consider the previous example. Imagine that instead of having participants walk in the same uniform direction, we had them walk in various directions all over the pool. This unsynchronized movement would create a great deal of turbulence in the water. Additionally, you can increase turbulent water flow around the body and its limbs by applying Newton's laws of motion and by increasing frontal resistance, changing the length of the lever or limb, and adjusting hand position. These principles are discussed in the sections that follow.

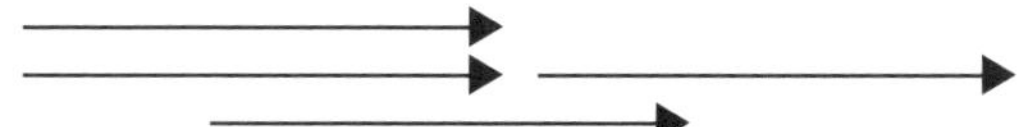

Figure 6.3 Streamlined flow.

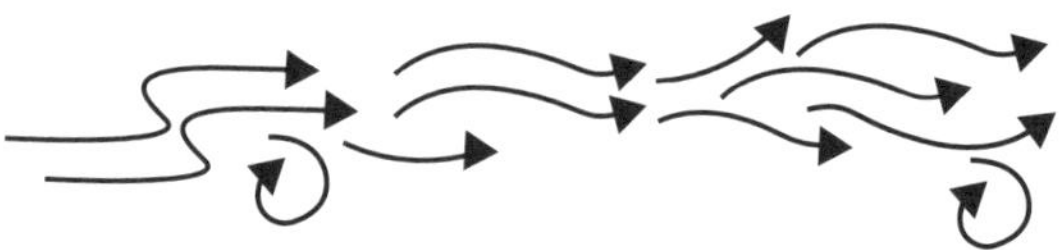

Figure 6.4 Turbulent flow.

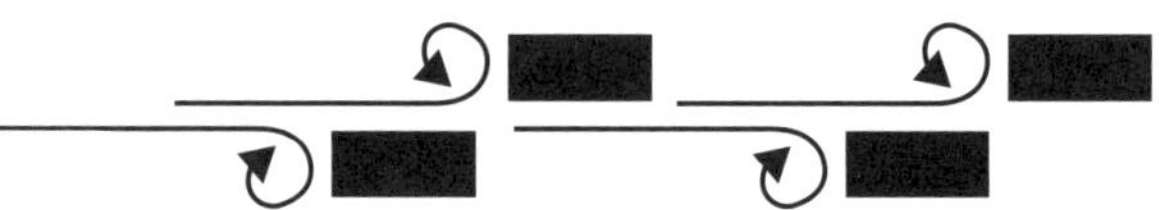

Figure 6.5 Eddies.

Drag

Movement in water is inherently slower than movement on land. **Drag**, the resistance you feel to movement in the water, is a function of fluid characteristics (viscosity), frontal shape and size, and the relative velocity between the participant and the water (how water is moving and how the participant is moving in the water). Drag creates different loading to the muscles during water exercise compared to land exercise. On land, muscle load decreases when you achieve a constant speed. In the water, you have a constant muscle load provided by the water through full range of motion. Drag is experienced with every movement and in every direction. Because of this, it can be used as a powerful tool for exercise progression and regression. To make exercises harder, we increase drag forces by altering the size (larger) or shape (less streamlined) of the body or body part and by increasing movement speed. To make exercise less intense, we can reduce surface area and movement speed and make the body or body part more streamlined. Drafting (where one participant moves in direct alignment with another person to shield drag forces) can also reduce overall resistance. If class participants travel in unison across the pool, drafting occurs. Those traveling in front will experience more drag, while those traveling behind other individuals will feel much less drag; thus, they will expend less energy to achieve the same speed.

Hydrostatic Pressure

Hydrostatic pressure is defined as the pressure exerted by molecules of a fluid on an immersed body. According to **Pascal's law**, pressure is exerted equally on all surfaces of an immersed body at rest at a given depth. Pressure increases with depth and the fluid density of the water.

This hydrostatic pressure affects internal organs of the body as well as the skin. Hydrostatic pressure can decrease swelling, especially in the lower extremities that are immersed more deeply. The pressure offsets the tendency of blood to pool in the lower extremities during exercise and aids venous return to the heart. Since this pressure is exerted on the chest cavity, it can also help to condition the muscles used to inhale deeply and forcefully. However, people who have respiratory disorders might have difficulty breathing when immersed in the water past the rib cage due to the hydrostatic pressure.

Although hydrostatic pressure has no direct relationship to intensity in water exercise, it does affect bodily systems and organs. As stated earlier, this pressure can affect the vascular and respiratory systems. It is believed that hydrostatic pressure might be at least partially responsible for lower working heart rates in the water.

Surface Tension

Surface tension is the force exerted between the surface molecules of a fluid. This creates a skin on top of the water that makes it more difficult to break through the surface. This characteristic of water may add a level of difficulty for some participants.

As a limb moves from under the water into the air, the effort required to break through the surface tension and deal with the changing viscosity between environments might result in stress to the joints involved (usually the shoulder), increasing the risk of overuse or acute injury. Movements should be performed either under the water's surface or above the water's surface, but not interchangeably between the two. Exceptions to this recommendation would include streamlined movements, such as the front crawl and back crawl swim strokes, or movements performed slowly to improve range of motion (rather than more powerful movements that improve muscular strength or endurance).

Newton's Laws of Motion

We exert forces every day to move objects, move our body, change direction, stand upright, and move against gravity. The forces that cause motion can be analyzed by applying Sir Isaac Newton's laws of motion: inertia, acceleration, and action and reaction. This section explores how these laws can be used to alter, progress, or regress aquatic exercises. All of the physical laws work together to allow us to use the water to its fullest potential. Combining the physical laws with teaching techniques, such as providing options and encouraging self-monitoring, allow people of different fitness levels to participate in the same class.

Law of Inertia

The law of **inertia** states that an object will remain at rest or in motion with constant velocity (speed and direction) unless acted on by a net external (unbalanced) force (Ostdiek and Bord 1994).

This law states that an object remains stationary unless a force causes it to move. When a force is applied that is greater than resisting forces, such as friction, the object will begin to gain speed in the direction of the applied force. If the object is moving at a constant speed in a particular direction, it will require a force to change either the speed or direction of the object. This tendency to resist changes in the state of motion is called an object's inertia. In other words, in order to change a movement in any way or to go from rest to exercise, a person must exert some effort. This effort must be strong enough to overcome inertia.

The mass of the object affects the amount of force required to change its speed or direction. Mass relates to both weight and inertia. On land, the force of gravity on a mass generates its resistance to change direction and speed. An object with more mass requires more force to overcome its inertia. An example of the effect of inertia on land is that it takes more force to push a car than a grocery cart because the car has more mass and friction. If the same force were applied to both, the grocery cart would move further and faster because it has less mass and friction than the car (figure 6.6).

In water exercise, three things are affected by the law of inertia: movement of the limbs (limb inertia), movement of the entire body (total-body inertia), and movement of the water (water inertia).

Limb Inertia

The primary resistance to land-based movement occurs when the motion is against gravity. On land, the muscular effort required to move a limb is caused by inertia—you must apply force to move the limb, change direction, and stop the movement. In flexion and extension of the hip, you start the motion, stop the motion, start the motion in the opposite direction, stop the motion, and repeat. As you perform this movement faster (such as during a jog), it requires more force and energy, as long as you maintain the same range of motion, because you are overcoming inertia more often. Air is not very viscous, and does not offer much resistance unless the movement speed is very fast.

The primary resistance to the limbs in the water is from drag, which relates to a combination of viscosity of the water and the relative speed of the motion between the limbs and the water. Because the water offers additional resistance, more force or energy is required to initiate, stop, and change movements. For example, force is applied to abduct the legs and the arms to initiate a jumping jack. Force is used to stop the movement, initiate adduction, and then stop adduction. Thus, additional energy is required to move the limbs from a state of rest.

Additionally, combining movements together (choreography) increases intensity through the law of inertia. Changing from a jumping jack to a cross-country ski movement causes the limbs of the body to change directions and planes of motion. It would be less intense to perform 16 jumping jacks than to perform 8 jumping jacks and 8 cross-country skis. Thus, more changes in choreography result in more intense exercise.

Total-Body Inertia

Total-body inertia can contribute to exercise intensity if traveling is incorporated into the choreography. It requires more effort to

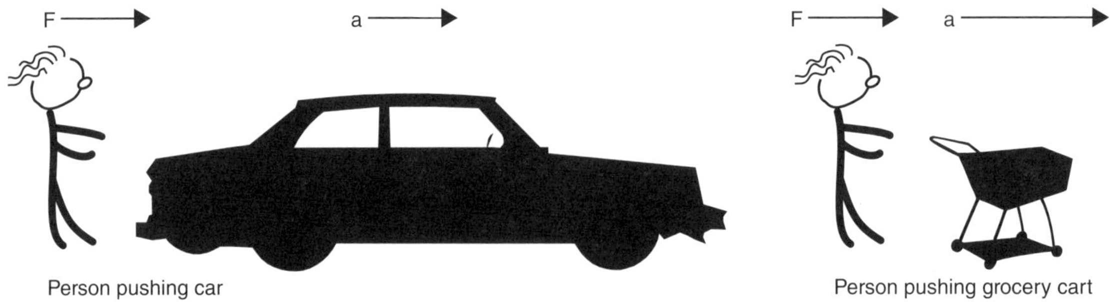

Figure 6.6 Force and acceleration. If the same force is applied to pushing a car and a grocery cart, the grocery cart will move further and faster because it has less mass and friction.

overcome inertia to start, stop, or change a movement for the entire body than it does to continue with the same movement. Think of a train. The engine must produce a great deal of force to get the train moving. Once the train is moving, the engine must provide only enough energy to overcome air and ground resistance from the wheels on the track. It takes more force to start or stop a train than it takes to keep it moving at a constant speed. In other words, the engine doesn't have to work as hard once the train is moving.

Similarly, it takes more force to start a body moving and stop the body from moving than it does to continue the same movement. Jogging 16 counts forward and backward requires force to initiate the jog forward, stop the jog, change the direction to move backward, and stop the jog. (Of course, limb inertia is happening as well.) This movement could be made more intense by jogging 8 counts forward, 8 counts backward, 8 counts forward, and 8 counts backward. This combination requires more force or energy because you would stop and change direction twice as often. By jogging 4 counts forward, 4 counts backward, 4 counts to the right, 4 counts to the left, and 8 counts in your own circle, you would be increasing intensity by overcoming inertia even more to start, stop, and change direction.

Water Inertia

If participants in class move in the same direction and then turn around, the group will feel that it is moving against the current. The water will have begun to move with the group. When the group turns, the inertia of the water makes it continue in the original direction at its previous speed. The group turns, but the water keeps going.

The water's inertia can be used to increase exercise intensity. If you take multiple steps forward in one direction, the water begins to move in that direction with you. When you reverse direction (turn around or walk backward), you will be trying to stop and then reverse the water's motion, just as you would have with the body's motion. Combined, this effect also increases exercise intensity. If you jog forward and then back, you are applying force to overcome not only body inertia but also the water's inertia as well. Incorporating traveling movements in your choreography increases energy expenditure by increasing total-body inertia and the water's inertia.

When using the law of inertia (total-body, water, and limb inertia) in exercise programming, consider two factors. The first is your participants. They must be reasonably fit and skilled at water exercise in order to follow more complicated patterns that change movements and directions. The second factor involves acoustics in your pool setting. Participants can become frustrated attempting to follow more complex patterns when they cannot understand the verbal cues. In poor acoustical situations, instructors are often more successful using traveling moves to overcome inertia. Traveling patterns with simple movement combinations are typically easier to cue with body language than complex combinations, although both options increase intensity based on the law of inertia.

Additionally, consider carefully when applying the law of inertia to deep water. If exercises are changed too quickly, body position and alignment may be compromised. You may use starting and stopping, changing direction, and varying movements to alter intensity; however, you should also pay attention to postural cues.

Instructors should know how to use the law of inertia to increase and decrease intensity for a multilevel class. A less-fit participant can be instructed to jog 24 counts in place to decrease intensity; participants with a higher fitness level can incorporate traveling to increase intensity. Understanding the law of inertia enables you to help participants individualize the program to meet their goals and abilities.

Using the law of inertia to increase or decrease exercise intensity comes down to one thing: change. If you change directions, exercises, or movement more frequently, the intensity increases (see table 6.1). Fewer changes in movement result in less intensity. Vary the number of repetitions, directional changes, and use of limbs to alter exercises so they are appropriate for your specific clients.

Table 6.1 Altering Intensity With Inertia

Knee lifts in place (limb inertia)	
Knee lifts in place combined with jumping jacks in place (limb inertia)	More intense
Knee lifts moving forward and backward combined with jumping jacks in place (limb, total-body, and water inertia)	More intense
Cross-country ski in place (limb inertia)	
Cross-country ski 8 counts moving forward and 8 counts moving backward (limb, total-body, and water inertia)	More intense
Cross-country ski with all class participants moving together in a circle for 32 counts, then turning and skiing in the opposite direction against the water's current (limb, total-body, and water inertia—water inertia is especially noticeable)	More intense

Law of Acceleration

According to the law of **acceleration**, the reaction of a body as measured by its acceleration is proportional to the force applied (in the same direction as the applied force) and is inversely proportional to its mass. Therefore, the rate of acceleration of an object is the result of any and all forces acting on that object.

Acceleration involves how fast an object will change its direction or speed when a force is applied. Acceleration is how quickly you change velocity. Velocity expresses the exact relation between force and acceleration. Many aquatic fitness professionals get confused, thinking that acceleration means simply increasing speed, like pressing the accelerator in your car. This is not completely true. Think about acceleration as applying more force to move your limb through a greater range of motion, or your body over a greater distance, at the same tempo.

For a given body or mass, a larger force causes a proportionally larger acceleration. All objects have mass. Objects with a larger mass require a greater external force to change speed at the same rate that a smaller object does. As mentioned previously, it takes a lot more force to push a car than to push a grocery cart because the car has more mass. The direction of the acceleration of an object is the same direction as the force acting on it (Ostdiek and Bord 1994). As an aquatic fitness professional, you must remember that not every participant has the same mass or the same ability to apply muscular force. When applied to water exercise, a heavier person applying the same force as a lighter person will not move as far or jump as high. The heavier person has more mass and thus must apply more force to move the same distance. On the other hand, muscular people may have a lot of mass but also be able to generate a lot of force to move their body mass effectively. Each participant will move differently in the water.

The law of acceleration can be used to alter aquatic exercise intensity in two ways. One involves pushing harder (applying more force) against the pool bottom to propel the body upward or through the water. The other involves pushing harder (applying more force) against the water's resistance with the arms or legs. These two applications may be used simultaneously to further increase the intensity level.

Let's first consider pushing off the pool bottom. The greater a vertical force applied to an object, the higher the object will go. When applied to aquatic exercise, the harder you push off the bottom of the pool, the higher you will be able to jump. You can use the law of acceleration to increase intensity by applying more force to the pool bottom to jump higher.

The concept of acceleration also applies to power tucks as described in chapter 8. More force is required to move the legs through a greater range of motion (tucking the knees to the chest) in the same period of time. One example is the difference between a regular jumping jack and a jumping jack in which the legs tuck up on the outward movement. To increase intensity even more, the participant could tuck the knees on both the outward and inward movements of the legs (figure 6.7).

Another example is seen when jumping forward and backward. More force needs to be applied to move the legs a greater distance on the bottom of the pool, as well as when jumping higher and tucking the knees. So, jumping forward and backward and increasing the distance between where the feet land on the pool bottom (while maintaining the same tempo) will increase intensity. Additionally, tucking the legs as if jumping over a log is more intense than jumping forward and backward with a normal bound (closer to the pool bottom) at the same tempo. In both options, more force is required to accelerate the legs through a greater range of motion at the same tempo. To make the exercise even more intense, have participants jump farther **and** tuck the knees to jump higher (figure 6.8).

Applying more force against the water's resistance provides strengthening benefits for the muscle groups performing the movement. It also requires more effort and energy expenditure. Consider the cross-country ski exercise: Gently swinging the arms requires less effort than pulling the arms forcefully along the sides of the thighs at a greater depth.

As previously mentioned, it requires more muscular force to move the same mass farther in the same period of time. For example, it requires more force or muscular effort to leap 6 feet (1.8 m) to the right every beat of music than to leap 3 feet (.9 m) to the right every beat of music. So, another way to increase intensity using the law of acceleration is to encourage participants to travel farther—leaping farther or taking larger steps—with each beat, applying more muscular force. You can see how this involves both pushing harder off the pool bottom with the feet and pulling the arms with more force against the water's resistance.

It is important to understand how to use the law of acceleration to both increase and decrease intensity. With acceleration, movements using less force against the water's

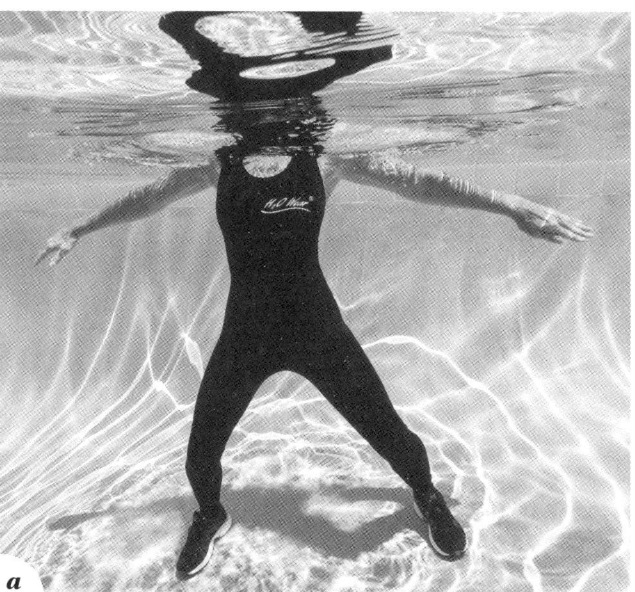

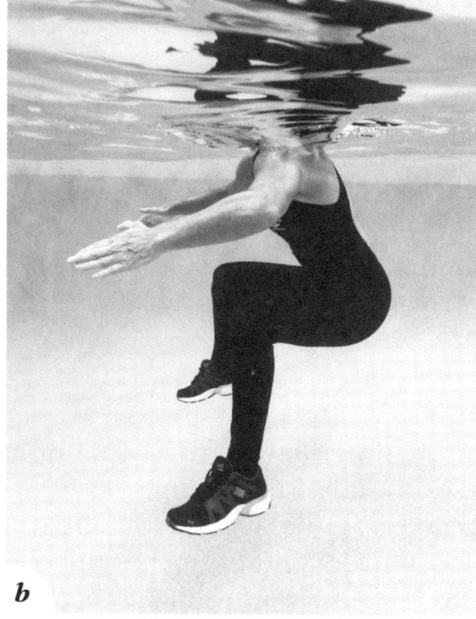

Figure 6.7 Acceleration in a jumping jack *(a)* with normal intensity and *(b)* adding more force to increase the intensity by tucking the knees (side view of tuck).

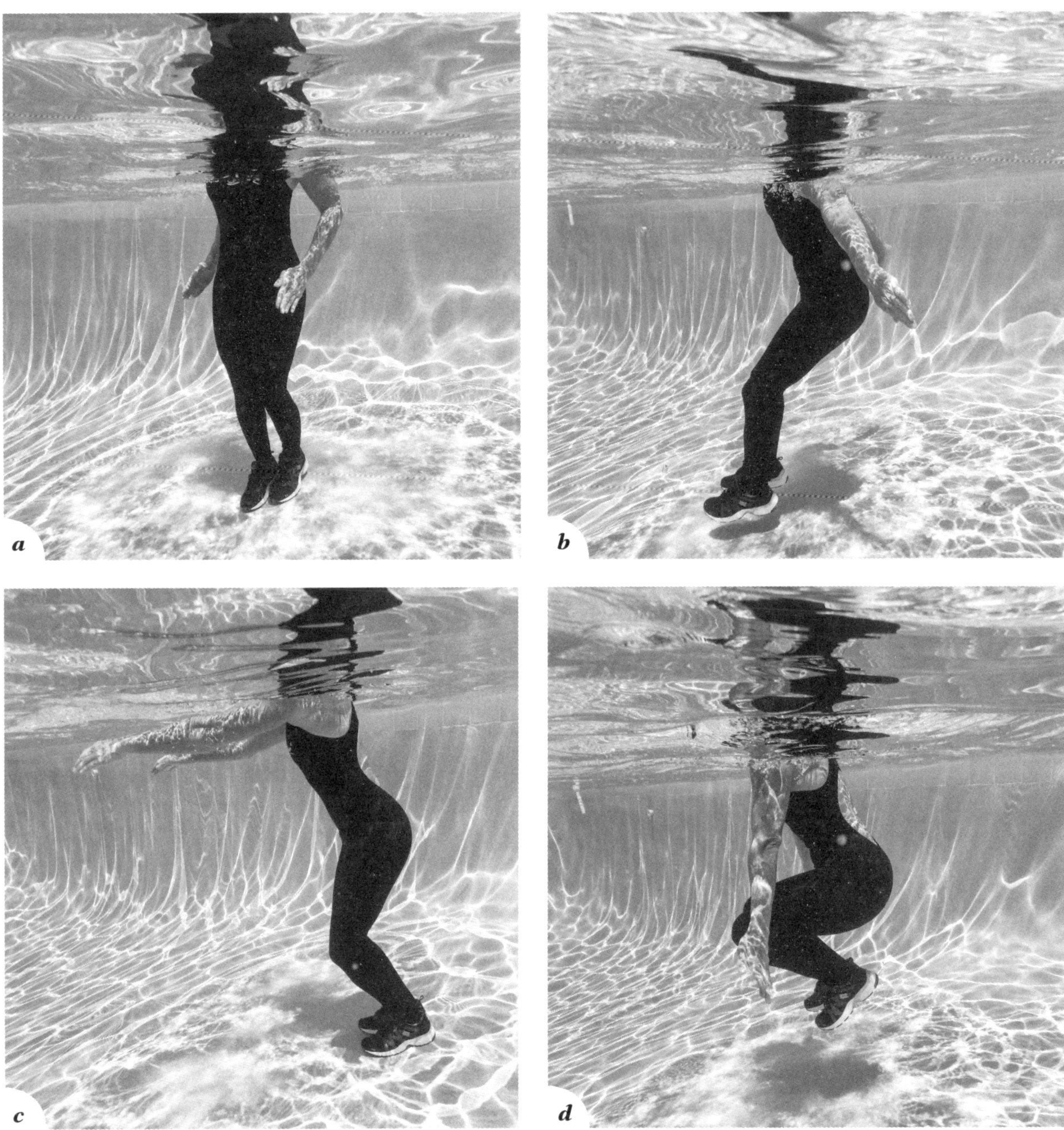

Figure 6.8 A forward and backward jump with more intensity; *(a)* start position, *(b)* forward jump, *(c)* backward jump, and *(d)* adding more force to increase the intensity by tucking the knees between each jump.

resistance or the pool's bottom at the same tempo require less effort. Examples for decreasing intensity include skimming the arms through the water, reducing range of motion while maintaining the tempo, taking smaller steps, or not pushing as hard against the pool bottom. Movements that position the limbs to work harder against the water's resistance and movements that require you to push harder off the pool bottom to jump higher or take larger steps at the same tempo will increase intensity. Ultimately, to use the law of acceleration, you must increase or decrease the amount of force applied. More force yields more resistance and less force results in less resistance. Acceleration can be used in deep or shallow water at any impact level (impact levels are discussed in detail in chapter 8). It is a great tool for adding variety and intensity to a class. Table 6.2 shows how a regular jumping jack can be made more intense using more force to increase acceleration.

Law of Action and Reaction

According to the law of **action and reaction**, for every action, there is an equal and opposite reaction.

Newton's third law makes an important statement about force. A force can be described generally as an interaction between two bodies. For example, you cannot play tug-of-war without people on the other end of the rope. There would be no force for you to pull against and no tension in the rope. If you want to play one-man tug-of-war, you could anchor the other end of the rope to a pole to provide the force to pull against. Another example is pushing against a wall. When you push against a wall, it pushes back with equal force. Forces occur in pairs, and Newton named these paired forces *action* and *reaction*.

When you push your feet against the bottom of the pool (action), the reaction is that your body pushes upward (opposite direction of the action). This is not unique to the water; the same reaction occurs when you push your feet against the ground on land. However, the properties of the water make action and reaction noticeable with every movement, which is not true of all actions and reactions in air. In the water, when you sweep your hands to the left (action), it results in the body moving to the right (reaction). When you push your arms forward (action), it results in the body being pushed backward (reaction).

In the aquatic environment, arm and leg patterns are a common and effective way

Table 6.2 Altering Intensity With Acceleration

Regular jumping jack with normal bound on the out and in movements	
Jumping jack with the legs tucked on the out movement and a normal bound on the in movement	More intense
or	
Jumping jack with a normal bound on the out movement and the legs tucked on the in movement	
Jumping jack with the legs tucked on both the out and in movements	Most intense
Jumping front and back with feet close to pool bottom	
Jumping front and back while tucking the knees, as if jumping over an object on the pool bottom	More intense
or	
Jumping front and back, covering more distance on the pool bottom	
Jumping front and back while tucking the knees *and* covering more distance on the pool bottom	Most intense
Regular jumping jack	
Jumping jack pulling the legs together (hip adduction) with more force	More intense
or	
Jumping jack pushing the legs apart (hip adduction) with more force	
Jumping jack pulling the legs together (hip adduction) *and* pushing the legs apart (hip adduction) with more force	Most intense
Leaping 4 times to the right and 4 times to the left	
Leaping 4 times to the right and 4 times to the left while pushing off the bottom with more force to cover more distance	More intense

to employ the law of action and reaction. Arm movements can be combined with leg movements to assist progress in the intended direction or impede progress in the intended direction of travel. Assisting patterns make the movement easier to perform, create less turbulence, and reduce resistance. Impeding patterns are more challenging and create more turbulence and increase resistance.

For example, using front crawl arms or sweeping the arms back assists forward movement of the body. Using back crawl arms or sweeping the arms forward assists backward movement of the body. Consider another example: Pushing both arms forward in front of the body while jogging forward makes forward movement more intense or difficult. The reaction of the body (based on the action of the arms) is to move backward; this opposes the reaction of the body to travel forward as the feet are pushed backward against the pool bottom while jogging.

The legs can also assist or impede traveling movement. For example, in a kick while traveling forward and backward, the upward and forward action of the leg causes a downward and backward reaction of the body. A front kick emphasizing the upward movement of the leg (hip flexion) assists traveling movement backward and impedes movement when traveling forward.

As with all of Newton's laws, consider the fitness level and abilities of your participants when using the law of action and reaction. If participants are not strong enough or skilled enough to use impeding arms to increase intensity while still maintaining body position and alignment, then assisting arms is a more prudent choice (see table 6.3 for examples of exercises that use the law of action and reaction to change intensity). Safety and alignment are primary considerations when combining arm and leg movements.

Additional Training Principles

Frontal resistance, lever length, and speed are additional principles that should be understood and considered when designing aquatic exercise programs. Each of these principles can be used to increase or decrease exercise intensity in both shallow and deep water.

Frontal Resistance

Movement in water is resisted in every direction. This resistance is due to the horizontal forces of the water resulting from the water's viscosity. **Frontal resistance** is a direct result of the horizontal forces of water, and noticeably increases effort of movement in the water. Since the force of gravity is offset by the water's buoyant force, the primary resistive force experienced in the pool is horizontal resistance. The intensity of aquatic exercise will be affected by adjusting frontal resistance.

In the water, **frontal surface area** represents the total area of the surface of an object moving against the resistance of the water. The size of an object presented against the water's horizontal resistance affects the amount of energy required to move the object through the water. Most boats are tapered in front so they can slice through the water,

Table 6.3 Altering Intensity With Action and Reaction

Knee tuck (net upward reaction) with arms pressing toward the pool bottom (net upward reaction) ⟶ Assisting arm and leg actions	
Knee tuck (net upward reaction) with arms pressing toward the surface of the water (net downward reaction) ⟶ Impeding arm and leg actions	More intense
Jog forward with breaststroke arms (assisting arm and leg actions)	
Jog forward with reverse breaststroke arms (impeding arm and leg actions)	More intense

creating less turbulence and fewer eddies. Reduced surface area allows for more streamlined movement and requires less energy to move the boat (6.9). In water exercise, presenting a smaller frontal surface area to the intended line of travel also makes movement easier. For example, the surface area of the side of the body is typically smaller than the surface area of the front of the body. Movement sideways thus creates less frontal resistance than moving forward. To further increase resistance by means of frontal surface area, you could walk forward with the arms out to the side and palms forward. Traveling forward with wide knee lifts (hips externally rotated) is more intense than traveling forward with front knee lifts because the wide knee lifts increase the width of the body's frontal surface area.

Note that during deep-water exercise, frontal resistance is even more prevalent since the body is submerged to neck depth. By maintaining a vertical body position during travel in deep water, the body can present maximum surface area against the water and increase intensity. Often due to lack of body awareness, unfamiliarity with water exercise, or lack of strength, participants will lean too far forward during deep-water exercise. This creates a more streamlined body position, leading to easier movement, reduced intensity, and diminished caloric expenditure. For these reasons, as well as the need to maintain ideal alignment and posture, repeatedly cue deep-water participants to maintain a vertical body position, with the body leaning forward no more than 10 degrees (figure 6.10). Research clearly indicates that maintaining proper vertical alignment in deep water significantly affects energy expenditure. In other words, the more vertical your participants are, the more calories they will burn.

An object or a body must be traveling to encounter frontal resistance. The total body is not affected by the water's horizontal resistance during a stationary exercise (e.g., jogging in place). However, the moving limbs are affected. Therefore, the frontal surface area of the limbs and hands moving against the water's resistance will influence the intensity of stationary exercises.

Frontal surface area created by the positioning of the hand while moving the arm through the water affects the amount of effort required from the associated working muscles. The hand can serve as a paddle to scoop more water, or can be positioned to minimize resistance. The size of the surface area of the hand as it moves through

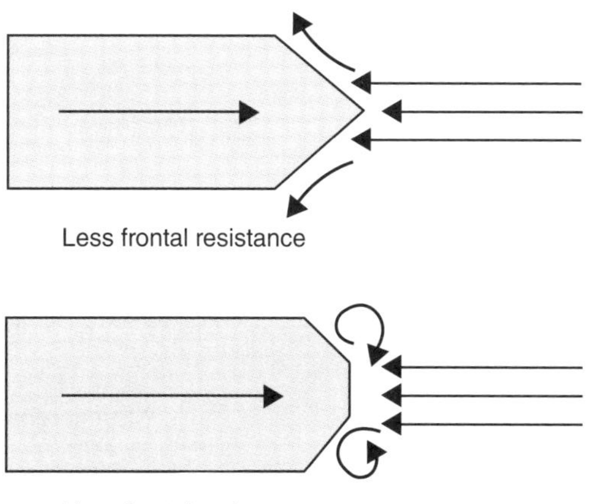

Figure 6.9 Frontal resistance.

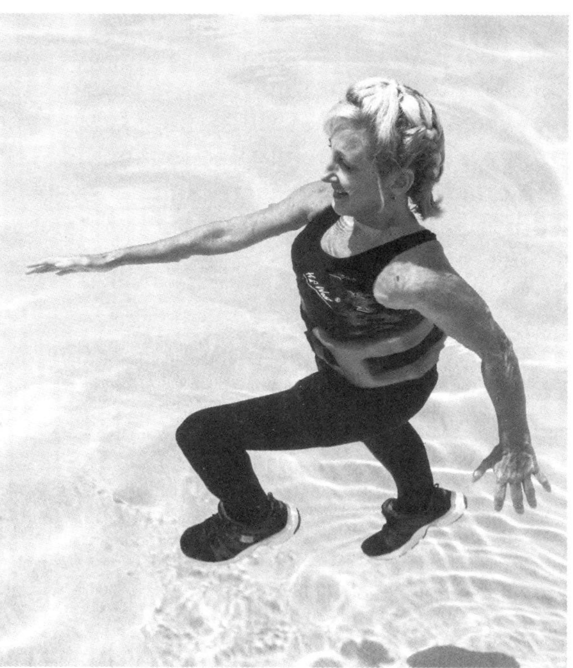

Figure 6.10 Maintaining a vertical position positively affects energy expenditure in deep-water exercise.

the water and its shape determine how much water the hand pulls and how much resistance it creates. A hand sliced sideways through the water creates minimal resistance. The hand position used for most swimming strokes (an open, slightly cupped hand with fingers relaxed and slightly spread) is the most effective at pulling water.

Many beginning aquatic exercisers ignore or do not understand hand positioning in the water and thus do not use the water most effectively. Teaching participants how to position their hands will increase the effectiveness of the workout. The basic progression of using the hands for frontal surface area resistance would be as follows:

Slice → Fist → Open hand with fingers together → Open hand with fingers slightly spread

Although more challenging hand positions can be beneficial for those seeking increased intensity, less demanding hand positions are useful for participants with weak upper bodies and core stabilizers, shoulder or joint problems, **arthritis**, or any other musculoskeletal condition that might be aggravated by adding resistance.

In deep water, as in shallow, hands can be used to alter resistance. In deep-water exercise, the hands are also more important for maintaining stability and balance as well as achieving proper form and technique. Additionally, hand positions play a vital role in helping the body to move in the desired direction when traveling during deep-water vertical exercise.

The principle of frontal resistance can be applied to all forms of water exercise, including shallow and deep formats as well as aerobic or strength training. When you increase the frontal surface area moving through the water, the intensity of the exercise increases (see table 6.4). The frontal surface area may relate to the full body, the limbs, or additional equipment being used, thus providing a practical tool for increasing and decreasing intensity with or without the use of equipment.

Levers

The limbs (arms and legs) can be used to increase or reduce the intensity of aquatic exercises by changing the length of the lever. As discussed in chapter 4, the amount of force required for movement is based on the length of the lever arm. Shorter levers (bent arms and legs) require less force to move than longer levers (straight arms and legs). A straight leg can be made even longer by plantar flexing the ankle. A straight arm can be made longer by holding the wrist in a neutral position with the hand open.

As you can see, the lever arm not only alters the amount of force needed due to mechanical aspects, but it also increases the amount of frontal surface area resistance the body will experience as the limb is moved through the water.

Table 6.4 Altering Intensity With Frontal Resistance

Front knee lifts traveling forward	
Wide knee lifts (hips externally rotated) traveling forward	More intense
Wide knee lifts with arms abducted and palms turned front traveling forward	Most intense
Jumping jacks traveling laterally	
Jumping jacks traveling backward	More intense
Cross-country ski with hands slicing	
Cross-country ski with palms leading in both directions	More intense

In exercise, the length of the moving limb affects intensity or the amount of energy required by the muscles to produce the desired movement. A knee lift requires less effort from the iliopsoas muscle than a straight-leg kick. In a knee lift, the water's resistance along the length of the limb from the hip joint to the knee joint must be overcome. In a kick, the amount of the water's resistance from the hip joint to the toes along the full length of the leg must be overcome. The same is true of movements performed with the arms. A lateral lift of the arms with the elbows bent requires less effort than a lateral lift of the arms with the elbows extended (figure 6.11). The principle of levers also means that a person with longer limbs must perform more muscular work than a shorter-limbed person to move the same range of motion in the same amount of time.

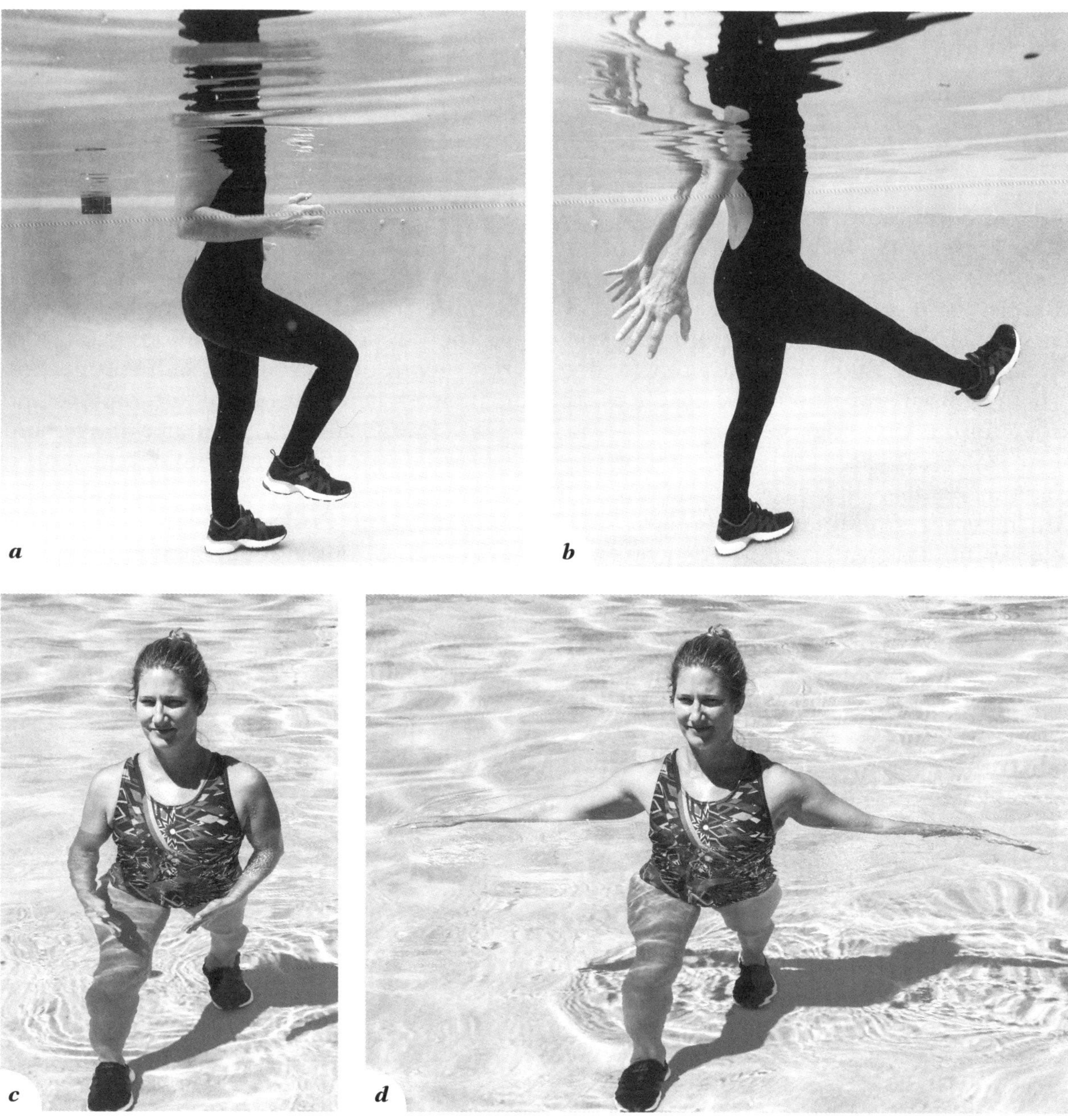

Figure 6.11 Lever arms: *(a)* knee lift with shorter lever arm, *(b)* front kick with longer lever arm, *(c)* lateral raise with shorter lever arm (shown at the beginning of the exercise), and *(d)* lateral raise with longer lever arm (shown at the end of the exercise).

Begin or warm up with shorter levers and then gradually progress to longer levers through the course of the workout to avoid excessive stress on joints. Although increasing the lever arm increases intensity (see table 6.5), there is no benefit to working with locked or hyperextended limbs. Maintaining a slight bend in the limb (soft joints) actually provides a slight training advantage by creating eddies, which in turn increase turbulence. Maintaining soft joints also reduces strain to the soft tissue in the joint and better ensures that the intended muscle will provide the effort.

Speed of Movement

The terms speed and velocity are often used interchangeably. But speed is not always the same as velocity. Technically, **speed** measures the rate at which we move or travel; **velocity** involves not only speed but also direction. In movements that involve only one direction, speed and velocity are practically synonymous; in this manual, we use the word speed for our discussions.

In water exercise, the resistance of the water increases with the speed of movement, which requires additional muscular effort and results in greater caloric expenditure (Pinto et al. 2011; Pöyhönen et al. 2000). Although increasing speed does increase intensity, it is only one of the many tools available in aquatic exercise design. The most effective and functional way to train a muscle is through its full range of motion. When speed is increased, range of motion and body position can be compromised. When you cue participants to go faster, they will often choose to reduce range of motion to achieve a faster speed, rather than adding force and maintaining range of motion. If the intensity modification, including increased speed, results in a reduced range of motion or compromised posture, it should be reconsidered. Design your programs to allow for a balance between increasing speed, improving overall function, and maintaining safety of your participants.

Interaction and Application

As you have probably noticed, many of the aquatic properties and principles, as well as the physical laws of motion, overlap or rely on one another. These same properties, principles, and laws allow instructors and participants alike to enhance movement beyond the possibilities of land. Let's look at a few examples of how these hydrodynamic considerations work together to heighten the effectiveness of the aquatic environment.

While jogging in chest-deep water, the body rebounds from foot to foot, overcoming limb inertia to begin and end each step. When you begin moving forward, the body

Table 6.5 Altering Intensity With Levers

Movement	
Knee lifts	
Straight front kick with ankle dorsiflexed	More intense
Straight front kick with ankle plantar flexed	More intense
Knee swing (hip flexion & extension with knee flexed)	
Leg swing (hip flexion & extension with knee extended)	More intense
Lateral arm lift with elbow flexed	
Lateral arm lift with elbow extended	More intense

must then overcome total-body inertia and the water's inertia. With each step forward, the body and the limbs are experiencing frontal resistance created by the water's viscosity. Drag resists the movement of the legs and arms as you push and pull the arms and legs from position to position. The action of the feet pushing down and back against the pool bottom causes the opposite reaction, which propels the body off the bottom and forward. The shorter levers of the bent legs allow for a greater speed of movement, while buoyancy offsets the impact experienced by the body. All of this is occurring with one simple jog that can be changed in a multitude of ways to alter the exercise's intensity and purpose.

Become familiar with the principles and physical properties of water in addition to the physical laws of motion, and use them to create safe and effective water exercise programs for all participants. Dynamic programming develops your skills as an instructor, which in turn enhances function and fitness levels for your participants. The best way to appreciate these laws and concepts is to feel them in the water. As you make the connection between reading this information and moving your body in the water, the laws will become something you can automatically apply to your class design.

Refer to table 6.6 to review the properties and laws of motion in the water that affect and determine muscular effort or intensity. It is important to learn and understand the options available when creating your choreography. Learning these principles and the effects they have on increasing or decreasing workload for each participant in your exercise program enhances the effectiveness of your instruction and serves as the cornerstone to effective vertical aquatic exercise.

Table 6.6 Increasing and Decreasing Intensity in Water Exercise

Law or principle	To increase intensity:	To decrease intensity:
Law of inertia *Total-body inertia, water inertia, and limb inertia*	Combine movements to start, stop, and change direction. Use fewer repetitions in a combination. Add traveling movements.	Repeat the same move for several repetitions. Remain in place (no travel).
Law of acceleration *Force and mass*	Push harder against the water's resistance or against the pool bottom to jump higher or take larger steps.	Skim the arms through the water, reduce range of motion, take smaller steps, or apply less resistance to the pool bottom or against the water.
Law of action and reaction *Opposing forces*	Use impeding arms, legs, or combinations.	Use assisting arms, legs, or combinations.
Frontal resistance—body and limbs *Frontal surface area*	Increase the size of the frontal surface area (body or limb) presented in the line of travel.	Decrease the size of the frontal surface area (body or limb) presented in the line of travel.
Frontal resistance—hand positions *Slice, fist, open, and cupped*	Cup the hand with the fingers slightly apart.	Slice the hand through the water or make a fist.
Levers *Long and short levers*	Use long levers with extended arms and legs.	Use shorter levers with flexed arms and legs.

Summary

Research supports the idea that immersion has a vast array of effects on many systems within the body that offer many beneficial outcomes during exercise. Each participant responds differently to immersion. Additionally, environmental factors and programming options influence the extent to which participants experience these effects.

In water, you are subjected to two opposing forces: the downward vertical force of gravity and the upward vertical force of buoyancy. Buoyancy reduces weight bearing to the body's joints and is based on the depth of the water. If the center of gravity and the center of buoyancy are vertically aligned, the body is relatively stable in the water.

Drag is the resistance to movement in the water. It is a function of fluid characteristics (viscosity), frontal shape and size, and the relative velocity between the participant and the water (how water is moving and how the participant is moving in the water). Drag is experienced with every movement and in every direction when immersed in the water.

Additional properties of water—viscosity, hydrostatic pressure, and surface tension—all influence submerged movement. These properties can be used to change, challenge, and adapt exercise for a wide range of participants.

Newton's three laws of motion are key elements in altering intensity of aquatic exercise. Using inertia (total body, limb, and water), acceleration, and action and reaction effectively will allow you to provide multilevel programming and allow for progression in training. The water's viscous properties make these laws more prevalent in program design for aquatic exercise as compared to land exercise.

Additional training principles can help you alter exercise intensity in aquatic programs, including frontal resistance, levers, and speed of movement. These interrelated concepts can help you modify exercises to meet the needs of a wide range of participants.

Review Questions

1. By adding the element of travel in aquatic choreography, you are increasing intensity using the law of ____________________.

2. Describe the two ways that the law of acceleration can be used to alter aquatic exercise.

3. Friction between the molecules of a liquid or gas is referred to as ____________________.

4. Which movement is more intense based on frontal resistance: an alternating wide jog traveling forward or an alternating wide jog traveling to the side?

5. List the three types of inertia that are experienced in water exercise.

6. Would pushing the arms forward while jogging forward in the water increase or decrease intensity?
7. Will you sink or float if you weigh more than the water you displace?
8. What is the primary force that causes resistance in the aquatic environment: buoyancy, gravity, or the water's viscosity and drag?
9. Incorporating impeding or assisting arm movements applies which physical law to alter exercise intensity in the water?
10. List the two important factors to consider when applying the law of inertia in aquatic exercise programming.

See appendix D for answers to review questions.

References and Resources

Cole, A.J., and B.E. Becker. 2004. *Comprehensive aquatic therapy*. Waltham, MA: Butterworth-Heinemann.

Denning, W., M. Eadric Bressel, D. Dolny, M. Bressel, and M.K. Seeley. 2012. A review of biophysical differences between aquatic and land-based exercise. *IJARE* 6(1).

Grolier Educational. 1990. *The new book of popular science*. Volume 3. Danbury, CT: Lexicon.

Kinder, T., and J. See. 1992. *Aqua aerobics: A scientific approach*. Peosta, IA: Bowers.

Masumoto, K., and J.A. Mercer. 2008. Biomechanics of human locomotion in water: An electomyographic analysis. *Exercise and Sport Sciences Reviews* 36(3):160-169.

Miller, F. 1977. *College physics*. 4th edition. New York: Harcourt Brace Jovanovich.

Ostdiek, V., and D. Bord. 1994. *Inquiry into physics*. 3rd edition. St. Paul: West.

Pinto, S.S., E.L. Cadore, C.L. Alberton, E.M. Silva, A.C. Kanitz, M.P. Tartaruga, and L.F.M. Kruel. 2011. Cardiorespiratory and neuromuscular responses during water aerobics exercise performed with and without equipment. *International Journal of Sports Medicine* 32(12):916.

Pöyhönen, T., K.L. Keskinen, A. Hautala, and E. Mälkiä. 2000. Determination of hydrodynamic drag forces and drag coefficients on human leg/foot model during knee exercise. *Clinical Biomechanics* 15(4):256-260.

Shoedinger, P. 1994. *Principles of hydrotherapy*. Aquatic Therapy Symposium. Charlotte, NC: Aquatic Therapy and Rehabilitation Institute.

Sova, R. 2000. *Aquatics: The complete reference guide for aquatics fitness professionals*. 2nd edition. Pt. Washington, WI: DSL.

Torres-Ronda, L., and X.S. del Alcázar. 2014. The properties of water and their applications for training. *Journal of Human Kinetics* 44(1):237-248.

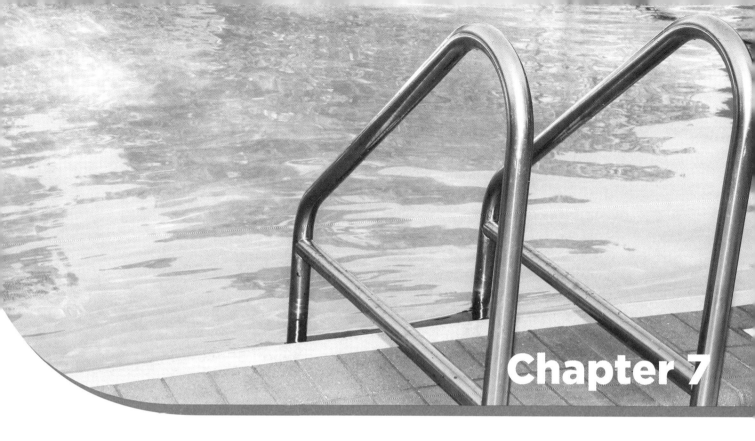

Pool Environment and Design

Introduction

Exercise professionals face many challenges when designing safe and effective programming for participants. As an aquatic fitness professional, you will have additional considerations unique to the pool environment, including water and air temperature, water and air quality, pool design and structure, and acoustic factors. You must learn to manage the aquatic environment as well as your class to maximize results and minimize associated risk.

Key Chapter Concepts

- Understand the recommended guidelines for water temperature, air temperature, and humidity levels to ensure a safe pool environment for aquatic exercise.
- Understand how the pool environment influences heat dissipation during aquatic fitness programs and how to adjust programs accordingly.
- Recognize water temperature ranges for programs that target specific populations and health conditions.
- Be aware of the importance of maintaining water and air quality for pool safety.
- Explain the influence of pool design—pool slope and depth, surfaces of the pool bottom and pool deck, gutters, designated entry and exit areas, and acoustic concerns—on safe and effective program design.
- Recognize the need for adequate pool space at the appropriate water depth and the value of wearing shoes in and around the pool area.

Water Temperature

Water temperature of 83 to 86 degrees Fahrenheit (28-30 °C) is considered comfortable for movement, and allows the body to react and respond normally to the onset of exercise and the accompanying increase in body temperature. Physiological changes caused by water temperature are minimal in this range. Cooling benefits are felt as body temperature increases with the level of activity, so there is little risk of overheating when exercising in this temperature range. For this reason, the Aquatic Exercise Association recommends the temperature range of 83 to 86 degrees Fahrenheit for most moderate- to vigorous-intensity programs.

In water below 78 degrees Fahrenheit (26 °C), physiological responses are altered (Cannon and Keatinge 1960; Chewning 2011; Gregson et al. 2011). Metabolic rate and heart rate decrease and the majority of the blood remains near the core of the body to keep the organs warm and functioning. When circulation is reduced to the extremities, the muscles become cold and inflexible, increasing risk of injury. Reduced circulation related to immersion in cold water also limits available oxygen for the muscles in the extremities, which may lead to muscle cramping.

Water temperatures at or above 90 degrees Fahrenheit (32 °C) also affect physiological responses, including increased internal body temperature, elevated metabolic and heart rates, and increased circulation and fluid distribution (Chewning 2011). This temperature is too warm for moderate- to vigorous-intensity exercise programs; overheating can occur as heat dissipation is hindered. This temperature is better suited for therapeutic-type activities, such as water massage or range-of-motion and strength and rehabilitation exercises for musculoskeletal injuries. This water temperature also works well for water tai chi, Ai Chi, Pilates, yoga, arthritis, and stretching programs.

Each participant will have a temperature preference and will respond differently to aquatic exercise. Encourage participants to self-monitor for comfort and intensity. If they are too warm, they should slow down; if they are too cold, they can increase activity or intensity levels. Also encourage participants to dress appropriately for the pool environment in order to remain comfortable no matter what the pool temperature.

Table 7.1 lists general recommended temperatures for various programs based on the **AEA Standards and Guidelines for Aquatic Fitness Programming**. Keep in

Table 7.1 Recommended Water Temperature From Aquatic Exercise Association Standards and Guidelines for Aquatic Fitness Programming

Competitive swimming	78-82 °F (25.6–27.8 °C)*
Resistance training	83-86 °F (28.3–30 °C): minimum range
Therapy and rehab	90-95 °F (32.2–35 °C)** Low function program—cooler temperatures might be more appropriate for higher intensity programs and specific populations
Multiple sclerosis	80-84 °F (26.7–28.9 °C)
Parkinson's disease	90-92 °F (32.2–33.3 °C): ideal temperature****
Pregnancy	83-85 °F (28.3–29.4 °C)
Arthritis	83-90 °F (28.3–32.2 °C)*** 91-94 °F (32.8–34.4 °C): may be allowed with special considerations***
Older adults	83-86 °F (28.3–30 °C): moderate to high intensity 86-88 °F (30–31.1 °C): low intensity
Children, fitness	83-86 °F (28.3–30 °C)
Children, swim lessons	84+ °F (28.9+ °C)* Varies with age, class length, and programming; ideal learn-to-swim program is best suited for 84-89 °F (28.9–31.7 °C) when available
Infant programs (4 and under)	90-93 °F (32.2–33.9 °C)*
Obese	80-86 °F (26.5–30 °C)

* USA Swimming

** Aquatic Therapy & Rehab Institute (ATRI)

*** AEA Arthritis Foundation Aquatic Program

**** American Parkinson Disease Association (APDA)

mind that variations to these recommendations are sometimes necessary, requiring you to make adjustments in class design and programming to ensure participant safety. Also, populations not listed might require specific water temperatures for safe and effective programming. See chapter 12 for more information on special populations and chronic conditions.

Many facilities have both a warm water therapy pool and a fitness pool. These facilities can offer a wide range of programming in the appropriate water temperature. Facilities with only one pool typically opt for midrange water temperature that can be used for many types of programs. This choice increases programming options that will, in turn, increase facility use and income. For example, a pool temperature of 84 degrees Fahrenheit (29 °C) is appropriate for both swimming and for shallow- or deep-water aerobics. This temperature is also acceptable for active arthritis programs, especially if participants wear clothing to conserve body heat, and falls within the range suggested for people with **multiple sclerosis**.

Air Temperature and Humidity

Ideal air temperature and humidity levels are not easily determined since many factors must be considered. The general recommendation for indoor pool air temperature is a range of 75 to 85 degrees Fahrenheit (24–29.5

°C); air temperature should not exceed 85 degrees Fahrenheit for the comfort of the aquatic professionals on the deck (USA Swimming 2017). The general recommendation for indoor pool air humidity is a range of 50 to 60 percent; lower than 50 percent relative humidity can cause a chilling effect on the participants when exiting from the pool (ASHRAE 2016).

Air temperature and humidity affect both the participants in the pool and the aquatic professionals working on the pool deck. Programming should be adjusted to all environmental conditions to provide safe training options for participants. When leading class from deck, take precaution to avoid overheating or dehydration. Dress appropriately, drink plenty of water, and incorporate a variety of effective cueing techniques to avoid overexertion. See chapter 10 for more information on safe deck instruction.

If you teach at an outdoor pool, you will have the challenge of facing unpredictable environmental conditions influenced by wind, humidity, and direct sunlight. High temperatures and full sun exposure contribute to overheating of the participants and the instructor on deck. High humidity levels can make conditions more extreme. Cool air temperatures, especially combined with wind, can contribute to chilling, even if the water is warm. When the air temperature is cool, advise participants to keep their heads dry and wear appropriate clothing, such as a neoprene vest or jacket. Additionally, avoid going from the pool to the deck to instruct the class; chilling will be more pronounced if you are wearing wet clothing while on deck. You must remain flexible and versatile to provide programming that works with fluctuating environmental conditions.

Heat Dissipation in the Aquatic Environment

Heat, a by-product of metabolism, is eliminated from the body through **radiation** (heat lost through dilation of the blood vessels at the surface of the body), **evaporation** (sweat evaporating from the skin, cooling the body), **conduction** (the transfer of heat to a substance or object in contact with the body) and **convection** (the transfer of heat by the movement of a liquid or gas between areas of different temperatures). All four methods of heat dissipation are involved during aquatic exercise.

Since participants are surrounded by water, which cools the body more efficiently than air, most will not experience the negative effects of heat when exercising vigorously in the pool. The water temperature of most aquatic programs is well below normal body temperature (98.6 °F / 37 °C), and thus facilitates cooling through conduction and convection. However, a great deal of heat is also dissipated from the head. Restricting heat dissipation (for example, through the use of bathing caps or shower caps) can lead to heat-related illness, especially in warmer water or with higher-intensity programming (chapter 13).

Observe participants—both for overheating and for chilling—and adjust programming and exercise intensity accordingly. To prevent chilling, have participants begin with large muscle movements as soon as they enter the pool to adjust from the change in air temperature to water temperature. Also, encourage participants to maintain movement to generate heat for the majority of time they are in the water. Even slight pauses will begin the cooling process. For example, during static stretching of the lower extremities, keep the upper extremities moving to generate heat, or vice versa. The amount of movement needed to maintain core temperature depends on the water temperature, the participant's body composition, and the type of clothing worn.

In situations where overheating is a concern, such as air or water temperatures above the recommended range, high humidity conditions, and direct sunlight, it may be necessary to add periods of reduced activity to allow the body to dissipate excess heat created by movement. At outdoor pools, protecting the head with loose-fitting hats can also be beneficial. Always encourage proper hydration to help prevent heat-related stress. Water consumption before, during, and after exercise is recommended but not always followed, since many participants do not want to be bothered with taking a bathroom break during class. Watch for signs of dehydration and heat-related illness, discussed more in chapter 13.

Water and Air Quality

Although maintaining water and air quality is usually not the responsibility of an aquatic instructor, it would be a good idea to have a basic understanding of both. Water and air quality can have an impact on your comfort, the comfort of your participants, and the success of your programs.

Water Quality

Public and private pools offering group fitness programs should be maintained by a licensed pool operator or manager with the appropriate credentials as designated by state, national, or international codes. These people are trained and licensed to keep the public safe in an aquatic environment. For more information on appropriate guidelines for the maintenance of pools and details on becoming a certified pool and spa operator, check with the National Swimming Pool Foundation (NSPF) at www.nspf.org.

Although you, as the aquatic fitness professional, may not be responsible for monitoring or maintaining water quality, you should still understand the general concept of maintaining a clean and safe pool environment. Swimming pools vary in size, shape, and location, but they all work in basically the same way. To provide a safe environment, pools require a combination of water filtration, circulation, and chemical treatment to continually clean a large volume of water.

Pool disinfectant systems are required for public health and are essential for four reasons:

- They eliminate dangerous pathogens, such as bacteria, viruses, and protozoa, which thrive in water. This reduces the potential for the spread of disease from bather to bather.
- They balance the chemistry of the water to avoid damage to various parts of the pool.
- They balance the chemistry of the water to avoid irritation to bather's skin, eyes, lungs, and mucous membranes.
- They balance the chemistry of the water to keep it clear.

Sometimes participants complain of throat or eye irritation, swimsuits fading, skin irritations, or their hair changing color from the pool water. When water quality is properly maintained, these concerns are minimized. Additionally, suggest that your participants shower before entering the pool. The shower water will be absorbed by their clothing, skin, and hair, which will reduce the amount of pool water absorbed. This practice also helps maintain stable water quality by washing off lotions and perfumes. They can also buy products that remove pool chemicals from swimsuits, skin, and hair.

Air Quality

Air temperature, humidity levels, and circulation are important issues for indoor pool facilities. They influence both comfort and safety for you and your participants; thus, they require constant monitoring. Every indoor pool has some sort of heating, ventilation, and air conditioning (HVAC) system. These systems control air temperature, airflow, and humidity. They do not remove contaminants from the air; however, they do remove air from the pool area and replace it with fresh outdoor air. Adequate ventilation is critical for maintaining proper humidity and removing chemical fumes from the pool area. Air quality for indoor pool facilities should be monitored according to the country, state, and local health department guidelines.

Pool Considerations

Pools come in many shapes, sizes, and depths. The depth of the water, as well as pool slope, pool gutters, and the surface of the pool bottom, can create additional programming considerations in aquatic exercise.

Arrive at least 10 minutes early for class to conduct a quick safety check. Inform participants of any problems or concerns that could result in injury, such as equipment on the pool deck that could cause a fall or a broken pool ladder needed for entry into the water. You should also record pool hazards in writing and forward your record to the facility manager or pool operator. Read more about legal considerations and responsibilities in chapter 15.

Pool Slope and Depth

A pool with a gradual slope is ideal for accommodating participants of varying heights in shallow-water programs. This will allow each participant to exercise within the recommended depth of mid-rib cage to midchest. Although this depth range may not work for all specialized programming, in general, it reduces impact and allows for proper alignment, control of movement, and sufficient training of all the major muscle groups against the water's resistance.

Almost all pools have some degree of slope. It is good practice for participants to face different directions while exercising. This helps offset musculoskeletal and alignment imbalances that can occur because of working on a sloped surface. A steep slope can cause slipping, uneven footing, equipment instability, and poor body alignment; such a pool may not be appropriate for shallow-water programs. Transitional or deep-water formats are more appropriate for this type of pool.

A section of the pool with a depth of 3.5 to 4.5 feet (1–1.4 m) is considered ideal for most shallow-water programs, but a slightly larger range of 3 to 5 feet (.9–1.5 m) comfortably accommodates most adult exercisers at the recommended water depth (figure 7.1). Water depth affects a participant's impact level, control of motion, and body alignment. Water that is too shallow (waist level or below) increases impact, limits the effective use of arms against the water's resistance, and reduces the cooling potential during exercise. Water that is too deep (above armpit depth) compromises control of motion, limits the ability to remain grounded on the pool bottom, and affects maintenance of proper body alignment.

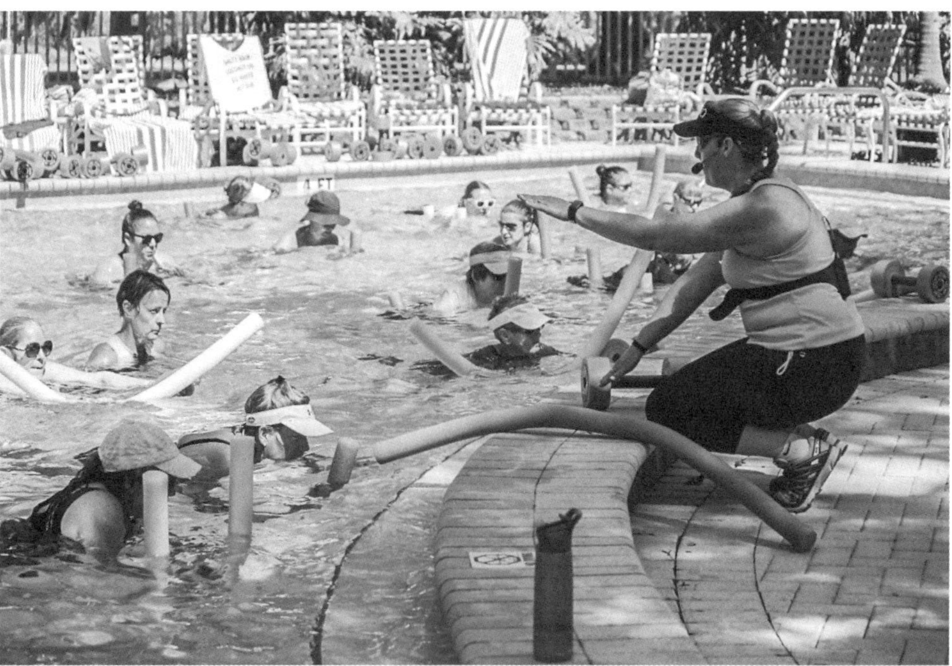

Figure 7.1 Having enough room for participants while keeping them close enough to see and hear the instructor is crucial in pool choice.

Deep-water exercise is most successful when the body can be suspended vertically, and is free to move in a full range of motion in any direction without experiencing impact or weight-bearing stress. A pool depth of 6.5 feet (2 m) or more provides the ideal environment for a deep-water class.

As a safety measure, inform participants of changes in pool depth, even when clearly marked on the pool or deck. This will help prevent a non-swimmer from getting into deep water and lower the risk of an unwanted rescue.

Pool Bottom

Pools are constructed of many types of materials, including concrete, ceramic tile, metal, vinyl, and plastic. The type of material used to construct the pool and how it is finished (i.e., painted or coated) determines the surface of the pool bottom. The pool bottom surface is of little concern to deep-water exercisers or swimmers. However, it can affect the quality of a shallow-water workout. Rough surfaces are abrasive to the participants' feet. If the surface is slippery, it becomes very difficult to push against the pool bottom to travel, change direction, land safely when jumping, or stabilize for grounded activities. For these reasons, water shoes are recommended for most shallow-water exercise programs. The benefits of wearing water shoes are discussed later in this chapter.

Also, consider the impact of where the pool bottom meets the pool wall. Pools that have a rounded slope may prohibit exercises that require participants to stand at the side of the pool; on the other hand, that slope might be great for doing a post-workout calf stretch.

Deck Surfaces and Pool Gutters

Deck surfaces can be slippery, especially when wet. Participants should be encouraged to wear shoes and reminded to use caution when entering and exiting the pool. Most pool deck surfaces are also made of materials that are nonresilient. When teaching from the pool deck, wear appropriate shoes, use a teaching mat, and limit high-impact demonstrations.

Pool gutters can affect how students enter and exit the pool and how they hold on to the side of the pool. They also provide options for toning and stretching exercises. Be aware of the pool's design, and do not include exercises or positions that might put participants at risk for possible injury.

Pool Entry and Exit

In accordance with the **Americans with Disabilities Act (ADA)**, fitness facilities, including swimming pools, that have been built or altered since 1990 in the United States must be accessible to people with disabilities. The U.S. Department of Justice published revised regulations in 2010, including the 2010 Standards for Accessible Design. The ADA Requirements: Accessible Pools Means of Entry and Exit establish two categories of pools: large pools with more than 300 linear feet of pool wall and smaller pools with less than 300 linear feet of wall. Large pools must have two accessible means of entry, with at least one being a pool lift or sloped entry; smaller pools are only required to have one accessible means of entry, provided that it is either a pool lift or a sloped entry.

Any pool that also has stair access should have safety handrails for the stair. The area around all entry and exit points should be free of potential hazards, such as exercise equipment, lane lines, and towels.

Acoustics

Acoustics in pool areas are generally poor, and can alter the quality of instruction. You might compete with echo from high ceilings and concrete walls as well as noise from fans, filtration systems, whirlpools, music, and other activities in the pool. It can be very difficult for the instructor to verbally communicate cues and instructions. Enhance your leadership skills by incorporating hand and arm signals and other nonverbal cueing techniques.

Experiment with different teaching locations around the pool. Due to pool construction or layout, it might be less noisy in one area than another. Your voice might carry more clearly from some locations than others. Sometimes students can hear you better when you instruct from deck; other times, they can hear you better when you are in the pool. Microphone systems are available for use in the aquatic environment; some are waterproof and can be worn in the water, others are designed for on-deck instruction only (figure 7.2). Often, these systems are a worthy investment for facilities and instructors because they enhance program quality and reduce your risk of **voice injury**.

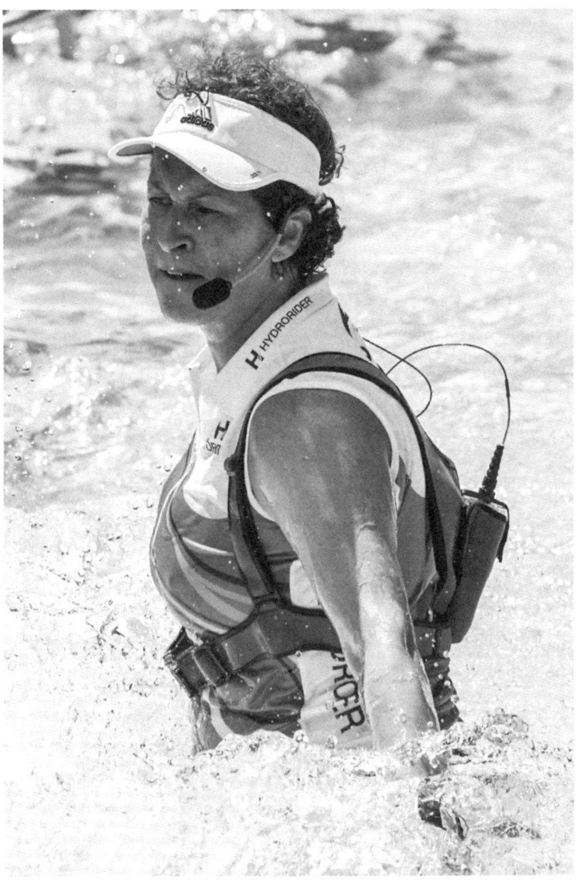

Figure 7.2 Waterproof microphones enable instructors to provide real hands-on teaching.

Music is motivating. It can help maintain proper cadence and intensity and assist with timing of training intervals. Consider the acoustics at your pool when selecting the type of music as well as the volume at which it is played.

Participant Considerations

In addition to being aware of your pool design and environmental concerns, you must always be attentive to the needs and safety of the participants.

Participant Workout Space

Ideally, allow a working space of 4 feet front to back by 8 feet side to side (1.2 × 2.4 m) per person during shallow-water cardiorespiratory programs. This space requirement of 32 square feet (9.8 m^2) may increase if equipment is being used. To determine the number of students for your pool, measure the square footage of the useable area (based on depth and bottom slope for shallow water), then divide by 32 if using feet or 9.8 if using meters.

The optimal working space for deep-water exercise is slightly larger than for shallow-water exercise because deep-water participants tend to drift. Ideally, each deep-water exercise participant should have 32 to 36 square feet (9.8–11 m^2) of working space depending on the level of the class, the type of programming, and equipment choices. A beginner-level class with predominantly stationary exercises requires less space than an advanced workout using traveling exercises. Participants can determine spacing by remaining vertical with arms abducted at the shoulders and turning in a circle; if they can move without touching other participants, they have enough space.

If optimal space is not available, you will need to plan exercises accordingly and be aware of positioning and spacing throughout the class.

Aquatic Shoes

Wearing shoes can be beneficial for aquatic fitness participants, providing safety when entering and exiting the pool and while walking on deck or in surrounding areas that could be slippery (figure 7.3).

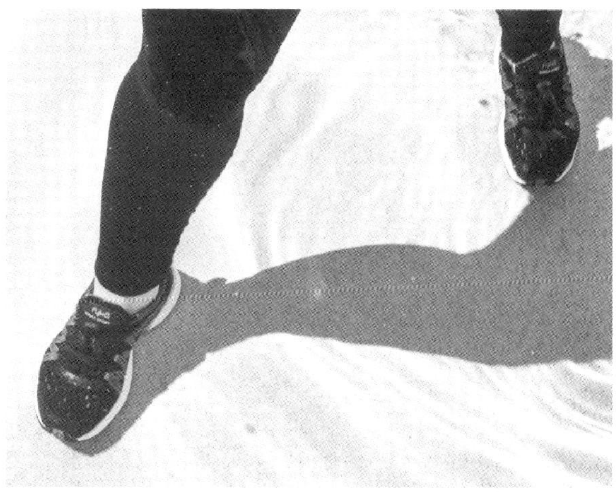

Figure 7.3 Specialty water shoes are a good investment for safety and for achieving a better in-pool workout.

For shallow-water programming, shoes provide extra shock absorbency, ensure good footing, and protect skin on the feet. Shoes reduce impact stress from bounding-type movements by providing cushioning and support. Shoes are beneficial for participants who have orthopedic problems or who need to wear orthotics even while exercising in the pool. Wearing shoes improves the quality of the workout by allowing for better footing and traction when moving and changing directions. Constant friction and impact can be harmful to the soles of the feet, especially for diabetic participants or those with delicate skin, circulation issues, or skin disorders. Shoes help protect the bottom of the feet from rough surfaces or objects on the pool bottom.

Deep-water programs eliminate contact with the pool bottom and shoes may hinder full range of motion at the ankle during long-lever leg movements. However, shoes can still add to the safety and comfort of participants in the dressing room, on the pool deck, and while entering and exiting the water.

Wearing shoes, in effect, adds resistance at the end of a long lever. Class design and exercise choice will determine if this is beneficial or if it creates unnecessary stress to the joints. Some shoes create additional weight that can assist participants with vertical alignment in deep-water vertical activities. Conversely, other shoes add significant buoyancy to the lower leg; participants with inadequate core strength may not be able to maintain proper vertical alignment. Participants should be aware of these potential challenges and use caution until accustomed to how their selected shoes influence movement in the water.

The AEA recommends that all aquatic fitness instructors wear shoes and use a mat while teaching on deck (figure 7.4). Wearing appropriate shoes for deck teaching is vital to instructor safety. If you teach completely on deck, wear appropriate athletic shoes to provide cushioning and support. If you teach on deck and in the water or if you enter the water to cool off, wear an appropriate water fitness shoe to minimize impact and provide the support needed for both environments.

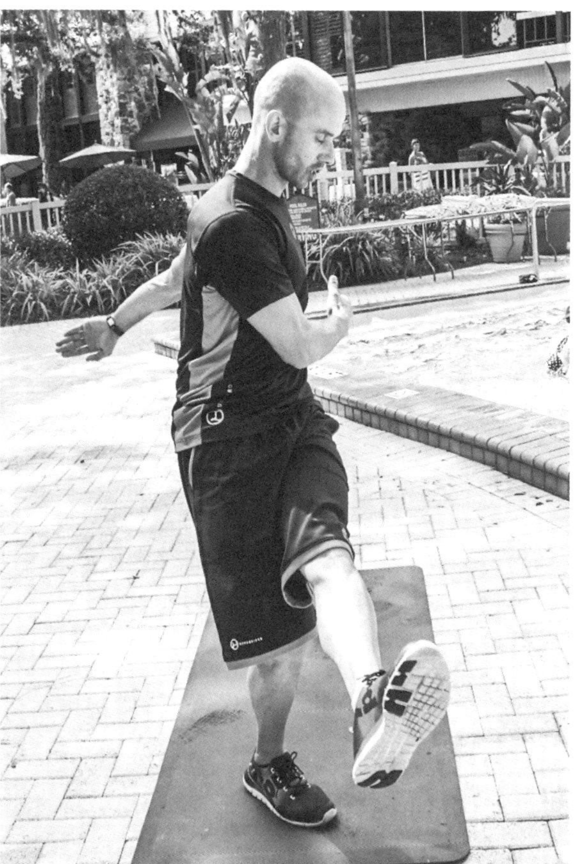

Figure 7.4 Nonslip cushioned mats are recommended for instructor safety when teaching on the pool deck.

Aquatic Fitness Program Checklist

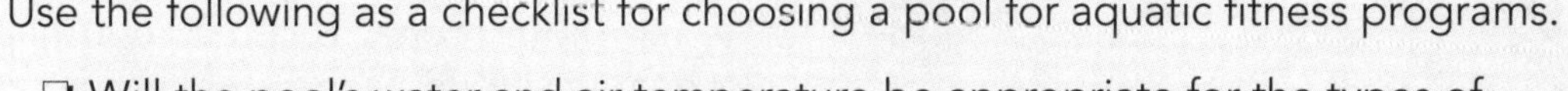

Use the following as a checklist for choosing a pool for aquatic fitness programs.

- ❑ Will the pool's water and air temperature be appropriate for the types of programs you wish to teach?
- ❑ Will air temperature and humidity levels allow you to safely teach and demonstrate from deck?
- ❑ What will be the maximum number of participants based on available space within the recommended water depth?
- ❑ Are the pool bottom and slope appropriate for the type of class you wish to teach?
- ❑ Is there adequate space for you to teach and demonstrate from the deck?
- ❑ Will your targeted class population be able to safely enter and exit the pool?
- ❑ Will the pool gutters and sides limit the type of programming you plan to conduct?
- ❑ Is the pool deck kept clean and free of hazards?
- ❑ Are the pool chemicals properly monitored and kept in accordance with the local board of health and state standards?
- ❑ Is the pool area properly ventilated?
- ❑ Will the pool acoustics work for the type of program you plan to teach?
- ❑ Do you have a microphone available?
- ❑ Are pool conditions conducive for any equipment you plan to use? Is adequate storage space available for the equipment? (For additional information on equipment, see appendix C.)
- ❑ Is a lifeguard on duty during your class? Does the pool area have appropriate life-saving equipment? (For additional information on water safety, see chapter 13.)

Chances are that not all of these parameters will be perfectly met. However, all of these factors will have some effect on the way you teach your aquatic program. Choose your facility and pool based on the parameters that are absolutely necessary for you to conduct a safe and effective class for the target population and type of programming you plan to teach. Or, adjust your programming to the pool environment. For example, if a pool meets your physical specifications, but acoustics are poor, experiment with different sound systems and placement, microphones, or types of music until you find a suitable option.

Summary

The pool environment creates unique challenges for program design and class leadership. Water and air temperatures, along with humidity, affect heat dissipation during exercise, which influences the comfort and safety of participants and instructors. Develop and modify programming to accommodate environmental changes. Appropriate clothing and proper hydration can also enhance comfort and minimize safety issues associated with the surrounding conditions.

The pool's structural design influences programming and safety considerations for both the participant in the water and the professional on deck. Be familiar with your pool. Pool slope and depth, the surface of the pool bottom and the pool deck, pool entry and exit, and acoustic factors all influence programming. Since you have little control over the pool structure, design a safe and effective program to fit the unique parameters of your pool.

Ensuring participant comfort and safety also requires attention to available workout space in the appropriate pool depth. Shoes offer safety in and around the pool area and can enhance the quality of exercise in shallow-water training.

Review Questions

1. How is radiation different from convection in relation to heat dissipation during exercise?

2. What are the concerns associated with performing vertical exercise in water 78 degrees Fahrenheit (26 °C) or below?

3. What is an ideal water temperature range for a typical cardiorespiratory aquatic fitness class?

4. What is the recommended water depth range for conducting a shallow-water aquatic fitness program?

5. The optimal working space for deep-water exercise is ____________ shallow-water exercise.

   a. slightly smaller than
   b. the same as
   c. slightly larger than
   d. twice as large as

6. The participant cannot dissipate heat by sweating when exercising in the water.

   a. True
   b. False

7. The general recommendation for indoor pool air temperature is a range of ______________.

8. List at least three benefits of wearing aquatic shoes during shallow-water exercise.
9. The acoustics in pool areas are generally poor. List three ideas that can help reduce instructor voice injury and enhance leadership skills.
10. Explain why it is generally recommended to exercise at mid–rib cage to mid-chest depth during shallow-water programs.

See appendix D for answers to review questions.

References and Resources

ASHRAE 2016. Standards and Guidelines. www.ashrae.org

Aquatic Exercise Association. 2015. *AEA Arthritis Foundation program leader: A training guide for exercise and aquatic programming.* Nokomis, FL: Author.

———. 2016. *Standards & guidelines for aquatic fitness programming.* Nokomis, FL: Author.

Cannon, P., and W.R. Keatinge. 1960. The metabolic rate and heat loss of fat and thin men in heat balance in cold and warm water. *Journal of Physiology* 154(2):329.

Chewning, J. 2011. *The effect of water temperature on aquatic exercise.* Nokomis, FL: Aquatic Exercise Association. https://aeawave.com/Portals/2/Research/IA_TheEffectofWaterTemperatureonAquaticExercise_Handout.pdf

Gregson, W., M.A. Black, H. Jones, J. Milson, J. Morton, B. Dawson, G. Atkinson, and D.J. Green. 2011. Influence of cold water immersion on limb and cutaneous blood flow at rest. *American Journal of Sports Medicine* 39(6):1316-1323.

Harris, T. 2002. How swimming pools work. *HowStuffWorks.com,* September 17. www.howstuffworks.com/swimming-pool.htm.

Howley, E.T., and D.L. Thompson. 2012. *Fitness professional's handbook.* 6th edition. Champaign, IL: Human Kinetics.

Lindle, J. 2001. Is your indoor pool equipment safe? *AKWA* 15(4):3-4.

Moor, F., E. Manwell, M. Noble, and S. Peterson. 1964. *Manual of hydrotherapy and massage.* Nampa, ID: Pacific Press Publishing Association.

Osinski, A. 1988. Water myths. *The AKWA letter* 2(3):1-7.

Sharkey, B.J., and S.E. Gaskill. 2013. *Fitness and health.* 7th edition. Champaign, IL: Human Kinetics.

Sova, R. 2000. *Aquatics: The complete reference guide for aquatic fitness professionals.* 2nd edition. Pt. Washington, WI: DSL.

U.S. Department of Justice. 2012. ADA requirements: Accessible pools—Means of entry and exit. www.ada.gov/pools_2010.htm.

USA Swimming Facilities Development Department, 2017. Build a Pool Conference. www.usaswimming.org/facilities

Part III

Instruction and Programming

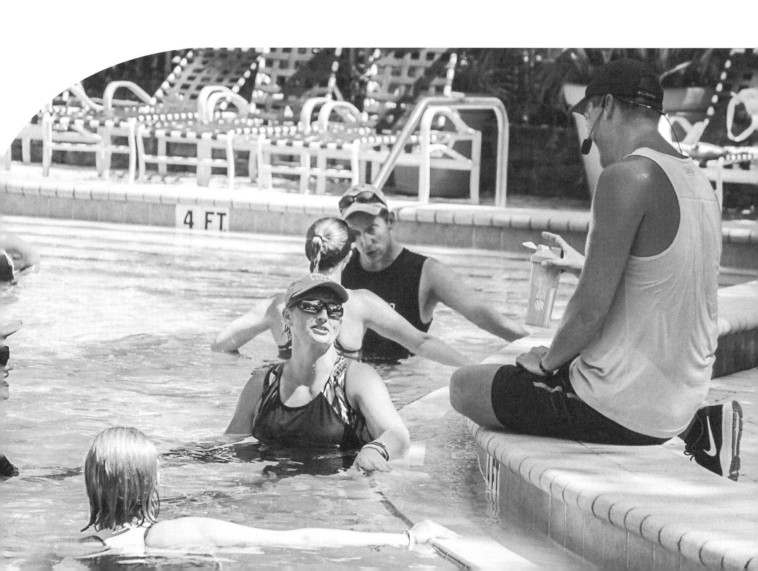

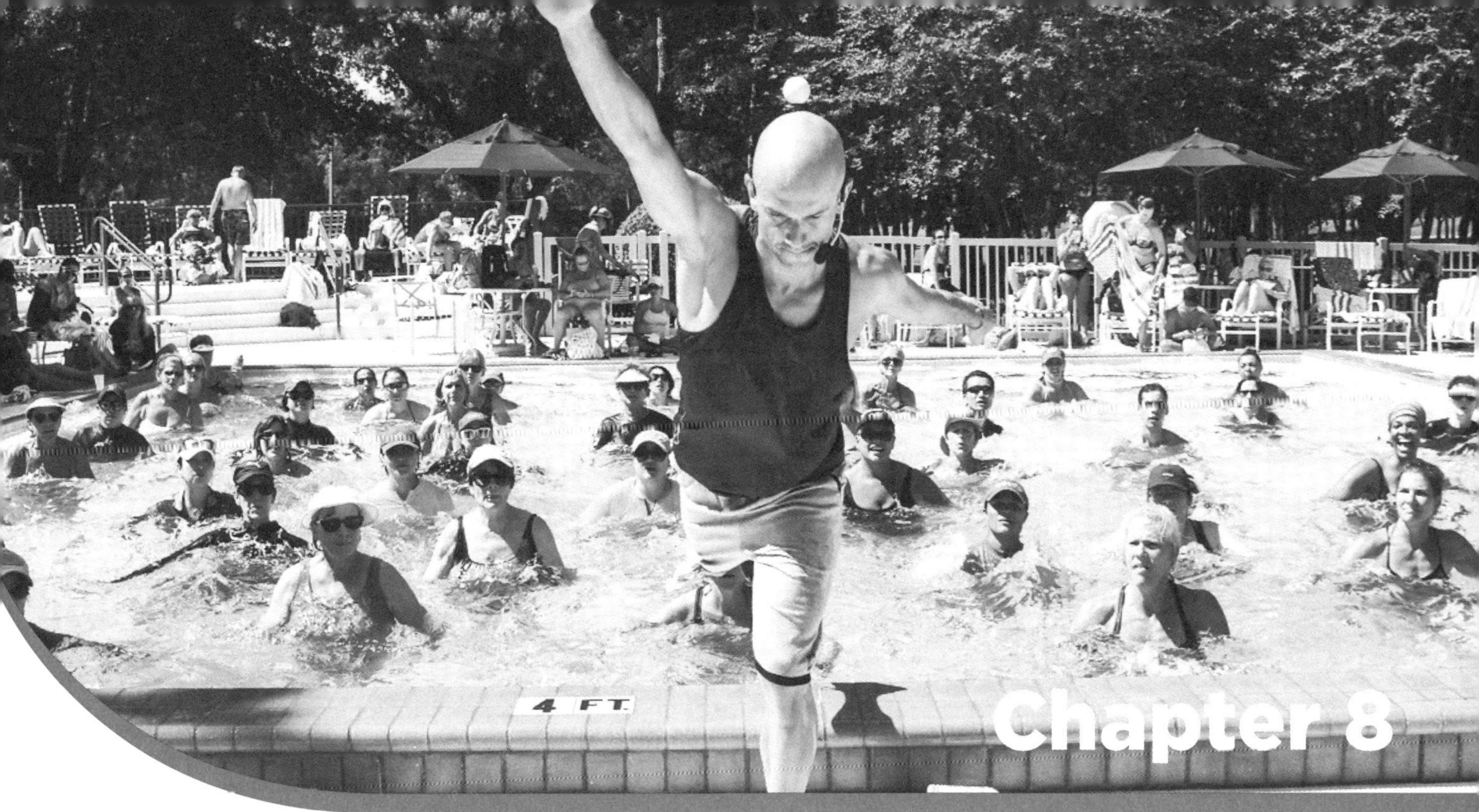

Shallow-Water Exercise

Introduction

Aquatic fitness instructors, whether working in a group setting or training one on one, will benefit from understanding how to use the unique properties of the water to provide a safe, effective, and enjoyable workout. In this chapter, we discuss lower-body base moves, arm movements and positions, various impact alternatives, and tempo for shallow-water aquatic fitness programs. Maintaining proper posture and alignment during shallow-water exercise is also covered.

Key Chapter Concepts

- Define shallow-water exercise.
- Learn evidence-based benefits of shallow-water exercise.
- Learn variations to the three types of lower-body base moves used in shallow-water exercise.
- Understand the five methods for creating safe and effective movements for the upper body.
- Discover impact options to accommodate the variety of fitness levels of participants in your classes.
- Understand the benefits of using land, water, and half water tempos, as well as cadence, to add variety to your aquatic programming and aid in safe transitions.
- Recognize how the aquatic environment influences posture and alignment, and understand the importance of proper demonstration and cueing to maintain neutral alignment.

Defining Shallow-Water Exercise

Shallow-water exercise is typically performed in water that ranges in depth from mid-rib cage to midchest. This provides the benefits of both reduced impact and grounding forces and allows participants to maintain proper alignment and control their movements. By using the properties of the water, training in shallow water allows for a wide variety of programming that can positively influence cardiorespiratory fitness, muscular strength and endurance, and flexibility.

Water below waist depth may require greater thought and planning due to increased impact and reduced cooling effects. Additionally, water exceeding midchest requires greater considerations due to the lack of grounding forces and greater immersion effects.

Pools with a depth range of 3.5 to 4.5 feet (1–1.4 m) are effective for most shallow-water fitness classes. Expanding the depth range to 3 to 5 feet (.9–1.5 m) will accommodate nearly all heights of participants and shallow-water program options. A gradual slope of the pool bottom is preferred for accommodating varying heights of participants.

Shallow-Water Exercise Research and Application

Shallow-water exercise is different than land-based exercise in that it provides resistance in every direction of submerged movement and has significantly less impact. All movements performed against the resistive force of the water (without added equipment) require concentric muscle actions and provide a better opportunity for muscle balance when compared to exercise performed on land. The aquatic environment allows people limited by the impact concerns of land-based training to exercise at an appropriate intensity for achieving improvements in all fitness components. It also allows people of higher fitness levels to train at greater intensities without experiencing increased musculoskeletal stress.

Research presented in chapter 1 indicates that aquatic exercise, when performed at an appropriate intensity, could result in improvements in cardiorespiratory fitness, muscular strength, flexibility, balance, functional capacity, and body composition. The research also supports the benefits of using heart rates (specifically the Kruel Aquatic Heart Rate Deduction) and rating of perceived exertion to monitor the intensity of shallow-water exercise. Additional research has shown that a properly designed shallow-water program can meet the ACSM's exercise prescription guidelines for achieving health benefits (D'Acquisto, D'Acquisto, and Renne 2001; Campbell et al. 2003). See chapter 1 for the ACSM's guidelines for exercise.

Shallow-water exercise is not just an effective mode of exercise. It has also been proven equivalent to land-based exercise in terms of energy expenditure provided that the intensity is similar. An average shallow-water exercise class results in an energy expenditure of 8 **kilocalories** per minute, or 480 kilocalories per hour (Nagle et al. 2013). Land-based classes average 3.9 to 12.3 kilocalories per minute, or 234 to 738 kilocalories per hour (Igbanugo and Gutin 1978). On land, caloric expenditure depends on the intensity of the class and the participant's body weight. Body size (surface area), experience with water exercise, and training intensity all influence the caloric expenditure of water exercise.

According to research, wearing shoes in shallow water may also influence caloric expenditure. A research study evaluated the performance of a 500-yard (457 m) shallow-water running test with and without shoes. The researchers found that wearing shoes resulted in significantly faster running times and higher predicted maximal oxygen uptake ($\dot{V}O_2max$; Clemens and Cisar 2006). This suggests that aqua shoes provide traction, allowing for a more intense workout that burns more calories.

Shallow-water exercise also shows comparable improvements in cardiorespiratory and muscular strength and endurance to those gained in land-based workouts. This is very beneficial for participants who may be limited by pain or discomfort during land-based training (Sardinha, Pinheiro, and Szejnfeld 2013). Studies have shown that people with arthritis have been able to tolerate shallow-water exercise, and some have reported a decrease in pain as a result of participation in water exercise (Batterham, Heywood, and Keating 2011).

Shallow-water exercise proves to be not just an acceptable alternative to land-based training. In some cases—depending on the person's health, fitness level, and exercise goals—it may be a preferred option.

Shallow-Water Base Moves

Movement variations begin with base moves. **Base moves** are the smallest parts or segments in choreography, and can be modified or changed to create intensity and variety. Base moves for exercise design typically focus on a movement of the lower body. In shallow water, the three options we build from include the following:

- Moves that land on alternating feet, e.g., knee lift or pendulum
- Moves that land on both feet (jump), e.g., cross-country ski or jumping jack
- Moves that land repeatedly on one foot (hop), e.g., knee swings or kick swings

Knowledgeable instructors use base moves and variations of base moves to create safe and effective workouts. Table 8.1 lists common variations of base moves for the legs. Refer to appendix A for descriptions and pictures of several of these moves. A clear understanding of the physical laws and the properties of water allows you to add variety to base moves without sacrificing safety or effectiveness. Traveling with a knee lift is an example of varying a base move to create more intensity through increased inertia. Base moves can also be combined to create patterns or combinations in choreography.

Many instructors design choreography based on lower-body movements and then add arm movements that are similar to the leg movements. Giving more consideration to arm movements can add variety and physical and mental challenges to any leg pattern. Table 8.2 lists common upper-body base moves (i.e., joint motions at the shoulders and elbows).

You can add variety to the upper-body base moves in five basic ways. The first is to change a specific arm move that is combined with a specific leg move. For example,

Table 8.1 Variations of Shallow-Water Base Moves for the Lower Body

Moves that land on alternating feet	Moves that land on both feet	Moves that land repeatedly on one foot
Narrow jog	Jump feet together	Single-leg hop
Wide jog	Jump feet wide	Knee swings
Jog out, out, in, in	Jumping jacks	Kick swings
Crossing jog	Cross-country skis	Cancan *(knee lift, bounce, front kick, bounce)*
Knee lifts	Moguls	Repeaters for one-footed moves *(performing multiple repetitions on one side before changing lead leg)*
Kicks	Front-back jumps	
Leg curls	Twist	
Ankle reach front	Propelled and plyometric jumps *(variations include hip abduction, hip adduction, knee tuck, heel tuck, frog [feet together and knees apart])*	
Heel reach behind		
Pendulum		
Rocking horse		
Leaps		
Side steps		
Mambo *(rock forward and then back on same side)*		
Cha-cha *(3 quick jogs and a pause)*		

Table 8.2 Base Moves for the Upper Body

Movement from the shoulder	Movement from the elbow and the forearm
Abduction (frontal and transverse planes)	Flexion
Adduction (frontal and transverse planes)	Extension
Flexion	Supination
Extension	Pronation
Hyperextension	
Rotation: medial and lateral	
Circumduction	

a typical jumping jack arm movement would be arm abduction and adduction as the legs are abducting and adducting. To add variety, try combining a jumping jack with arm movements in the transverse plane, such as transverse abduction and adduction, or in the sagittal plane, such as shoulder flexion and extension. You can also vary the movement in the frontal plane by crossing the arms forward, crossing the arms behind the body, alternating a front or back cross, or moving the arms in opposition to the legs (when the legs abduct, the arms adduct).

A second way to add variety is to create a combination focusing on the upper body instead of the lower body. In this option, the leg movement might stay the same but the arm movements vary in a designated pattern (table 8.3).

A third way to add variation is to use the arms above the water's surface (figure 8.1). Arm movements above the head represent a functional range of motion (e.g. reaching to a shelf above your head or turning on a ceiling fan), and are acceptable in water exercise programs. In general, arms should stay either in the water or out of the water throughout the combination or pattern. If you need to make the transition from out of the water to in the water, consider using short levers to avoid stress on the shoulder and elbow joints. Limit the number of repetitions of overhead arm movements and combine overhead movements with stationary lower-body movements

Table 8.3 Arm Patterns

Jumping jack with arm pattern								
Water tempo	1	2	3	4	5	6	7	8
Legs	Out	In	Out	In	Out	In	Out	In
Arms	Abduct	Transverse adduct	Transverse abduct	Adduct	Abduct	Transverse adduct	Transverse abduct	Adduct
Front kick with arm pattern								
Water tempo	1	2	3	4	5	6	7	8
Legs	Right	Left	Right	Left	Right	Left	Right	Left
Arms	Push L forward and R back	Push R forward and L back	Push L forward and R back	Push R forward and L back	Adduct both arms	Abduct both arms	Adduct both arms	Abduct both arms

that allow for better spinal alignment to protect the back. Note that greater intensity may be experienced while keeping the arms submerged and using the resistance of the water.

A fourth option is to keep the arms in a neutral position. Neutral arm positions neither assist nor resist leg movements. Since the upper body cannot assist with stability, the core muscles must work harder. With this option, you lose the benefit of training the upper body against the water's resistance, but you experience more intense core training. Examples of neutral arms would be arms at the sides, hands on the hips, arms crossed in front of the chest (figure 8.2), or hands behind the head. You should always consider your participants' needs and abilities when deciding to incorporate neutral arm positions into your classes.

A fifth option would be to have the arms merely float (or rest) in the water during activity (figure 8.3) or use the arms in a sculling

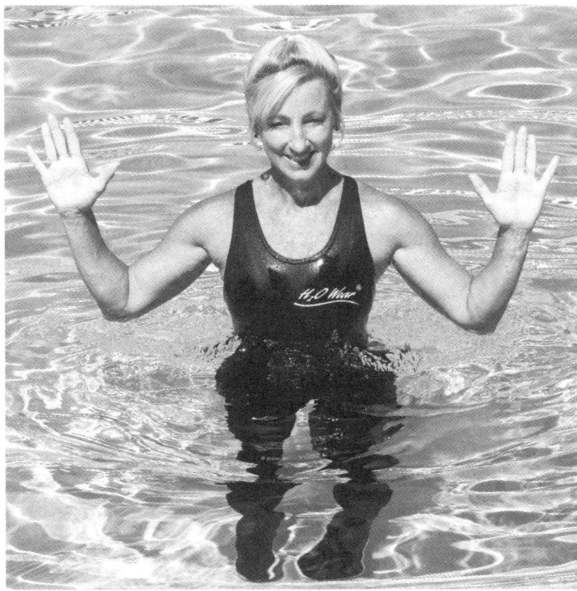

Figure 8.1 Arms out of water.

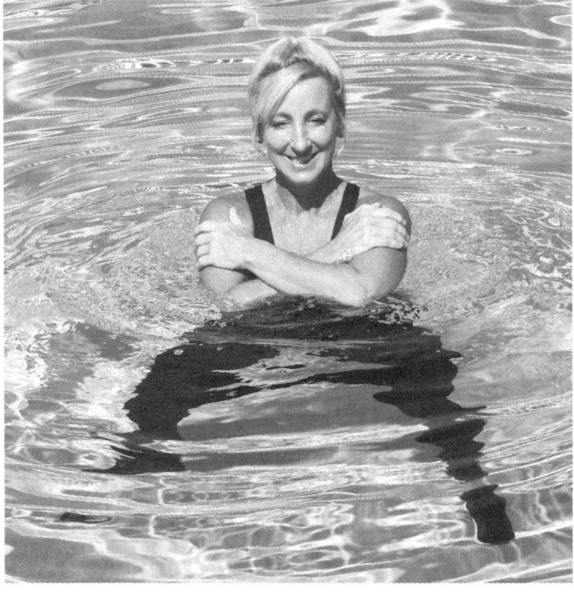

Figure 8.2 Arms in neutral position.

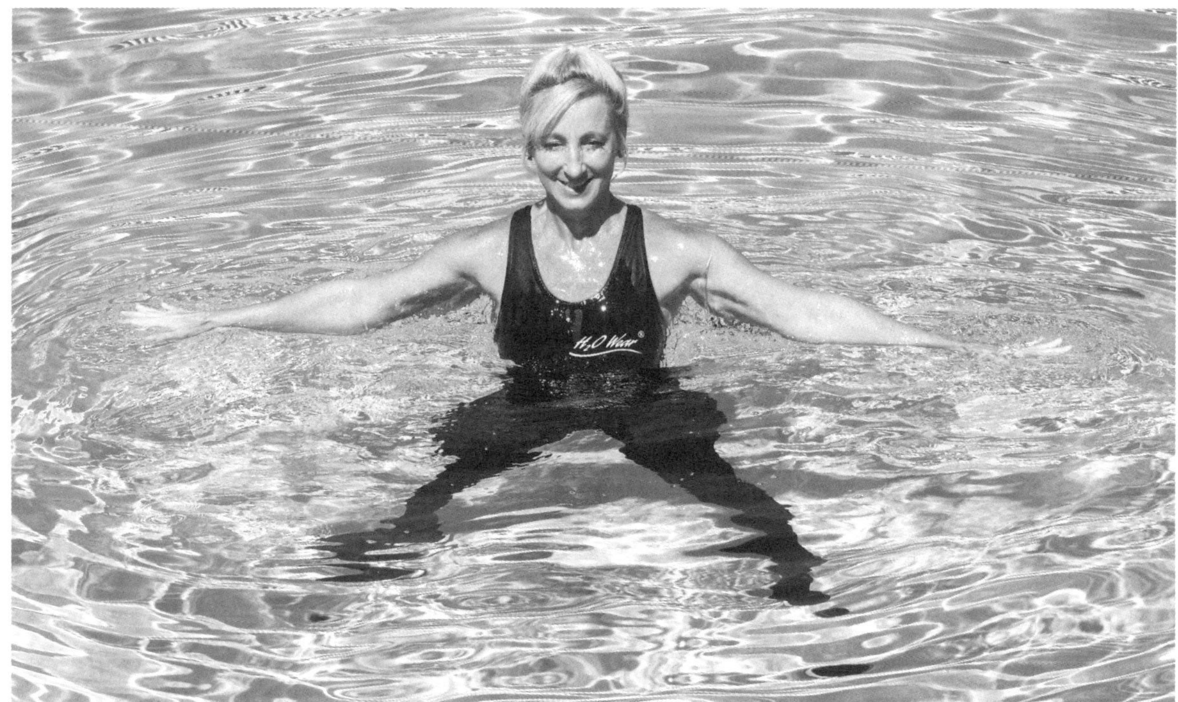

Figure 8.3 Floating arms.

motion under the water. This makes it easier for the participants to maintain proper body position, alignment, and balance, and it can help people who have difficulty with maintaining balance and who require extra assistance during exercise. It can also help beginning exercise participants become acclimated to the aquatic environment. However, this option may be a disadvantage for fit participants because the core muscles are not as actively engaged to support and stabilize the body.

In designing your shallow-water programs, common sense must rule when it comes to arm movements. Consider the individual needs of your participants and offer a variety of arm movements and positions to provide appropriate challenges. Arms can be used to assist movement, impede movement, assist balance, or create a more challenging core workout. Arms can be used in or out of the water to create variety in choreography. Just remember, any arm movement repeated for a long period in one position might push the limits of safety. Observe participants; if form is not maintained, consider making the arm patterns less challenging or allowing time for recovery. Table 8.4 provides examples of the arm movements or positions used in shallow-water exercise.

Impact Options for Shallow-Water Exercise

Shallow water is an excellent medium for exercise because of the reduced gravitational forces experienced by the body when partially submerged. Thus, shallow water provides a lower-impact alternative to land-based programming. Even within the aquatic realm, we can modify the impact forces created by the workout. Keep this in mind because participants may be able to handle increasing the intensity of their workout but physically unable to increase the impact. Many participants choose the water specifically for a lower-impact exercise alternative.

The depth of the water directly affects the amount of impact transferred through the musculoskeletal system. Moving in deeper water decreases the impact for a given exercise, while moving to shallower water increases the impact for the same exercise.

Table 8.4 Examples of Arm Use for Shallow-Water Exercise

1. Change typical arm and leg patterns.	Combine jumping jack legs with shoulder transverse abduction and adduction. Combine cross-country ski legs with shoulder abduction and adduction.
2. Create arm combinations or patterns. Keep the leg movement the same, but change the arms.	Jogging legs with arm combination, where both arms move together: Count 1 = Elbow flexion Count 2 = Elbow extension Count 3 = Shoulder flexion Count 4 = Shoulder extension *See table 8.3 for more examples.*
3. Use the arms above the water's surface.	Clap overhead with a jumping jack. Reach forward out of the water with a cross-country ski.
4. Hold the arms in a neutral position; neither assist nor impede the leg movement while adding challenge to the core muscles.	Cross the arms on the chest while water walking. Place hands on hips as legs perform a rocking horse.
5. Float the arms on the surface of the water or scull the arms under the water to assist with balance and stability.	Rest arms on the surface of the water while performing a leg swing front and back.

Exercising without touching the pool bottom, as in deep-water exercise, actually creates a non-impact workout. See chapter 9 for more information on deep-water exercise.

Shallow-water exercises can be performed at various impact levels. Many movements can be performed in the water with either a bounding (e.g., jogging) or a non-bounding (e.g., walking) style. (Note: It is difficult to perform non-bounding moves when exercising in water that is armpit depth or greater.) Incorporating both techniques allows for greater variety in your programming while letting participants choose the option that works best for their ability level. We can take the bounding moves a step further and make them plyometric in nature by pushing forcefully off the pool bottom to propel the body up and out of the water. This increases both intensity and impact. Following are basic impact variations typically used in shallow-water programming.

Levels I, II, and III

Aquatic programs that include various levels of impact provide additional movement opportunities for your participants. Impact variations for levels I, II, and III use the buoyant properties of the water to provide training options for different ability levels, achieve specific goals, and add variety to your classes.

Level I movements (figure 8.4) are performed in an upright position. They involve impacting movements where both feet are off the pool bottom for a brief period of time and then land or rebound. Level I movements may use acceleration to push participants up and out of the water, increasing both intensity and impact. All of the shallow-water base moves can be performed at level I.

Level II movements (figure 8.5) are performed by flexing the hips and knees to submerge the body to shoulder depth while executing the move. As with level I movements, both feet are off the pool bottom for a brief period of time. However, since the shoulders remain at the water's surface, the level of immersion is increased. This significantly reduces impact forces and requires the core muscles and upper body to work harder against the horizontal forces of the water.

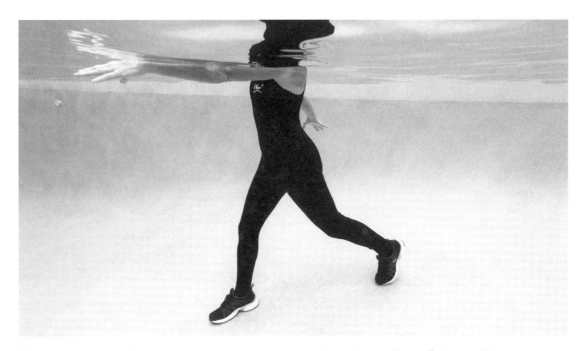

Figure 8.4 A level I cross-country ski where the body is rebounding off the pool bottom.

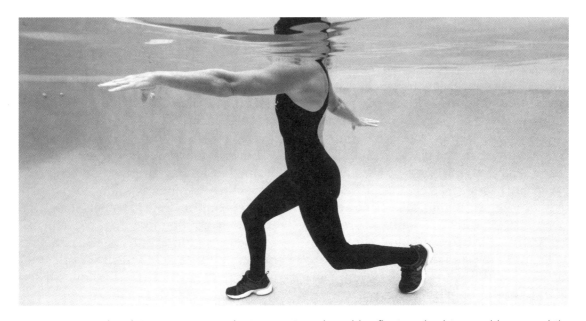

Figure 8.5 A level II cross-country ski; impact is reduced by flexing the hips and knees, while submerging the body to shoulder depth.

Creating more horizontal force against the water's resistance increases intensity without the momentum and vertical force experienced with level I. Participants need to be properly instructed and encouraged to create this force in order to gain the benefits of level II movement. Many of the shallow-water base moves for the lower body can be performed at level II, such as jogging, jumping jacks, cross-country skis, and moguls. Level II movements are low-impact exercise options.

Level III movements (figure 8.6) are performed without touching the pool bottom.

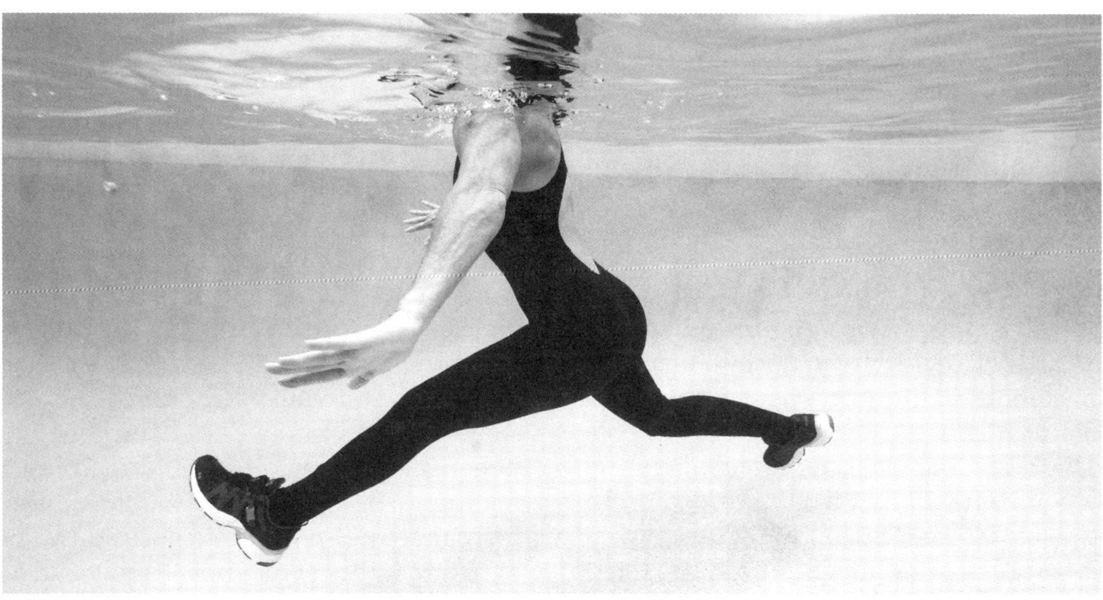

Figure 8.6 A level III cross-country ski where the body is suspended off the pool bottom, which eliminates impact.

The body is submerged to the shoulders, as in level II, while the movement is performed suspended. Impact is completely eliminated and workload is shifted to the upper body (keeping the head above water) and the torso (stabilization and alignment), since the movement is executed against the horizontal forces of the water. Jumping jacks and cross-country skis are common movements performed at level III. The challenge of level III movements is determined in part by body size and composition. A lean, muscular participant needs to expend more energy to remain afloat as compared to a more buoyant participant. As with level II movements, participants will need to be encouraged to exert additional force against the water's horizontal forces and to use full range of motion to maintain intensity. Participants uncomfortable with taking their feet off the bottom of the pool can be encouraged to perform the movement at levels I or II.

Power tucks (figure 8.7) are variations of movements performed in levels I, II, and III that increase intensity and add variety. Power tucks use acceleration to emphasize movement under the water to increase the muscular effort. The knees pull forcefully toward the chest (tucking the knees toward

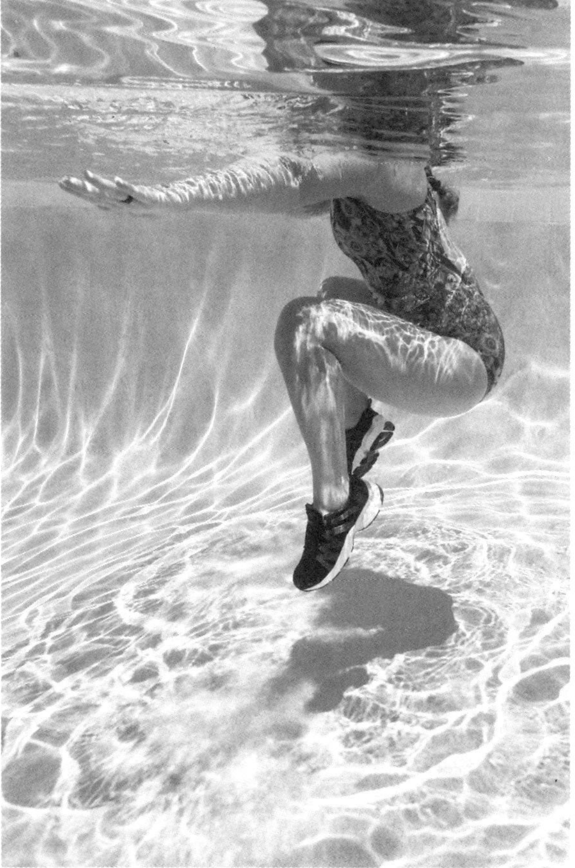

Figure 8.7 Power tucks are movement variations that tuck the knees as the legs transition during the exercise.

the body) and then the legs push forcefully away and toward the pool bottom. Power tucks may or may not alter the impact level; in level I, power tucks increase impact, but in levels II and III, the impact is not altered.

Grounded Movement

Like level I movements, **grounded movements** are performed in an upright position, but one foot remains in contact with the pool bottom at all times. Grounded movements use drag resistance to provide a challenging yet low-impact workout in shallow water. In addition to the benefit of creating variety and a low-impact option for participants, most grounded movements are taught easily by the instructor from deck. Participants in the water can mimic the movement in the same manner as you demonstrate on the pool deck.

Let's look at some examples. A grounded jack could be performed as a half-jack (the right leg moving out and in followed by the left leg moving out and in), or as a side-step squat (one leg stepping out to perform a squat before returning center). A grounded cross-country ski could be performed by moving the right leg front and back for several repetitions, and then switching to the left leg. Another variation of a grounded cross-country ski is a front or back lunge (stepping one foot front or back, lowering into a lunge, and then returning to the start position). One-footed moves can also be grounded. In a grounded knee lift, since one foot remains firmly planted, the movement becomes a march.

Repeaters, or performing several repetitions on one side before switching the lead leg, offer one method for creating intensity in grounded movement. Performing multiple repetitions on one leg while the other foot is grounded increases the need for stabilization and balance, thus increasing the intensity of the exercise. With a little creativity, you can offer an entire grounded class or incorporate grounded movements into almost any shallow-water format.

Propelled Movement

Plyometrics, or jump training, is a technique for improving jumping ability and power by using the **stretch reflex** to facilitate recruitment of additional muscle **motor units**. Plyometric training uses the eccentric muscle action created prior to the jump to generate elastic energy (the stretch reflex) that provides power for the jump. As the body lands from one jump, that eccentric muscle action will again generate power for the next jump. Research has shown that there are many benefits of adding plyometric training to an aquatic program when gains in motor performance and power are desired (Martel et al. 2005; Miller et al. 2007; Reddy and Maniazhagu 2015; Robinson et al. 2004; Stemm and Jacobson 2007).

Plyometrics performed in the water can be referred to as **propelled movements** (figure 8.8). The reduced gravity in the water provides for reduced motor unit recruitment through the stretch reflex. However, jumping in the water can enable the participant to recruit more motor units from the water's drag, surface tension, viscosity, and resistance proper-

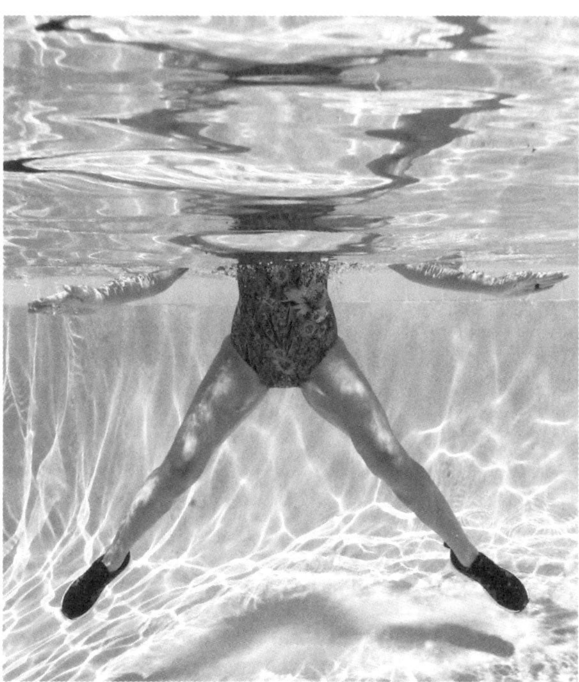

Figure 8.8 Example of propelled movement.

ties. One of the advantages of aquatic jump training is the increased resistance in all directions of submerged movement. Plyometric training on land is very high impact. High impact training can increase risk of injury to weight-bearing musculoskeletal structures, especially when landing. Plyometric or propelled movements in the water do not result in the same impact as land-based training. Aquatic jump training represents a safer, more efficient alternative because the water's resistance creates additional workload and allows for increased motor unit recruitment with decreased impact, thereby reducing risk of injury and delayed onset muscle soreness (Triplett et al. 2009).

Propelled movements are high-intensity exercises, but they can be used in a typical group class or sport-specific training. Performing propelled movements in chest-deep water, combined with lower-impact options for less-fit participants, reduces the risk of injury and allows all participants to be successful. Using the laws of inertia, acceleration, and action and reaction to propel movements upward, forward, or backward can add variety to movement and increase intensity.

Shallow-Water Tempo Options

An effective shallow-water exercise class includes movements performed at various tempos to ensure that proper intensity is maintained during the aerobic portion of the workout while allowing for full range of motion. Tempo options offer variations for each movement. For example, a knee lift can be performed at **land tempo**, **water tempo**, or **half water tempo** (either as a double knee lift or with a bounce center). The tempos can also be combined for additional variety. An example of a combined-tempo knee lift is performing two water tempo knee lifts followed by one knee lift at half water tempo (often cued as "single-single-double").

Land Tempo (LT)

Some instructors chose to increase intensity simply by increasing speed. Although this is effective, the quality of movement often deteriorates and range of motion decreases as tempo increases. Land tempo, sometimes cued as "double time," is the same speed of movement used on land (table 8.5). Impact or movement occurs at each beat, making movements quick, often with limited range of motion. Since a muscle is worked most effectively through its full range of motion, the muscle conditioning effectiveness of the exercise could be limited. These quick movements with limited range of motion also increase the risk of injury.

Well-placed land tempo movements can add variety and fun to aquatic choreography. Combine land tempo movements with water and half water tempo movements (discussed in following sections) in such a way that allows for slower, safer transitions in neutral alignment. When considering using land tempo moves, keep the following recommendations in mind:

- Use sparingly—no more than 15 percent of your programming.
- Use short-lever, one-footed moves, simple two-footed moves, or reduce the range of motion.

Table 8.5 Land Tempo (LT) Movements

Move	Beat 1	Beat 2	Beat 3	Beat 4	Beat 5	Beat 6	Beat 7	Beat 8
Jumping jack	Out	In	Out	In	Out	In	Out	In
Cross-country ski	Right	Left	Right	Left	Right	Left	Right	Left
Knee lift	Right	Left	Right	Left	Right	Left	Right	Left

**8 land tempo beats

- Remain stationary; traveling with fast movement might increase injury risk. An exception to this would be sprinting.
- Do not perform movements that combine environments. Keep the arm movement either completely under the water or above the water.
- Do not sacrifice alignment or joint integrity.

Water Tempo (WT)

Water tempo allows for full range of motion, balanced muscular conditioning, and additional time for safe transitions needed in the aquatic environment. Water tempo involves movement on every other beat of the music at the recommended 125 to 150 **beats per minute (bpm)** as shown in table 8.6. Long-lever movements can be safely achieved at the lower end of the recommended bpm range, while movements with short levers may be appropriate for the higher end of the bpm range. Most of your aquatic programming exercises should be made up of water tempo movements combined with half water tempo movements.

Half Water Tempo (1/2 WT)

Half water tempo is simply performing water-tempo movements with a bounce on every other water beat. In other words, a movement (including the bounce) requires four beats of the music. Half water tempo adds variety to aquatic exercises. The bounce can be used to transition from one move to another while remaining in neutral alignment. (Transitions are discussed in detail in chapter 10.) This tempo option allows for more focused muscular force in all directions of movement and encourages a greater range of motion.

Options exist for the placement of the bounce depending on the move (see table 8.7). A 1/2 WT jumping jack is performed by jump-

Table 8.6 Water Tempo (WT) Movements

Move	Beat 1	Beat 2	Beat 3	Beat 4	Beat 5	Beat 6	Beat 7	Beat 8
Jumping jack	Out		In		Out		In	
Cross-country ski	Right		Left		Right		Left	
Knee lift	Right		Left		Right		Left	

**8 land tempo beats

Table 8.7 Half Water Tempo (1/2 WT) Movements

Move	Beat 1	Beat 2	Beat 3	Beat 4	Beat 5	Beat 6	Beat 7	Beat 8
Jumping jack	Out		Bounce out		In		Bounce in	
Cross-country ski (double ski)	Right		Bounce right forward		Left		Bounce left forward	
Cross-country ski (ski bounce center)	Right		Bounce center		Left		Bounce center	
Knee lift (double knee)	Right		Bounce right up		Left		Bounce left up	
Knee lift (knee bounce center)	Right		Bounce center		Left		Bounce center	

**8 land tempo beats

ing out, bouncing at the out position, jumping in, and bouncing at the in position (cued as a "double jack"). A cross-country ski could be performed by jumping the feet apart front to back, bouncing in this position, jumping and switching the feet front to back, and bouncing in this position (cued as a "double ski"). A 1/2 WT ski can also be performed by jumping the feet apart front to back, jumping and bringing the feet together to bounce center, jumping with the opposite feet front to back, and then jumping to land with the feet together again (cued as a "ski bounce center"). Most one-foot moves can be performed at half water tempo. For example, a 1/2 WT knee lift can be performed by lifting the right knee, bouncing with the right knee lifted, switching to the left knee lifted, and bouncing with the left knee lifted (cued as a "double knee lift"). The knee lift can also be performed by lifting the right knee, bouncing center with both feet, lifting the left knee, and bouncing center with both feet (cued as a "knee bounce center").

Cadence

For **cadence training**, you begin with a set movement speed (cadence) and then increase or decrease the rate of that cadence to adjust the exercise intensity. Cadence training is a popular training method with deep-water running and is now being used in multiple formats in both shallow and deep water. The use of cadence is very effective in increasing exercise intensity as long as the range of motion and proper form are maintained. See chapter 9 for more details on cadence training.

Combined Tempos

You can offer even more variety by combining tempos within your exercise session and within movement patterns. Table 8.8 outlines a few examples of combined-tempo movements.

The more experience you gain as an instructor, the easier it will be to successfully incorporate these tempo options into shallow-water programming. Regardless of the choice of tempo or the combination of tempos, maintaining alignment is always important.

Posture and Alignment With Shallow-Water Exercise

Exercise is most effective when the body is in neutral alignment. Posture and alignment can easily be compromised during shallow-water exercise. The feet are in contact with the pool bottom, so the body has a point of reference for alignment. However, the multidirectional resistive forces and buoyancy of the water can make it difficult to maintain alignment. These factors may also influence the participants' ability to perform movements efficiently, especially for those who lack body awareness or experience with water exercise. Participants will require additional time to learn how to maintain neutral spine and perform movements efficiently in the water, so begin with stationary movements before progressing to traveling movements.

The center of buoyancy becomes more of a factor as water depth increases. Keeping the center of buoyancy and the center of gravity aligned will promote better balance and body control in the water. Unless participants are performing an exercise specifically targeting balance or proprioception, center of buoyancy and center of gravity should remain aligned. See the section on body awareness in chapter 9 for additional information on alignment and efficient movement.

You must properly demonstrate all movements and cue participants to maintain neutral alignment throughout the class. Some participants will have difficulty maintaining alignment due to a lack of core strength and body awareness. The resistance of the water and buoyancy may encourage participants to flex their hips and bring their upper body forward to make their bodies more streamlined to allow for easier movement through the water. You should provide visual and verbal cues by demonstrating neutral alignment and reminding participants to keep their ears over their shoulders, their shoulders over their hips, their hips over their knees, and

Table 8.8 Land Tempo (LT) Movements Combined With Water Tempo (WT) and Half Water Tempo (1/2 WT) Movements

Combined moves	Beat 1	Beat 2	Beat 3	Beat 4	Beat 5	Beat 6	Beat 7	Beat 8	Beat 9	Beat 10	Beat 11	Beat 12	Beat 13	Beat 14	Beat 15	Beat 16
4 WT knee lifts with 8 LT leg curls (LC)	R KL		L KL		R KL		L KL		R LC	L LC	R LC	L LC	R LC	L LC	R LC	L LC
4 LT jumping jacks (JJ) with 2 1/2 WT cross-country skis (CC)	O JJ	I JJ	O JJ	I JJ	O JJ	I JJ	O JJ	I JJ	R CC		BC		L CC		BC	
1 1/2 WT cross-country ski (CC) & 2 LT jumping jacks (JJ) & 4 WT leg curls (LC) For the next repetition, begin with a L ski.	R CC		BC		O JJ	I JJ	O JJ	I JJ	R LC		L LC		R LC		L LC	

**16 land tempo beats

R = right; L = left; O = out; I = in; BC = bounce center; KL = knee lift; LC = leg curl; JJ = jumping jack; CC = cross-country ski their knees over their ankles. The addition of equipment will require participants to make even more adjustments to their alignment. Always provide options for participants who are unable to maintain alignment when using equipment.

Consider all of these factors when designing programs and incorporating instructional cues to assist participants with maintaining alignment during shallow-water exercise. For more information on posture and alignment, see chapter 4.

Summary

Pools with a depth range of 3.5 to 4.5 feet (1–1.4 m) are effective for most shallow-water fitness classes. Expanding the depth range to 3 to 5 feet (.9–1.5 m) will accommodate nearly all heights of participants and shallow-water program options.

Research supports shallow-water exercise as an appropriate alternative for land-based training and as a viable mode of cross-training.

Shallow-water movement patterns are built around variations of one-footed moves that land on alternating feet, two-footed moves that land on both feet simultaneously, or hopping moves that involve landing repeatedly on one foot. Understanding the physical laws and properties of water allows you to add variety to the base moves without compromising safety or effectiveness.

There are five primary ways to use the arms in shallow-water aquatic programming. These arm movements may provide greater muscular effort for the upper body or greater muscular effort for the torso. They can also challenge balance and stability. Using the arms out of the water may be appropriate for a limited time; however, a more effective workout may be achieved when using the arms against the resistive forces of the water.

Various impact options are available for shallow-water exercise, including levels I, II, and III, and grounded and propelled movements.

Shallow-water moves can be performed at land tempo, water tempo, or half water tempo. Class design should be primarily water tempo and half water tempo to allow for safe and effective movements. Land tempo should be used sparingly because it does not always allow for full range of motion. Cadence training is also becoming more popular in shallow-water programs.

Lack of core strength and body awareness can make it difficult to maintain neutral alignment during shallow-water exercise. Instructors should visually and verbally cue for proper alignment throughout the class.

Review Questions

1. Pendulum, rocking horse, and side steps are variations of which lower-body base move?

   a. Moves that land on both feet
   b. Moves that land repeatedly on one foot
   c. Moves that land on alternating feet
   d. None of these

2. Arm movements above the head represent a functional range of motion, but are not recommended in a shallow-water exercise class.

   a. True
   b. False

3. What tempo does the following chart represent?

Beat: 8 land tempo beats	1	2	3	4	5	6	7	8
Front kick	R		L		R		L	

4. Level II movements are considered to be ________________.

   a. high impact
   b. low impact
   c. non-impact
   d. suspended

5. Power tucks are variations of movements performed in levels I, II, and III that always increase the impact level.

   a. True
   b. False

6. Land tempo, sometimes cued as ________________, is the same speed of movement used on land.

   a. double time
   b. doubles
   c. bounce center
   d. half time

7. Crossing the arms over the chest while water walking is an example of using the arms in what manner?

   a. Changing typical arm and leg patterns
   b. Creating arm combinations or patterns
   c. Neutral arm position
   d. All of these

8. You can add variety to arm patterns in five basic ways. Which option makes it easier for participants to maintain proper alignment?

9. _______________movements are performed in an upright position, and involve impacting movements where both feet are off the pool bottom for a brief period of time.

   a. Grounded
   b. Level I
   c. Level II
   d. Level III

10. Plyometrics performed in the water can be referred to as _________.

   a. suspended movements
   b. double-time movements
   c. propelled movement
   d. level III movements

See appendix D for answers to review questions.

References and Resources

Batterham, S., S. Heywood, and J. Keating. 2011. Systematic review and meta-analysis comparing land and aquatic exercise for people with hip or knee arthritis on function, mobility and other health outcomes. *BMC Musculoskeletal Disorders* 12:123.

Campbell, J., L. D'Acquisto, D. D'Acquisto, and M. Cline. 2003. Metabolic and cardiovascular response to shallow water exercise in young and older women. *Medicine & Science in Sports & Exercise* 35(4):675-681.

Clemens, C.A., and C.J. Cisar. 2006. The effect of footwear on the reliability of the 500-yard shallow water run as a predictor of maximal aerobic capacity ($\dot{V}O_2$max). *AEA Aquatic Fitness Research Journal* 3(1):36-39.

D'Acquisto, L., D. D'Acquisto, and D. Renne. 2001. Metabolic and cardiovascular responses in older women during shallow-water exercise. *Journal of Strength and Conditioning Research* 15(1):12-19.

Denomme, L., and J. See. 2006. *AEA instructor skills*. 2nd edition. Nokomis, FL: Aquatic Exercise Association.

Fleck, S., and W. Kraemer. 2003. *Designing resistance training programs*. 3rd edition. Champaign, IL: Human Kinetics.

Howley, E.T., and D.L. Thompson. 2012. *Fitness professional's handbook*. 6th edition. Champaign, IL: Human Kinetics. Igbanugo, V., and B. Gutin. 1978. The energy cost of aerobic dancing. *Research Quarterly. American Alliance for Health, Physical Education and Recreation* 49(3):308-316.

Kinder, T., and J. See. 1992. *Aqua aerobics: A scientific approach*. Peosta, IA: Bowers.

Kravitz, L. 1994. The effects of music in exercise. *IDEA Today magazine* 12(9):56-61.

Lindle, J. 2002a. *Turn up the heat*. Instructor training workshop. West Harrison, IN: Fitness Learning Systems.

———. 2002b. *Waved water choreography*. Instructor training workshop. West Harrison, IN: Fitness Learning Systems.

Martel, G., M. Harmer, J. Logan, and C. Parker. 2005. Aquatic plyometric training increases vertical jump in female volleyball players. *Medicine & Science in Sports & Exercise* 37(10):1814-1819.

Miller, M., C. Cheatham, A. Porter, M. Ricard, D. Hennigar, and D. Berry. 2007. Chest-and waist-deep aquatic plyometric training and average force, power, and vertical-jump performance. *International Journal of Aquatic Research and Education* 1(2): 6.

Nagle, E., M. Sanders, A. Shafer, B. Barone Gibbs, J. Nagle, A. Deldin, B. Franklin, and

R. Robertson. 2013. Energy expenditure, cardiorespiratory, and perceptual responses to shallow-water aquatic exercise in young adult women. *The Physician and Sportsmedicine* 41(3):67-76.

Reddy, H., and D. Maniazhagu. 2015. Effects of low intensity of aquatic and land plyometric training on speed. *International Journal of Physical Education Sports Management and Yogic Sciences* 5(1):16-19.

Robinson, L., S. Devor, M. Merrick, and J. Buckworth. 2004. The effects of land vs. aquatic plyometrics on power, torque, velocity, and muscle soreness in women. *Journal of Strength & Conditioning Research* 18(1):84-91.

Sardinha, U., M. Pinheiro, and V. Szejnfeld. 2013. Comparison of the effectiveness of exercise practice in and out of the water on the knee muscle strength of women with rheumatoid arthritis. Research poster presentation at the International Aquatic Fitness Conference, Palm Harbor, FL, May 14-18, 2013.

See, J. 1997. *Successful strategies*. Instructor training workshop. Nokomis, FL: Innovative Aquatics.

———. 1998. *Teaching with a full deck*. Instructor training workshop. Nokomis, FL: Innovative Aquatics.

———. 2002. *Get decked*. Instructor training workshop. Nokomis, FL: Innovative Aquatics.

Sova, R. 2000. *Aquatics: The complete reference guide for aquatic fitness professionals*. 2nd edition. Pt. Washington, WI: DSL.

Stemm, J., and B. Jacobson. 2007. Comparison of land-and aquatic-based plyometric training on vertical jump performance. *Journal of Strength & Conditioning Research* 21(2):568-571.

Triplett, N., J. Colado, J. Benavent, Y. Alakhdar, J. Madera, L. Gonzalez, and V. Tella. 2009. Concentric and impact forces of single-leg jumps in an aquatic environment versus on land. *Medicine & Science in Sports & Exercise* 41(9):1790-1796.

Wilmoth, S. 1986. *Leading aerobics dance exercise*. Champaign, IL: Human Kinetics.

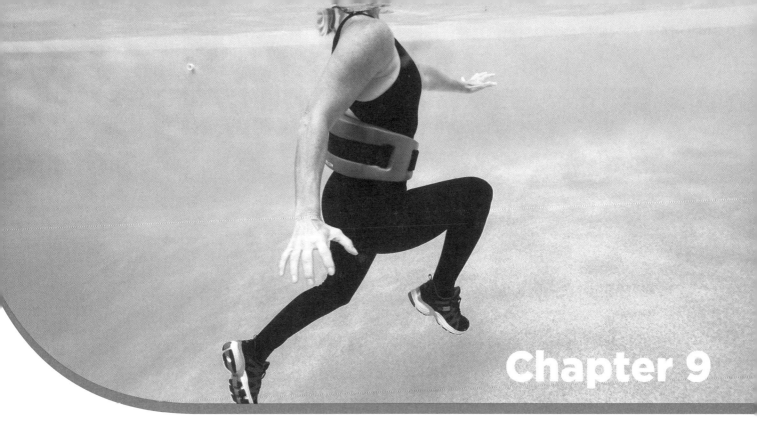

Chapter 9

Deep-Water Exercise

Introduction

This chapter is devoted to **deep-water exercise**—non-impact training that can offer a full range of exercise challenges. Aquatic programming in deep water has evolved from the most basic deep-water running programs to very popular and creative formats that use effective equipment options and serve a range of target markets. Deep water provides an excellent training modality for all ages and abilities and is well supported by a growing body of research. Specialized programming can be geared toward older adults, people with back problems, obese participants, and marathon runners, to name just a few. Deep water is both an enjoyable and an effective aquatic training medium for a full range of participants.

Key Chapter Concepts

- Define deep-water and transitional depth training.
- Understand current deep-water training research relating to cardiorespiratory effects, effort and energy expenditure, and form.
- Learn variations to the three lower-body base moves used in deep water and how these differ from shallow-water exercise.
- Understand the various methods for incorporating safe and effective upper-body movements in deep water.
- Recognize non-impact exercise variations achieved through body positioning.
- Define and apply the various deep-water tempo options.
- Recognize the key concepts that set deep-water, non-impact training apart from shallow-water exercise.
- Recognize the importance of participant evaluation for deep-water safety and understand how to teach vertical recovery techniques.

Defining Deep-Water Training

Deep-water exercise is traditionally defined as an exercise program performed suspended in water at a depth that allows the participant to remain vertical while not touching the bottom of the pool. This type of aquatic exercise is normally conducted in water ranging from 6.5 to 10 feet (2–3 m) deep; however, various depths can work for different clients. The term deep water may be a little misleading because most deep-water exercises can be performed in water that is a few inches *less* than the participant's height, since the body is suspended with the head above the water's surface. Water depth should allow the body to move freely through range of motion and intensity variations without the feet contacting the pool bottom. A flotation device is typically worn for neutral buoyancy, which allows the participant to concentrate on working against the drag properties of the water as opposed to trying to stay afloat. Participants can move freely in all three planes of motion, creating a total-body workout, muscle balance, and a substantial challenge for the core muscles without impact stress to the joints.

Some facilities cannot accommodate deep-water exercise; however, they may have areas of **transitional water depths**. Transitional water depth is too deep for typical shallow-water exercise, yet too shallow for conventional deep-water exercise. **Transitional depth training** is not considered traditional shallow-water programming because the participant is not rebounding off the pool bottom. It is not considered traditional deep-water exercise because the participant touches the bottom of the pool during some movements (similar to level II movements but with less hip and knee flexion). Thus, the term transitional describes water exercise performed in pools with water depths between 4 and 6 feet (1.2–1.8 m). Flotation equipment may be used, and shoes are recommended because there is some contact with the pool floor. Options for transitional pool depths can include altering lever length, range of motion, or arm patterns to achieve desired intensity.

Deep-water training gained popularity in the 1980s and 1990s as an alternative for athletes who had sustained an injury and were trying to maintain their fitness level. Interestingly enough, injury continues to be the primary factor for athletes entering the water for workouts; however, now it is for prevention as well as recovery. From this foundation, deep-water exercise has grown in popularity for both the athletic and general populations. Its growth has propelled research into its effectiveness. Although the majority of deep-water research investigates deep-water running, other areas of suspended exercise have been explored.

Deep-Water Exercise Research and Application

Two primary considerations make deep-water exercise different from shallow-water exercise: the level of immersion and lack of contact with the pool bottom. These two variables create a ripple effect in physiological changes that manifest throughout the body. Heart rate response, body mechanics, and immersing and offloading the joints establish new parameters for the instructor to consider. The following sections discuss the application of current research results for safe and effective deep-water programming.

Cardiorespiratory Effects

Research indicates that deep-water exercise, when performed at the proper intensity and duration, produces favorable health benefits and serves as a viable training option for maintaining or improving physical fitness (Killgore 2012). With this in mind, some cardiorespiratory considerations should be accounted for when designing and implementing a deep-water exercise program.

Heart Rate

Notable changes in heart rate response during deep-water exercise are due to heat dissipation as well as the effects of hydrostatic pressure and lack of gravitational forces. Generally, when compared to land-based training, deep-water heart rate response is lower during both maximal and submaximal exercise. There is a larger discrepancy in heart rate during maximal exercise than submaximal exercise. In fact, some studies support the idea that submaximal exercising heart rates remain consistent with heart rates during exercise on land (Killgore 2012).

This is important if you use heart rate to gauge exercise intensity or if your participants use heart rate monitors. If you are using heart rate to determine intensity, then the target heart rate may be lower than that experienced on land. Consider using the Kruel Aquatic Heart Rate Deduction (see appendix E) to individualize participants' target heart rates. For participants using heart rate monitors, explain the effects of the water on heart rate to help them understand possible discrepancies between land and water heart rate responses. At the same time, reassure them that similar fitness results are achieved in water.

Oxygen Consumption ($\dot{V}O_2$)

Oxygen consumption ($\dot{V}O_2$) is a direct measure of how well your body uses oxygen. It is the best measurement of cardiorespiratory, or aerobic, fitness. Although this measurement is not commonly used for group fitness classes, it is frequently used to measure cardiorespiratory fitness during research. Therefore, it provides us with an understanding of changes in fitness from deep-water exercise. (Maximal oxygen uptake, $\dot{V}O_2max$, is discussed in chapter 1.)

As with heart rate response, $\dot{V}O_2$ during deep-water training is markedly lower for maximal exercise and similar for submaximal exercise when compared to land training. However, with appropriate exercise design, $\dot{V}O_2$ can be maintained (athletes and very fit populations) or improved (sedentary or less fit populations). These findings hold true only if the level of exercise is appropriate. You should plan programming that demands greater levels of effort to gain improvements in cardiorespiratory fitness ($\dot{V}O_2$). As an example, training sessions for an athlete should closely resemble the intensity, duration, and frequency of land-based training or should incorporate a similar training volume in the combination of land and water training.

Effort, Perceived Effort, and Energy Expenditure of Deep-Water Exercise

Effort, or conscious exertion, can be measured by physical or subjective means. Heart rate and $\dot{V}O_2$ are two physical ways of measuring effort, while rating of perceived exertion (RPE) is a subjective method for measuring effort. (RPE is discussed in more detail in chapter 1.) Research supports the effectiveness of using the RPE scale for gauging intensity and effort during deep-water exercise. However, some studies report a higher RPE value for deep water when compared to the same intensity on land (DeMaere and Ruby 1997; Dowzer et al. 1999; Frangolias and Rhodes 1995; Killgore et al. 2006). It is suggested that RPE values could be 1 to 3 points higher during deep-water exercise than during land-based training (Killgore 2012). This increase in perceived effort might be due to higher blood lactate levels, a key marker for muscular fatigue, in addition to the added multidirectional resistance exerted by the water (Frangolias and Rhodes 1995; Glass et al. 1995; Michaud et al. 1995; Svendenhag and Seger 1992). It is hypothesized that working the arms and legs against the water's resistance might create more anaerobic energy use and explain the higher RPE in both trained and untrained subjects.

When teaching deep-water classes, be aware of the increased perception of work (higher RPE) and the possible accumulation of lactic acid that may reflect as muscle fatigue. You might want to incorporate active recovery periods to allow for lactic acid removal; thus, an interval format is one method that works well for deep-water training.

Energy expenditure is closely connected with effort. The harder participants work, the more calories they will burn. During deep-water exercise, caloric expenditure varies between 8.8 (lower intensity) and 18.9 (higher intensity) kilocalories per minute, or 528 to 1,134 kilocalories per hour, for most cardiorespiratory class formats (Coad et al. 1987; Demaere and Ruby 1997). On land, caloric expenditure is highly dependent on body weight as well as intensity and duration. In comparison, most land-based group fitness classes average between 3.9 and 12.3 (Igbanugo and Gutin 1978) kilocalories per minute, or 234 to 738 kilocalories per hour. In relation to energy expenditure, weight loss and favorable changes in body fat and girth have been shown with the inclusion of deep-water exercise (da Silva Medeiros et al. 2016; Pasetti, Gonçalves, and Padovani 2012).

Form

Form, otherwise known as biomechanics, is an area of concern for all varieties of exercise. Form can be compromised during deep-water exercise due to many different variables. Deep-water exercise is very different in relation to **proprioception** (the body's ability to sense internal and external changes and to initiate appropriate responses), grounding forces, and overall body mechanics.

When fully suspended, some people may not have adequate body awareness for maintaining the appropriate posture. This could be from the lack of physical contact with the pool bottom, which results in reduced proprioceptive feedback from the gravity-impacted joints. The absence of compressive forces (non-impact) doesn't allow the joints to assist in providing proprioceptive information as they would on land (Mergner and Rosemeier 1998) or in shallow water. This means that the body has to create a new method of understanding where it is and how it is moving (Roll et al. 1998). Therefore, allow an adaptation period for new participants in deep-water exercise. During this time, participants should learn the biomechanics and proper form of the exercises without focusing on intensity.

Form is not only an important attribute for safety considerations, it also has been found to be a contributing factor in caloric expenditure. Because the density of water is 800 times that of air (Di Prampero 1986), the water provides greater resistance to movement; this resistance can be increased with the speed and surface area (Di Prampero 1986; Shanebrook and Jaszczak 1975) of the moving object. Many studies have illustrated that an experienced deep-water participant is able to elicit a greater caloric expenditure, produce a more comparative heart rate and $\dot{V}O_2$ to land exercise, and even mimic land-based patterns with greater effectiveness (Chu and Rhodes 2001; Frangolias and Rhodes 1995, Reilly, Dowzer, and Cable 2003) than a novice deep-water exerciser.

Deep-Water Base Moves

Most exercises that are performed on land or in shallow water can be performed in deep water as well. A key difference is lack of contact with the pool bottom and the inability to rebound. However, in deep water, you will still use the pool bottom to reference correct body alignment and foot placement.

As discussed in chapter 8, the three primary categories of lower-body base movements are focused on how the body lands or makes contact with the pool bottom. In deep water, participants will not land on their feet. Instead, you will instruct participants to move into the desired position using the pool bottom as a reference for foot placement. Thus, deep-water base movements can be categorized as the following:

- Moves that use an alternating foot pattern
- Moves that use a double-foot pattern: Both legs or feet simultaneously perform the same (e.g., deep-water jack) or opposition (e.g., cross-country ski) action
- Moves that use a repeated single-foot pattern

Table 9.1 demonstrates common variations of base moves for the legs appropriate for deep water. Refer to appendix B for a description and pictures of several of these moves.

Deep-water base moves can be used to create fun and challenging choreography, construct exciting interval workouts, target muscular resistance, and achieve a multitude of other program goals. Because there is no contact with the pool bottom, cueing to achieve the correct body position is very important. Movements of the arms and hands can provide assistance with maintaining or achieving appropriate alignment. For this reason, you must give careful thought to selecting upper-body movements.

The base moves or joint actions of the shoulders and elbows are the same in deep water as in shallow water (refer back to table 8.2). Using the arms in various ways (see table 9.2) can promote a wide range of benefits. However, additional considerations should be taken when designing arm-focused exercises for deep water.

- Ensure that participants have the body control to perform specific arm and leg actions simultaneously. Some participants may need to rely on the arms for stabilization and body alignment.

Table 9.1 Variations of Deep-Water Base Moves for the Lower Body

Moves with alternating foot pattern	Moves with double-foot pattern	Moves that use a repeated single-foot pattern
Narrow jog	Deep-water jacks	Knee swings
Wide jog	Cross-country skis	Kick swings
Jog out, out, in, in	Modified hurdles	Cancan *(knee lift, return to neutral, front kick, return to neutral)*
Crossing jog	Flutter kicks	Repeaters for one-footed moves *(performing multiple repetitions on one side before changing lead leg)*
Knee lifts	Moguls	
Kicks	Tuck front to back *(tuck knees and shoot legs forward, then tuck knees and shoot legs behind, as if jumping over a log)*	
Leg curls		
Ankle reach front		
Heel reach behind		
Cha-cha *(3 quick jogs and a pause)*		

Table 9.2 Examples of Arm Use for Deep-Water Exercise

Change typical arm and leg patterns.	Combine cross-country ski legs with transverse shoulder abduction and adduction.
Create arm combinations or patterns. Keep the leg movement the same, but change the arms.	Jogging legs with arm combination, where both arms move together: Count 1 = Shoulder flexion Count 2 = Shoulder transverse abduction Count 3 = Shoulder transverse adduction Count 4 = Shoulder extension
Use the arms above the water's surface.	Flutter kick with alternating single-arm reach overhead.
Hold the arms in a neutral position neither assist nor impede the leg movement.	Cross-country ski legs with the arms crossed on the chest.
Float the arms on the surface of the water or scull under the water to assist with body position, alignment and balance.	Moguls legs while arms scull to maintain balance.

- If the arms are taken above the water's surface, the participant will find it challenging to maintain neutral buoyancy on most exercises. The action of lifting the arms up out of the water pushes the body downward; this may result in the participant's head going under the water. Unless actively counteracting the downward force with a specific lower-body exercise, such as a whip kick or flutter kick, using the arms above the water's surface may not be an appropriate choice for all participants.

Non-Impact Water Exercise

All deep-water movements are suspended; thus, all exercises are non-impact. However, we can vary the body positions and mimic shallow-water impact options. This can be especially helpful when instructing a class where some participants are in deep water, while others are in shallow water.

Let's look at a cross-country ski for a comparison of movements.

- Performing the ski in deep water with the body aligned and vertical with longer levers and soft joints is similar to the shallow-water level I body position. Remember that in deep water, there will be no impact.
- Maintaining proper alignment but with exaggerated hip and knee flexion in deep water is similar to shallow-water level II body positioning, again, without the impact.
- Two options exist for providing a deep-water option similar to shallow-water level III exercises that require more core and upper-body involvement. Option 1: Maintain the flexed hip and knee positioning, but add more emphasis on upper-body movement (such as powerful sculling). Attempt to lift the body higher in the water—bring the shoulders above the water's surface. Option 2: Maintain the flexed hip and knee positioning, but lift the hands out of the water. This requires more core stability and more powerful movements of the legs to keep the body positioned and the head above water.
- Although grounding is not possible during deep-water exercise, you can mimic shallow-water grounded exercises by visualizing contact with the pool bottom. With the cross-country ski example, one leg remains vertically extended (as if standing on the pool bottom) while the other performs the ski action. This adds more focus to the stabilization musculature of the lower body and core, and is a good option for repeated single-leg movements.

• Plyometric movements are impossible in deep water due to the lack of contact with the pool bottom. However, you can still use acceleration to propel the body upward by using the limbs to apply force against the water, similar to shallow-water propelled movements. For the cross-country ski, instruct your participants to drive the legs together as quickly as possible to create an upward movement (popping out of the water).

• Power tucks are performed the same way in deep water as in shallow water, using acceleration to emphasize movement under the water to increase the muscular effort. The knees pull forcefully toward the chest (tucking the knees toward the body) and then the legs push forcefully away and toward the pool bottom while moving in the cross-country ski action.

Deep-Water Tempo Options

As with shallow-water exercise, deep-water training has a variety of tempo options. Land tempo, water tempo, half water tempo, and cadence are all used in deep water (see chapter 8 for further explanation of tempos). These tempo options in deep water have similarities and differences when it comes to exercise execution. Form and body mechanics remain the primary consideration when selecting movement tempo.

Land Tempo (LT)

Land tempo (see table 9.3), or pairing an action with every beat of the music, is performed exactly in deep water as it would be in shallow-water exercise. This tempo can be both fun and effective when participants can maintain correct form and alignment. Use short-lever movements or movements with a purposeful reduction in range of motion when performing exercises at land tempo. You should also consider movement transitions for safety and alignment (refer to chapter 10 for details on safe transitions).

Water Tempo (WT)

Water tempo (see table 9.4) involves movement on every other beat of the music. It is the primary tempo used for both shallow-water and deep-water exercise. This tempo ensures the ability to move against the water's resistance with good alignment and through the entire joint range of motion. This is even more important in deep-water exercise. With the body suspended in the water,

Table 9.3 Land Tempo (LT) Movements

Move	Beat 1	Beat 2	Beat 3	Beat 4	Beat 5	Beat 6	Beat 7	Beat 8
Deep-water jack	Out	In	Out	In	Out	In	Out	In
Cross-country ski	Right	Left	Right	Left	Right	Left	Right	Left
Knee lift	Right	Left	Right	Left	Right	Left	Right	Left

**8 land tempo beats

Table 9.4 Water Tempo (WT) Movements

Move	Beat 1	Beat 2	Beat 3	Beat 4	Beat 5	Beat 6	Beat 7	Beat 8
Deep-water jack	Out		In		Out		In	
Cross-country ski	Right		Left		Right		Left	
Knee lift	Right		Left		Right		Left	

**8 land tempo beats

it is not necessary to fully extend the hip or knee to support the body; thus, participants are more likely to reduce range of motion.

Half Water Tempo (1/2 WT)

In shallow-water exercise, half water tempo can be performed in two ways: with a center bounce between movements (e.g., cross-country ski with bounce center) or a holding bounce or a double movement (e.g., cross-country ski, bounce in that position, switch legs, bounce in that position). Although you can't perform a bounce in deep water, you can add a pause (see table 9.5).

In our cross-country ski example, instead of the center bounce, you could perform the ski with the right leg forward, bring both legs together in a neutral position and pause for a single count, ski with left leg forward, and then return to neutral for the pause. This pause clearly engages the core muscles to stabilize the body in an upright position. Alternatively, you could perform the ski with the right leg forward, tuck both knees center (pause), ski with left leg forward, and tuck both knees center (pause). We also have the option to use half water tempo in deep water with a double movement (e.g., ski with right leg forward and pause, switch leg positions and pause with the left leg forward). On this double move, you may choose to include a gentle pulse on the pause. This tempo requires greater stabilization and helps to emphasize greater range of motion for the lower body, specifically the hips and knees.

Cadence

Cadence, or the rate of movement, is commonly used for deep-water running, but it can be employed for a variety of movements. Whether using the music's beat, a metronome, or a self-selected cadence, the general concept is that you begin with a set cadence and then increase or decrease the rate of that cadence. When music is used, participants can execute the movements using either the LT beat or the WT beat. Having your music stored on a smartphone or other device allows you to use an app to adjust the beats per minute (bpm). You can gradually increase or decrease the bpm as appropriate. Or you may choose to use a metronome. Consider an example: Ask participants to begin jogging to a set metronome cadence of 80 bpm; every 30 seconds, increase that cadence by 2 bpm until reaching 100 bpm.

Another option allows participants to self-select a starting cadence. In this case, the participants count their repetitions performed during a set time period, for example, 10 seconds. You would then ask your participants to increase their cadence by a specified number (e.g., 1, 2, 3). During the next 10-second interval, their goal would be to

Table 9.5 Half Water Tempo (1/2 WT) Movements

Move	Beat 1	Beat 2	Beat 3	Beat 4	Beat 5	Beat 6	Beat 7	Beat 8
Deep-water jack	Out		Pause out		In		Pause in	
Cross-country ski (double ski)	Right		Pause right forward		Left		Pause left forward	
Cross-country ski (ski pause center)	Right		Pause center, legs vertical		Left		Pause center, legs vertical	
Cross-country ski (ski pause center)	Right		Pause center, knees tucked		Left		Pause center, knees tucked	
Knee lift (double knee)	Right		Pause right up		Left		Pause left up	
Knee lift (knee pause center)	Right		Pause center		Left		Pause center	

**8 land tempo beats

increase repetitions accordingly. Performing more repetitions over the same period of time requires moving at a faster cadence. This self-selected option allows for participants with a wide variety of fitness levels to reach their potential during any cadence drill.

The use of cadence is very effective in increasing the effort of the exercise being performed as long as the range of motion is maintained. It is imperative to cue and to continue cueing participants to maintain the range of motion throughout the variations in cadence. Remember, if you are using cadence for longer lever movements, the cadence will be slower due to the longer levers.

Deep-Water Considerations

The following sections discuss applications that differentiate deep-water training from shallow-water formats. Although all aquatic formats share many similarities, several important concepts set deep-water, non-impact training apart.

Total Immersion

The most basic principle to remember is that the body is immersed in a predominantly unnatural environment. Total immersion (to neck depth) is not a normal placement for the body, and yet it is the very first part of the deep-water experience. Everything slows down; the body takes longer to begin a movement pattern, sustain repetitions, and make any kind of change. Because there is no contact with the pool bottom, neurological processes must find new pathways for successful completion of tasks, from the simplest one of staying vertical to the potentially complex movement patterns of the exercises. Instructors should not ignore the moment of immersion. It is the first step into deep water, and factors significantly in the teaching of deep-water alignment and exercise technique.

A learning curve is associated with exercising in this new environment. Familiarization sessions allow new participants to acclimate to deep water and to learn how their body reacts to total immersion (Azevedo et al. 2010; Kilgore et al. 2010). During this familiarization period, participants are instructed on how to move without concentrating on intensity. By concentrating on form, body mechanics, and alignment without focusing on exertion level, participants can learn how to move safely and effectively with little risk of injury. The number of exercise sessions needed to gain familiarity with suspended movement and comfort in deep water will be different for each person. People accustomed to water (previous swimmers or shallow-water exercisers) may require less time to acclimate, while those who have not participated in aquatic activities will probably require more time.

Body Awareness

Humans are bipedal, and the erect stance is fundamental to function. Regardless of exercise modality, improved functional capacity on land must be at the top of the list of goals. Placing the body in a vertical position in water maintains a familiar organizational strategy for spatial orientation (figure 9.1). Head above shoulders, shoulders above hips,

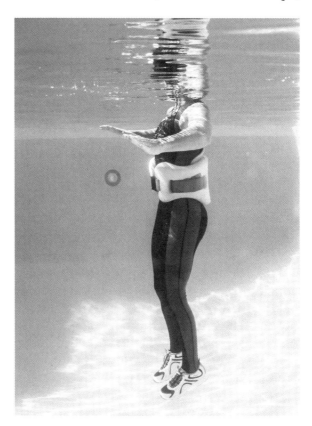

Figure 9.1 Correct deep-water alignment.

hips above knees, and knees above ankles is normal human body orientation. Maintaining this upright position helps the body deal with the unfamiliar characteristics of deep-water immersion, including lack of contact with the pool bottom and the diminished effect of gravity.

When cueing for this upright body position, you are referencing the five bony landmarks of neutral postural alignment. However, instructors rarely call out "mastoid process over acromion process." Instead, instructors say, "ears in line with shoulders," replacing the anatomical language with everyday words that will help participants achieve the same result.

In deep water, the vertical working position should reflect the exact same alignment, but the positioning is typically taught in a dynamic, rather than static, setting. For instance, if the legs are moving in an alternating jogging action, the instructor needs to cue the placement of the legs so they maintain vertical alignment (figure 9.2). For a stationary jogging action, cues would include the following:

- Raise each knee toward the chest in front of the body.
- Bend the knee so the ankle is posterior of (behind) the knee.
- Fully extend each leg so it returns to the vertical line.

Common mistakes to look for and correct include:

- Collapsing the chest toward the hips. Practice elongating the body and give cues for maximum space between the pelvis and the rib cage.
- Kicking the heels up behind the body, which might cause a compensatory anterior pelvic tilt and resultant lower-back arch because the body is falling forward. Correct this by asking for a higher lift of the knees in front and placement of the ankle posterior of the knee (but not behind the body).
- Lifting the knee with the foot in front of the knee and not returning each leg to the fully extended position under the body. In this scenario, participants feel that they are falling backward, and will probably curl forward and project the chin to compensate. Although the degree of hip flexion is good, cue for more knee flexion so the heel is posterior to the knee. Reinforce hip and knee extension so the body returns to the vertical line with each repetition.

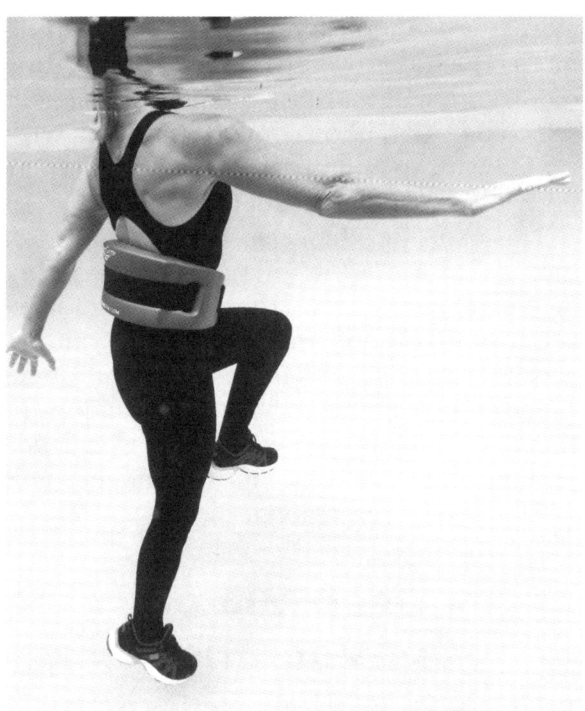

Figure 9.2 Correct leg action for deep-water jogging.

The deep-water jack, another commonly used movement, should reflect a similar movement pattern and alignment as a jumping jack performed in shallow water or on land. The hips and shoulders abduct and adduct while the body remains vertical. Although this exercise can be performed with arms and legs moving through abduction and adduction simultaneously, the body tends to bob up and down, especially when greater force is applied against the water. Thus, participants may prefer moving the arms and legs in opposition (i.e., abducting the arms while the legs are adducting) to maintain neutral buoyancy (figure 9.3).

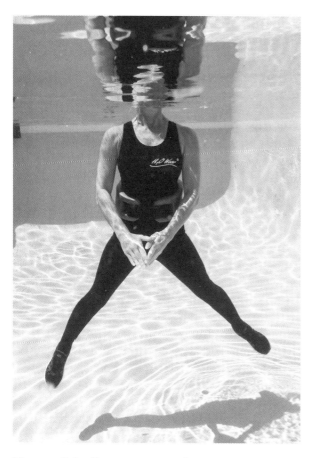

Figure 9.3 Deep-water jack using opposition arms and legs.

With these concepts in mind, cues for a deep-water jack may include the following:

- Begin with the legs together and the arms abducted and near the water's surface (T position).
- As the legs abduct, the arms adduct. Then, reverse the movement.
- Keep the shoulders, hips, knees, and ankles in line when the legs are together.
- Engage the core muscles to keep the body tall.
- Maintain a slight bend at the knees and elbows.

Of course, you may not use all of these cues at one time; instead, select cues that can assist and correct any mistakes you may be observing. Some of the common mistakes to watch for include the following:

- Flexing at the hips and allowing the legs to come in front of the body, which will look like a seated jack. Cue participants to extend the hips so that the ankles and feet are directly aligned with the shoulders, hips, and knees.
- Bending the knees and elbows too much. This reduces the effort of the movement. Unless the participant needs to reduce intensity, encourage long limbs but soft joints.
- Allowing the legs to drift behind the body so that the heels are behind the hips. This results in hyperextension of the lower back. Cue participants to engage the core, contract the gluteal muscles, and bring the ankles and feet below the hips.
- Not completing the full movement (i.e., limiting the range of motion during hip abduction and adduction). This reduces the overall training effect and limits the physical gains at the joints being worked. Cue participants to move through a full range of motion with good alignment, reducing the movement speed if necessary.
- Leaning the upper body forward. Often due to lack of postural muscle strength, this can lead to excess strain on the back, hips, and neck. Reinforce tall posture, engaged abdominals, and lengthened spine.

These alignment issues are unique to deep water because the feet do not touch the pool bottom. In shallow water, it is easier to maintain alignment because participants naturally bring the foot down under the body, just as they do on land.

Dynamic Stabilization

Dynamic stabilization is the body's ability to maintain neutral, or near neutral, postural alignment (a stable position) while moving. In the majority of activities performed, a structurally safe position for the core of the body is attempted before overload is added. Neutral postural alignment is a position that places the spine in its strongest, safest alignment. This vertically aligned position in deep water allows a centering from which other movements are possible without causing injury. The lack of contact with the pool bottom in deep water causes the body to use a totally new neuromuscular strategy to achieve this neutral postural alignment.

This process translates into the following guidelines:

- At the beginning of class, allow time for the participants to establish the dynamic stabilization strategy through the postural muscles. This means offering non-traveling exercises at the start of class and gradually progressing to moving patterns while giving postural corrections to achieve neutral alignment.
- Frequently revisit neutral postural alignment, especially before challenging exercises in which high-intensity resistance is loaded on any of the limbs.
- To maximize stability, use basic transitions that pass through neutral position (as discussed in chapter 10).
- Make sure that the flotation belt or other equipment does not hinder a participant's ability to achieve neutral postural alignment.

Center of Buoyancy and Diminished Gravity

The diminished effect of gravity also plays a vital role in achieving good alignment for deep-water exercise. Remember that the force of gravity is still present; otherwise, the water would not stay in the pool. For the moving body, this means that we still have a center of gravity (the center of a body's mass) through which the body maintains equilibrium. On land, the body's center of gravity is located between the pelvic region and belly button. In shallow-water classes, participants can still maintain a base of support and keep the center of gravity low and within the base. As the water gets deeper, center of buoyancy (the center of a body's volume) starts to influence equilibrium and balance more than center of

Deep-Water Posture Strategy

On land and in shallow water, the proprioceptive mechanism by which you know whether you are standing upright and balanced primarily works through the ankle joints and actual contact with the ground. From a standing position, the brain receives continuous messages through the ankles. These messages to the central nervous system initiate a loop of proprioceptive feedback that control muscle tone and generate reflex responses. In simple terms, sensory receptors in the muscles, joints, and connective tissues gather information about the body's position, process that information, and enable the central nervous system to make the appropriate response. For example, when you are falling, proprioception allows the brain to know that the fall is occurring, activate the correct strategies to regain balance, and send the messages to the muscles to contract and avoid the fall. The muscles in the legs and feet contract to adjust positioning and regain balance.

In deep water, you can no longer use this strategy of proprioceptive feedback. The body now must use a different system to know if it is vertical and balanced. The messages to the brain no longer come through the feet and ankles. Instead, the core postural muscles play the key role in the new strategy for balance and correct alignment of the body. These muscle groups are active 100 percent of the time in deep water. Their activity is discreet but constant. Continuous contraction of the core muscles is the main reason why marked postural improvements are seen in people who regularly attend deep-water classes. Core stabilization also occurs in shallow water, but it is much more dynamic in deep water. You must understand this dynamic stabilization process to teach deep-water exercise effectively.

gravity does. We no longer have the feet in contact with the pool bottom or within the base of support.

Center of buoyancy is located in the chest region close to the pockets of air created by the lungs. In deep water, there is an interplay between the center of gravity and center of buoyancy. Gravity is a downward force and buoyancy is an upward force, so when a body is immersed in water, the two opposing forces are acting on the body. If you entered deep water and did nothing at all, the center of buoyancy and center of gravity would most likely place the body horizontal, facedown. When participants are asked to be in a vertical working position, the center of buoyancy and center of gravity move into vertical alignment. As the two centers line up, participants have a feeling of balance and equilibrium. Watch participants carefully as they make these alignment adjustments. Look for anything that might be causing difficulty, such as body composition, placement of flotation equipment, or the type of flotation used.

Placement of Flotation Equipment

A key issue in alignment considerations is the placement of flotation equipment on the immersed body. The addition of buoyancy affects equilibrium. Ultimately, the center of buoyancy and center of gravity relate to one another and determine if the participant is able to maintain a vertical position. Buoyancy belts and other flotation equipment promote better alignment of the center of buoyancy and center of gravity. When these points are aligned, appropriate posture and biomechanics are more easily maintained (Killgore 2012). Without appropriate buoyancy, people have the tendency to rely on the upper body for maintenance of body position and propulsion while reducing the exertion in the lower body (Killgore et al. 2010; Wilber et al. 1996).

The AEA Standards and Guidelines for Aquatic Fitness Programming (see text box) encourage flotation attached to the trunk or upper arms for optimal safety. Flotation belts are the most popular choice of flotation equipment for deep-water exercise. A variety of belts are sold that differ in buoyancy amount and distribution. Participants may need to try various types of belts before finding one that meets their needs.

- Participants with higher body fat might need a belt with a smaller amount of buoyancy or may not need a belt for flotation at all. These clients may need additional assistance with proper alignment.
- Muscular participants might need a belt with greater buoyancy, multiple belts (one fitting on the back and one fitting around the front overlapping one another), or additional flotation.
- Consider altering location of buoyancy to accommodate body fat distribution.

A well-fitting flotation belt will allow the participant to maintain the head above the water level with the body in a relaxed, motionless, vertical position. During inhalation and exhalation, the body will naturally rise and fall as air pressure changes within the lungs. During inhalation, the body rises slightly; it then sinks slightly on exhalation. When proper neutral buoyancy is established, this change in level is minimal. Also, the more relaxed participants remain and the more evenly and consistently they breathe, the easier it is for them to maintain the proper level in the water. Stabilizing the core while maintaining proper breathing patterns assists with correct alignment.

Adding equipment, such as submerged buoyant hand bars for upper-body strengthening exercises, also affects the established equilibrium. Recall that center of gravity and center of buoyancy are dynamic; they change when the body moves. When buoyancy equipment is added to an exercise, the participant must adapt by stabilizing and conforming to the changes related to the position of the body and the equipment. As in any type of water exercise, the participant's ability level will determine if additional resistance equipment is advisable. Carefully consider the participant's ability to stabilize and

AEA Standards and Guidelines for Aquatic Fitness Programming

Equipment Considerations

The AEA recommends that deep-water exercise be performed with flotation equipment attached to the trunk of the body (flotation belt or vest) or the upper arms (flotation upper arm cuffs specifically designed for water exercise). With proper progression and training, ankle cuffs may be an appropriate flotation option for some people. In deep water, flotation equipment that is attached to the body eliminates the potential for letting go of the buoyancy assistance device, even if the participant becomes panicked. Flotation equipment that requires the participant to hold on to the device, such as a noodle, a kickboard, or a set of hand bars, can create a false sense of well-being and could lead to a water rescue. The participant's swimming skills, core strength, and personal comfort in deep water should all be considered when choosing floatation equipment.

Handheld buoyancy equipment may be used for additional upper-body resistance in both shallow- and deep-water programs. If handheld buoyancy equipment is used, the AEA recommends providing options for participants who lack the ability or fitness level to use the equipment appropriately. Periods of training with the equipment submerged should be limited and frequent breaks should be incorporated into the workout. Cue participants to maintain neutral alignment of the wrists and avoid tight gripping of the equipment. Carefully observe and cue to make sure that proper alignment of the shoulder girdle is maintained, including scapular depression and retraction. The same recommendations apply if handheld flotation equipment is used for suspended training in shallow water.

maintain the appropriate body mechanics prior to introducing equipment other than the primary flotation device.

Balance

Balance is key in deep-water movement. Even without anchor points for the feet on the bottom of the pool, each movement still requires an end point. When you perform a cross-country ski, how do the legs know when to change direction? They are limited by personal range of motion and controlled by the movement and rhythm demonstrated by the instructor. If each leg is placed equidistant between the front and back of the body, the movement feels balanced. Symmetrical exercises are easier to perform because both sides of the body match. Thus, a deep-water jack feels comfortable because both legs do the same movement pattern at the same time. Symmetrical alternating exercises, such as running and cross-country skiing, are also balanced because both sides of the body performs the same action, just in an alternating sequence. See appendix B for deep-water exercise descriptions and photos.

Asymmetrical moves are more challenging because the uneven placement of the limbs in deep water often causes the trunk to shift away from a vertical position. For example, moguls, in which both legs are placed to one side of the body and then switched across to the other side, are more challenging to perform because the movement is asymmetrical (figure 9.4).

When the legs push to one side, the body naturally leans to the opposite side. As participants feel the body going off balance, they will attempt to maintain a vertical,

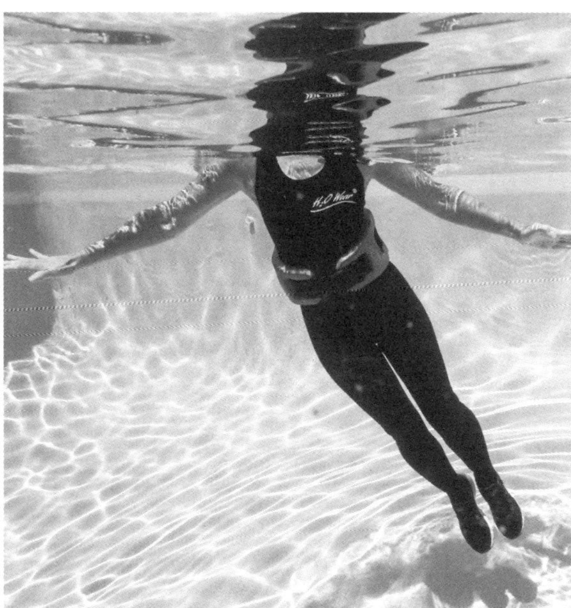

Figure 9.4 Correct form for a mogul.

balanced position, requiring the postural muscles of the trunk to work harder. Instructors can offer asymmetrical exercises with the intention of developing core strength; however, compromised body alignment is discouraged. Take care to select exercises that are appropriate for the population. Less-accomplished participants may react with uncontrolled or ballistic movements, potentially overstressing the postural muscles, particularly in the lower back.

Evaluate each exercise for postural integrity and decide if the move is suitable for the level of your participants. Including movement progressions and regressions is important when teaching a group with various levels of ability and fitness. Controlled, precise movements at an appropriate tempo with safe transitions will assist in maintaining balance and proper alignment.

Participant Evaluation and Safety

The aquatic environment offers a safe means to exercise for a wide variety of populations, yet it includes an inherent risk: water. Exercising in deep water adds a level of safety concern that should be addressed prior to entering the pool. You should evaluate each client's ability to participate in deep-water exercise comfortably and safely. You must consider their basic abilities regardless of the intensity level of your deep-water classes.

Since participants will not be touching the pool bottom, perform a quick assessment by asking each new participant a few simple questions:

- How comfortable are you in the water?
- What kind of experience do you have with water and water exercise?
- Can you swim?

These questions can give you important information to help determine if deep-water exercise is appropriate for participants, if extra evaluation is in order, or if they will require additional guidance before beginning the class.

In addition to these questions, discuss and practice vertical recovery techniques with all participants. Vertical recovery techniques allow participants to regain upright alignment in a safe and efficient manner. When participants do not have adequate body control or core strength, or if additional equipment hinders proper alignment, the result is often an unplanned prone or supine body position. Recovery from the prone position (lying facedown) involves three simple steps: (1) Tuck the knees into the chest, (2) extend the neck to look up, and (3) use the arms to assist the body upright (shoulder flexion) (figure 9.5). Similarly, recovery from the supine position (lying face up) requires three steps: (1) Tuck the knees into the chest, (2) tuck the chin to the chest, and (3) use the arms to assist the body upright (shoulder extension) (figure 9.6). Practicing these recovery techniques under controlled circumstances, possibly in shallow water first, affords a greater level of comfort to participants and the safety team (i.e., lifeguard, aquatic director, pool manager, instructor).

Table 9.6 covers some common problems and solutions related to deep-water exercise that should be evaluated and discussed with participants before starting.

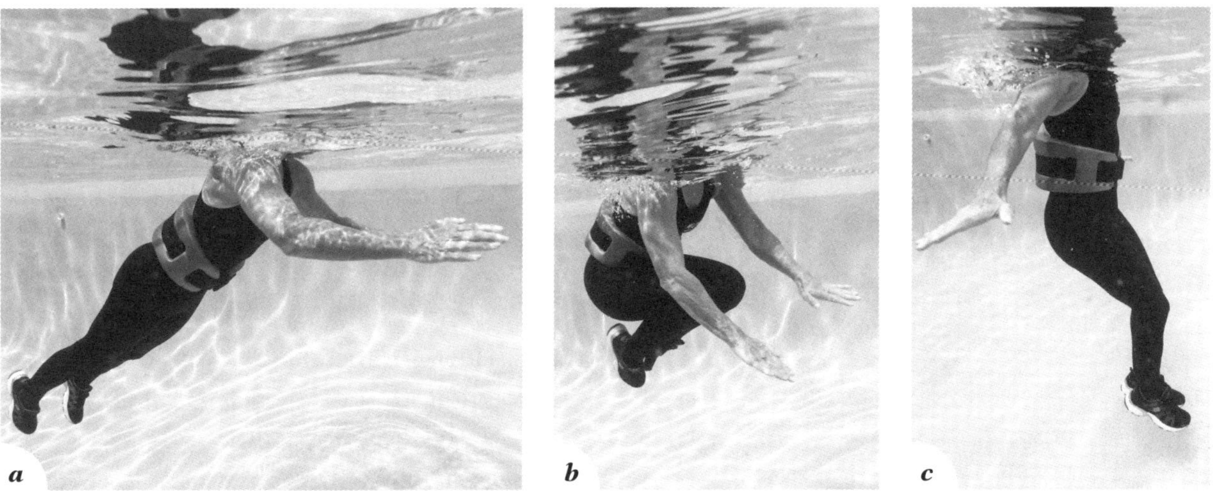

Figure 9.5 To recover from *(a)* the prone position, *(b)* tuck the knees into the chest and *(c)* use the arms to assist the body into an upright position.

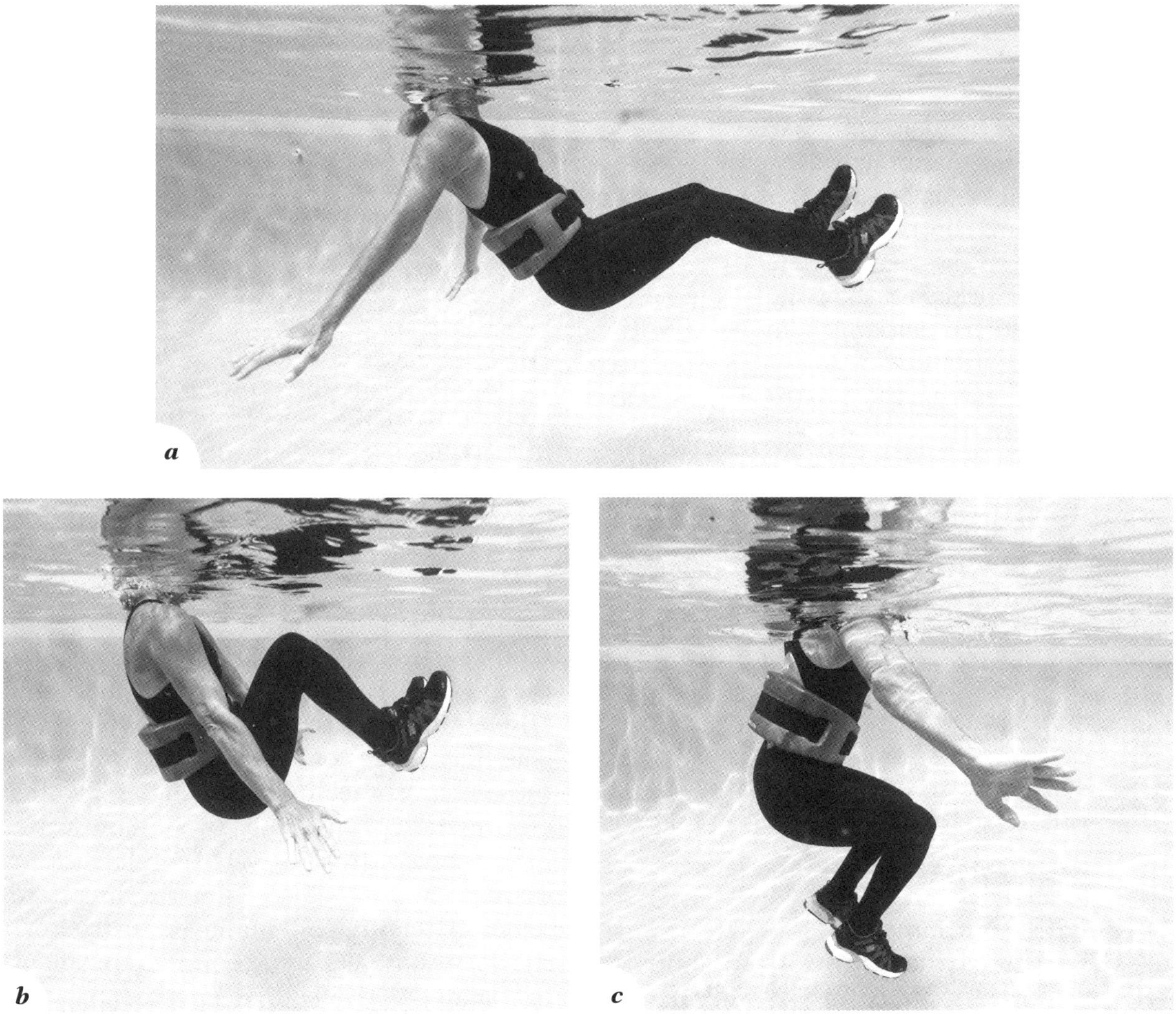

Figure 9.6 To recover from *(a)* the supine position, *(b)* tuck the knees to the chest, tuck the chin to the chest, and *(c)* use the arms to assist the body into an upright position.

Table 9.6 Concerns and Solutions for Deep-Water Exercise

Concern	Solution
Maintenance of vertical alignment	**Core stabilization:** Participants need both core strength and endurance. **Body awareness:** Participants will need an adaptation period to learn new strategies for posture maintenance. **Equipment:** Selection of flotation device and proper placement on the body will assist with vertical alignment.
Pool entry and exit	**Education:** Explain safe entry and exit options for the pool, including operation of chair lifts if needed. Participants should not jump or dive into the pool while wearing attached flotation equipment.
Participant is a non-swimmer or is uncomfortable in deep water	**Equipment:** Ensure that flotation equipment is properly fitted and provides ample buoyancy. Additional support equipment, such as a noodle, may provide comfort and stability. **Location:** Have the participant stay close to the pool wall for comfort. Or, consider beginning in a transitional depth and progressing to deep water when comfortable. **Education:** Teach vertical recovery techniques. **Introductions:** Introduce the safety team and show the participant where the lifeguard and you will be stationed during the class.

Participants who are not ready to directly enter a deep-water class could prepare for class integration with the following methods.

- Rehearse deep-water activities in shallow water. Introduce deep-water moves with buoyancy assistance in shallow water. Controlled opportunities to experience impact-free exercise can help participants overcome fears while becoming familiar with moves and equipment.
- Encourage development of trunk stabilizer muscles. Participation in shallow-water exercise or other core-strengthening programs can help participants strengthen the trunk stabilizers that will be required for a successful experience in deep water.
- Empower participants with self-rescue techniques. Teach them how to return to vertical from a back float and from a prone position. Explain how to control panic symptoms (e.g., "Lie back and relax until you are able to return to an upright position.").

Properly preparing participants for deep-water exercise will create a more enjoyable class experience, minimize safety issues, and increase program benefits.

Summary

Deep-water training is an exercise program performed suspended in water at a depth that allows the participant to remain vertical and yet not touch the bottom of the pool. Transitional depth training describes exercise performed in pools with water depths between 4 and 6 feet (1.2–1.8 m). In this type of training, flotation equipment may be used, although there is some contact with the pool floor.

Two primary considerations make deep-water exercise different from shallow-water exercise: the level of immersion and lack of contact with the pool bottom. Apply current research specific to deep-water exercise to develop safe and effective programming. Key areas of applicable and available research include cardiorespiratory effects; effort, perceived effort, and energy expenditure; and biomechanical considerations (form).

Three primary categories of lower-body base movements are used in deep water: moves that use an alternating foot pattern, moves that use a double-foot pattern, and moves that use a repeated single-foot pattern. Although there is no contact with the pool bottom, and rebound is eliminated, deep-water exercise still uses the pool bottom to reference correct body alignment and foot placement. Movements of the arms and hands can provide assistance with maintaining or achieving appropriate alignment.

All deep-water movements are suspended; thus, all exercises are non-impact. However, we can vary the body positions in deep-water exercise to mimic shallow-water impact options. Not only does this add variety to deep-water programs, these options can also assist when instructing classes that incorporate both water depths.

Deep-water tempo options are similar to those used in shallow-water exercise: land tempo, water tempo, half water tempo, and cadence. However, there are important differences in the performance of the movements since the feet do not touch the pool bottom.

The most basic principle of deep-water exercise is that the body is immersed in a predominantly unnatural environment where neurological processes must find new pathways for successful completion of tasks. In deep water, the vertical working position should reflect the exact same alignment as in land-based movement, but the positioning is generally taught in a dynamic, rather than static, setting (dynamic stabilization). Since deep-water exercise lacks contact with the pool bottom, the body must learn to use a totally new neuromuscular strategy to achieve neutral postural alignment.

As the water gets deeper, the center of buoyancy (the center of a body's volume) starts to influence equilibrium and balance more than the center of gravity. A feeling of balance and equilibrium is noticed when the center of buoyancy and the center of gravity are vertically aligned. The addition of buoyancy, including flotation belts, also affects equilibrium and balance.

Symmetrical exercises are easier to perform because both sides of the body are performing the same movement, either together (e.g., deep-water jack) or in an alternating sequence (e.g., cross-country ski). Asymmetrical moves (e.g., moguls) are more challenging because the uneven placement of the limbs in deep water often causes the trunk to shift away from vertical.

It is important to evaluate a client's ability to participate in deep-water exercise comfortably and safely. Discuss and practice vertical recovery techniques with all participants. Consider the basic abilities of your participants regardless of the intensity level of your classes.

Review Questions

1. With transitional depth training, participants do not rebound off the pool bottom. However, they may touch the bottom of the pool during some movements.

    a. True
    b. False

2. When compared to land training, deep-water training shows higher oxygen consumption ($\dot{V}O_2$) for maximal exercise and submaximal exercise.
   a. True
   b. False
3. Form is not only an important attribute for safety considerations, it also has been found to be a contributing factor in ____________________.
4. Deep-water base movements can be categorized as moves that use an alternating foot pattern, moves that use a double-foot pattern, and moves that use a repeated single-foot pattern.
   a. True
   b. False
5. ____________________________is the body's ability to maintain neutral, or near neutral, postural alignment (a stable position) while moving.
   a. Dynamic stabilization
   b. Dynamic training
   c. Suspended stabilization
   d. Vertical alignment
6. In deep water, the core postural muscles play the key role in maintaining balance and correct alignment of the body.
   a. True
   b. False
7. A well-fitting flotation belt will allow the participant to maintain the head above the water level while ________________________________.
8. Which of the following would be considered an asymmetrical move in deep-water exercise?
   a. Deep-water jacks
   b. Moguls
   c. Cross-country skis
   d. Jogging
9. Half water tempo (1/2 WT) moves cannot be performed in deep water because you cannot bounce on the pool bottom.
   a. True
   b. False
10. For optimum safety in deep-water exercise, vertical recovery techniques should be discussed and practiced ____________________ .
   a. with non-swimmers only
   b. with non-swimmers and participants fearful of the water
   c. with all participants
   d. only if there is not a lifeguard on duty

See appendix D for answers to review questions.

References and Resources

Azevedo, L.B., M.I. Lambert, P.S. Zogaib, and T.L. Barros Neto. 2010. Maximal and submaximal physiological responses to adaptation to deep water running. *Journal of Sports Sciences* 28(4):407-414.

Burns, S.S., and T.D. Lauder. 2001. Deep water running: An effective non-weightbearing exercise for the maintenance of land-based running performance. *Military Medicine 166*:253-258.

Bushman, B.A., M.G. Flynn, F.F. Andres, C.P. Lambert, M.S. Taylor, and W.A. Braun. 1997. Effect of 4 wk deep water run training on running performance. *Medicine and Science in Sports and Exercise* 29(5):694-699.

Chu, K.S., and E.C. Rhodes. 2001. Physiological and cardiovascular changes associated with deep water running in the young. *Sports Medicine* 31(1):33-46.

Coad, D., R. Storie, H. Perez, and J. Wygand. 1987. The energy cost of treadmill vs. hydroexercise. *Medicine and Science in Sports and Exercise* 19:63.

da Silva Medeiros, N., A. Schraiber Colato, F. Guichard de Abreu, L. Silva de Lemos, L. Cabral Fraga, C. Funchal, and C. Dani. 2016. Influence of different frequencies of deep water running on oxidative profile and insulin resistance in obese women. *Obesity Medicine* 2(2016):37-40.

DeMaere, J.M., and B.C. Ruby. 1997. Effects of deep water and treadmill running on oxygen uptake and energy expenditure in seasonally trained cross country runners. *Journal of Sports Medicine and Physical Fitness* 37(3):175-181.

Di Prampero, P.E. 1986. The energy cost of human locomotion on land and in water. *International Journal of Sports Medicine* 7(2):55-72.

Dowzer, C.N., T. Reilly, and N.T. Cable. 1998. Effects of deep and shallow water running on spinal shrinkage. *British Journal of Sports Medicine* 32(1):44-48.

Dowzer, C., T. Reilly, N. Cable, and A. Nevill 1999. Maximal physiological responses to deep and shallow water running. *Ergonomics* 42(2):275-281.

Frangolias, D.D., and E.C. Rhodes. 1995. Maximal and ventilatory threshold responded to treadmill and water immersion running. *Medicine and Science in Exercise and Sport* 27(7):1007-1013.

Glass, B., D. Wilson, D. Blessing, and E. Miller. 1995. A physiological comparison of suspended deep water running to hard surfaces. Journal of Strength and Conditioning 9(1):17-21.

Hertler, L., M. Provost-Craig, P. Sestili, A. Hove, and M. Fees. 1992. Water running and the maintenance of maximum oxygen consumption and leg strength in women. *Medicine and Science in Sports and Exercise* 24:S23.

Igbanugo, V., and B. Gutin. 1978. The energy cost of aerobic dancing. *Research Quarterly. American Alliance for Health, Physical Education and Recreation* 49(3):308-316.

Killgore, G. 2006-2008. Research conducted in thesis work. Professor of Human Performance, Linfield College, McMinnville, OR. Founder/CEO, AQx, Inc.

Killgore, G.L. 2012. Deep-water running: A practical review of the literature with an emphasis on biomechanics. *Physician and Sportsmedicine* 40(1):116-126.

Killgore, G.L., S.C. Coste, S.E. O'Meara, and C.J. Konnecke. 2010. A comparison of the physiological exercise intensity differences between shod and barefoot submaximal deep-water running at the same cadence. *Journal of Strength and Conditioning Research* 24(12):3302-3312.

Killgore, G.L., A.R. Wilcox, B.L. Caster, and T.M. Wood. 2006. A lower-extremities kinematic comparison of deep-water running styles and treadmill running. *Journal of Strength and Conditioning Research* 20(4):919-927.

Kravitz, L., and J. Mayo. 1997. *The physiological effects of aquatic exercise: A brief review.* Nokomis, FL. Aquatic Exercise Association.

Mergner, T., and T. Rosemeier. 1998. Interaction of vestibular, somatosensory and visual signals for postural control and motion perception under terrestrial and microgravity conditions—a conceptual model. *Brain Research Reviews* 28(1):118-135.

Michaud, T.J., D.K. Brennan, R.P. Wilder, and N.W. Sherman. 1995. Aquarunning training and changes in cardiorespiratory fitness. *Journal of Strength and Conditioning Research* 9:78-84.

Pasetti, S.R., A. Gonçalves, and C.R. Padovani. 2012. Continuous training versus interval training in deep water running: Health effects for obese women. *Revista Andaluza de Medicina del Deporte* 5(1):3-7.

Reilly, T., C.N. Dowzer, and N.T. Cable. 2003. The physiology of deep-water running. *Journal of Sports Science* 21(12):959-972.

Richie, S.E., and W.G. Hopkins. 1991. The intensity of exercise in deep-water running. *International Journal of Sports Medicine* 12:27-29.

Roll, R., J.C. Gilhodes, J.P. Roll, K. Popov, O. Charade, and V. Gurfinkel. 1998. Proprioceptive information processing in weightlessness. *Experimental Brain Research* 122(4):393-402.

Rudzki, S., and M. Cunningham. 1999. The effect of a modified physical training program in reducing injury and medical discharge rates in Australian army recruits. *Military Medicine* 164(9):648-652.

Shanebrook, J.R., and R.D. Jaszczak. 1975. Aerodynamic drag analysis of runners. *Medicine and Science in Sports* 8(1):43-45.

Sova, R. 2000. *Aquatics: The complete reference guide for aquatic fitness professionals*. 2nd edition. Pt. Washington, WI: DSL.

Svedenhad, J. and J. Seger. 1992. Running on land and in water: comparative exercise physiology. *Medicine and Science in Sports and Exercise* 24(10):1155-1160.

Whitley, J.D., and L.L. Schoene. 1987. Comparison of heart rate responses: Water walking versus treadmill walking. *Physical Therapy* 67:1501-1504.

Wilber, R.L., R.J. Moffatt, B.E. Scott, D.T. Lee, and N.A. Cucuzzo. 1996. Influence of water run training on the maintenance of aerobic performance. *Medicine and Science in Sports and Exercise* 28:1056-1062.

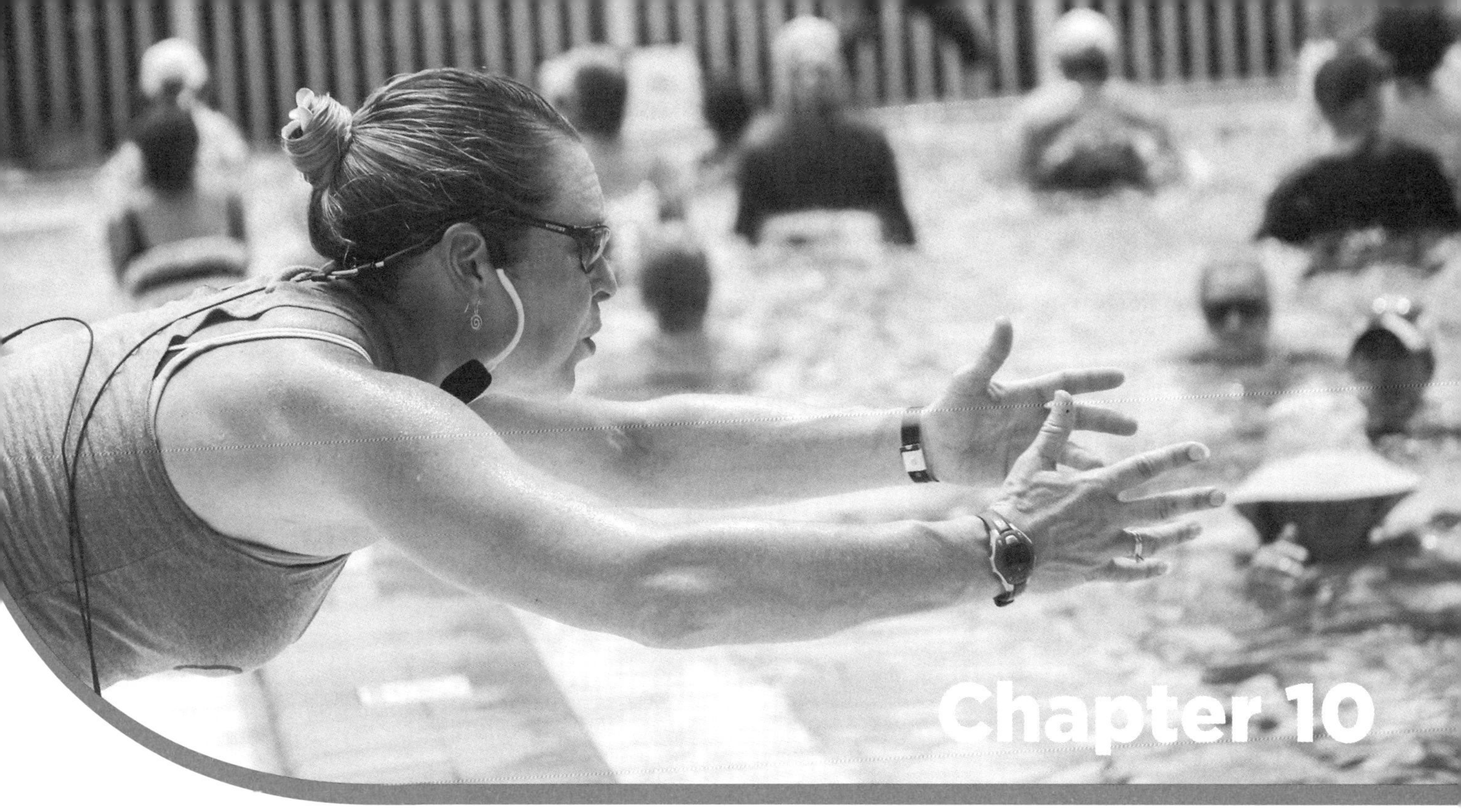

Aquatic Exercise Leadership

Introduction

In this chapter, we discuss the key skills of aquatic exercise leadership. As an aquatic fitness professional, you serve as a role model to participants by demonstrating and developing proper form and alignment. You incorporate well-planned cues, smooth transitions, and effective movement patterns to guide participants safely through any type of aquatic program with confidence, all while achieving desired results. You explore the effective use of music to enhance classes, motivate participants, and improve training results. Additionally, you lead classes in a manner that provides optimal results safely while maintaining a level of professionalism at all times.

Key Chapter Concepts

- Recognize the importance of demonstrating, teaching, and reinforcing proper posture and alignment.
- Explain the purpose of different types of cues—form and safety, motivational, transitional, imagery, feedback, and relaxation—and differentiate between the various types of transitional cues.
- Understand the three methods for delivering cues in your class: audible, visual, and tactile.
- Understand the differences and similarities between the three primary categories of transitions for shallow-water and deep-water exercise.
- Define the common terms associated with choreography as well as the various choreography styles.
- Understand how to use music effectively in aquatic programming, including the recommended tempo for various class formats.
- Explain the advantages and disadvantages of teaching from in the water, on the pool deck, or with a combination of both locations.
- Recognize the attributes associated with professionalism for aquatic fitness instructors.

Instructor Form and Alignment

A good example is the best teacher. As an aquatic fitness professional, your form and alignment while leading class or coaching clients should exemplify what you want your participants to achieve (figure 10.1). By demonstrating proper alignment, you encourage participants to do the same. Maintain correct body alignment, good posture, precise and controlled movements, and proper tempo at all times, whether you are in the pool or on the deck. Correct body alignment, from a side view, requires the ears to be centered over the shoulders, the shoulders over the hips, hips over the knees, and knees over the ankles. The chest should be open and the rib cage lifted, abdominal muscles pulled inward and upward, and shoulders back yet relaxed. For a review of neutral body alignment and neutral spinal alignment, refer to chapter 4.

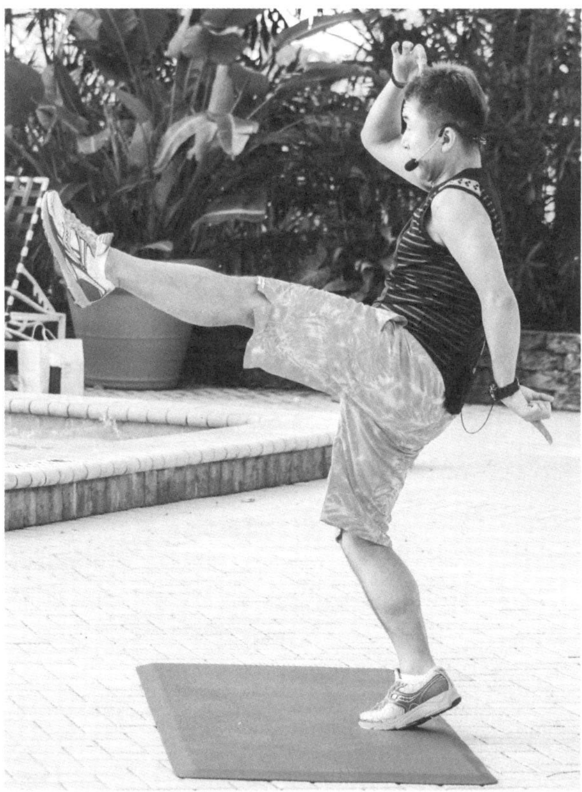

Figure 10.1 The best teachers provide clear directions on how to maintain proper form.

Your cueing and transition skills (discussed later in this chapter) will also assist participants in their ability to perform exercises with proper form and alignment. General alignment and form factors to demonstrate and to watch for in your participants include the following:

- Move with purpose and control.
- Avoid excessive twisting of the knees in relation to the foot. The knees should remain in line with the toes. When doing twisting movements, rotate from the waist while keeping the hips and legs stationary and properly aligned or allow the body to move as a unit while keeping the knees in line with the feet.
- When performing a leg curl, avoid forced overflexion of the knee, which places significant stress on the joint. To better target the hamstrings, the hip remains extended during the leg curl; in other words, the knee will be pointed toward the pool bottom rather than lifted in front of the body (figure 10.2).
- When performing exercises in shallow water, focus on foot mechanics. The entire foot should make contact with the pool bottom, either rolling heel to toe or toe to heel on takeoff and landing. Proper aquatic footwear will provide support for the foot and the ankle.

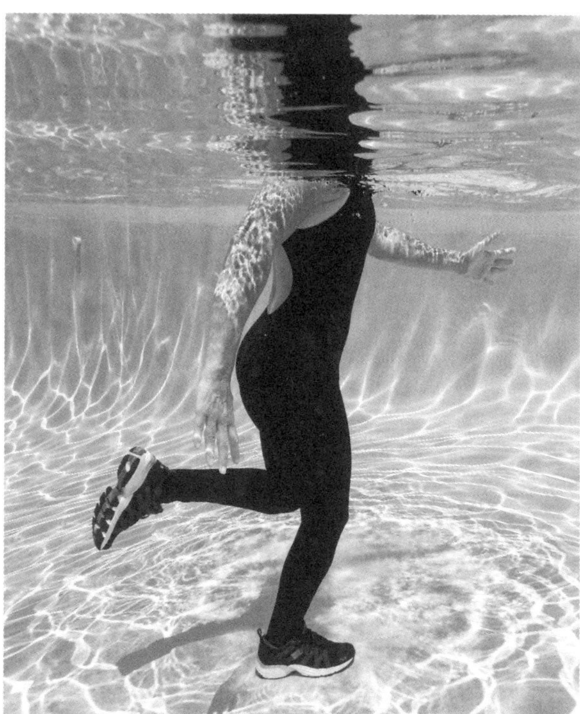

Figure 10.2 Proper form for performing an underwater leg curl.

- Emphasize proper alignment of the shoulder girdle (e.g., avoid elevating the scapulae, which brings the shoulders toward the ears). This is especially important during upper-body exercises, with or without added equipment.
- Movements should be performed without pain and without forcing the body into positions of discomfort.

Cueing

A cue is a specialized form of communication. **Cueing** is the act of communicating information to initiate action. Effective cueing allows the class to flow smoothly from one move to another in a seamless manner. Learning to use different types of cues and mastering various delivery methods take practice and experience. However, these important instructor skills are well worth striving for in your aquatic fitness career.

Cues serve several purposes, including those listed here:

- **Form and safety cues** address proper posture, safe joint action, appropriate levels of force and intensity, breathing techniques, and muscle focus. It is generally preferable to use positive rather than negative form cues, such as, "Brace the abdominals and align the spine" rather than, "Don't arch your back."
- **Motivational cues** encourage participants to act in a positive manner, both mentally and physically. An example is, "Looking good—you've got this combination!" Participants should feel positive about their capabilities and eager to challenge themselves within safe boundaries and without the stress of competition.
- **Transitional cues** inform participants that a change is about to take place and explain how to make that change safely and effectively. Timing is very important. Transitional cues should be delivered early enough to communicate the move but not so early that the timing of execution is confusing. Read more about transitions and transitional cues later in this chapter. The following are specific methods of cueing transitions:

* **Directional cues** communicate the desired direction you want your participants to travel or the direction you want them to move their bodies. Examples include moving forward, backward, to the corner, to the side, or in a circle.
* **Numerical cues** communicate the desired repetitions of each movement or the number of repetitions remaining before a change, such as, "Let's do 8 more."
* **Movement or step cues** tell participants the basic movement being performed (e.g., jumping jacks, rocking horse, jog, kick).
* **Footwork cues** describe specifically how the lower body should be used; typically expressed as "right" and "left."
* **Rhythmic cues** express the musical counts used during movement. Tempo changes and complex counts are considered rhythmic cues (e.g., land tempo, water tempo, half water tempo, single-single-double). See more on movement tempos in chapters 8 and 9.

- **Imagery cues** use vivid descriptions that appeal to one or more of the senses (sight, hearing, touch, smell, and taste) to help participants achieve a desired goal in exercise. This type of cue might be used during intense movement to help participants become more focused, possibly allowing for a higher intensity for a longer period of time. For example, you could say, "Don't quit yet, the finish line is just before you. . . . you are almost there!" They can also be used to facilitate relaxation and stretching, as in, "Imagine you are floating in warm water with the sun on your face, the sound of birds calling quietly as they fly overhead . . . "
- **Feedback cues** are used to maintain an open line of communication between the instructor and the participants. Often phrased as questions, they are designed to get a response from participants (either verbal or visual feedback). Inquiring about participants' level of fatigue, comprehension of the described movement, alignment, muscle focus, and so on gives the instructor valuable information for modifying the daily class plan and class goals. Examples might include, "Can you feel your shoulder blades pull together when we do this exercise?", and, "The water is warmer than normal today. Do you need to take the intensity down? If so, you know it is okay to adjust your workout!"
- **Relaxation cues** bring awareness to muscle tension versus muscle relaxation. Relaxation cues can be used at any point during the class to initiate proper body mechanics or alignment. For example, you may ask your participants to tense their shoulders (lifting up toward the ears) and then relax them before beginning an upper-body exercise to bring awareness of proper alignment of the shoulder girdle.

Delivering Cues

After considering the purpose of the cue, consider how to deliver it. You can deliver your cue in three primary ways: audible, visual, and tactile.

Audible Cueing

An **audible cue** is any cue received through hearing, including spoken words (verbal) and sounds, whistles, claps, musical changes, and bells. This is generally the most common method of cueing by group exercise instructors. Make the most of each word spoken when using verbal cues. Use your voice sparingly to avoid **vocal cord** damage. Verbal cueing is most effective when it

- is given early enough to allow for reaction time,
- is limited to one to three carefully chosen words,
- is spoken at a rate that can be easily understood, and
- varies in tone.

When you are counting a **combination** for participants (i.e. using a numerical transition cue), consider counting backward, such as "8, 7, 6, 5, 4, 3, 2, 1." On the last two counts, tell participants the planned change. Since "3" rhymes with "where they want to *be*," this is a good memory trigger for a new instructor. Leaving the last two counts for a transitional cue gives participants forewarning that the combination is about to change or progress. Some instructors also do this by counting forward, saving counts 7 and 8 for the verbal cue. This technique might make participants pay attention and listen for something new that is about to happen.

Visual Cueing

Visual cues might not be used as often as audible cues, but are often the type of cue that most participants notice (figure 10.3). Pool acoustics (water splashing, ventilation systems, high ceilings) often make it difficult for participants to understand spoken words or hear other audible signals. Thus, visual cueing is an important skill to learn.

Visual cues include hand signals, eye contact, facial expressions, posture, physical demonstration, and body language. Adding emphasis or exaggeration to movements can assist participants in understanding your planned exercise and movement execution, such as where to add force, overall intensity, alignment tips, and breath awareness. Observe participants; if you see the action you desire from your participants, then your visual cue was effective and successful. If not, you may need to adjust your demonstration. Video recording your visual cueing while instructing a class and practicing in front of a mirror are both great ways to evaluate and improve your technique. See table 10.1 for examples of audible and visual cueing techniques.

Tactile Cueing

Tactile cues (touch cues) are less common than audible and visual cueing. The tactile learner learns best by doing. A tactile person practices the movement and masters an awareness of how that movement feels in the body. Helping these participants improve alignment and execution through tactile cueing can increase the movement's effectiveness and facilitate the learning process. An example of a tactile cue would be gently touching the muscle that the exercise is targeting to bring awareness to the correct movement (figure 10.4). Another option might be to explain the range of motion for a given exercise, such as holding a noodle under the

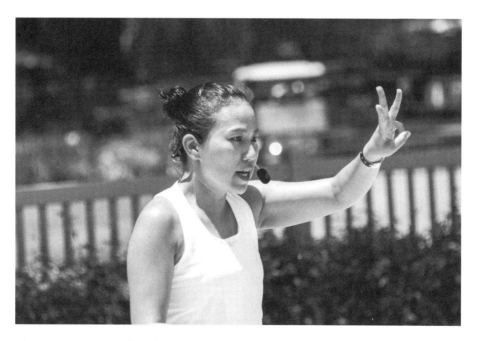

Figure 10.3 Use clear hand signals to help cue participants so as not to miss important information.

Table 10.1 Examples of Audible and Visual Cueing Techniques

Movement	Audible cue	Visual hand cue
Walk	"Walk"	Two-finger wag
Knee lift	"Knees"	Thumbs-up
Heels up	"Heels"	Thumbs point over shoulders
Rocking horse	"Rock"	Wave side, palm front then down
Jumping jack	"Jack"	Hands together, then arch hands up and out, up and in to show jump out and in
Straight-leg kicks	"Kick"	Use extended arm to demonstrate kick in desired direction
Pendulum	"Pendulum"	Raise one arm to the side and back down as the other arm repeats to the opposite side
Turn	"Turn"	Move the hand in a circle overhead
Repeat entire combination	"From top"	Tap top of head with one hand and then lift hand up away from the head

water and asking participants to bring their knees to touch the noodle with each repetition of a tuck jump. This option could also allow for self-monitoring or for participants to work in pairs to provide tactile cues to achieve the goal.

Learn to use touch appropriately and effectively. Tactile cueing is used more frequently in **personal training** than in group exercise. An instructor or personal trainer should always ask permission before touching participants to avoid offending or startling them. Never manipulate a participant into a movement or force a joint beyond its pain-free range of motion.

Additional Cueing Tips

Using all three methods to deliver cues will allow you to reach a wide range of partici-

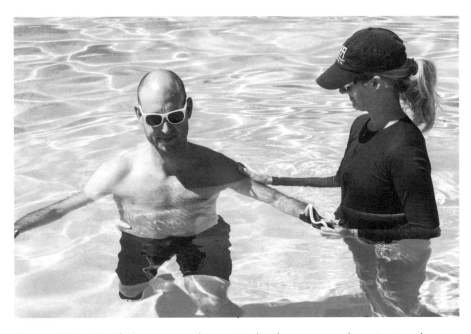

Figure 10.4 Tactile learners can be assisted with movement by using touch cues.

pants and engage all learning styles. You will need to practice the movements and plan out the audible, visual, and tactile cues to use during class.

Write down the cues you want to use and when to incorporate claps or whistles, body movement, arm or hand signals, or facial expressions. Lesson plans can assist in organizing the verbal, nonverbal, and tactile cues associated with each movement or combination and keep you on track with your class schedule. A sample lesson plan is located in appendix E.

Cueing in the water is a little different than cueing land-based exercise because movement speed and **reaction time** are reduced when the body is submerged. Practice delivering cues before participants need them. Cueing with the rhythm of the music sometimes helps with this timing. Develop good cueing skills from the start; this is easier than breaking ineffective habits.

If you develop a pattern that you use often, you can make cueing easier by giving the pattern a name. For instance, you might name a specific 32-count combination with only one word. Consider this example: Jump forward 8 counts, leap right for 8 counts, jump back for 8 counts, and leap left for 8 counts. Because this movement pattern creates a box made up of four 8-count movements, you can name—and cue—this pattern as "box." This one-syllable word simply and effectively reflects the entire combination and limits stress to your voice. Teach the pattern elements and directions to participants and then gradually reduce the cue to one word.

Consistency with cues will help participants learn and retain the information needed to perform exercises correctly. For example, if you use a visual signal of one hand up with palm forward to indicate you want participants to stop traveling, do not also use that same hand signal to indicate backward travel—it will be confusing. Additionally, it might be advisable for the entire aquatic exercise staff within a facility to use the same verbal and visual cues. This makes it easier for participants to join different classes and assists substitute instructors in leading effective classes.

Another great cueing technique is signaling participants to "watch me." If you are not sure how to cue something or if the change is difficult to articulate, this simple reference that a change is coming will help prepare participants for the next step.

To observe and to maintain a personal connection with participants, aquatic fitness professionals often teach by **mirror imaging** (figure 10.5). With mirror imaging, you face the participants while leading the exercises; when you cue, "Left," you are physically demonstrating with your right side. When teaching a more complicated foot pattern or a combination that involves various directions, you may find it easier to have participants follow from behind (you face the same direction as the participants). You can look over your shoulder to check on them and maintain visual contact. When participants have mastered the pattern, you can turn around to mirror image them. However, if an additional lifeguard is not on duty while you are instructing, it is recommended not to turn your back to the participants.

After the class has mastered the entire combination through the cueing techniques described in this chapter, you can then start to challenge participants intellectually. See if they can perform the movements using only verbal cues. Then try using only visual cues. Finally, see if participants have paid enough attention to perform the entire combination with no visual or verbal cues from you.

Once choreography and cues are designed, practice presenting all this information in front of a mirror or in front of fellow instructors. Analyze the use of eye contact, body language, precision and control, and energy and enthusiasm. Eye contact is necessary for creating trust, confidence, and sincerity between instructor and student. Visual contact is also valuable for giving feedback and other cueing information. Body language can convey energy, encourage performance, and express empathy and concern for the participants.

Cueing style is personal and it develops over time. Some instructors find the drill sergeant command-based style effective, whereas others find expressive cueing gets

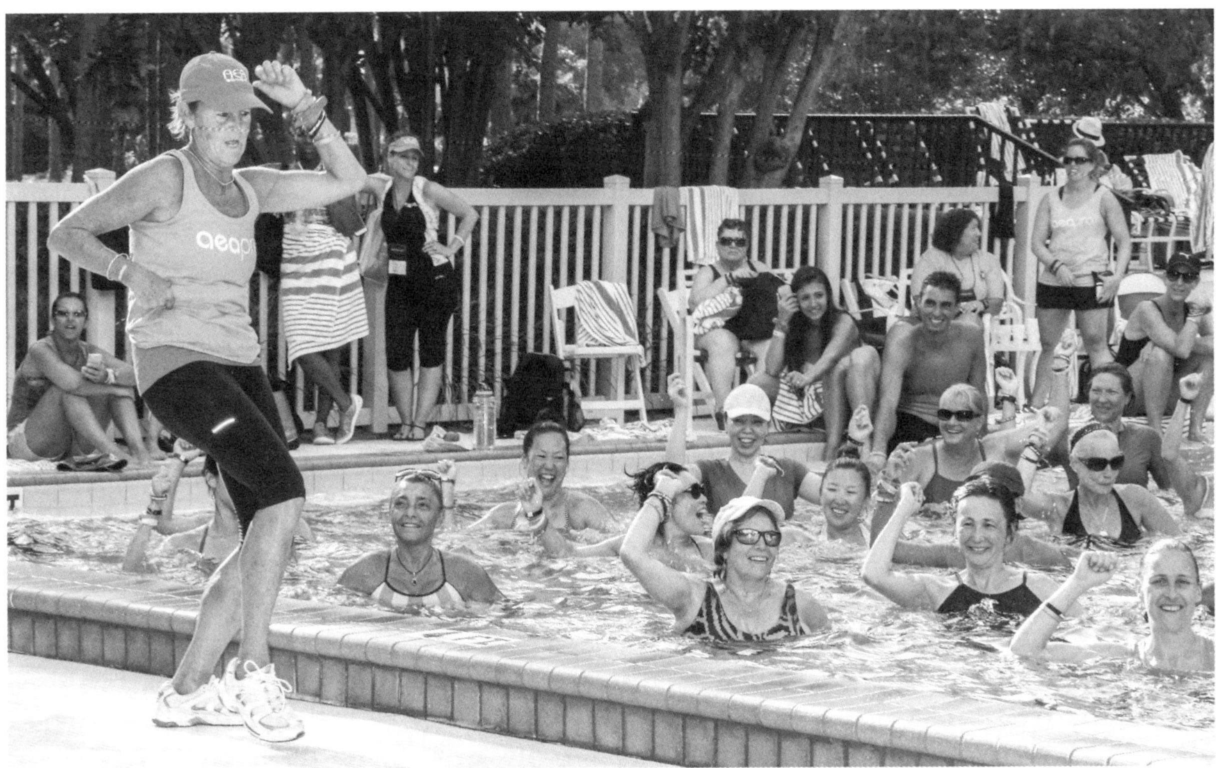

Figure 10.5 Mirror imaging can help participants master a combination more easily.

better results. Depending on your teaching personality and the personality of the class, a blending of styles usually creates an effective level of communication. If a class thrives on strong leadership, a command-based style might prevail. A class of aggressive, strong-willed, independent participants might be offended by commands. Experimenting with various styles will help you quickly identify the cueing styles that highlight your teaching personality and that are appropriate for your classes. Practice until you can customize your cueing style to match the needs of each class.

Transitions

A **transition** occurs when there is a change from one move to another move. Smooth transitions are critical in designing a well-balanced and enjoyable workout. The performance of movements, as well as the reaction time for changing movements, is slower when exercising in the water. Although this allows additional time to prepare for the next exercise or combination, it also means that transitional cues must be given earlier than in a land-based routine.

As previously discussed, various types of transitional cues can be given for any movement. For example, to cue a "Rocking horse 3 and turn," you can incorporate any of the following:

- Directional—cueing for the direction the body is moving: "Up, back, up, up."
- Numerical—cueing the number of repetitions before change: "4, 3, 2, 1" or counting up "1, 2, 3, 4."
- Footwork—cueing which foot the weight should be on: "Right, left, right, right,", or " Left, right, left, left."
- Movement or step—cueing to describe the actual move: "Rock, rock, rock, hop-turn."
- Rhythmic—cueing based on the tempo or the rhythm of the movement: "Single, single, double."
- A mixture of transitional cues might be more effective than relying on a single method, such as "Rock, 2, 3, hop-turn" or "4, 3, 2 and turn."

Be especially cautious on transitions in which direction of travel is altered or when moving the limbs from one plane to another. These types of transitions might temporarily take the body out of normal alignment and cause added musculoskeletal stress. All transitions should feel fluid, allowing change from one move to another, or one direction to another, without interrupting the flow of the class. The water's buoyancy allows participants to perform transitions that might be awkward or considered high risk on land. Even though the water is a forgiving environment, risk of injury still increases when the body is out of alignment.

Shallow-Water Transitions

Shallow-water transitions fall into three primary categories: basic, intermediate, and advanced. Your class population, the goal of your class, and the class **format** help determine which transitions are most applicable.

A **basic transition** is a transition in which the next move begins where the previous move ended or passes through neutral alignment (ears, shoulders, hips, knees, and ankle are vertically aligned). It is simple to cue and easy for all levels of participants to perform with good form. A basic transition passes from:

- a one-footed move to a one-footed move in the same plane
- a one-footed move to a two-footed move or vice versa with a center bounce
- a two-footed move to a two-footed move with a center bounce

For example, a water tempo (WT) knee lift to a WT front kick is a transition that occurs from a one-footed move to a one-footed move, and both movements are in the sagittal plane. Continuing with the alternating leg movement offers a transition that flows smoothly and allows you to maintain neutral alignment with minimal coordination and core strength. An example of a basic transition between two-footed moves is seen with a 1/2 WT cross-country ski center bounce to a WT jumping jack; each move passes through neutral by landing with the feet together. Finally, let's consider a basic transition between a one-footed move (knee lift) and a two-footed move (cross-country ski). The moves must pass through neutral alignment. Since a WT knee lift ends with one foot down and the other foot lifted, add a center bounce after each repetition (i.e., change to a 1/2 WT knee lift bounce center; see figure 10.6). Ending the knee lift with a center bounce allows the transition into the cross-country ski to begin from neutral alignment (table 10.2).

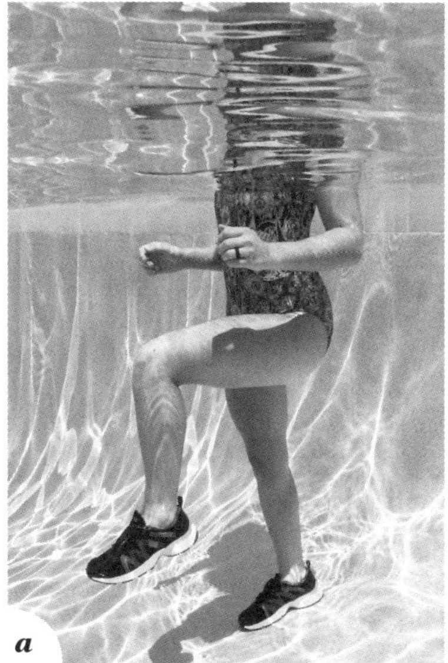

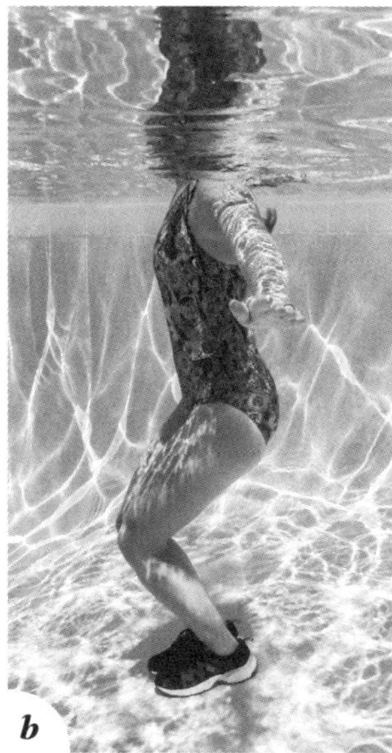

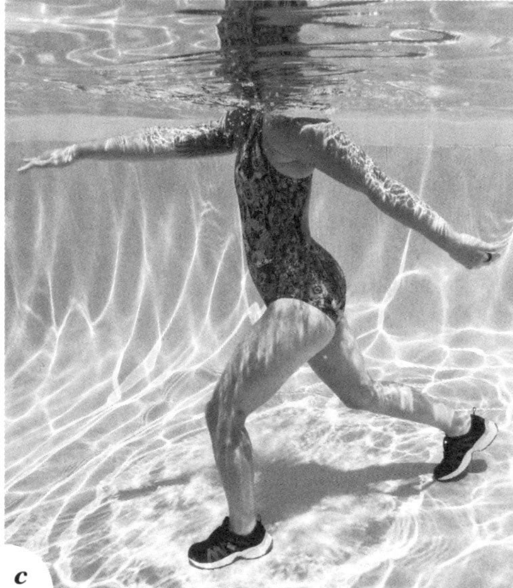

Figure 10.6 Example of a basic transition: *(a)* 1/2 WT knee lift, *(b)* performed with a bounce center where the body is in neutral alignment, into *(c)* a cross-country ski.

Novice instructors might find it easier to use a **transitional move**. This involves returning to a simple move (typically a bounce in shallow water) before transitioning to another move. This method allows more time for the instructor and participants to prepare for the next component of the pattern and reinforce or regain alignment.

An **intermediate transition** requires a little more coordination and core strength to maintain safe alignment; the arms assist with balance as needed. This type of transition is safe for experienced participants, but may be challenging for people with musculoskeletal limitations or medical conditions. An intermediate transition requires additional cueing skills and choreography planning in order to maintain class flow.

Generally, an intermediate transition passes from:

- a one-footed move to a one-footed move in a different plane
- a one-footed move to a two-footed move (or vice versa) without a center bounce
- a two-footed move to a two-footed move without a center bounce

Let's explore examples of each. An intermediate transition between one-footed moves in different planes can be seen when changing from a WT straight-leg back kick (sagittal plane) to a WT pendulum (frontal plane). The kick ends with the weight on right leg and left leg lifted behind the body; initiating the wide jog requires the left leg to swing forward and out into the frontal plane. With practice, this is not difficult to achieve, but it does require more coordination and core strength. In the example of a one-footed move to a two-footed move in the same plane without a center bounce, consider a WT knee lift to a WT cross-country ski. The knee lift ends with the right foot down and the left knee lifted. While tightening the core, you transition directly into a cross-country ski with left foot forward by jumping and placing the left foot forward and the right foot back (figure 10.7). Since the transition does not pass through neutral alignment, this is an intermediate transition (table 10.2). We also have an intermediate transition when changing between two-footed moves without a center bounce, as seen in a 1/2 WT (double) cross-country ski to a mogul. The ski exercise will end with one foot in front and the other foot back. It requires good core strength to pull the legs together and simultaneously jump them both out to one side to begin the mogul.

An **advanced transition** can be considered in choreography designed for experienced aquatic participants and fit people or athletes. This transition requires additional

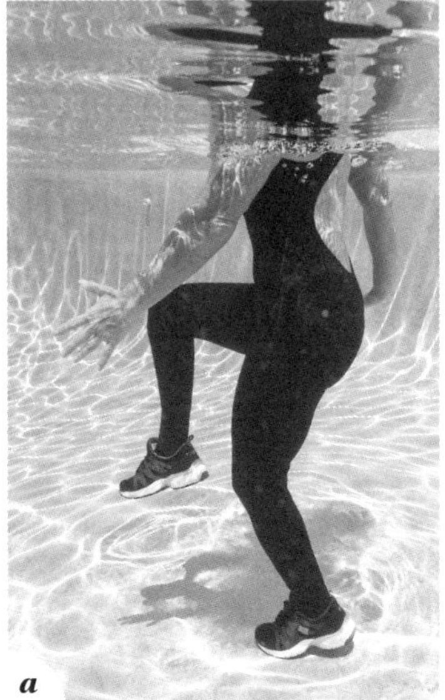

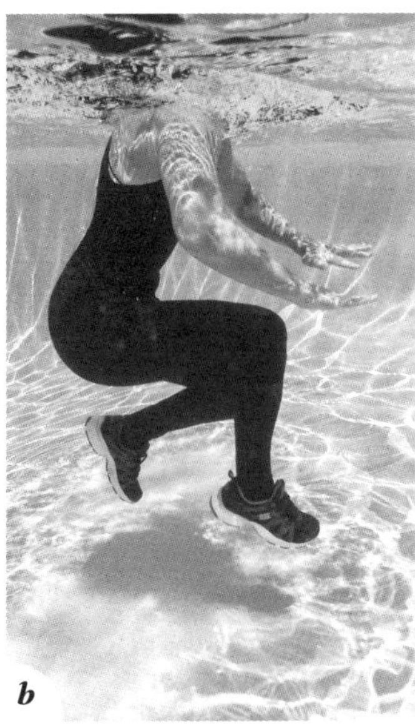

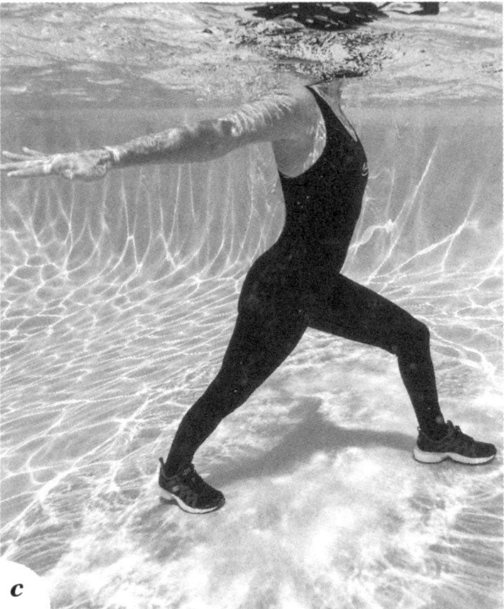

Figure 10.7 Example of an intermediate transition: *(a)* WT knee lift, *(b)* transition which involves core and upper-body strength, *(c)* into a WT cross-country ski.

core strength and coordination to pass through the transition safely. An advanced transition passes from:

- a one-footed move to a two-footed move (or vice versa) with a change in impact level (impact levels are discussed in chapter 8)
- any transition that involves a change in plane *and* a change in impact level

Again, consider each scenario. First, let's look at a level I knee lift transitioning to a level III cross-country ski (table 10.2). The knee lift ends in a tall upright posture with the left knee lifted and weight on the right leg. Transitioning to a level III cross-country ski requires the body to flex quickly at the hips and knees while leaning forward slightly and using the upper body to help lift both feet off the pool bottom. The core muscles must remain engaged to protect the lumbar spine. This transition requires more coordination. Our second advanced transition scenario involves a change in both movement plane and impact level, such as a level III cross-country ski to a level I pendulum. The ski is suspended off the bottom of the pool with the legs moving front and back in the sagittal plane. The transition requires transitioning the weight to one foot on the pool bottom while pushing the body into an upright position and abducting the opposite leg (frontal plane) to initiate the pendulum (figure 10.8). Significant core strength, coordinated movements,

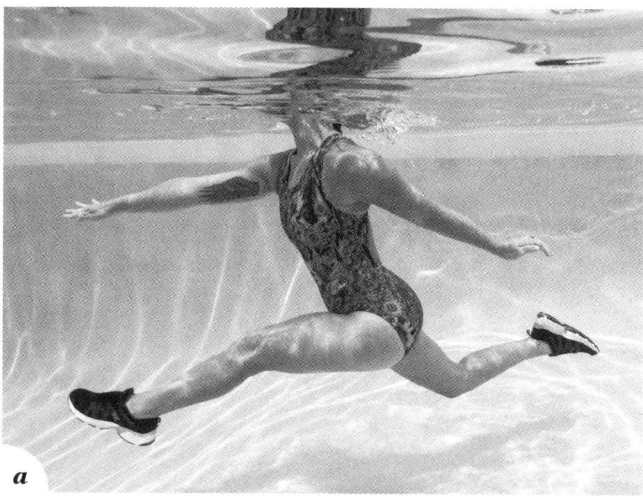

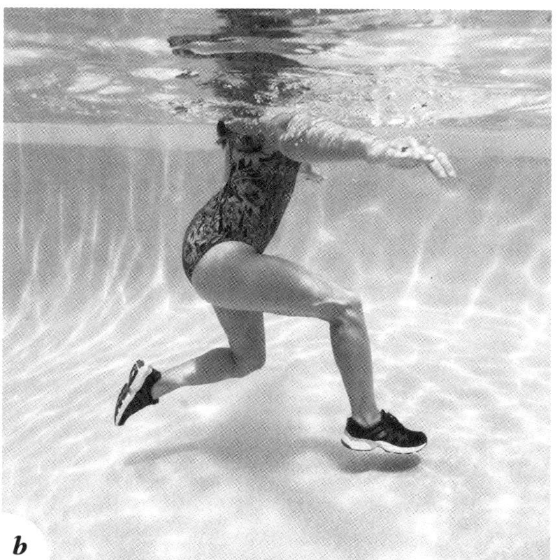

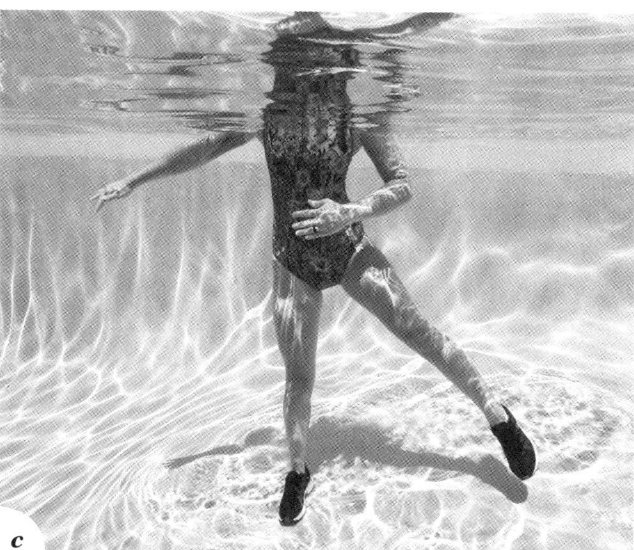

Figure 10.8 Example of an advanced transition: *(a)* level III cross-country ski, *(b)* transition which involves a change in impact and planes, into *(c)* a level I pendulum.

Table 10.2 Shallow-Water Transition Examples

R = right L = left BC = bounce center

Note that the counts are designated in water tempo beats.

Knee lift to a cross-country ski—basic transition								
Water tempo beat	1	2	3	4	5	6	7	8
1/2 WT knee lift bounce center	R knee	BC	L knee	BC	R knee	BC	L knee	BC
Water tempo beat	9	10	11	12	13	14	15	16
WT cross-country ski	R ski	L ski	R ski	L ski	R ski	L ski	R ski	L ski
Knee lift to a cross-country ski—intermediate transition								
Water tempo beat	1	2	3	4	5	6	7	8
WT knee lift	R knee	L knee	R knee	L knee	R knee	L knee	R knee	L knee
Water tempo beat	9	10	11	12	13	14	15	16
WT cross-country ski	L ski	R ski	L ski	R ski	L ski	R ski	L ski	R ski
Knee lift to a cross-country ski—advanced transition								
Water tempo beat	1	2	3	4	5	6	7	8
WT knee lift	R knee	L knee	R knee	L knee	R knee	L knee	R knee	L knee
Water tempo beat	9	10	11	12	13	14	15	16
WT cross-country ski—level III	R ski suspended	L ski suspended	R ski suspended	L ski suspended	R ski suspended	L ski suspended	R ski suspended	L ski suspended

and planned use of the upper body are all required for safely achieving this advanced level transition.

Develop your ability to cue transitions to facilitate flow and exemplify professionalism in your class. If you are just starting as an aquatic fitness professional, keep your shallow-water transitions simple and safe. Consider using a transitional move to give participants an opportunity to safely catch up if you cue late or forget to cue, or plan basic transitions. More experienced instructors can incorporate intermediate and advanced transitions to expand choreography options and offer training challenges as appropriate for the class population.

Deep-Water Transitions

As mentioned, transitions that involve changes in direction of travel or planes of movement can temporarily take the body out of alignment. During these types of transitions, injury is more likely to occur when the body is impacting. Thus, the potential for injury is somewhat reduced in deep water.

In deep-water exercise, we do not have the considerations of impact changes during transitions.

However, since the body is totally suspended, the participant cannot push off the pool bottom to assist with the transition. It must be feasible to transition from one move to the next without any additional leverage, which often requires more core strength and stability, as well as upper-body strength. Deep-water transitions should focus on reestablishing vertical posture and allow participants to feel balanced.

Because of these differences, deep-water transitions are categorized differently than shallow-water transitions. Deep-water transitions are referred to as either a basic transition, a transitional move, or a **tempo transition**.

A **deep-water basic transition** is similar to that in shallow water: A new move begins where the previous move ended. Consider the following deep-water pattern where basic transitions provide a safe and effective option:

- Knee-high jog—short lever in sagittal plane
- Cross-country ski—lengthen the legs but remain in the same plane
- Vertical flutter kick—similar move with reduced range of motion
- Front kicks—same plane of motion
- Ankle reach front—similar move with added rotation of hip and flexion of the knee
- Straddle jog—maintaining short lever, moving smoothly to frontal plane
- Knee-high jog—maintaining the jog while returning to sagittal plane

A **deep-water transitional move**, often a jog or vertical flutter kick, allows more time to prepare for the next movement in a pattern. This may be needed to change planes or direction of travel, or simply to stabilize the body in the water. Because the feet are not in contact with the pool bottom, the body experiences a greater level of instability. Transitional movements allow participants to regain body alignment and maintain control. In the basic transition sample combination, transitional moves are not required because you can flow from one move to the next by stabilizing with the core and the upper body while repositioning the legs. The knee-high jog moves easily into the cross-country ski, the ski action passes right through the position for the flutter kick, the flutter kick is a good position for moving into front kicks, and so on.

You need to follow the pathway of the exercise to see if the limbs can go directly to the next move or you need to insert a transition move. Consider this deep-water pattern that benefits from several transitional moves (TM):

- Knee-high jog
- Straddle jog
- (TM) Knee-high jog—to prepare for change in planes
- Cross-country ski
- (TM) Knee-high jog—to prepare to initiate travel
- Running backward
- (TM) Knee-high jog—to prepare for a change in direction of travel
- Running sideways
- (TM) Knee-high jog—to stop and stabilize the body
- Front kicks

Although an accomplished deep-water exerciser could manage these changes without a transitional move, when working with a mixed-level group, it is safest to add a transitional move. This ensures that all participants are neutrally aligned as they pass through the transition without compromising intensity.

Here are some general guidelines regarding transitional moves.

- When changing the plane of motion, a transitional move is usually needed unless the body comes back to neutral postural alignment within the movement repetition.

Straddle jog to cross-country ski requires a transitional move. Cross-country ski (half water tempo ski, pause at the center) to jacks is a basic transition although there is a change in planes because both moves pause in the center.

- When continuing travel in the same direction, a transitional move is typically not needed. For example, deep-water running forward to a traveling cross-country ski forward is a basic transition.
- Changing the direction of travel generally benefits from a transitional move because the body is immersed to the neck; there is no contact with the pool bottom to assist with the change. The water's inertia will challenge your participants' body position with any directional changes in deep water. Observe your participants; if their alignment is being compromised, add a transitional move before starting the new direction of travel.
- When making a change in arm patterns to a different plane of motion, consider using a transitional move. For instance, suppose you are performing a cross-country ski with an alternating arm swing in the sagittal plane and you would like to maintain the ski pattern for the legs but change the arms to horizontal abduction and adduction. The change will be smoother if the legs come together and perform four counts of a flutter kick while the arms reposition. Then, you can continue the cross-country ski with the new arm pattern.

You can also use a **deep-water tempo transition** to facilitate changes from one move to another while suspended. Just as in shallow water, half water tempo (1/2 WT) movements in deep water will facilitate smooth transitions into most other moves because the ending position is in neutral alignment. In deep water, a one-count return to the center position (a pause center) or the use of a center tuck will replace the bounce center used in shallow water. You can also incorporate doubles as a method of half water tempo in deep-water training. The following pattern benefits from using tempo transitions to move through neutral alignment:

- 6 cross-country skis (WT)
- 1 cross-country ski (1/2 WT with pause center)
- 4 front kicks (1/2 WT with pause center)
- Moguls R, L, R & center tuck hold (WT, WT, 1/2 WT with center tuck)
- Moguls L, R, L & center tuck hold (WT, WT, 1/2 WT with center tuck)
- 4 deep-water jacks (WT)
- 7 modified hurdles (WT)
- Shoot legs down to center

Well-planned transitions in the deep water certainly add to the quality and effectiveness of your workout while reducing the risk of injury. Including a variety of transitional methods enhances your movement combinations as well as your teaching skills. Beginners benefit from transitions in neutral alignment. Accomplished deep-water exercisers can typically handle patterns with fewer transition moves. As always, alignment should not be compromised.

Choreography

Although the term **choreography** might bring to mind a variety of images, it simply means the arrangement or written notation of a series of movements. Well-planned choreography can make every aquatic class or workout exciting. At the same time, choreography should provide a balanced workout that promotes both safety and effectiveness. The following common terms allow an easier understanding of aquatic choreography.

Component or move: The smallest part or segment in choreography. A knee lift, kick, or jumping jack is considered a *move*, or basic component of choreography.

Pattern or combination: A pattern or combination is two or more moves linked together in sequence.

Choreography style: Different methods of linking together moves to create combinations.

Transition: A transition occurs when there is a change from one move to another move.

Cue: A cue is a signal to class participants. It is the act of communicating information to instigate action.

Music beat: The beat is the steady pulse of a song. Beats can be found in music or created by a metronome or other device or the instructor.

Music tempo: The rate of speed at which the beats occur in music; designated as beats per minute (bpm).

Water tempo: A rate of speed appropriate for the aquatic environment that allows for slower reaction time and full range of motion; every other beat of the music tempo when using the recommended bpm range.

Just as in land-based exercise, aquatic fitness programs use a variety of **choreography styles** to create safe, effective, and enjoyable workouts. The following are the most common styles of choreography that work well for water exercise. Individual moves are described in appendices A and B.

Freestyle Choreography

Freestyle is a style of choreography in which a series of moves are performed without a predictable pattern. The instructor generally continues through a long list of moves until the class is finished, with or without repeating any given component. Although this choreography has no repeatable patterns, it does require planning to deliver a balanced workout with safe and effective transitions.

Example:

8 rocking horses right, 8 rocking horses left

16 jogs with knees high

8 leg curls bounce center

8 cross-country skis bounce center

16 jumping jacks

16 pendulums

Pyramid Choreography

In **pyramid choreography**, the number of repetitions for each move in a combination is gradually decreased or increased. The instructor might use 16 repetitions each of four different moves and then repeat those same moves in groups of 8, then 4, and then 2. It is also possible to reverse back to the original pattern by repeating the combination in a series of 4, 8, and finally 16 repetitions.

This style works well for teaching a more complex combination that would be confusing if initially shown in the final format. By building a broad base of repetitions for each movement, the participants can learn the pattern with correct technique. Then, with a gradual decrease in the number of repetitions while maintaining the pattern, the workout becomes more challenging, both physically and mentally.

Example:

16 kicks to the front

16 side leg lifts

16 kicks to the back

8 bounces in place

8 tuck jumps

next . . .

8 kicks to the front

8 side leg lifts

8 kicks to the back

4 bounces in place

4 tuck jumps

next . . .

4 kicks to the front

4 side leg lifts

4 kicks to the back

2 bounces in place

2 tuck jumps

finally . . .

2 kicks to the front

2 side leg lifts

2 kicks to the back

1 bounce in place

1 tuck jump

Add-On Choreography

Add-on choreography is a way of building patterns gradually while providing positive reinforcement through repetition as the sequence is learned. It is sometimes called the memory or building block method. After one move is established (A), another move is taught (B), and then added on to the first move (A + B). More moves follow, one at a time, to develop a combination, either simple or quite intricate, depending on the instructor's leadership skills and the level and interest of participants.

This style allows the participants to work out while learning; there is no disruption of the flow of the class while teaching the combination.

Example:

Teach and practice A . . .

8 jogs forward with heels high

8 jogs backward with knees high

then teach and practice B . . .

cross-country ski 3 bounce center

put together A-B and practice . . .

8 jogs forward with heels high

8 jogs backward with knees high

4 sets of cross-country ski 3 bounce center

then teach and practice C . . .

jazz kick (or football punt)

put together A-B-C and practice . . .

8 jogs forward with heels high

8 jogs backward with knees high

4 sets of cross-country ski 3 bounce center

16 jazz kicks (or football punt)

Patterned Choreography

In **patterned choreography**, a set pattern of moves is initially taught in its final form. Participants learn by repeating the total combination over and over. The number of repetitions needed to learn the pattern depends on its complexity. This style works well with less intricate patterns, more advanced participants, or dance-style classes. Patterned choreography is often used when the instructor choreographs a specific routine to each different song. In this case, the pattern might also include slight variations to accommodate the music (e.g., always performing a portion of the combination during the chorus).

Example:

4 leaps to the right

7 rocking horses right, and turn to the front

8 pendulums

4 leaps to the left

7 rocking horses left, and turn to the front

8 pendulums

Repeat pattern over and over

Layer Technique

The **layer technique** begins with a pattern that can be repeated. The pattern can be taught first through pure repetition or with add-on or pyramid choreography. When participants are comfortable with the pattern, instructors can gradually superimpose modifications (e.g., turns, tempo adjustments, impact changes) or replace existing moves with new moves, one at a time in the pattern. The instructor can also un-layer the sequence if desired, returning to the original pattern.

Example of move substitution (*denotes the change):

Begin with . . .

4 wide steps right, 4 wide steps left

4 sets of jumping jacks in 3s

8 ankle touches to the front

4 front kick bounce center

Change to . . .

4 wide steps right, 4 wide steps left

4 sets of jumping jacks in 3s

8 ankle touches to the front

*2 sets of knee swing 3 bounce center

Change to . . .

4 wide steps right, 4 wide steps left

4 sets of jumping jacks in 3s

*8 leg curls

2 sets of knee swing 3 bounce center

Change to . . .

4 wide steps right, 4 wide steps left

*8 jumping jacks with ankle cross

8 leg curls

2 sets of knee swing 3 bounce center

Finally, end with . . .

*8 slides to the right, 8 slides to the left

8 jumping jacks with ankle cross

8 leg curls

2 sets of knee swing 3 bounce center

Example of movement modification (*denotes the change):

Begin with . . .

4 jumping jacks

Rocking horse single-single-double (R, L, RR)

Rocking horse single-single-double (L, R, LL)

8 straight-leg front kicks

8 jogs

Change to . . .

*4 jumping jacks with 1/4 turn as feet land together

Rocking horse single-single-double (R, L, RR)

Rocking horse single-single-double (L, R, LL)

*8 straight-leg back kicks

8 jogs

Change to . . .

4 jumping jacks with 1/4 turn as feet land together

Rocking horse single-single-double (R, L, RR)

Rocking horse single-single-double (L, R, LL)

8 straight-leg back kicks

*8 football jogs (out, out, in, in, out, out, in, in)

As an instructor, you are not limited to the five styles of choreography discussed. You can use other styles or methods or blend two or more styles together. However, the styles discussed in this section are relatively simple and work well in the water. Often, instructors become proficient and comfortable using one style of choreography. Participants also have different learning styles or preferences. Teaching freestyle choreography might be easy for the instructor and appeal to some participants because of its nonrepeating style. However, it might be frustrating for those who like order and patterns. By stepping outside your comfort zone and introducing a variety of choreography styles to your class, you might reach and motivate a greater number of participants.

Varying your choreography can add to your participants' overall feelings of satisfaction and enjoyment. Different styles of choreography can make old moves feel new and fresh. You can expand your leadership skills by introducing new methods of choreography as well as new movements and combinations. You and your participants will enjoy the change!

Music

Music can be used for motivating participants, maintaining tempo, and achieving a desired intensity. Although music is not required for aquatic fitness programming, you might want to take advantage of the positive reinforcement that music can provide. According to Dr. Len Kravitz in "The Effects of Music on Exercise" (1994), music can provide many benefits to exercise. Participants perceive better performance when music is a part of their fitness program, although actual performance may not show improvement. Music can positively affect the attitude of participants during exercise, so proper music selection is important. Music tends to evoke pleasant associations with the fitness program.

Three primary things relating to music have been identified that can possibly influence exercise performance (Santos 2016):

1. Our tendency to move in time with synchronous sounds (e.g., tapping your toes to the beat of a song)

2. Music's ability to increase arousal (e.g., the desire to move rather than to sit)
3. Music's ability to distract from the discomfort related to exercise (e.g., sweating, labored breathing, muscle soreness)

In situations where the pool acoustics are poor, adding music might create an environment in which it is more difficult to learn and teach. For example, participants with limited hearing capabilities might find that music prohibits them from understanding the instructor's verbal cues. Or, teaching in a multi-use facility where other activities are taking place simultaneously may limit the use of music. Instrumental selections might be a better option because your verbal cues will not have to compete with lyrics of the music. Additionally, instrumental music often appeals to intergenerational classes.

When using music, the AEA suggests using approximately 125 to 150 bpm at half tempo for traditional shallow-water aerobics activities and 100 to 135 bpm at half tempo for most deep-water training formats. Half tempo (also referred to as water tempo) simply means counting every other beat. Music in these tempo ranges motivates participants and allows for full range of motion and long-lever movements. This speed of execution also enables participants to fully benefit from water's unique properties. Other considerations for tempo selection include the class format, the use of equipment, and the water depth.

When selecting tempo, also consider your participants' ability levels and program goals. A tempo that is too slow may restrict participants from working to their potential. One shallow-water exercise study showed that

AEA Standards and Guidelines for Aquatic Fitness Programming

Music Tempo

The following are general guidelines for music tempo (beats per minute, or bpm) in various types of aquatic programs (table 10.3). The slower reaction time of submerged movement benefits from the music being utilized at half tempo (i.e. every other beat of the music) in most situations.

Table 10.3 AEA Standards and Guidelines for Music Tempo

Class format	Recommended bpm
Shallow water cardiorespiratory	125-150
Deep water cardiorespiratory	100-135
Aquatic kick boxing	125 – 132 Basic techniques or skills and drills 128 – 140 Cardio combinations or advanced level
Muscular conditioning	115 – 130
Interval—Shallow water	125 – 150 Interspersed with higher or lower tempos
Interval—Deep water	100 – 130 Interspersed with higher or lower
Circuit training	125 – 150 Aerobic segments – shallow water 100 – 135 Aerobic segments – deep water 115 – 130 Resistance training segments

increasing music tempo created an increase in the physiological responses of rating of perceived exertion (RPE) at maximal heart rate achieved, percentage of maximal theoretical heart rate estimated, and blood lactate concentration (Barbosa et al. 2010). The researchers suggested that music tempo should be selected "according to the goals of the session they are conducting to achieve the desired intensity" (224). Tempo that is too fast may hinder some participants from achieving their full range of motion. As cadence increased (from 120 bpm up to 180 bpm) with a shallow-water jumping jack, a corresponding decrease in upper-body range of motion (ROM) was noticed, although lower-body ROM remained consistent (Costa et al. 2011). Faster tempos may be appropriate for higher-intensity classes to motivate participants to work harder, provided that they maintain full range of motion. Slower tempos may be more appropriate for less-fit participants, participants with functional limitations, or less intense classes. Choice of tempo should be based on the ability of the participants and the goal of the class.

Safe and Effective Instruction

Instructors have three options for positioning while teaching an aquatic fitness class:

- From on the pool deck
- From in the pool
- Going back and forth between the deck and pool

Advantages, disadvantages, and safety concerns exist for each of these methods. This section outlines the pros and cons of each teaching position, offering tips for each method and alerting you to safety concerns.

Teaching From the Pool Deck

The AEA considers deck instruction as the preferred method of leading aquatic fitness in most situations. See the sidebar AEA Standards and Guidelines for Deck Instruction for more information.

Advantages

- You are highly visible to participants.
- You can use your whole body to provide visual cues.
- Often, but not always, you can be better heard from on deck.
- You have better visibility of your class. You can see what participants are doing. This is especially important if you are expected to be both lifeguard and instructor. See chapter 13 for AEA Standards and Guidelines for Aquatic Fitness Programming—Lifeguard recommendations.
- Some movements, because of their complexity, can be explained and demonstrated only from the deck where participants can see what your whole body is doing.
- Complex choreography is better explained and demonstrated from the deck.
- New participants can usually follow deck instruction best because the instructor is more visible.
- It is easier to change or adjust your music from the deck.

Disadvantages

- You are exposed to the elements (heat, humidity, sun, wind).
- You are leading from a hard surface without the support and buoyancy of the water.
- You increase your risk for injury caused by slipping or impact.
- Your participants might be in prolonged neck hyperextension looking up at you on deck.
- The tempo and execution of movements (air and gravity) must be altered to approximate water conditions (viscosity and buoyancy).
- It can be difficult to demonstrate movements unique to the water, such as suspended training, or high-impact options, including propelled moves.

AEA Standards and Guidelines for Aquatic Fitness Programming

Deck Instruction

The AEA recommends deck instruction as the preferred method of leading aquatic classes in most situations. Deck instruction provides the highest level of safety for the participants by allowing better observation and quicker response to emergency situations. Deck instruction also provides greater visibility of the aquatic fitness professional to the participant and the participant to the aquatic fitness professional. The AEA recommends that the aquatic fitness professional remain on deck when there is no additional lifeguard on duty, when there are new participants in the program, or when new movements are being demonstrated.

The safety of the aquatic fitness professional does not have to be compromised if proper precautions are taken. Suggestions for safe deck instruction include the following:

- Avoid high-impact movement demonstration.
- Use a chair for low-impact demonstrations and balance needs.
- Consider non-impact teaching techniques.
- Wear proper footwear for deck instruction.
- When available, use a teaching mat to reduce impact stress.
- Wear appropriate clothing for the environment in which you work.
- Drink sufficient water to stay hydrated and protect your voice.
- Use a microphone when available or incorporate non-verbal cues.
- Position the music source where it provides the least interference with vocal cueing.
- Use caution when utilizing any electrical source, including sound systems, near a pool due to potential hazard of electrical shock.
- Lead the workout rather than participate in the workout.
- Train for endurance, strength, flexibility, and balance within your personal workout program to assure the ability to perform safely on the deck.

Movement Execution and Weight Transfer

Safe and effective demonstration of impact options for various moves and combinations is one of the toughest challenges an instructor faces when teaching from the deck. On deck, the instructor needs to demonstrate grounded, propelled, and level I, II, and III movements at an appropriate tempo with gravity and without the benefits of buoyancy. Needless to say, this requires careful planning as well as the assistance of teaching tools, such as chairs, stools, and walls. Here, we discuss three deck instruction options: full impact, low impact, and non-impact.

Full (high) impact. Many moves, such as jumping jacks, cross-country skis, jogs, knee lifts, kicks, turns, leaps, and rocks, can be demonstrated with full impact on deck (see figure 10.9). With modification to a slower tempo, full impact is most similar to the actual mechanics of the movement as it is to be performed in the water.

Deck demonstration provides challenges that make full-impact instruction precarious. Most pool decks are made of a hard surface, such as concrete or tile, and might

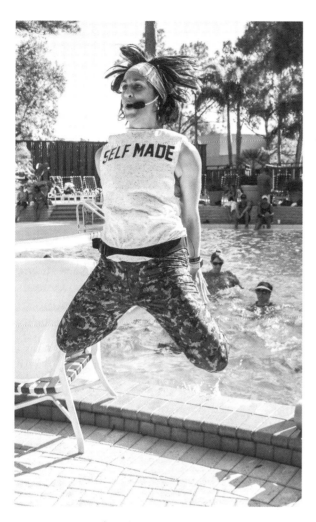

Figure 10.9 If a slower tempo is used, full impact instruction most closely resembles the actual exercise being taught.

be slippery, especially when wet. Leading a class with full impact increases your risk for overuse and acute injuries. Most aquatic fitness professionals choose low-impact or non-impact demonstrations to save wear and tear on their musculoskeletal system. You can reduce slipping and impact stress by wearing a supportive pair of shoes and using a nonskid cushioned mat on deck. Full impact should be used only sparingly to demonstrate the first few repetitions of a movement, set a pace, or motivate the class.

Reduced (low) impact. Reduced impact demonstration protects your musculoskeletal system when leading from the pool deck. It is often the preferred method of deck instruction for most movements because of its versatility and safety (figure 10.10). However, reduced impact demonstrations are not without challenges.

Since your actual demonstration might not show the intended impact level, you must otherwise cue participants immersed in the water to perform the desired impact. Consider the use of clear vocal cues, hand signals, or even printed signs (e.g., "jump", "propel", or, "tuck"). You might also refer to a participant in the pool with proper mechanics for others to observe and imitate.

Low-impact demonstrations can also challenge your balance skills. The use of a pole, wall, or chair for support can help with balance on deck. Maintaining a wide base of support (feet at shoulder width or slightly wider) and lowering your center of gravity (slight squat position) improves stability and balance and makes many movements easier to perform on deck at the appropriate tempo.

If you march on deck, participants will generally march in the pool. However, if you

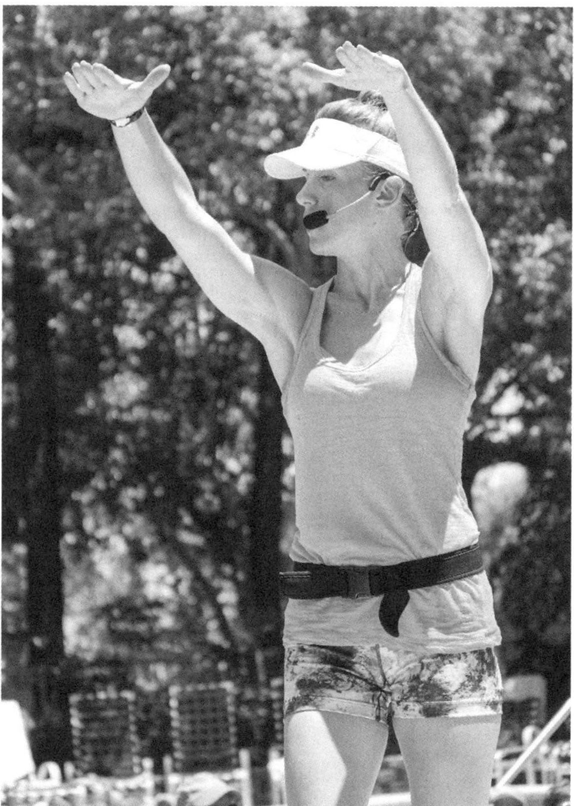

Figure 10.10 Reduced impact instructing from the deck is often the preferred method.

wanted them to jog in the water, your visual cue was not successful. The problem lies with your demonstration of weight transfer. Adjust your teaching technique while still keeping a low-impact option by quickly shifting the weight from one foot to the other, while enhancing your demonstration with exaggerated visual cues. Plantar flexing at the ankle and rolling from the ball of the foot to the heel to quickly shift weight from one foot to the next gives more of the appearance of jumping from foot to foot to perform a jogging motion. This technique helps motivate participants to perform the desired movement with proper intensity.

You may also incorporate a chair or stool for a low-impact teaching alternative. While seated, you can demonstrate one-footed and two-footed moves with less impact because most of your body weight is supported by the chair or stool, yet the feet do contact the pool deck with each move. The drawback is that participants may assume that the movement is at level II, even if the exercise should be performed at level I in the water. To make this more effective, add a verbal cue, a hand signal, or possibly even a cue card to clarify.

Non-impact. Some instructors, by necessity or choice, teach from the deck with non-impact techniques. This requires the instructor to become more skilled at verbal and nonverbal cueing techniques to motivate participants and guide them through transitions and move changes.

One method of non-impact deck instruction employs a chair, bench, or stool to elevate the feet off the pool deck (figure 10.11). Sitting allows you to demonstrate many leg movements without impact. Drawbacks of this include the fact that you are seated. As mentioned previously, if the desired body position for the exercise is standing (level I), then you must convey this through other cueing techniques. This method also requires strong hip flexor muscles to perform the movements and strong abdominal muscles to support the lower back. Although chairs are readily accessible, they might not be as versatile as a stool. With a 32- to 36-inch (81-91 cm) stool, the instructor can demonstrate moves with less hip flexion. A more extended leg might give participants a better idea of how the move should be performed in a standing position. Because the stool has no back or arms, it is easier to demonstrate turning or movements that require directional change. Although the mechanics demonstrated on deck are not identical to what is desired,

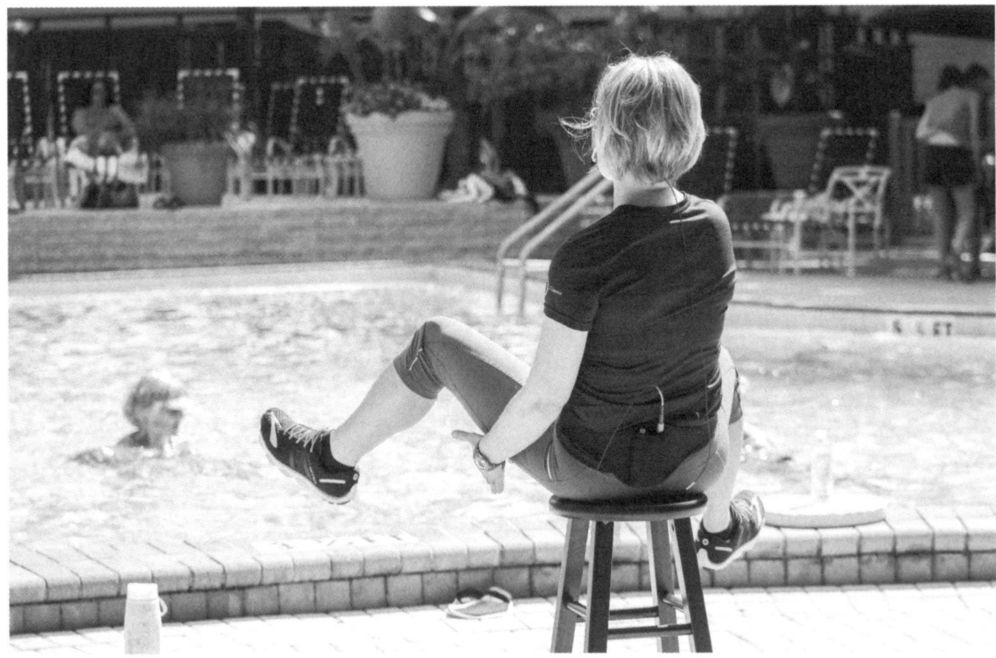

Figure 10.11 A stool can provide a safe option for deck instruction.

with additional verbal and visual cueing, the movements taught from a chair or stool can ensure that participants achieve the correct movement in the water.

Another effective and widely used method of non-impact instruction from the deck involves the use of the arms to demonstrate leg movements. To emphasize the demonstration, cue, "My arms are your legs," or place shoes on your hands to drive home the visualization. Using your arms to demonstrate the out and in movements of a jumping jack or the front-to-back movement of a cross-country ski works quite well. It is also very easy to convey proper tempo and weight transfer without balance or impact issues. Combining use of the arms with verbal and nonverbal cueing can effectively guide most movements with minimal stress to your body.

Well-inflected and well-timed verbal cueing can also be effective in conveying water movements from deck. You might feel comfortable using a high-impact or a low-impact demonstration for a few repetitions and then shifting to all-verbal cueing once participants have caught on. Although verbal cueing can save wear and tear on the musculoskeletal system, vocal injury becomes a risk. The instructor should take precautions to reduce risk of vocal injury, as discussed in chapter 13.

Teaching From Within the Pool

There may be times when teaching from within the pool is the preferred option. In order to provide the participants with a safe and effective workout, you must make several considerations. Just as with deck instruction, it requires practice to develop good instructor skills for teaching in the pool.

Some instructors cannot easily teach from the deck because of physical limitations. An instructor who has chronic back pain or arthritis flare-ups or is in the later stages of pregnancy might prefer to teach in the water. Many water instructors have their roots in aquatic programming as enthusiastic and dedicated participants who were recruited and encouraged to instruct. Transitioning to the pool deck may be initially uncomfortable or intimidating. Additionally, some class formats or those requiring specialized equipment may be more effectively demonstrated from in the water (see figure 10.12). Keep in mind participant safety, such as having a lifeguard on deck.

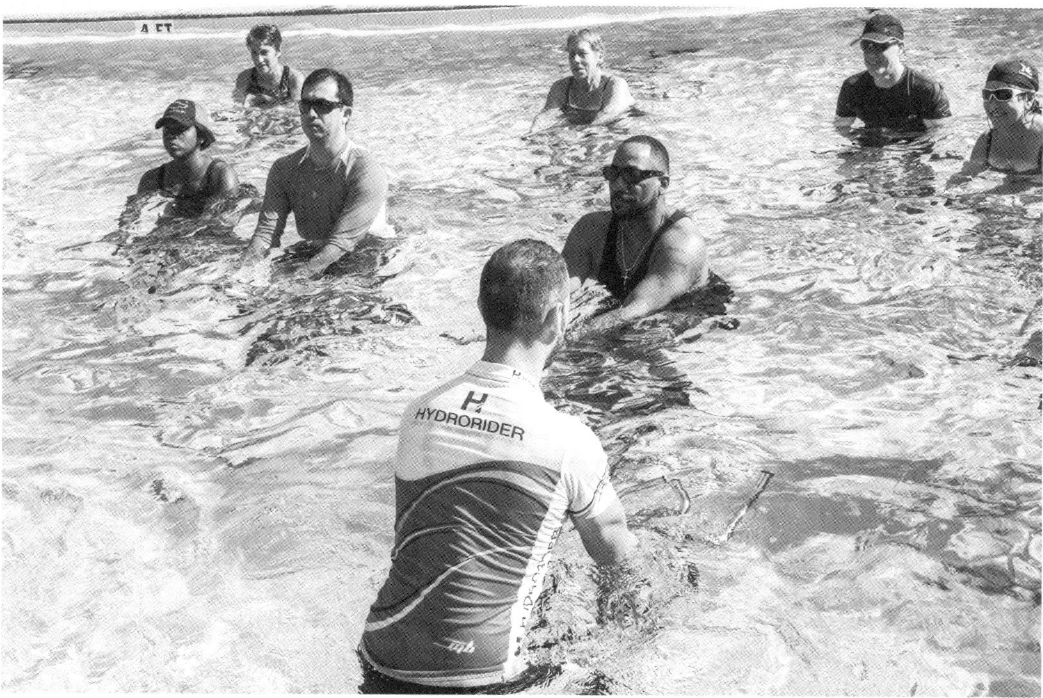

Figure 10.12 The use of certain equipment requires teaching from within the pool.

Advantages

- You are not exposed to the elements (heat, humidity, sun, wind), and have the benefit of the cooling effect of the water.
- You benefit from the support, cushioning, and reduced impact stress offered by the water.
- You can move around your class giving one-on-one feedback and interaction. You can use tactile cueing when appropriate.
- You can feel the movement in the same way as the participants. This may enable you to better motivate them and also allows you to more precisely adjust intensity for some movements.
- It is easier to demonstrate with proper tempo and weight transfer from in the water.
- It allows you to connect with your class.

Disadvantages

- It is very difficult for participants to see what you are doing. If you have a large class or several new participants, teaching from in the pool can be very challenging.
- Visual cueing is very limited. Because many participants are visual learners, some might get frustrated when they cannot see what they are supposed to do.
- It might be more difficult for participants to hear or understand you.
- Some movements are difficult to explain from in the pool, such as a complicated leg pattern involving turns.
- It is more challenging for you to monitor your participants.
- From a safety standpoint, you should teach from on deck if there is no lifeguard available so you can easily recognize a water rescue situation.

It is possible to be an effective instructor from in the water. Adjustments need to be made to cueing and choreography based on class participants. If you have a large number of participants who are new to the water or your class, you will need to use intentional verbal cueing and simplified choreography and move through the class to help new participants. If you have a group that has been with you for several programs, you might be able to introduce more advanced choreography.

When teaching from in the pool, consider the following tips:

- Place more importance on verbal cueing, inflecting your voice and explaining the same move in several different ways. Because you may at times be facing away from some participants, a waterproof microphone is highly recommended.
- Change your positioning in the pool throughout class. You can use a circle format with you in the middle or alongside participants in the circle, or you can remain in the center of the pool and have participants form groups on your right and left. Position newer participants where they can see you best. Wear dark-colored tights so participants can easily see your leg movements under water.
- Maintain eye contact as much as possible with participants. Sometimes participants' facial expressions can tell you who is having difficulty. Eye contact also opens the door to verbal communication. Give participants the opportunity to ask for help. Phrases such as "Who can I help?" or "Does anyone need assistance?" encourage participants to ask for help when they don't understand.
- Use the buddy system. If you have a large class with new participants, ask seasoned participants to buddy up with newer participants. They can help by explaining and demonstrating moves. You might even offer reduced class fees to class ambassadors in exchange for assisting new participants.
- If your pool design allows, you can move to shallower water to demonstrate moves. This way, the class can see more clearly what you are doing and observe visual cues for form and alignment. Remember safety factors because impact increases in shallower water.

- Start with basic moves and gradually develop choreography patterns. Building block choreography works well. Also, consider teaching a combination from a stationary position before adding the element of travel. Develop patterns with travel elements that move participants in the pool so you can visit with everyone.
- Show leg movements with your fingers, arms, and hands. Demonstrate arm movements above the water's surface and then do the movement submerged. Use props to help with instruction, for example, have cue cards at different places around the pool deck to hold up for visual aids.

Teaching From On Deck and in the Pool

This method combines the advantages of on-deck and in-pool teaching and reduces the disadvantages of both locations. Of course, safety issues are associated with moving from pool to deck. If your pool does not have easy access, you might choose to teach the first half of class from the deck to familiarize participants with all the moves. Then you might get into the pool for the second half of the class and use those moves to create combinations and patterns and add travel. This minimizes the number of times you have to get in and out of the pool. A good pair of water shoes is essential. You want a pair that cushions impact, reduces slipping, and allows you to go safely from the deck to the pool.

Knowing how to teach both on deck and in the pool expands your choreography and programming options. You can introduce and teach just about any movement. Your marketability as an instructor expands as your teaching skills expand, allowing you to teach a greater variety of formats.

Leading the Workout

There is a difference between leading the workout and getting a workout. Though there is no question that certain physical and psychological benefits are obtained whenever an instructor teaches, there is a significant difference between teaching to the group's level of fitness and performing at the instructor's level. A class can most effectively be taught to the midrange ability of that particular group. Choose the level where the majority of participants will be challenged (beginner, intermediate, or advanced) and teach to that range while offering modifications to increase or decrease intensity to address everyone's needs. Keep in mind that this level might not necessarily be your personal ability range.

Your primary role as an instructor is to provide a well-balanced fitness experience for your participants. This involves providing a safe, effective, and enjoyable experience that motivates your participants to continue coming to class. Leading the workout means you are not matching the participants repetition for repetition; rather, you are observing the participants and cueing for alignment, safety, and motivation.

Always remember that the class belongs to the participants. It is important to reserve enough time and energy for your personal workout; avoid using your class as your training session. Participate in someone else's class or develop a personal workout routine to increase your level of fitness. This is also an excellent way to model the benefits of variability or cross-training.

Professionalism

What makes a great instructor? Many combined qualities create someone who is capable of leading an aquatic fitness class that safely provides optimal results, creates a feeling of success for all participants, and promotes camaraderie in an enjoyable environment. Strive to present yourself as an exercise professional in your appearance, attitude, and behavior.

Dress for exercise as opposed to sun bathing or swimming. Supportive clothing that allows you to remain modest while moving on deck or entering and exiting the pool portrays professionalism and sets the tone that you are here to teach an exercise class (figure 10.13). Proper aquatic attire for instruction includes the following:

- Professional clothing appropriate to your teaching environment, such as a supportive bathing suit, tights, or bike shorts worn over or under the suit to provide modesty; shorts-style swim trunks for men; or another combination of acceptable, professional aquatic fitness attire
- Support bra for women and an athletic supporter for men
- Supportive, nonslip aquatic exercise shoes
- A hat, sunglasses, and sunscreen if teaching outdoors

Arrive early enough to class to be able to properly set up, prepare for your class, and greet participants. Establish a preclass ritual that creates a positive mind-set. Some instructors meditate in the car before entering the fitness facility, some listen to a certain song, and others recite a favorite quote before starting class. A positive mind-set and attitude translates to a positive class environment. For consideration of other instructors, properly clean up and put away equipment after your class. Follow facility procedures for taking time off or recruiting substitute teachers if you are ill or can't teach a class. Know and understand posted emergency procedures and follow facility procedures for documenting events requiring medical attention and processing class registrants.

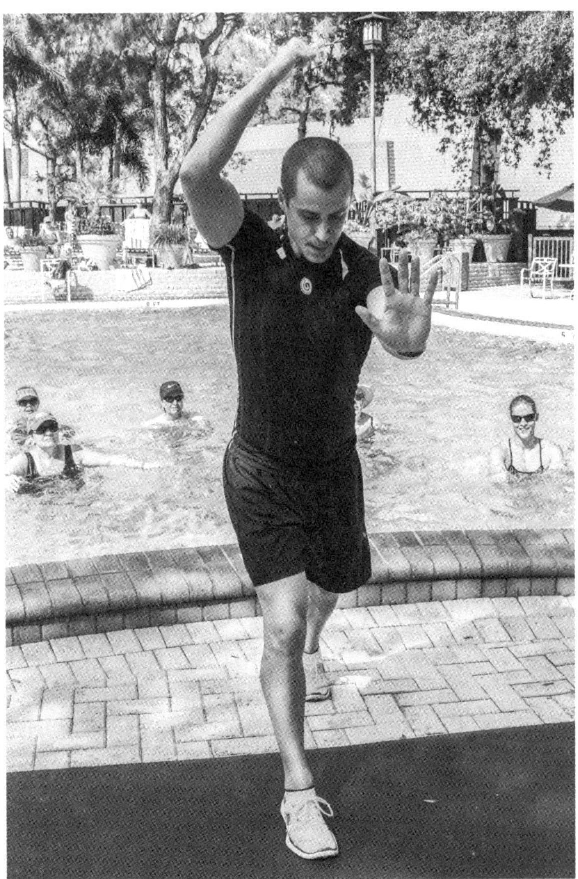

Figure 10.13 How instructors dress can set the tone for a safe and professional class.

Qualifications that employers look for in an aquatic fitness instructor include the following:

- Education and knowledge. Employers might require you to have a professional certification or equivalent. You should be able to demonstrate a reasonable understanding of the principles of water, exercise principles, and choreography and cueing, and have a willingness to continue learning.
- Experience. Many employers seek instructors with teaching experience. If you do not have experience, many employers recruit instructors to serve in a mentoring or training program to receive practical experience before teaching.
- Energy and enthusiasm. Employers are looking for instructors who are excited about teaching and convey that excitement to participants.
- Motivation. As an instructor, you need to be self-motivated and able to motivate others. A motivated and motivating instructor retains and recruits participants for programs.
- Good interpersonal skills. To be a group fitness instructor, you need to have a friendly, compassionate personality.
- Adaptability. The aquatic environment is seldom stable. You need to be able to adapt to environmental and facility changes.
- Responsibility and consistency. Employers want instructors who consistently show up and teach a good class.
- Sincerity. You need to show that you care and are there to serve the clients.

Becoming an outstanding instructor is a continuous process. You need to be open to learning and improving, not just for yourself but also for the participants who look to you and your skills to help them reach their fitness goals.

Summary

As an aquatic fitness professional, your form and alignment should exemplify what you want your participants to achieve during class. Your cueing and transition skills also assist participants in performing exercises with proper form and alignment.

Cueing, a specialized form of communication, allows the class to flow smoothly from one move to another. Cues are used to serve several purposes, including proper form and safety, motivation, transitions between moves, imagery to enhance performance, feedback between you and the participants, and relaxation for body awareness.

Cues may be delivered by audible, visual, and tactile methods. Using all three methods will allow you to reach a wide range of participants and engage all learning styles.

Well-planned transitions are important for safe programming. Transitions fall into three primary categories for shallow-water and deep-water exercise. For shallow water, your class population, the goal of your class, and the class format help determine which transitions are most applicable. With deep-water programming, the category of transition is primarily dependent on the ability to reestablish vertical posture and maintain balance.

Choreography simply means the arrangement or written notation of a series of movements. Aquatic fitness programs use a variety of styles of choreography to create safe, effective, and enjoyable workouts. Learning to use and blend the various styles will enhance your leadership skill and motivate participants.

Music, although not required, can be used for motivating participants, maintaining tempo, and achieving a desired intensity in your aquatic classes. Selecting the best style for your population and the appropriate tempo for the class format will enhance the workout experience.

There are three options for instructor positioning while teaching an aquatic fitness class, each with advantages, disadvantages, and safety concerns for both you and your participants. Carefully consider your teaching location: from on the pool deck, from in the pool, or a combination of both.

Strive to present yourself as an exercise professional in your appearance, attitude, and behavior. Your goal is to safely lead aquatic fitness classes that provide optimal results, create a feeling of success for all participants, and promote camaraderie in an enjoyable environment.

Review Questions

1. ____________________ is a specialized form of communication designed to instigate action.
   a. A cue
   b. Choreography
   c. Imagery
   d. Motivation
2. _________________________are used to maintain an open line of communication between the instructor and participants.
   a. Imagery cues
   b. Feedback cues
   c. Transitional cues
   d. Tempo cues
3. Cueing "right, left, right, right" is an example of what type of transitional cue?
4. A(n) _________cue is any cue received through hearing, including spoken words (verbal) and sounds, whistles, claps, musical changes, and bells.
   a. visual
   b. tactile
   c. feedback
   d. audible
5. Which type of shallow-water transition requires the greatest degree of core strength and coordination to safely execute?
6. The AEA recommends deck instruction as the preferred method of leading aquatic classes in most situations.
   a. True
   b. False
7. _____________________ is a style of choreography in which a series of moves are performed without a predictable pattern.
   a. Patterned
   b. Pyramid
   c. Add-on
   d. Freestyle
8. List four qualifications employers might look for in an aquatic instructor.

9. A ____________________, often a jog or vertical flutter kick, allows more time to prepare for the next movement in a pattern that may be needed to change planes or direction of travel or simply stabilize the body in the water.

   a. deep-water basic transition
   b. deep-water advanced transition
   c. deep-water transitional move
   d. deep-water tempo transition

10. ________________________________is an example of a non-impact deck instruction technique.

   a. Using the arms to demonstrate leg movements
   b. Using a stool or chair to demonstrate leg movements without touching the feet on the pool deck
   c. Performing a march instead of a jog.
   d. A, B, and C
   e. A and B only

See appendix D for answers to review questions.

References and Resources

American College of Sports Medicine. 2018. *Guidelines for exercise testing and prescription*. 10th edition. Baltimore: Lippincott, Williams & Wilkins.

American Council on Exercise. 2007. *Group fitness instructor manual*. 2nd edition. San Diego: Author.

Bandy, W.D. 2001. The effect of static stretch and dynamic range of motion training on the flexibility of the hamstring muscles. *Journal of Orthopaedic & Sports Physical Therapy* 27(4):295-300.

Barbosa, T.M., V.F. Sousa, A.J. Silva, V.M. Reis, D.A. Marinho, and J.A. Bragada. 2010. Effects of musical cadence in the acute physiologic adaptations to head-out aquatic exercises. *Journal of Strength & Conditioning Research* 24(1):244-250.

Clemens, C.A., and C.J. Cisar. 2006. The effect of footwear on the reliability of the 500-yard shallow water run as a predictor of maximal aerobic capacity (VO_2max). *AEA Aquatic Fitness Research Journal* 3(1):36-39.

Costa, M.J., C. Oliveira, G. Teixeira, D.A. Marinho, A.J. Silva, and T.M. Barbosa. 2011. The influence of musical cadence into aquatic jumping jacks kinematics. *Journal of Sports Science and Medicine* 10:607-615.

Denomme, L., and J. See. 2006. *AEA instructor skills*. 2nd edition. Nokomis, FL: Aquatic Exercise Association.

Fowles, J.R., D.G. Sale, and J.D. MacDougall. 2000. Reduced strength after passive stretch of the human plantar flexors. *Journal of Applied Physiology* 89(3):1179-1188.

Howley, E.T., and D.L. Thompson. 2012. *Fitness professional's handbook*. 6th edition. Champaign, IL: Human Kinetics.

Innovative Aquatics. 2008. *Personal pool programming*. Nokomis, FL: Personal Body Trainers.

Kravitz, Len. 1994. The effects of music on exercise. *IDEA today* 12.(9): 56-61.

Santos, J. 2016. Music: How to be a TOP instructor! *Akwa* 29(5):10.

Sova, R. 2000. *Aquatics: The complete reference guide for aquatic fitness professionals*. 2nd edition. Pt. Washington, WI: DSL.

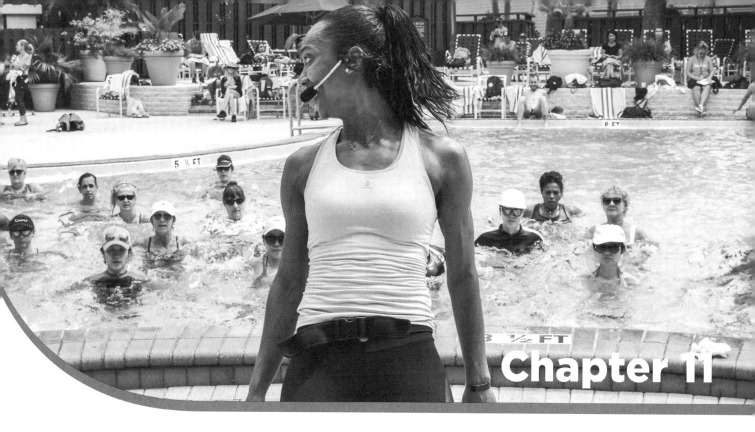

Chapter 11

Aquatic Exercise Programming

Introduction

The aquatic environment lends itself to a diverse array of programming options. This chapter explores the basic recommendations for developing safe and successful aquatic programming for both group fitness and personal training. It considers various class formats while emphasizing the versatility of water exercise.

Key Chapter Concepts

- Explain the purpose for the main class components (warm-up, conditioning, cool-down, and stretch), and recognize how to adapt each for the aquatic environment.
- Understand how to create variations of the conditioning phase of class to achieve various goals and accommodate the needs and abilities of your participants.
- Learn how to incorporate general recommendations for class components into numerous programming formats that provide training variety and motivate a wide range of participants.
- Recognize movements in the aquatic environment that may require greater consideration to use them safely and effectively in class.

Class Components

Whether the aquatic exercise session occurs in shallow or deep water, includes strength or aerobic exercise, or involves kids, baby boomers, or older adults, the basic program formatting will have many similarities. Program **format**, or the way that the class is arranged, is designed around a multitude of factors, including the needs and ability of the class, size and shape of the pool, equipment availability, purpose of the session, water temperature, and many other elements relating to the program, the participants, and the environment in which the class takes place. Although these factors will help you to determine the appropriate class formatting for your situation, the basic components of the class or training session will remain somewhat consistent.

The components of a training session based on the recommendations of the ACSM include a warm-up, conditioning or sport-related exercise, cool-down, and stretching (2018). The purpose of class formatting is to steadily progress the body into an exercise state and then gradually return it to a pre-exercise state. Each component serves a physiological purpose to enhance the training process while minimizing risk. Table 11.1 provides guidelines for adjusting class components to the aquatic environment to ensure a safe and effective workout in the pool.

A seasoned instructor uses a variety of methods to create interesting program formats while maintaining the key elements of each training component. Frequently changing the format creates opportunity for adaptation. Most participants enjoy variety in class format, music choices, and exercise selection. Variety in programming allows participants to advance in fitness and assists with long-term exercise adherence. Regardless of the class format, remember the purpose for each training component and follow the general recommendations for the fitness industry.

Warm-Up Component

The warm-up serves the following purposes:

- Allows the body to adjust to the changing demands of the exercise session (transitioning from rest to work)

Table 11.1 AEA Recommendations for Program Design

Class component	Considerations	Duration range
Warm-up	Purpose of class Water temperature	5-15 minutes
Conditioning	Purpose of class Available equipment Participant ability Participant needs and goals Water temperature Water depth	20-120 minutes
Cool-down	Purpose of class Intensity of class Water temperature	5-15 minutes
Stretching	Purpose of class Muscles targeted during class Participant needs and goals Participant ability Water temperature	

- Prepares the musculoskeletal system by increasing tissue extensibility, improving muscle contraction, and increasing joint range of motion (ROM)
- Increases blood flow to working tissues
- Increases metabolic rate (Gray, De Vito, and Nimmo 2002)
- Allows acclimation to the exercise environment
- May reduce risk of injury
- Improves performance (Bishop 2003)
- Provides physiological preparation for exercise (Ladwig 2013)

The aquatic warm-up consists of a thermal warm-up, prestretch, and cardiorespiratory warm-up and lasts at least 5 minutes. Two necessary (thermal and cardiorespiratory) warm-up segments and one optional (prestretch) segment can be instructed in a variety of ways to allow for the warm-up period to fit the specific needs of your program.

The first fundamental warm-up segment is the **thermal warm-up**. The thermal warm-up is made up of rhythmic movements that generate body heat while allowing for acclimation to the aquatic environment. Movements performed during this portion of the warm-up may include water walking the length of the pool, marching in place, or jogging combined with various arm movements, such as reaching forward, side-to-side, up, down, and across the body. The water temperature will partially determine the duration of this portion of the warm-up. If exercising in cooler water (80-83 °F or 27-28 °C), the thermal warm-up might need to be lengthened by 5 to 10 minutes to ensure that adequate body heat is generated before progressing. On the other hand, if exercising in warmer water (greater than 86 °F or 30 °C), this portion of the warm-up may be condensed since the water temperature will assist in thermally preparing the body.

The second part of the warm-up is the optional **prestretch**. Depending on the temperature of the water and the purpose of your class, you may choose not to include a prestretch at all or to modify it by using dynamic (rhythmic) stretching instead of static stretching. Studies indicate that static stretching can reduce muscle contraction ability and performance (Simic, Sarabon, and Markovic 2013). Thus, a dynamic stretch might be more appropriate if the exercise session is focused on power, strength, or agility, such as athletic training formats. Dynamic stretching is generally preferred for athletic precompetition and prepractice, and assists with power-focused or high-intensity training sessions. Some instructors prefer dynamic stretching to static stretching because it is easier to maintain core body temperature; however, it is imperative not to overstretch. Dynamic stretches are incorporated into whole-body movement. Instead of holding the stretch, use slow, large range-of-motion movements to stretch the muscles (e.g., slow transverse shoulder abduction, adduction to stretch pectorals and posterior deltoids, slow kicks front to stretch hamstrings, or slow kicks back with knee flexed to stretch hip flexors and quadriceps).

Both dynamic and static stretching are important aspects of exercise design, but good judgment on the part of the fitness professional is necessary to determine which technique is most appropriate for the population, the program format, and the environment. Whichever method you choose, be sure to keep the core temperature elevated and the limbs warm. If class time is limited and flexibility is not your primary goal of the session, you can omit the prestretch and instead stretch at the end of the class.

The third part of the warm-up is the **cardiorespiratory warm-up**. Its primary purpose is to elevate the heart and respiration rates gradually in preparation for more strenuous exercise. The cardiorespiratory warm-up allows the body to perform more efficiently during strenuous exercise and makes the transition much more comfortable. It is recommended to include this phase of the warm-up process even if the main segment of the class does not target aerobic training. All forms of exercise benefit from increased blood flow, increased oxygen levels, and joint lubrication.

Some instructors use the cardiorespiratory warm-up as a preview of coming attractions. New choreography can be taught at a slower pace. This might also be a time to include a social element, such as partnered water walking. Additionally, this portion of the warm-up should highlight the specific movements and intensities that will be performed during the class. Specificity during the warm-up will allow the body to appropriately prepare for the workout to follow. Table 11.2 provides examples of warm-up activities appropriate for various program goals.

Conditioning Phase

The conditioning phase of a class format consists of the primary exercise mode. This could be cardiorespiratory, strength or muscular endurance, flexibility, neuromotor exercise,

Table 11.2 Example Warm-Ups

Class focus	Example warm-up	Purpose
Cardiorespiratory fitness—*shallow water*	• 2 minutes: Walk forward and backward using alternating arm pattern • 1 minute: Increase stride length • 1 minute: Side step, traveling laterally with arms abducting and adducting • 1 minute: Increase side step cadence • 1 minute: Front kicks with pause to stretch at the top • 1 minute: Heel high jog with pause to stretch at the top • 1 minute: Cross-country ski, increasing effort • 1 minute: Knee high jog, increasing effort • 1 minute: Jumping jack, increasing effort	Thermally warm up the body while increasing heart rate and respiration rate with the walk and side step. Prestretch the body using dynamic stretching with front kick and heel high jog. Prepare the cardiovascular system for the class by increasing the effort or intensity with the cross-country ski, knee high jog, and jumping jack.
Cardiorespiratory fitness—*deep water*	• 2 minutes: Jog forward and backward using alternating arm pattern • 1 minute: Add breaststroke with forward jog and reverse breaststroke with backward jog • 1 minute: Wide jog traveling laterally while scooping the water with the arms to assist with travel • 1 minute: Increase wide jog cadence • 1 minute: Front kicks with pause to stretch at the top • 1 minute: Heel high jog with pause to stretch at the top • 1 minute: Cross-country ski, increasing effort • 1 minute: Knee high jog, increasing effort • 1 minute: Deep water jack, increasing effort	Thermally warm up the body while increasing heart rate and respiration rate with the jog and wide jog. Prestretch the body using dynamic stretching with front kick and heel high jog. Prepare the cardiovascular system for the class by increasing the effort or intensity with the cross-country ski, knee high jog, and jumping jack.
Strength	• 2 minutes: Long strides forward and backward with breaststroke arms • 2 minutes: Crossing side step with arms crossing and opening • 2 minutes: March progressing to a jog with arms pushing left to right (trunk rotation) • 2 minutes: Cross-country ski progressing in intensity with arms in opposition swinging front to back • 2 minutes: Jog forward and backward with impeding arms (backstroke with forward jog and front crawl with backward jog)	Thermally warm up the body while preparing for total-body movement and full range of motion in various planes. Prepare the cardiovascular system as well as the musculoskeletal system with large movements, core stabilization, and progressive intensities.

or skill-related training. The conditioning phase may include a mixture of two, or even all five, options, depending on the purpose of the class as well as your participants' needs and abilities.

Cardiorespiratory Endurance Training

Cardiorespiratory endurance training can be structured as continuous, interval, or circuit formats. Each format challenges the cardiorespiratory and metabolic systems differently. To review these differences, refer to chapter 1.

The way that the cardiorespiratory component of the class is arranged should reflect the purpose of the class, the ability level of your class participants, as well as the environmental factors of your pool (see the sidebar Programming Ideas for Cardiorespiratory Endurance Training). The ACSM recommends a minimum of 20 minutes of vigorous intensity conditioning or 30 minutes of moderate

Class focus	Example warm-up	Purpose
High-intensity intervals	• 2 minutes: Walk forward and backward using alternating arm pattern • 1 minute: Increase stride length • 1 minute: Side step traveling laterally with arms abducting and adducting • 1 minute: Increase side step cadence • 30 seconds: Ankle hops (2-footed movement with the primary hopping motion coming from the feet and ankles; knees and hips stay soft but straight while the ankles plantar flex and dorsiflex) • 1 minute: Knee high jog increasing effort • 30 seconds: Level II tuck jumps • 1 minute: Wide jog increasing effort • 30 seconds: Tuck jumps alternating knees together and then wide • 1 minute: Cross-country ski increasing intensity • 30 seconds: Rocking horse with exaggerated jump forward and back	Thermally warm up the body while increasing heart rate and respiration rate with the walk and side steps. Prepare the cardiovascular system and increase intensity to prepare the body for a higher level of work and potentially greater levels of impact with the variations in hops, jumps, and more intense cardiorespiratory exercises.
Flexibility and mobility	• 2 minutes: Walk forward and backward using alternating arm pattern • 1 minute: Increase stride length • 30 seconds per side: Lunge stretch for hip flexors and gastrocnemius • 30 seconds: Hold right lunge position, clasp hands in front of body, and stretch the shoulder girdle • 30 seconds: Hold left lunge position, open the arms (transverse abduction), reaching the fingertips back to stretch the chest • 1 minute: Side step, traveling laterally with arms abducting and adducting • 1 minute: Increase side step cadence • 30 seconds per side: Side lunge stretch for hip adductors and groin • 30 seconds per side: Leg swings forward and back • 1 minute: Jog 5 steps forward then heel toe raises; jog 5 steps backward then heel toe raises	Thermally warm up the body while increasing heart rate and respiration rate with the walk and side steps. Prestretch the body using static (lunges, shoulder, and chest) and dynamic (leg swings, toe raises) stretching. Prepare the cardiovascular system for the class by increasing the effort or intensity with the increased stride length, cadence, and jogging patterns using inertia.

intensity conditioning. Adjustments in class format can reflect these time variations. Classes may range in duration from 30 minutes to well over an hour, and the length of the cardiovascular component will depend on the abilities of the participants and the purpose of the class. For example, moderate intensity training needs to occur at least five days per week and needs to include between 30 and 60 minutes of cardiovascular exercise per session. More intense training needs to occur at least three days per week and needs to include between 20 and 60 minutes of cardiovascular exercise per session.

Movements can range from simple isolated movements to complex combinations and patterns. Of course, you want to consider your class population and the purpose of the movement in relation to the class' goals. Using large muscles and performing movements at an intensity to promote oxygen consumption will assist in improving cardiorespiratory fitness and caloric expenditure. Additionally, application of the physical laws creates a workout that effectively uses the principles of water while enhancing participant outcomes. Monitoring for appropriate intensity, as well as offering alterations to make exercises more or less challenging, helps to ensure that all participants reach their fitness potential.

Nearly any movement can be performed to train the cardiorespiratory system. Some examples might include jumping jacks, jogging forward with breaststroke arms, cross-country ski elevating out of the water, and straight-leg kicks moving forward. Please refer

Programming Ideas for Cardiorespiratory Endurance Training

- Traditional fitness format (combinations of base-move variations and impact levels using the aquatic principles to alter intensity)
- Dance-oriented programs (specific styles such as ballroom, ballet, hip-hop, and various ethnic rhythms such as African and Latin)
- Water striding or jogging, including aquatic treadmill
- Martial arts
- Boot camp
- Sport-specific training
- Aquatic step
- Aquatic cycling
- Aquatic trampoline
- Aquatic pole

Many of these formats can also be modified for special populations and health considerations, including perinatal, older adults, children, obese populations, arthritis, and cardiac rehabilitation. See chapter 12 for more information.

These programs have the potential for many variations.

Training format:

- Continuous training
- Interval training
- Circuit training

Equipment:

- No equipment
- Drag equipment
- Buoyancy equipment
- Rubberized equipment
- Specialized equipment
- Flotation equipment

Water depth:

- Shallow water
- Deep water
- Transitional water depth
- Both shallow and deep

to appendices A and B for more examples of shallow-water and deep-water exercises. Along with the countless variety of movements, these exercises can be grouped, organized, or assembled in many different formats, creating endless opportunities for variety.

Muscular Fitness Training

Muscular fitness training includes exercises performed with or without equipment to target specific muscles, muscle groups, or body segments (upper body, lower body, or trunk). The intention is to overload muscles or muscle groups to improve muscular endurance or strength. You can employ greater force, additional resistance (equipment), or increased repetitions to improve muscular fitness during water exercise.

Remember the principle of progressive overload when beginning a muscular training program. Do more repetitions with less resistance to promote endurance gains and use higher resistance with fewer repetitions to promote muscular strength gains. The ACSM recommends two to four sets of 8 to 12 repetitions each for strength and power and one or two sets of 15 to 20 repetitions for endurance. The aquatic environment lends well to stimulating and cultivating muscular endurance. With the added drag forces and multidirectional resistance from the water, the body immediately experiences the need for greater effort to create movement. This results in muscular endurance gains. Achieving adequate resistance to elicit strength gains in the water can be a challenge for very fit populations. However, by using the resistance of the water along with the application of acceleration (force) and equipment, any participant can become stronger in the pool (Colado et al. 2009). As with all types of exercise, progressions must be made in order for the body to continue to adapt and become stronger. Altering lever length or hand position, increasing the speed and force of the movement (Colado, Tella, and Triplett 2008), and adding or advancing equipment (e.g., larger surface area or greater level of buoyancy) are methods for progressing muscular resistance training in the aquatic environment.

Programming Ideas for Muscular Fitness Training

- Target muscle isolation activities as the primary component of class with a series of exercises that will provide a balanced workout for all of the major muscles groups.
- Incorporate muscular endurance into a continuous training format.
- Combine muscular conditioning with cardiorespiratory circuit stations.
- Use muscular conditioning for the recovery cycle in an interval class.
- Choose muscular conditioning exercises with a specific focus:
  - Targeting muscular strength with more intense resistance equipment and working to voluntary muscle fatigue
  - Targeting muscular endurance with moderate resistance and more repetitions
  - Targeting core musculature with the water's resistance or added equipment to improve stabilization and enhance posture
  - Muscular strength or endurance exercises mimicking functional, daily activities or sport performance
  - Use an aquatic step or aquatic pole as a tool for specialized muscular training activities
  - Choose Pilates programs adapted for the aquatic environment.

Programming for muscular strength and endurance can be formatted in a variety of ways. Muscular fitness conditioning stations can be alternated with cardiorespiratory stations in a circuit workout. You can also create a class format that uses only muscular fitness conditioning exercises. Some instructors incorporate muscle isolation with full-body movement as an active rest component in an interval work and rest cycle. More simply, muscular strength or endurance may be the focus of the class or just a small component (5-10 minutes). As is true for cardiorespiratory training, there are several format options for muscular fitness training, and various water depths can successfully be employed See the sidebar Programming Ideas for Muscular Fitness Training.

Muscular Flexibility, Mobility, and Range-of-Motion Training

A third option for the endurance phase of a class format is to target muscular flexibility, mobility, and range of motion. These programs can be performed with slow, broad movements that emphasize full range of motion with minimal resistance, functional movements that highlight mobility needed for daily skills, or various types of stretching exercises.

Participating in regular stretching and mobility exercises promotes better range of motion and may prevent or reduce risk of injury and muscle soreness. Positive changes in flexibility can be observed immediately following a stretching session and long-lasting flexibility can be obtained after less than four weeks (Garber et al. 2011). It is easy to forget the importance of range of motion in a fitness regimen and the role of flexibility as a primary component of fitness.

You must still consider the importance of the thermal warm-up and the principle of progressive overload when choosing this type of class format. An effective thermal warm-up and maintenance of warm muscles throughout this type of class are essential because flexibility exercises are safer and more effective when the body is warm. Because some of this programming may be slower in nature, water temperature may need to be a little warmer for participant comfort as well as optimal program outcome. Recommendations for water temperature are between 85 and 90 degrees Fahrenheit (30-32 °C). Progressive overload, or gradually increasing the amount of stress placed on the body over time, relates to all classes, including flexibility-based programs. Trying to push into a stretching position that

Programming Ideas for Muscular Flexibility, Mobility, and Range-of-Motion Training

- Tai chi programs adapted for the aquatic environment
- Ai Chi programs
- Yoga programs adapted for the aquatic environment
- Pilates programs adapted for the aquatic environment
- Extended final stretch segment to focus on flexibility
- Use of buoyant, weighted, and flotation equipment to enhance range of motion
- Weightless deep-water range-of-motion programs
- Interval-based class using flexibility, mobility, or range of motion (ROM) exercises as the recovery
- Programs for special populations and health conditions (e.g., arthritis, chronic pain; see chapter 12 for more information.)

the body is not yet ready for may result in injury, such as a muscle strain or tear.

The sidebar Programming Ideas for Muscular Flexibility, Mobility, and Range-of-Motion Training provides some options for highlighting muscular flexibility, mobility, and range-of-motion training into your aquatic classes.

Yoga and tai chi programs have become very popular in land fitness. Aquatic fitness has reflected this same trend; tai chi, Ai Chi, yoga, and stretching and relaxation programs are very popular in the pool. Many exercisers want this option for variety and to augment more vigorous cardiorespiratory and muscular fitness training. These programs also meet the needs of participants who prefer lower-intensity exercise or need added mobility and range of motion to complete their daily tasks. These class formats open the door to less-active people and to those who enjoy more gentle exercise and desire physical activity in a group environment.

Water adds a new dimension to range-of-motion and relaxation class formatting. As long as the water is warm and comfortable, buoyancy offers assisted stretching and the component of floating to enhance relaxation. Many facilities with warm-water pools are able to offer these class formats. Facilities without warm water pools may be able to offer these programs by adding full-body movement or dynamic stretching segments to keep body temperature elevated.

Neuromotor Exercise or Functional Fitness Training

Neuromotor exercises are those that require greater amounts of balance, coordination, agility, and proprioception. Often called **functional fitness training**, neuromotor exercises can be incorporated into a short segment of the class or can be the primary focus of the endurance component.

Incorporation of these types of exercises results in improvements in balance, agility, and muscular strength, while reducing fall risk (Garber et al. 2011; Nelson et al. 2007). This information provides clear reasoning for including neuromotor exercises for older adults; however, younger, athletic clientele also show improvement through reduced injury rates (Garber et al. 2011). As with any type of exercise, the training stimulus must present a challenge in order to yield improvements. For example, clients who lack balance, coordination, and agility may find walking with their arms in a neutral position (e.g., crossed at the chest) to be challenging, while those who are more proficient may

Programming Ideas for Neuromotor Exercise or Functional Fitness Training

- Functional fitness programs
- Tai chi programs adapted for the aquatic environment
- Ai Chi programs
- Yoga programs adapted for the aquatic environment
- Pilates programs adapted for the aquatic environment
- Walking challenge format (combining water walking with other skills, such as balance or agility) or gait training classes
- Interval-based classes with neuromotor exercises used as the recovery
- Circuit training that includes neuromotor exercise stations
- Programs for special populations (e.g., arthritis, chronic pain) that include a balance training component

need a bigger challenge, such as walking in tandem using a unilateral (one side only) arm pattern. The sidebar Programming Ideas for Neuromotor Exercise or Functional Fitness Training shares aquatic programming ideas for incorporating neuromotor exercises.

Skill-Related Training

Although skill-related components of physical fitness are commonly associated with athletes, they are important for everyone. Skill-related components can be incorporated into portions of any class or can be offered as stand-alone programming. Skill-related drills and exercises may be integrated into any class format and within any program focus.

Agility, or the ability to rapidly and accurately change body position, can be incorporated into aquatic fitness classes by using challenging footwork patterns at varied speeds. Static and dynamic balance can be targeted in your classes in a number of ways: through neuromotor exercises, as a recovery from a challenging interval, or in choreography. Coordination, or integration of senses with movement, can be improved by performing a separate drill, including complex choreography, or altering any expected pattern (such as mixing a jumping jack leg pattern with cross-country ski arm movement) to make it more challenging for your participants to perform. Power production, or the culmination of speed and strength, fits perfectly into a muscular strength or plyometric-based class, but it can be added to other class formats as well. One important thing to note with performing power-based movements is that an appropriate warm-up and preparation are essential. When moving with speed and strength, the body should be fully prepared. Reaction time can be paired with agility, coordination, or even speed when planning class activities. For participants to truly practice their reaction time performance, make certain they can hear you or see your cues. Speed, or how fast a movement is performed, is discussed in various sections of this manual. Stationary movements can be performed more quickly or travel can be accomplished at a shorter time interval. All of these skill-related components of physical fitness are important for every population that we serve.

Cool-Down Component

A cool-down serves the following purposes:

- Provides gradual recovery from the endurance phase of exercise
- Allows for the gradual recovery of heart rate and blood pressure (ASCM 2018)
- Enhances venous return, reducing the potential for blood pooling in the extremities and resultant dizziness or fainting (Fletcher et al 2001)
- Facilitates the dissipation of body heat
- Removes lactic acid produced during exercise
- Promotes flexibility in the poststretch

In most aquatic fitness programs, the cool-down consists of two parts: the **cardiorespiratory cool-down** and the **poststretch**. The cardiorespiratory cool-down follows the conditioning segment and consists of 5 to 10 minutes of slow, lower-intensity, controlled movement to help the body recover to preexercise values. The movements will be based on the focus of the conditioning segment, and may include walking or other low-impact movements or lower-intensity muscular conditioning movements. Neuromotor activities, dynamic stretching, or mobility exercises are all appropriate for this segment of class as well.

In addition to the slowed movement, the cooling effect of the water often assists with recovery. If the water temperature is cooler than the body, then the body will dissipate heat into the cooler environment and the cool water will assist in reducing the body temperature. Because of this heightened cooling effect, water temperature has a large effect on what activities can be performed during the cool-down. In cooler water, where chilling may become an issue, a more dynamic cool-down may be necessary. In warmer water, where body temperature may take longer to return to normal, the cool-down may need to be prolonged. In this case, pair slower movements with static stretching.

Exercise is a series of muscle contractions, or shortening of the muscle tissue. It is important to stretch after exercisc to retain and promote flexibility. The poststretch may consist of 5 to 10 minutes of stretching exercises to return muscles to a pre-exercise length. As mentioned before, water temperature will dictate a static or dynamic poststretch. Combining dynamic movement of one part of the body to statically stretch another is a good way to take advantage of water's buoyancy and resistance. Using a combination of static and dynamic stretching may be the perfect complement to the end of your class. See table 11.3 for examples of cool-downs for different classes.

Aquatic Program Formats

Using the general recommendations for class components, you can design numerous formats to keep aquatic classes engaging, provide training variety, and motivate a wide range of participants. This section discusses some of the most common aquatic formats, many of which can be modified for shallow, deep, or transitional water depths.

Table 11.3 Example Cool-Downs

Water depth	Example cool-down	Purpose
Shallow water	• 2 minutes: Review new combinations from the cardiorespiratory component at slower tempo	Begin to return heart rate to pre-exercise level with slower movements and reinforce new movement patterns.
	• 3 minutes: Dynamic balance drills: forward and backward tandem walking and side step traveling laterally with neutral arms	Include neuromotor activities that focus on balance while maintaining body temperature during dynamic drills.
	• 5 minutes: Dynamic stretching for major muscles, such as front–back knee swing for gluteals and hip flexors and side-to-side knee swings for hip rotator muscles	Conduct poststretch of the major muscles through dynamic flexibility while continuing to reduce heart rate.
	• 4 minutes: Static stretching interspersed with water walking	Continue with poststretch, performing static stretches to promote ROM and water walking to maintain warmth.
	• 1 minute: Deep breathing with rhythmic upper-body and core movements, such as figure-8 arm sweeps with spinal rotation and transverse shoulder abduction and adduction with spinal flexion and extension	Combine deep breathing for relaxation with rhythmic movements to maintain warmth.
Deep water	• 5 minutes: Combined upper-body stretches with gentle leg movements in various planes	Conduct poststretch of the upper body while beginning to return heart rate to pre-exercise level, maintaining warmth with lower-body movements.
	• 5 minutes: Dynamic lower-body stretches alternating with a static hold, e.g., gentle full-ROM front kick for 8 reps then a static stretch hamstring stretch for 20 seconds on each side	Continue with poststretch of lower-body muscles with a combination of dynamic (maintain warmth) and static stretches.
	• 1 minute: T-position (arms abducted at water's surface, legs vertically extended) with eyes closed and deep breathing.	Use deep breathing for relaxation with focus on maintaining vertical body alignment and core engagement. Closing the eyes helps improve body awareness.

Circuit Training

Circuit training is often referred to as station training. The stations can be cardiorespiratory, muscular fitness, flexibility, neuromotor, or any combination. The circuit format can be **instructor guided**, where everyone in the class is performing each station at the same time. You lead the group as each participant performs the same moves and uses the same equipment (if being incorporated) at the same time. The circuit can also be **self-guided**, with individuals or small groups rotating from station to station. A **combination circuit** combines these two options into one class; you lead the class in a cardiorespiratory segment and then the participants move individually or in small groups to various stations. Circuit training is very versatile, and is limited only by your creativity with the equipment available, your pool design, and your participants (figure 11.1). See appendix F for a sample shallow-water circuit-training workout.

Interval Training

Interval training is composed of a series of training cycles that include high-intensity (work) and low-intensity (rest) segments. Both work and rest are planned and functional. The work–rest ratio sets the foundation for interval training. Intervals can be aerobic or anaerobic in nature, resulting in different fitness outcomes for your class participants or clients.

Aerobic intervals would be arranged in a 1:1 (equal work and rest) or 1<1 (work is longer than rest) ratio. During the work phase of aerobic intervals, encourage participants to exercise moderately hard to hard. The rest phase is active, meaning that participants continue to exercise but at a lower level of effort. For an anaerobic interval, the work–rest ratio is usually 1:2 or 1>2 (where work is shorter than rest). During anaerobic intervals, cue participants to work at or near maximal effort. Recovery can include light activity or total rest. During both aerobic and anaerobic intervals, heart rates will undulate, going up with the work interval and down during the rest interval.

Some very specific interval ratios include HIIT and Tabata. HIIT, or high-intensity interval training, is designed for participants to exercise at or above their maximal capacity; rest periods vary depending on the goals of the class. Tabata is a very specific set of eight intervals (20 seconds of maximal effort

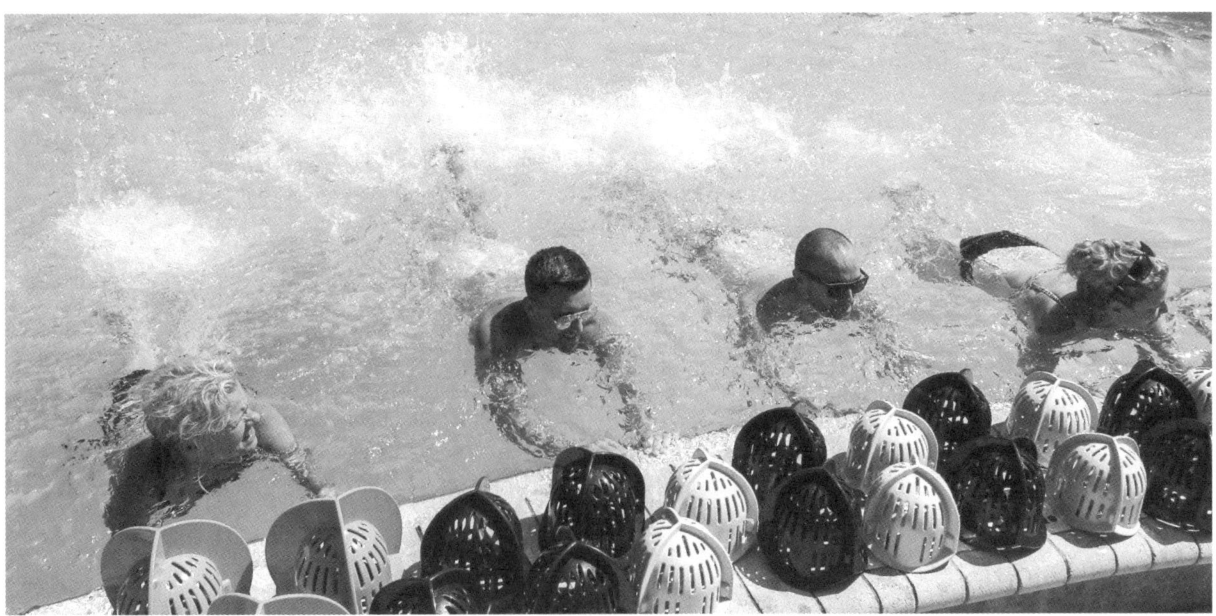

Figure 11.1 Circuit training in the water, as on land, is only limited by your creativity with equipment and space.

Table 11.4 Interval Training Examples

Interval type	Example
Aerobic interval 1:1 ratio	2 minutes hard cross-country skis (work): 2 minutes steady wide jogs (recovery)
Anaerobic interval 1:3 ratio	20 seconds maximal white water run (work): 1 minute easy march (recovery)
HIIT 1:4 ratio	20 seconds maximal level III jumping jacks (work): 80 seconds shifting weight from side to side (rest)
Tabata 2:1 ratio	20 seconds maximal high knee run (work): 10 seconds float or stand (rest) *Repeat 8 times*

followed by 10 seconds of complete rest) completed in rapid succession. See appendix F for a sample deep-water HIIT workout. Examples of various types of intervals are included in table 11.4.

Dance-Oriented Programs

Some aquatic programs are geared to more highly developed choreography sequences of dance-oriented movements. The class components remain similar; the difference is found in the level of complexity in choreography, which challenges the participants both physically and mentally. A variety of dance-oriented classes target specific styles of dance, such as ballroom, ballet, and hip-hop, or various ethnic rhythms, such as African and Latin. All of these styles can be mixed and incorporated into your classes as appropriate for your participants. When introducing this type of class, more simplistic choreography patterns are recommended. Once your participants begin to look and feel confident in the movements and transitions, greater complexity can be added. It is also helpful to teach segments of the combinations during the warm-up to prepare participants for what is ahead. This prevents unwanted decreases in intensity levels during the cardiorespiratory segment of class. Using choreography styles such as pyramid or add-on can help ensure that your participants understand the pattern as you progress.

Striding (Walk and Jog)

Striding can be incorporated as a warm-up or cool-down for other class programs, or the entire class format may be designed around striding patterns. This format easily adapts to all water depths and pool shapes and sizes (figure 11.2). The choreography or movement patterns are typically simple, making the choreography easy to follow and easy to instruct. These classes can provide a great opportunity to work on walking patterns, proficiency, balance, and range of motion. Striding programs can encourage social interaction among participants while providing a chance to improve fitness. With simple modifications of intensity and impact, this format can be designed for all levels of participants. Underwater treadmills offer more options for classes that center around walking

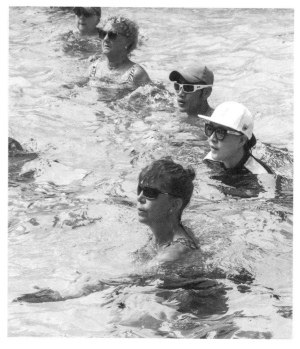

Figure 11.2 A practical benefit of water walking is that it can easily adapt to all depths and sizes of pools.

and jogging activities. See appendix F for a sample shallow-water striding workout.

Cycling

Stationary bikes designed specifically for the pool have become a popular training option for group exercise, personal training, and rehabilitation (see figure 11.3). With proper instruction, aquatic cycling can be a safe and effective option for all ability levels. Although similar to stationary cycling on land, pedaling while immersed takes advantage of the benefits of the aquatic environment. Resistance is determined by the unique design of the bike that increases drag resistance when pedaled; this resistance is adjustable on most styles of aquatic bikes. Resistance is also influenced by pedaling speed or revolutions per minute and by altering the body position on the bike. Aquatic cycling can achieve cardiorespiratory goals with continuous or interval training, or the goals may be more focused on muscular endurance or even strength. If your facility has a limited number of bikes, they can be set up as part of a circuit-training workout.

Step

Step training is a fitness program that incorporates a step (a bench or a platform) to step up and down during a portion of the class. This kind of training can be performed safely and effectively in the pool with aquatic-specific equipment and an appropriate environment. To prevent the step from moving excessively, the pool slope should be gradual. Adequate space is required; the amount depends on the size of the step and the movements that will be performed. Additionally, a good indication of appropriate water depth is to have water level at the elbows when participants stand on the bench. This means about chest depth when standing on pool bottom. Aquatic step formats can focus on muscle conditioning, cardiorespiratory training, or neuromotor activities. The step can be used for an entire class or for a section of the class.

Pole

This unique type of fitness training uses a vertical pole as a training tool. Poles specifically designed for aquatic training

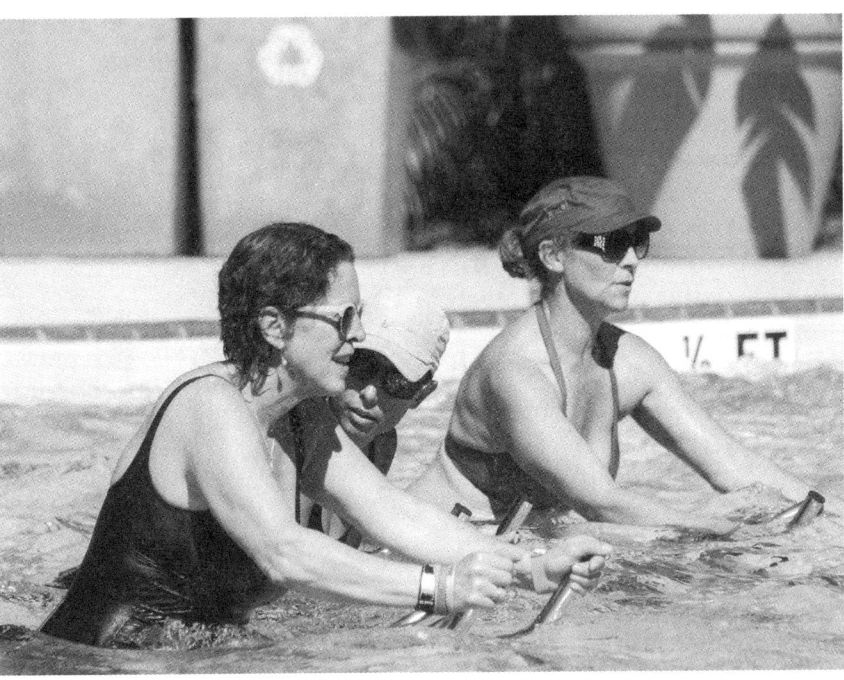

Figure 11.3 Stationary bikes designed for the aquatic environment have become popular.

have opened this format to many more participants (figure 11.4). According to the International Pole Dance Fitness Association (IPDFA), today's pole dancing has evolved into an exercise format practiced by performers as well as fitness participants, both men and women alike. Various protocols include training for improved posture, rehabilitation, muscular strength and toning, and choreographic techniques to challenge cardiorespiratory endurance, agility, coordination, and overall fitness (Thielen 2014). According to the IPDFA, modern-day pole dancing is actually a combination of centuries-old techniques, and has evolved into a format that relies heavily on dance as well as fitness skills.

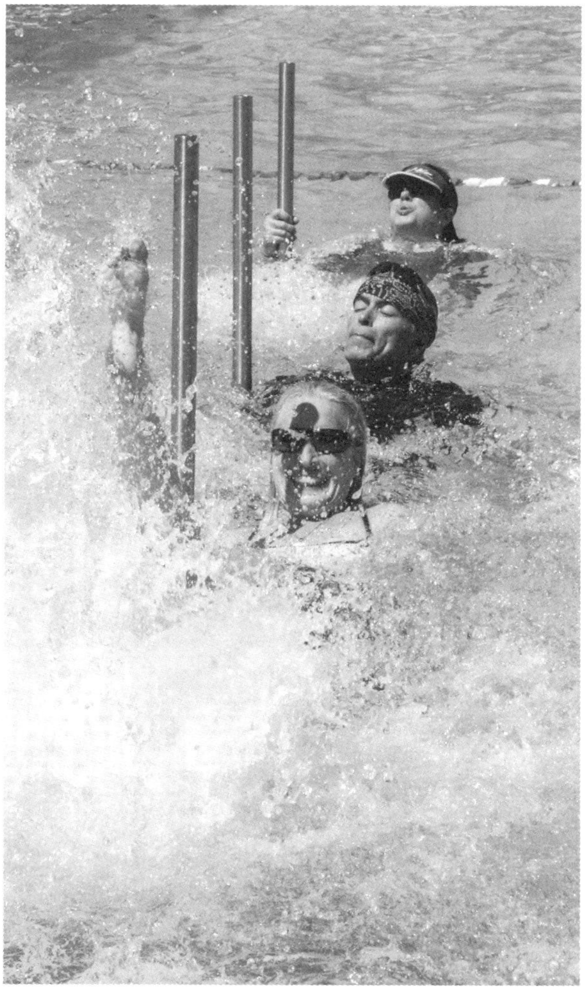

Figure 11.4 Exercise poles designed for the pool provide another training option.

Trampoline

Another type of exercise equipment that has transitioned from land to pool is the mini trampoline (figure 11.5). This training format is often referred to as rebounding. Although many exercises involve jumping, the elastic nature of the trampoline offers a low-impact exercise option. Additionally, the unstable surface of the trampoline causes the core muscles to be actively engaged during all movements. From cardiorespiratory training to core strengthening and balance skills, the mini trampoline can offer a unique workout. Moving the trampoline into the aquatic environment provides an element of comfort for participants concerned about falling.

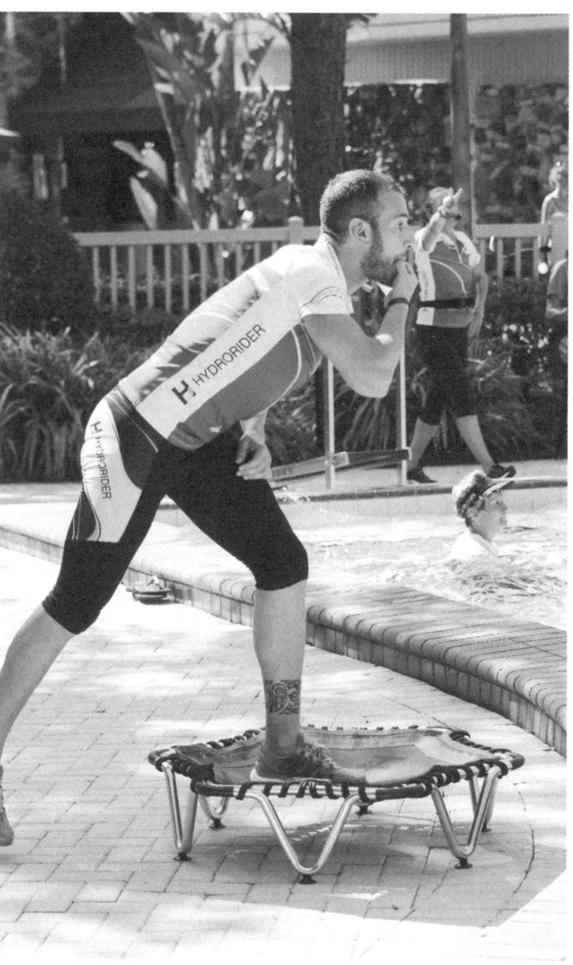

Figure 11.5 Trampolines can benefit both those who need low-impact workouts as well as balance training.

Muscular Conditioning

This type of training focuses on muscular strength and endurance, as well as stretching activities for flexibility. It may be incorporated as a segment of another program or as an independent class format. Muscular conditioning programs often employ additional equipment or use force and speed to promote added resistance for continued overload to the muscular system (figure 11.6). The key to this type of training is using precision and control to target isolated muscle groups or to provide functional movements. Some classes focus primarily on muscle conditioning, whereas others use muscle conditioning for specific segments, such as stations of a circuit training class or as part of the cardiorespiratory cool-down.

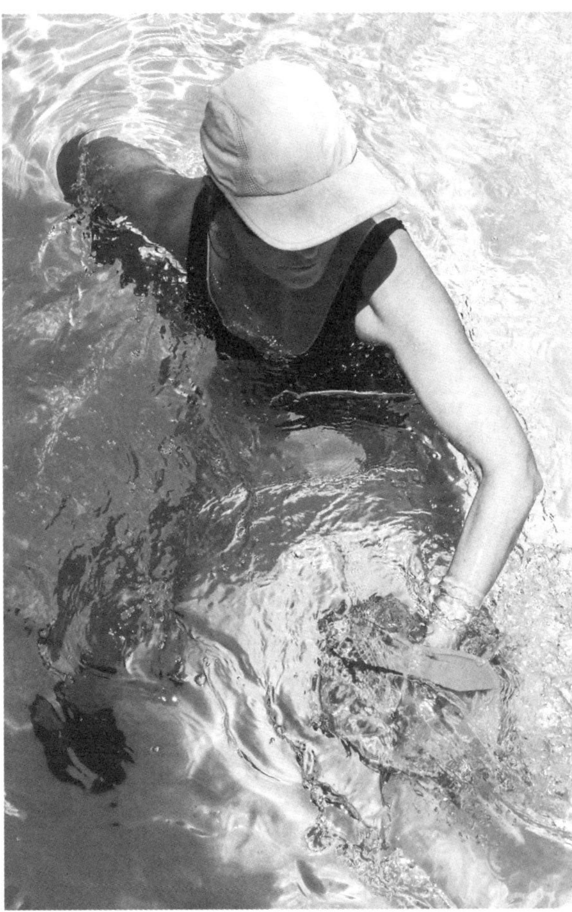

Figure 11.6 Incorporating equipment into a conditioning class adds resistance for improved fitness.

Martial Arts

A variety of martial arts have been adapted for water fitness programs (figure 11.7). Kickboxing, tae kwon do, jiujitsu, and traditional boxing, as well as combinations of these styles, are commonly seen in the pool. Martial arts–style classes normally use an interval workout altering speed and resistance to create effective training cycles. Transferring martial arts training techniques and movement patterns (kicks, punches, and blocks) into the water creates a high-intensity, highly resistive, yet lower-impact exercise option. By using the unique properties of the water, in particular buoyancy and drag forces, an optimal cross-training program can be created for group exercise participants and personal training clients. Specific equipment

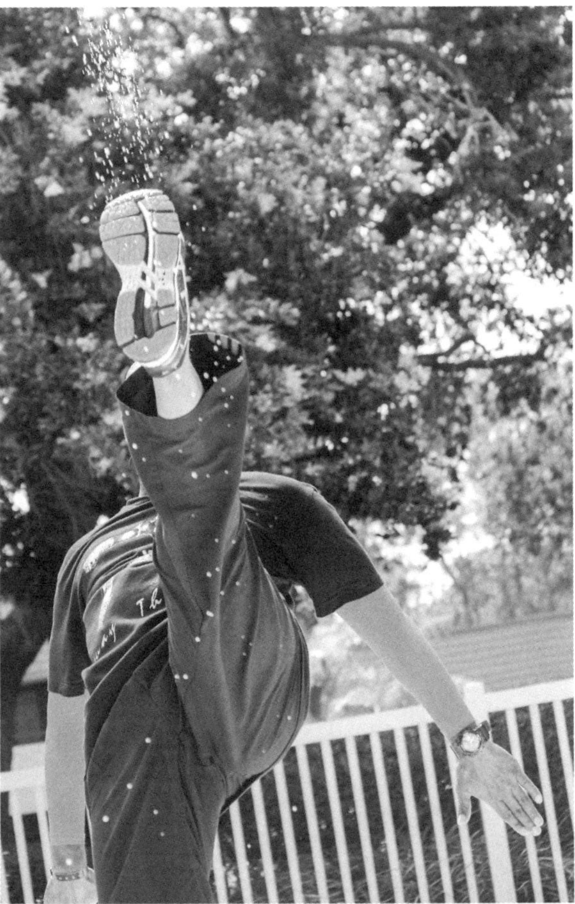

Figure 11.7 Aquatic martial arts combines the intensity of land training with low impact movements.

has been designed for the aquatic environment, including boxing gloves and training bags mounted on poles to serve as targets. See appendix F for a sample shallow-water kickboxing workout.

Boot Camp

Boot camp classes use a combination of muscular strengthening exercises, cardiorespiratory exercises, power or plyometric movements, and range-of-motion activities in a circuit or interval format to challenge overall strength and conditioning.

Some land-based boot camp classes include skills and drills that mimic activities used in military training programs while maintaining a sense of camaraderie and including an element of fun. Many of these same exercises and activities can be effectively adapted for the pool with the proper equipment and knowledge of the properties of the water. Boot camp formats are designed to achieve the physical benefits associated with higher-intensity workouts and the psychological benefits associated with achieving a specific goal. The supportive and resistive nature of the water allows participants who may be limited with land-based programs to successfully participate in a boot camp format. See appendix F for a sample deep-water boot camp workout.

Ai Chi

Ai Chi was created in Japan in the early 1990s by Jun Konno. This aquatic exercise and relaxation program employs a combination of deep breathing and slow, broad movements of the arms, legs, and torso with an inward-directed focus. Performed in warm, chest-deep water, the circular movement creates harmony, promotes a malleable body, and increases range of motion (figure 11.8). The flowing, continuous patterns of Ai Chi are facilitated by warm water and air temperatures. Ai Chi Ne, an extension of Ai Chi, involves working with partners. Both Ai Chi and Ai Chi Ne can be offered as unique class formats or used during the cool-down or as the rest component in interval training.

Pilates, Tai Chi, and Yoga

Yoga postures, tai chi movements, and Pilates exercises adapted for the aquatic environment have grown in popularity and

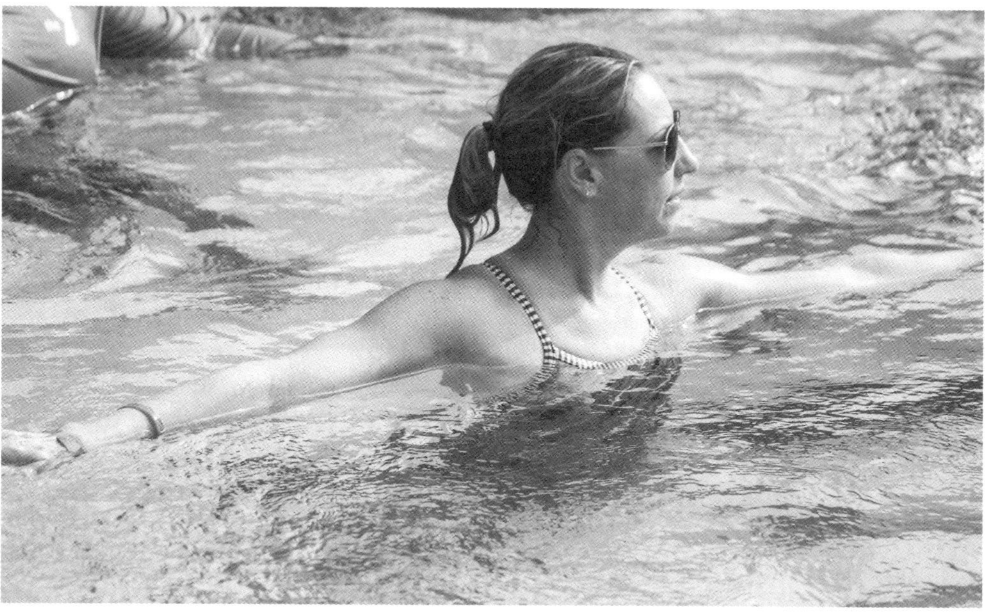

Figure 11.8 The warm environment of the pool can facilitate the flow of Ai Chi exercises.

variety (figure 11.9). These techniques have been incorporated into aquatic exercise in a variety of ways, including using them for strength-focused or muscle endurance classes, within an interval either as the work (strength) or recovery (range of motion or flexibility), or as circuit components, combination classes, or stand-alone classes. Breathing techniques, core strength, muscle activation, body alignment, and flexibility, which are important techniques for all class participants and instructors to learn, are the primary focus of these three modalities.

Pilates is a nonimpact program of strengthening and stretching exercises that involve precise muscle initiation and breath control. Land-based Pilates was developed by Joseph Pilates to target the stabilizing musculature with primary emphasis on the torso, referred to as the body's powerhouse. Every movement is controlled, precise, and performed with a purpose.

Tai chi is typically classified as a form of traditional Chinese martial arts. With its flowing and graceful movement patterns, tai chi transfers well into an aquatic environment as long as the water and air temperatures are appropriately warm. Benefits of aquatic tai chi include balance, coordination, agility, flexibility, and mental focus.

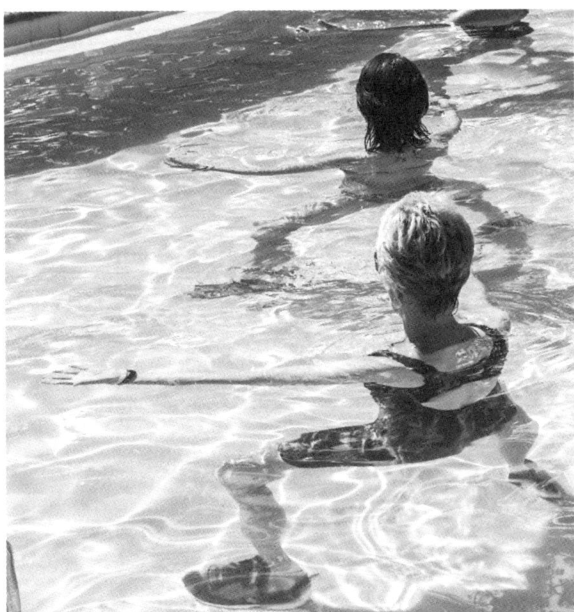

Figure 11.9 The precise, controlled nature of Pilates and yoga postures work well with the added support that an aquatic environment provides.

Yoga programs typically focus on alignment and lengthening of the spine while coordinating movement with breath. Many styles of yoga are performed on land, including hatha, Iyengar, vinyasa, and ashtanga. Postures, or asanas, are intended to quiet the mind, enhance focus, build strength, improve balance, and promote respiratory strength. Adapting yoga to shallow or deep water can allow for greater ability to perform the postures due to support from the water, while challenging the stabilization musculature from the undulating movements of the surrounding aquatic environment.

Functional Training

Functional training helps provide participants with the strength, flexibility, power, and endurance to move effectively and efficiently through the day. Specific activities vary depending on the participant's needs and daily activities. For instance, participants may desire to walk up and down stairs more efficiently or have more energy when playing with their grandchildren. Goals should be realistic and achievable and should guide the exercises selected for training. Exercises to improve mobility, stability, and balance are needed to improve or maintain functional independence. The buoyancy and resistance of the water make the pool an excellent place for functional training. Since the goal of functional training is the ability to perform daily activities with greater ease and the majority of our day is spent in a gravitational environment (on land), cross-training on land is essential. See appendix F for a sample functional training workout.

Sport-Specific Training

Sport-specific classes that have been adapted for the pool can have two purposes. People with sports performance goals can challenge

Periodization

The basic idea of periodization is to look at the bigger picture. This could be a semester, a calendar year, or a specified number of exercise sessions. When using periodization, first consider the goal of the exercise plan. If your goal is to increase overall fitness, you should incorporate both the health-related and skill-related fitness components. On the other hand, if strength is your primary focus, you should highlight it throughout the planning and programming process.

Once the goal has been established, the general focus for each week or set of weeks can be created. For example, if the primary goal is general fitness, then the focus of the first 4 weeks of training in a 12-week periodization plan might emphasize cardiorespiratory endurance training. Other components of fitness would also be included, but they would not be the primary focus. An example class might include a 10-minute warm-up, 20 minutes of continuous training (aerobic endurance), 10 minutes of strength-focused work, 10 minutes of continuous training, and a 10-minute cool-down with a focus on flexibility. During the course of the 4 weeks, the duration or intensity of the aerobic endurance segments would increase to add the new training stress necessary for improving the area of focus (aerobic endurance).

Of course, we cannot keep increasing effort and intensity without adding in rest. Rest should also be planned into the programming. A basic idea on how to include rest is the three up, one down paradigm. In this paradigm, programming increases in intensity over the course of 3 weeks and then is reduced in both intensity and volume for a week. Some classes may not need a full week of rest, but including at least one active rest day per month is recommended. Planning progresses in this fashion for the set length of time until complete, and then another periodization plan would be initiated.

In summary, periodization involves the following actions:

- Determine the length of time (e.g., 12 weeks, 6 months, a full year).
- Determine the goal (e.g., general fitness, specific fitness parameter).
- Create a training plan based on the goals.
- Design the individual workouts.
- Incorporate rest sessions.

the body through sport-specific training (e.g., running, jumping) without experiencing the impact stress of training on land. Pool facilities may partner with a local team (soccer, volleyball, football) to offer programs that meet the training needs of their athletes. These programs will provide intensities and activities or exercises that would satisfy the training requirements of the team's periodization schedule. **Periodization** is a way to structure a series of workouts to help ensure that fitness gains are created and overtraining is avoided. It is integral for athletic competitions but can also have very positive results for all participants hoping to improve in one or many areas of physical fitness.

People not necessarily interested in competition can participate in a challenging yet fun workout that includes movements that are typically performed during athletic events. You may choose to offer a sport-specific

Aquatic Personal Training and Small-Group Fitness

Personal training and small-group fitness formats are gaining popularity in the pool, giving aquatic fitness professionals an opportunity to expand their careers. **Personal training** offers individualized and customized fitness programs that meet the needs and goals of a specific client. Sessions are designed to enhance overall health, wellness, or fitness based on the individual. **Small-group fitness** is defined as two to five people working under the guidance of a fitness professional to achieve health and fitness benefits through a more intimate and personal setting than group exercise classes. With small-group fitness, the participants often have similar goals and abilities. Many applications exist, including the transition from rehabilitation or therapy to group exercise, as well as programming adapted to specific populations or conditions (e.g., pre- and postnatal women, people with **musculoskeletal considerations**, and obese individuals), age groups (e.g., seniors, teens, and children), or goals (e.g., tennis, golf, and skiing).

To begin aquatic personal training, the AEA recommends that fitness professionals hold a nationally or internationally recognized personal training certification to gain the necessary knowledge regarding fitness assessments and testing, business considerations, and interpersonal skills. Additionally, fitness professionals should hold the AEA Aquatic Fitness Professional certification to gain the necessary knowledge regarding the principles of water, aquatic equipment and muscle action, effective programming for pools, and water safety.

class to add variety to your regular aquatic schedule, or just for an occasional class option. Activities can be designed to mimic movements used during athletic events: dribbling or shooting in basketball or soccer, jumping to shoot baskets or hit volleyballs, running the bases in baseball, diving to catch balls, or balance skills for surfing. Creative applications of the properties of water and aquatic equipment can allow for a fun class that gives participants the opportunity to perform activities that they may not be able to perform on land.

Movements Requiring Greater Consideration

The water is a very versatile and forgiving exercise medium, but don't assume that this means participants will be able to safely perform movements exactly as instructed or intended. When planning your classes, consider the participants, the purpose of the movement, the purpose of the class, and the modifications or options you will need to offer. All movements, combinations, intensities, drills, and formats should be rehearsed and evaluated for safety and effectiveness before incorporating them into your class.

As a general rule, very few movements are contraindicated for aquatic fitness programs. Some movements may involve greater consideration, special cueing, and possibly modifications for some participants, yet be completely safe and effective for others. The following sections list some exercises that should be given extra consideration.

Very Fast Movements

It is acceptable to use speed to provide variety or adjust intensity, but remember that range of motion may be compromised with speed, and the water's benefits are often minimized. When fast movements are being introduced, consider using short levers (such as knee lifts and leg curls) and performing the movements in place (as opposed to traveling). As participants become accustomed to faster movements, it may become appropriate to introduce longer levers and travel, but this will depend on the participant, class style, and purpose. It is not acceptable to teach all, or even the majority, of a class at a very fast speed like land tempo. To achieve a well-rounded program, it is more effective to blend a variety of tempos with the laws and principles of the water discussed in chapter 6.

Extended Use of Arms Overhead

Ideally, every joint should be strengthened and stretched throughout its full ROM. Thus, overhead movements of the arms should be included when it is appropriate for the population, no shoulder injury or impingement is present, and the exercise has benefit. However, extended use of the arms overhead can lead to fatigue and poor form, possibly resulting in injury.

Overhead arm movements can be replicated by placing the body supine or prone in the water or hinging at the hips to position the torso parallel with the pool bottom. These body positions use the beneficial properties of the water while still achieving full shoulder ROM. Incorporating both vertical overhead activities and modified overhead activities can benefit participants in fitness goals and activities of daily living.

Very-High-Impact Exercises

Propelled jumps, which propel the body upward and out of the water, can be very useful for developing power in the lower body. These exercises are commonly used in athletic populations but can also be used for the general population. If you choose to include some of these moves in your class, be sure participants are at an appropriate water depth (at least mid-rib cage), cue for proper alignment and form, and include appropriate rest. Provide lower-impact alternatives that achieve similar results for participants with compromised joints or a lower fitness level. For example, many plyometric exercises can be simulated at level II or level III with modifications.

Modified Prone Activities

Modified prone activities are performed in a prone position with the head out of the water (figure 11.10). This position, achieved by holding on to the wall or a piece of flotation equipment or by sculling with the hands,

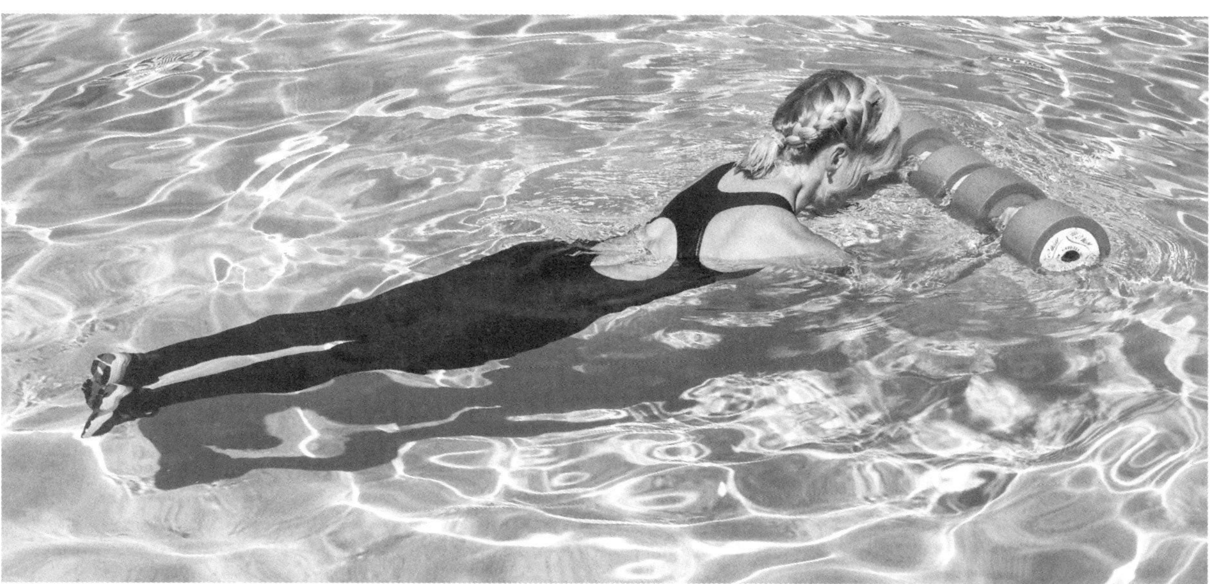

Figure 11.10 Consider adding equipment to assist with proper alignment in modified prone activities.

can lead to hyperextension of the lumbar spine, the cervical spine, or both. Although controlled extension and hyperextension are functional, these body positions should not be maintained for an extended period of time. This is particularly true for participants who may not be completely comfortable in the water (e.g., non-swimmers). The tension in the muscles due to unease can alter body position and make it much more challenging to maintain proper alignment. Consider other options such as adding equipment for support, altering the body angle, or performing the movement vertically.

Wall-Hanging Exercises

Exercises that require participants to hang for extended periods of time at the pool wall can be very stressful to the shoulder, wrist, hand, or finger joints. Hanging from the elbows with the back against the side of the pool may compromise the shoulder girdle and shoulder joints. Grasping the edge of the pool can strain the hands, wrists, and fingers in the attempt to maintain the position.

Most wall-hanging exercises can be performed in a vertical position in deep water (with flotation at the torso), modified to a standing position in shallow water, or achieved with additional flotation (such as a noodle). If you choose to incorporate wall-hanging exercises, limit the position to 1 or 2 minutes before returning to standing. Include options for those unable to exercise in this position.

Abdominal Conditioning

Aquatic fitness instructors should provide a variety of options for strengthening the abdominal muscles, both isometrically and isotonically, to improve fitness as well as function. Many of the movements that are categorized as abdominal exercises result in stabilization of the abdominal muscles while the hip flexors create the movement. Supine and vertical exercises that require the knees to move closer to the chest are initiated by the hip flexors while the abdominal muscles stabilize the torso.

Training the abdominal muscles to stabilize during movement is very beneficial in terms of fitness and functional mobility. However, overworking the iliopsoas, as with repeated hip flexion, can cause stress to the lower back. Since the majority of movements in an aquatic exercise class involve hip flexion (e.g., jogging, cross-country skiing, tuck jumps), the use of the hip flexors during abdominal work should be limited. Instead, focus on exercises that result in spinal flexion (e.g., supine or standing curls) or abdominal stabilization without hip flexion (e.g., spinal rotation exercises).

Summary

Program format must consider the needs and ability of the class, size and shape of the pool, equipment availability, purpose of the session, water temperature, and many other elements relating to the program, the participants, and the environment in which it takes place.

The components of a training session based on the recommendations of the American College of Sports Medicine (ACSM) include a warm-up, conditioning or sport-related exercise, cool-down, and stretching.

An aquatic fitness class warm-up consists of a thermal warm-up, prestretch (optional), and cardiorespiratory warm-up lasting at least 5 minutes. These segments may be instructed in a variety of ways to fit the specific needs of your program.

The conditioning phase consists of the primary exercise mode: cardiorespiratory, muscular strength or endurance, flexibility, neuromotor exercise, skill-related training, or any combination of these.

In most aquatic fitness programs, the cool-down consists of two parts: the cardiorespiratory cool-down and the poststretch.

Using the general recommendations for class components, numerous formats can be designed to keep aquatic classes engaging, provide training variety, and motivate a wide range of participants.

Although the water is a versatile and forgiving exercise medium, not all participants will be able to safely perform movements exactly as instructed or intended. Consider the participants, the purpose of the movement, the purpose of the class, and the possible modifications or options when planning programs.

Review Questions

1. The purpose of class formatting is to steadily progress the body into an exercise state and then gradually return it to a pre-exercise state.
   a. True
   b. False
2. Which of the following statements is *not* true regarding the warm-up component of class?
   a. Prepares the musculoskeletal system by increasing tissue extensibility
   b. Allows acclimation to the exercise environment
   c. Promotes more rapid removal of lactic acid
   d. May reduce risk of injury
3. The ______________________ is made up of rhythmic movements that generate body heat while allowing for acclimation to the aquatic environment.
   a. prestretch
   b. thermal warm-up
   c. cardiorespiratory warm-up
   d. poststretch
4. Cardiorespiratory endurance training can be structured as continuous, interval, or circuit formats.
   a. True
   b. False
5. _________________________ includes exercises performed with or without equipment to target specific muscles, muscle groups, or body segments (upper body, lower body, or trunk).
   a. Cardiorespiratory training
   b. Skill-related training
   c. Muscular fitness training
   d. Neuromotor exercise

6. A thermal warm-up is not needed for a class that targets muscular flexibility during the conditioning component since the moves are gentle and the water is warm.

   a. True
   b. False

7. In most aquatic fitness programs, the cool-down consists of two parts:_ ________________________________

   a. the cardiorespiratory cool-down and the prestretch
   b. the cardiorespiratory warm-up and the poststretch
   c. the cardiorespiratory cool-down and the poststretch
   d. the cardiorespiratory warm-up and the prestretch

8. ______________________ is often referred to as station training.

   a. Sport-specific training
   b. Tabata training
   c. Interval training
   d. Circuit training

9. Sport-specific training formats are applicable only to athletes due to the intensity of the workout.

   a. True
   b. False

10. If you choose to include very-high-impact moves, such as plyometric training, in your class, be sure to:

    a. Ensure that participants are at an appropriate water depth (at least mid-rib cage)
    b. Cue for proper alignment and form
    c. Include appropriate rest
    d. A, B, and C
    e. A and B only

See appendix D for answers to review questions.

References and Resources

American College of Sports Medicine. 2013. *ACSM's resources for the personal Trainer.* 4th edition. Baltimore: Lippincott, Williams and Wilkins.

_________. 2018. *Guidelines for exercise testing and prescription.* 10th edition. Baltimore: Lippincott, Williams and Wilkins.

American Council on Exercise. 2016. *ACE group fitness instructor handbook.* San Diego: Author.

Bishop, D. 2003. Warm up I. *Sports Medicine* 33(6): 439-454.

________. 2003. Warm up II. *Sports Medicine* 33(7):483-498.

Bandy, W.D. 2001. The effect of static stretch and dynamic range of motion training on the flexibility of the hamstring muscles. *Journal of Orthopaedic and Sports Physical Therapy* 27(4):295-300.

Clemens, C.A., and C.J. Cisar. 2006. The effect of footwear on the reliability of the 500-yard shallow water run as a predictor of maximal aerobic capacity (VO_2max). *AEA Aquatic Fitness Research Journal* 3(1):36-39.

Colado, J., V. Tella, and N.T. Triplett. 2008. A method for monitoring intensity during aquatic resistance exercises. *Journal of Strength and Conditioning Research* 22(6):2045-2049.

Colado, J., V. Tella, N.T. Triplett, and L. González. 2009. Effects of a short-term aquatic resistance program on strength and body composition in fit young men. *Journal of Strength and Conditioning Research* 23(2):549-559.

Denomme, L., and J. See. 2006. *AEA instructor skills.* 2nd edition. Nokomis, FL: Aquatic Exercise Association.

Fletcher, G., G. Balady, E. Amsterdam, B. Chaitman, R. Eckel, J. Felg, V. Froelicher, A. Leon, I. Pina, R Rodney, D. Simons-Morton, M. Williams, and T. Bazzarre. 2001. AHA Scientific Statement. Exercise standards for testing and training. A statement for healthcare professionals from the American Heart Association. *Circulation* 104:1694-1740.

Fowles, J.R., D.G. Sale, and J.D. MacDougall. 2000. Reduced strength after passive stretch of the human plantar flexors. *Journal of Applied Physiology* 89(3):1179-1188.

Garber, C., B. Blissmer, M. Deschenes, B. Franklin, M. Lamonte, I.-M. Lee, D. Nieman, and D. Swain. 2011. American College of Sports Medicine position stand. Quantity and quality of exercise for developing and maintaining cardiorespiratory, musculoskeletal, and neuromotor fitness in apparently healthy adults: Guidance for prescribing exercise. *Medicine and Science of Sports and Exercise* 43(7):1334-1359.

Gray, S., G. De Vito, and M. Nimmo. 2002. Effect of active warm-up on metabolism prior to and during intense dynamic exercise. *Medicine and Science of Sports and Exercise* 34(12):2091-2096.

Howley, E.T., and D.L. Thompson. 2012. *Fitness professional's handbook.* 6th edition. Champaign, IL: Human Kinetics.

Innovative Aquatics. 2008. *Personal pool programming.* Nokomis, FL: Author.

Ladwig, M. 2013. The psychological effects of a pre-workout warm-up: An exploratory study. *Journal of Multidisciplinary Research* 5(3):79.

Nelson, M., W. Rejeski, S. Blair, P. Duncan, J. Judge, A. King, C. Macera, and C. Castaneda-Sceppa. 2007. Physical activity and public health in older adults: Recommendation from the American College of Sports Medicine and the American Heart Association. *Circulation* 116(9):1094.

Simic, L., N. Sarabon, and G. Markovic. 2013. Does pre-exercise static stretching inhibit maximal muscular performance? A meta-analytical review. *Scandinavian Journal of Medicine and Science in Sports* 23(2):131-148.

Sova, R. 2000. *Aquatics: The complete reference guide for aquatic fitness professionals.* 2nd edition. Pt. Washington, WI: DSL.

Thielen, S. 2014. Acquapole® more than a pole in the pool. *Akwa* 28(4):5-6.

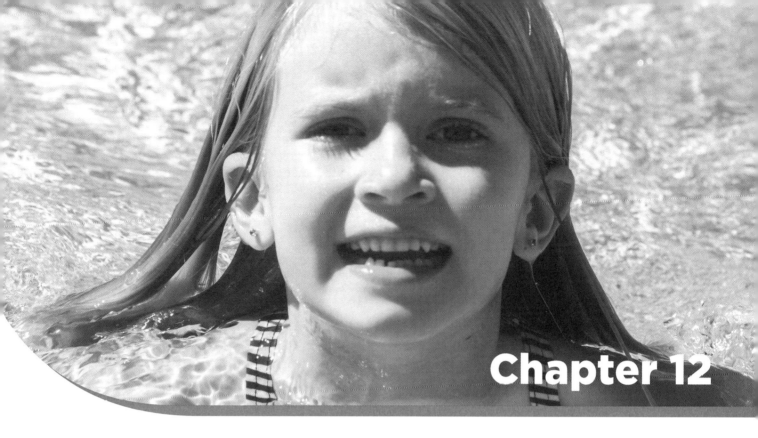

Special Populations and Health Conditions

Introduction

This chapter provides a brief overview of **special populations** (groups of people with similar characteristics, health conditions, or common age range) that benefit from exercise in the aquatic environment. Participants from the populations discussed may find the water a more manageable, comfortable, and enjoyable environment in which to exercise, thus promoting better health and overall wellness.

It is important to recognize your limitations as a fitness professional and to refer participants to a more qualified instructor, trainer, or health professional as necessary. Participants should be aware of their personal limitations and follow specified guidelines provided by their physicians during group exercise classes and personal fitness sessions. You can assist participants in following their medical recommendations by encouraging self-monitoring and providing exercise modifications where appropriate.

The information in this chapter is provided to make you aware that various populations have unique considerations in exercise programming. If you are working with clients or participants who require specialized considerations, you should seek additional resources, education, and training to assist you in developing safe and effective programming. This chapter is not all-inclusive for the various populations discussed, nor does it qualify you to be a specialist or prepare you to provide any level of therapy or medical advice.

Key Chapter Concepts

- Define special populations.
- Recognize your limitations as a fitness professional and when to refer participants to a more qualified instructor, trainer, or health professional.
- Be aware of how the specific properties of water, including hydrostatic pressure, buoyancy, and drag, allow for the adaptations associated with aquatic exercise programs.
- Identify special populations that are most commonly encountered in an aquatic exercise setting and understand general characteristics, exercise guidelines, and programming considerations for each.

The specific properties of water, including hydrostatic pressure, buoyancy, and drag, allow for the adaptations associated with aquatic exercise programs (Barbosa, Garrido, and Bragada 2007; Rahmann 2010). As discussed in chapter 6, hydrostatic pressure applies constant pressure to the body. This may aid in venous return (Becker 2009) and reduce swelling (Hartmann and Huch 2005; Rahmann 2010). As a result, the joints experience decreased swelling and can perform at a greater range of motion. Due to buoyancy, the aquatic environment allows aerobic and resistance exercises to be performed with less joint overload (Wang et al. 2007). For many participants, this means less joint pain.

In addition to all of the physical benefits that water exercise has to offer, the structure of a group exercise class can effectively increase motivation by providing social support. The camaraderie of the group can improve exercise adherence while alleviating loneliness, depression, and anxiety. Both the physical and psychological aspects of aquatic group fitness classes can promote improvements in health and well-being for many special populations.

The following sections outline the special populations most commonly encountered in an aquatic exercise setting. Many people will need a medical evaluation prior to initiating an exercise program and may have specific guidelines to follow in terms of frequency, intensity, time, and type of exercise. Medical clearance is recommended for special populations when initiating an exercise program or beginning a new exercise format (e.g., changing from shallow-water walking to land-based running), or should changes occur in the participant's physical condition.

Older Adults

Aging is a natural and gradual physiological process characterized by a decrease in functional capacities. Although many countries have accepted the World Health Organization's definition for the terms elderly or older person as a person with a chronological age of 65 years or more, it is important to understand that the rate of physical decline will vary from person to person (figure 12.1). Functional age is the level of physical independence, while chronological age is measured in years. Although both are relevant to programming, chronological and functional ages do not always align. Many older adults might have an advanced chronological age but a young functional age, and the reverse is possible as well.

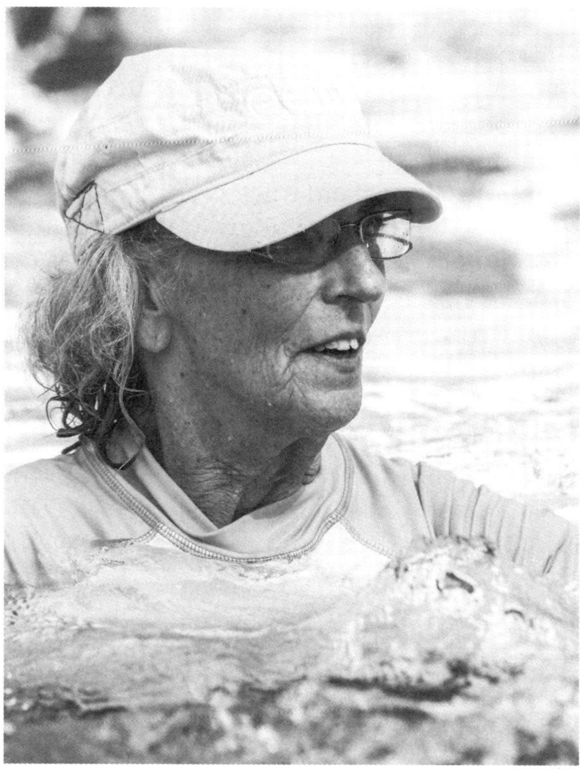

Figure 12.1 Many adults may be chronologically older, but they function like people much younger than themselves.

General Characteristics

The American Medical Association's Committee on Aging (www.ama-assn.org) found that it was almost impossible to distinguish between the effects of aging and the effects of physical inactivity. Low energy, weakness, poor muscular strength, stress and tension, high cholesterol, diabetes, stiffness, constipation, hypertension (high blood pressure), obesity, insomnia, back problems, and decreased range of motion are all common issues associated with both aging and physical inactivity. The good news is that research shows that participation in regular exercise at any age can help improve many of these conditions and reduce the risk for developing them.

Physical changes occur as part of the aging process. The degree to which these changes occur varies from person to person, and may be influenced by lifestyle choices.

Sensory Changes

- Decreased visual sharpness and perception, smaller visual field, and impaired judgment of the speed of moving objects
- Decreased hearing sharpness and reduced ability to discriminate among different sounds
- Reduced sensitivity to touch
- Decreased communication between muscles and nerves and decreased reaction time, leading to altered mobility, response time, spatial awareness, and balance

Physical Changes

- Decreased height, partially due to spinal compression
- Decreased bone density, with increased risk of fractures
- Decreased fitness levels (cardiorespiratory endurance, muscular strength and endurance, and flexibility)

Physiological Changes

- Enlarged heart with reduced function, decreased ability to contract, reduced pumping capacity, and reduced maximum attainable heart rate
- Reduced elasticity and diameter of blood vessels; increased blood pressure
- Decreased response of the immune system and ability to fight infection
- Decreased function of the respiratory system and reduced breathing capacity

Psychological Changes

Although psychological changes are harder to document, many older adults experience depression, anxiety, insomnia, and other psychological conditions.

Exercise Guidelines

The ACSM guidelines for older adults are similar to the general recommendations provided in chapter 11, with additional suggestions regarding the time and intensity of training. Older adults will benefit more by using perceived exertion to monitor exercise intensity (ACSM 2018). Instructors should select aerobic activities that do not create orthopedic stress, choose weight training or weight-bearing movements to target muscular fitness, and employ slow movements that pause in a sustained stretch to enhance flexibility. Programs should also include neuromotor exercises to both improve balance and reduce the risk of falling.

Exercise programs for older adults should focus on the physiological and psychological changes associated with the aging process, while also respecting the individual needs of the participants. A specific class for seniors should do the following:

- Promote musculoskeletal health, joint function, bone strength, muscular strength and endurance, posture
- Improve physical fitness and physical function: cardiorespiratory endurance, muscular strength and endurance, flexibility, body composition, power, coordination, and agility
- Assist with fall prevention: lower-body strength, balance, and walking skills
- Improve mental health: self-esteem, social interaction, sense of achievement and productivity, memory, and motivation

Programming Considerations

Safety. Five minutes spent before class acclimating new students to the pool surroundings can prevent accidents and alleviate the need for rescue or emergency assistance. Make sure participants are familiar with pool lifts, ramps, and accessible ladders for the shallow and deep ends as well as for changes in pool depths. Because of possible limitations with balance and reaction time, vision, and hearing, deliver instructions in a manner that is easy for participants to hear, see, and understand.

Programming. Many of the aquatic program formats discussed in chapter 11 can be adapted for an older adult population, including continuous, interval, and circuit training for both shallow and deep water. Offer low-impact options for participants who cannot safely or comfortably perform high-impact activities, even in the aquatic environment. Use all three planes for movement to encourage increased range of motion and better enhance performance of activities of daily living (ADLs). Include movements that change direction to improve balance and coordination. Transitional moves allow time to readjust body alignment during changes in movement planes or directions of travel. Plan movements that target muscular balance in both strength and flexibility, focusing on common areas of misalignment, such as rounded shoulders (scapular protraction) and forward head posture.

Leadership skills. Incorporate both audible and visual cues to accommodate participants with sensory limitations. Older adults benefit from eye contact and instructor interaction, both of which also allow you to monitor student comfort (e.g., becoming chilled, overheated, fatigued) and understanding of exercise technique. Encourage socialization and interaction among participants through planned activities. This can help maintain control of the class and minimize unwanted talking during times when the focus needs to be directed to intensity, form, alignment, and safety. Consider the pool acoustics when determining music use; participants must be able to hear your audible cues during class. If you incorporate music, choose an appropriate tempo for the population, class format, and water depth. Base the music style on the preferences of the participants.

Equipment. Upper-body drag equipment, especially gloves or mitts that do not require gripping, can be easier for older adults to use safely and effectively. The resistance level can be individualized and based on the participant's capacity to apply force against the water. Gloves should fit loosely to prevent a reduction in blood circulation. When using buoyancy equipment, remember that older adults may have a lower body density and a high level of buoyancy due to body composition. Choose buoyancy equipment that does not compromise body alignment and stability or the participant's capacity to apply force against the water. People who are not completely comfortable in the aquatic environment, as well as those with balance issues or limitations with walking, may benefit from using equipment for support, such as holding a noodle or kickboard on the surface of the water.

Children and Adolescents

The pediatric population includes infants, children, and adolescents or, chronologically speaking, those ranging from birth to 18 years (figure 12.2). This population is extremely diverse, both physiologically and psychologically, and programming should reflect this diversity. As discussed in the section on older adults, chronological age and physiological age are two very different things. This is an important consideration when working with the pediatric populations as well. Children mentally and physically develop at varying rates, and this developmental process affects their ability to perform exercises or skills within your aquatic classes.

General Characteristics

As children develop and grow, so do their various body systems. The cardiovascular, respiratory, musculoskeletal, and all of the

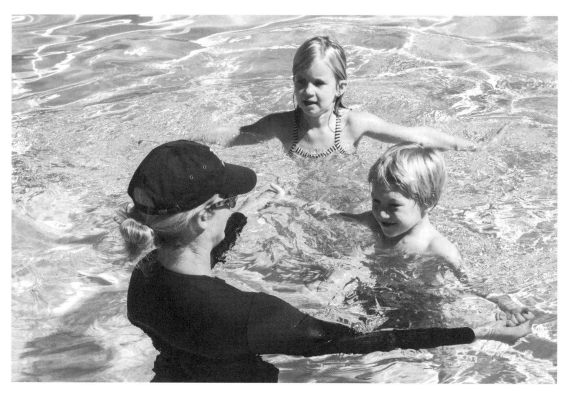

Figure 12.2 Children of all ages naturally add an element of playfulness and fun to aquatic exercise programs.

other systems mature to meet the needs of the developing body. Within each stage of development, physical abilities, characteristics, and traits emerge and advance. Developmental changes occur rapidly; as a result, so do sensory abilities and perceptions.

Sensory Changes

- Vision is blurry at birth and near vision advances before far vision. As age progresses, vision normalizes.
- Hearing develops prior to birth and sensitivity to sounds evolves with age.
- Pure reflexes advance to controlled motor sequences that become more complex with age. Gross (large) motor skills develop before fine (small) motor skills, large muscles develop before the smaller muscles, and basic development migrates from the head to the toes (head control before body control before walking).

Physical Changes

- Heart rate is higher in younger children and gradually decreases or normalizes with age.
- Respiration rate is higher in younger children and gradually decreases or normalizes as the child reaches adolescence.
- Infants and very young children may lack a developed coughing mechanism, thus increasing their risk around water.
- Infants and young children have poorly developed abdominal and upper respiratory muscles that negatively affect postural stability while promoting diaphragmatic breathing.

Physiological Changes

- The younger the child, the smaller the heart. This results in less blood pumped and, therefore, a higher heart rate. With age, the heart grows and so does the heart volume; the heart rate gradually decreases.
- Immune system: The immune system is not fully developed, making younger children more susceptible to infection.
- Children have increased respiration rate (faster breathing cycle) due to smaller airways, smaller lung volume, lungs that are not fully developed for oxygen and carbon dioxide exchange, respiratory muscles that fatigue faster, and abdominal muscles and upper respiratory muscles that are not fully developed. As the child develops, the respiratory system advances and the respiration rate slows, becomes more fatigue resistant, and experiences greater control from the upper respiratory muscles.
- The smaller the person, the greater the ratio of surface area (skin) to size. Thus, children have a proportionately larger body surface area compared to adults. This results in a diminished ability to regulate temperature that can result in excessive loss of heat or fluids.
- Metabolic rate is higher in children, and gradually slows with age.

Psychological Changes

- Psychological growth can play a major role in program outcomes. Keep your participants in mind when you design programs: Age, attention span, and general interests can promote participant and program success.
- Remember that development is a process associated with major cognitive advancements. Memory, problem solving, language, and reasoning abilities are just a few areas of development that are continually advancing throughout childhood. With these changes comes a need for alterations within programming.

Exercise Guidelines

The ACSM recommends at least 60 minutes of daily moderate- to vigorous-intensity activities, with at least three of those days focusing on vigorous levels. Cardio exercise should be enjoyable and age appropriate. Muscle- and bone-strengthening activities are also important to include within the 60-minute daily exercise allotment. The pool's fun factor can encourage children and adolescents to make daily exercise a lifelong choice.

Programming Considerations

Safety. A few minutes spent before class acclimating new participants to the pool surroundings and the rules associated with the aquatic environment can prevent accidents and alleviate the need for rescue or emergency assistance. Make sure participants (and parents of younger children) are familiar with the shallow and deep ends, as well as changes in pool depths. Water depth may be one of the challenges when working with young children; consider using submersible platforms or zero-depth entry areas for classes. Parent-partnered classes are good options for infants or children who cannot achieve optimal water depth for exercise. Since the ability to control body temperature is reduced in children, warmer water and air temperatures may be more suitable for lower-intensity exercise. Additionally, consider drink and bathroom breaks, as well as the use of swim diapers when working with very young children.

Programming. Exercise programs for pediatrics should focus on the main developmental changes while respecting the individual needs. Generally, programs for children should be focused on promoting fitness, enhancing social skills, improving motor skills, and advancing healthy habits. Movement patterns should begin simple and gradually progress to more advanced and coordinated patterns; movement tempo should also gradually progress as the participants progress.

Consider these various concentrations when working with different age groups:

Birth to 2 Years

- Water introduction classes
- Parent-paired or family inclusive classes
- Short-duration, mixed, and repeated activities
- Exercises emphasizing motor skills, hand–eye coordination skills, and body awareness and control

Ages 3 to 5 Years

- Preparation for play
- Short-duration, high-interest activities
- Avoid downtime by using quick transitions from one activity or exercise to another
- Emphasize gross- and fine-motor skills, hand–eye and foot–eye coordination, and agility
- Imagination and pretending games
- Alternating between high- and low-intensity activities
- Movement exploration
- Structured rest

Ages 6 to 9 Years

- Games
- Structured exercises interspersed with play
- Group interaction exercises
- Circuit training
- Relays or races
- Learned skill activities
- Swim programming
- Introduction to sports skills
- Exercises focused on balance, body control, and body mechanics
- Interval-type exercises and activities (start–stop and go fast–go slow games)

Ages 9 to 12 Years

- Exercise sessions and activities with structure
- Exercises focused on muscular strength and endurance, bone strengthening, as well as cardiorespiratory fitness and flexibility
- Form and mechanics
- Group and interval activities and exercises
- Socialization opportunities
- Gender-specific classes and games
- Circuit training
- Interval training

Adolescents

- Activities that build success
- Socialization opportunities
- Strength- and aerobic-focused exercises
- Bone-building exercises (higher impact or greater force production)
- Confidence-building activities
- Circuit training
- Interval training
- Functional training

Leadership skills. Consider delivery style when working with various age groups. Appropriate vocabulary, voice tone, and motivation can create a successful program. The use of verbal and visual commands, as well as instructions for parents on how to provide tactile cues with young participants, can all be effective with this population. Additionally, the use of appropriate music, themes, or toys during certain aspects of the class may provide motivation and stimulation.

Equipment. Attached flotation equipment such as a life jacket may provide comfort and assistance during child-focused programming. Other equipment use can be considered by addressing physical abilities, coordination, strength, and body control.

Pregnancy and Postpartum

The recommendations of the American Congress of Obstetricians and Gynecologists (ACOG) leave no doubt as to the benefits of physical activity and exercise during pregnancy. Activity promotes physical fitness and may prevent excessive gestational weight gain. Exercise may reduce the risk of gestational diabetes, preeclampsia, and the need for cesarean deliveries, as well as a wide variety of other pregnancy-related risks.

Beyond the sense of well-being and reduced body weight, studies have shown that the practice of aquatic exercise during pregnancy can provide many benefits, including the relief of lower-back pain (Granath, Hellgren, and Gunnarsson 2006; Waller, Lambeck, and Daly 2009) and improved or maintained physical function in regard to conducting daily tasks (Smith and Michel 2006). Buoyancy has been associated with reduced mechanical load on the spine, due to reduced weight in water (de Brito Fontana et al. 2012). This is especially relevant because discomfort related to weight gain and resulting changes to the center of gravity and body alignment are common among pregnant women. Submerged movement provides a massaging effect, and the hydrostatic pressure and the upward force of buoyancy contribute to improved venous return and peripheral circulation. A reduction of edema (swelling) is also noticed with water exercise (Kent et al. 1999; Hartmann and Huch 2005).

Group activities, especially when offered in the relaxed surroundings of the water, also provide a favorable psychological component for pregnant women, including improvement of mood (Polman, Kaiseler, and Borkoles 2007) and self-image (Smith and Michel 2006). Classes geared specifically to pregnant and postpartum women also promote interaction among participants, who are all experiencing similar physical and emotional changes (figure 12.3).

General Characteristics

A woman's body goes through many changes during the three trimesters of pregnancy. Physiological changes occur in many organs and systems to supply the fetus with proper nutrients and remove waste. Many structural changes occur to accommodate the fetus. For most pregnant women, exercise is a healthy choice that better enables the body to adapt to these changes. Many physiological and structural changes persist for 4 to 6 weeks postpartum. The general categories of change associated with pregnancy and the postpartum phase are as follows:

Cardiorespiratory Changes

- Increased heart rate, both at rest (10-15 % increase) and during exercise.
- Decreased lung capacity because of an increase in size of the uterus.

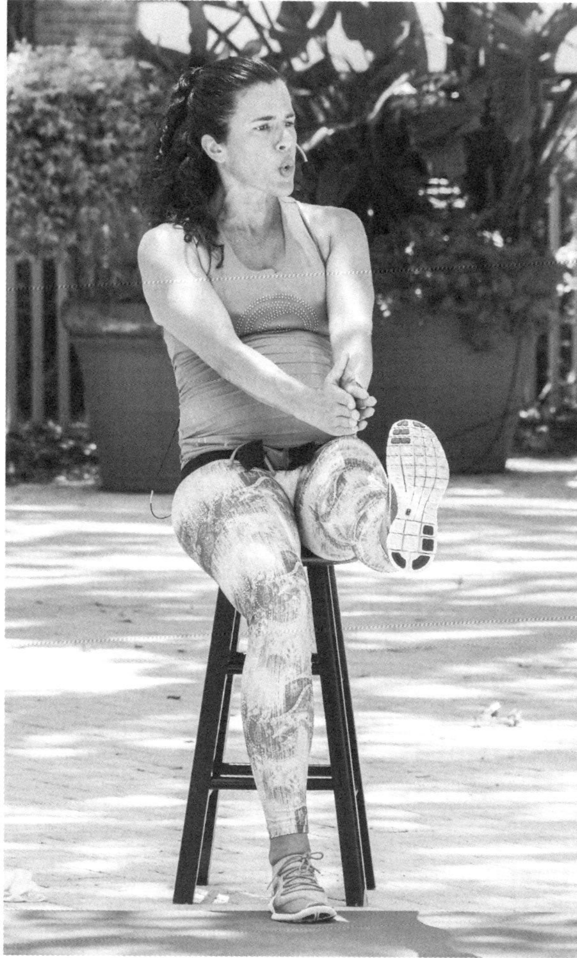

Figure 12.3 Pregnancy provides unique challenges to exercise, but the aquatic environment can be a gentler option.

- Increased blood volume and cardiac output. Increased blood volume is a partial cause for the swelling, cramping, and supine hypotension (abnormally low blood pressure while supine), and may also cause dizziness with sudden changes in movement.
- Softened and enlarged blood vessels result in varicose veins, hemorrhoids, swelling, decreased venous return, and increased potential for edema.
- Possible increased blood pressure.
- Possible development of preeclampsia (hypertension during pregnancy associated with significant amounts of protein in the urine) from 20 weeks gestation up to 6 weeks postpartum.

Postural and Anatomical Changes

- Increased size and weight of uterus. The uterus also moves from a pelvic position to an abdominal position.
- Increased size of abdomen and breast tissue influence posture (progressive increase in lumbar lordosis and pelvic rotation over femur; thoracic kyphosis and forward head) and body awareness.
- Altered center of gravity and center of buoyancy affect stability and balance.
- Increased external hip rotation.
- Decreased joint mobility (mainly at the ankles and wrists) due to increased water retention.

Metabolic and Hormonal Changes

- Increased basal metabolic rate requiring more calories (300-500 per day) to sustain the mother and the developing fetus.
- Increased heat production.
- Increased risk of hypoglycemia (low blood sugar).
- The hormone, relaxin, is released throughout the pregnancy to soften ligaments and loosen joints. This continues 6 to 12 months postpartum. Relaxin prepares the body for childbirth but also makes the musculoskeletal system vulnerable to injury due to joint instability. Abrupt, uncontrolled, and power movements should be avoided.

Exercise Guidelines

The ACSM (2018) recommends that pregnant women who were physically active and who are not experiencing medical complications follow the exercise recommendations for healthy adults; they should accumulate 150 minutes of moderate intensity aerobic exercise or 75 minutes of vigorous intensity aerobic exercise each week. Women who were previously inactive and who are not experiencing medical complications should begin with 15 minutes of aerobic exercise three days per week at an appropriate intensity and progress to 30 minutes of aerobic exercise on most days of the week. Women who are obese, hypertensive, or experiencing some type of medical complication should consult their physician for exercise guidelines.

The exercise program should be directed at supporting or creating conditions for a healthy, comfortable pregnancy and postpartum phase. The program should take into account musculoskeletal health, reduced joint compression, pain relief, postural awareness and education, and prevention of associated medical complications, while promoting social interaction and a healthy lifestyle. Additionally, exercise during pregnancy may help women prepare for the postpartum phase and may prevent depression.

Studies have shown that cardiorespiratory exercise at moderate intensity is generally safe for both the mother (including previously sedentary women) and the fetus (Cavalcante et al. 2009; Silveira et al. 2010). Additionally, women who have participated in exercise prior to pregnancy may be able to include greater intensities and program variations safely with medical clearance. However, women with the specific conditions or pregnancy complications listed here should not exercise during pregnancy (ACOG 2016).

The ACOG (2016) recommends that women with the following conditions avoid aerobic exercise during their pregnancy: certain types of heart and lung diseases, cervical insufficiency, or cerclage (a procedure in which the cervical opening is closed with stitches to prevent or delay preterm birth); being pregnant with twins or triplets with risk factors for preterm labor, placenta previa (a condition in which the placenta lies very low in uterus, so that the opening of the uterus is partially or completely covered after 26 weeks); preterm labor or ruptured membranes (water has broken) during the pregnancy; preeclampsia or pregnancy-induced high blood pressure; or severe anemia.

Pregnant women should stop exercising when fatigued and should not exercise to exhaustion. The ACOG (2016) also recommends that pregnant women avoid standing still (which causes the blood to pool in the legs and feet) or lying supine (the uterus presses on the large vein that returns blood to the heart). Both of these positions may cause blood pressure to decrease for a short time. The ACOG (2016) also suggests that women experiencing any of the following symptoms during exercise discontinue exercise: vaginal bleeding, dizziness, or shortness of breath before exercise, chest pain, headache, muscular weakness, calf pain or swelling; regular, painful contractions of the uterus, or fluid leaking from the vagina.

During pregnancy, the ability to maintain body temperature within normal limits is reduced. Thus, during aquatic exercise, water temperature above 89.6 degrees Fahrenheit (32 °C) should be avoided for aerobic activity to prevent dehydration, overheating, and a drop in blood pressure.

Programming Considerations

Safety. A physician's approval to begin, or continue exercise is recommended for all pregnant woman. Typically, a woman can continue with her prepregnancy workouts with her health care professional's approval (ACOG 2016). Classes should be self-paced, and each participant should pay careful attention to how she feels during exercise. Encourage proper hydration before, during, and after exercise and plan your classes to include bathroom breaks and water breaks. Include educational components in the class; for example, the ACOG website (www.acog.org) has materials for pregnancy and postpartum, such as *Exercise During Pregnancy (FAQ119)*. Promote an open line of communication. Be sure that your pregnant clients are sharing important information with you that may relate to the exercise program. Also, encourage them to speak with their doctors about any concerns they may have throughout their pregnancy.

Programming. Provide exercise options that accommodate the anatomical and physiological changes according to each trimester of pregnancy. For example, consider balance issues—traveling patterns interspersed with pauses offer excellent options for training core stability and balance. Due to the participants' enlarging abdomen, be aware of the degree of hip flexion with sagittal plane lower-body movements. In this case, low front kicks may be preferred over high kicks, or a heel high jog may be more comfortable than a knee high jog. To limit joint stress, grounded, level II and level III movements may be preferred to high-impact level I options. Avoid working at maximum range of motion, even when stretching, due to the laxity of the joints during pregnancy. Explore options for relaxation techniques appropriate to the water and air temperatures. Offer supplementary exercises such as core strengthening, hip mobility, and pelvic floor exercises. Since the need for oxygen increases during pregnancy, and shortness of breath may be experienced due to the uterus pushing against the diaphragm, include deep breathing exercises.

Leadership skills. Provide well-timed transitional cues due to balance and coordination changes. You should also regularly deliver additional posture and body awareness cues. Create an exercise environment that is open to self-monitoring (i.e., rating of perceived exertion scale) and self-pacing, while providing opportunities for participants to ask questions and socialize.

Equipment. When choosing equipment, take into account the risk-to-benefit ratio. Gloves are the most suitable equipment choice for this population, since they limit joint overload and allow greater freedom of movement with the use of hands for balance and propulsion in the water. Buoyant equipment, such as hand bars, may compromise body control for some people; additionally, this type of equipment may add too much stress to the wrist and finger joints during pregnancy. With deep-water classes, flotation equipment is still recommended, but placement and amount of buoyancy may need to be adjusted through the pregnancy. Flotation belts must not be too restrictive on the abdomen; flotation vests or upper arm cuffs (designed for water exercise, not inflatable swim cuffs) may be more comfortable options.

Obesity

In the United States in 2014, more than 68 percent of adults were classified as **overweight** or **obese**, and 6 percent were classified as extremely obese (ACSM 2018). **Obesity** is a multifaceted health issue that results from various contributing factors, including behaviors (e.g., dietary patterns, physical activity), genetics, the community environment, as well as disease and medications.

Lifestyle modification should target three key components: diet, exercise, and behavior therapy (Wadden, Butryn, and Byrne 2004). This section focuses on the aspect of exercise.

Exercise is beneficial to the obese participant in many ways. It helps promote negative energy balance (burning calories) and aids in weight loss efforts. With exercise, there is a higher likelihood that the weight lost is fat weight, and muscle weight is spared or improved. Additional benefits include the following:

- Reduced risk for chronic disease
- Improved circulation
- Stronger heart and lungs
- Increased stamina, strength, and endurance
- Lower resting blood pressure and heart rate
- Improved body composition
- Increased life span
- Increased self-confidence
- Positive changes in mood
- Relief of depression and anxiety
- Increased mental well-being
- Positive coping strategies

General Characteristics

Obese people are at a greater risk for many serious diseases and health conditions than those with a normal or healthy weight, including the following:

- High blood pressure
- Unbalanced cholesterol ratios
- Type 2 diabetes

- Coronary heart disease
- Stroke
- Gallbladder disease
- Osteoarthritis
- Sleep apnea and breathing problems
- Some types of cancer
- Depression and anxiety
- Pain and impaired function

Adapted from CDC, *Adult Obesity Causes & Consequences*

Exercise Guidelines

People who are overweight or obese should strive to exercise at least five days per week, including aerobic, muscular resistance, and flexibility activities. The duration of exercise should gradually progress, with a goal of 300 minutes of weekly activity, or about 60 minutes per day. The initial level of intensity should be moderate, progressing to vigorous activity as the individual is able.

For a general weight loss program, the ACSM recommends a reduction of 3 to 10 percent of initial weight over 3 to 6 months by an intervention of moderate- to vigorous-intensity aerobic exercise, resistance training, and behavior intervention (ACSM 2018). Note that vigorous exercise may provide additional health benefits, but it also has associated risks; thus, it should be encouraged for those participants who are able and willing to exercise at this level of exertion. A 3 to 10 percent weight reduction can have large effects on general health and well-being. As an example, for people with knee osteoarthritis, a weight reduction of 1 kilogram (2.2 lbs) has been associated with a knee load reduction of 4 units per step, a clinically meaningful reduction when considering how many steps are performed each day (Messier et al. 2005).

Obesity may offer a greater risk of falling in older adults (Himes and Reynolds 2011). This, coupled with the additional mechanical overload to the body, may make aquatic exercise an excellent choice for obese people to begin an exercise program. Additionally, since most of the body is submerged under water during exercise, many larger adults feel less self-conscious when exercising. Water exercise has fewer restrictions than land exercise. Repeated high-impact movements, excessive side-to-side movements, and activities that require extended periods of single-leg support may be too challenging and thus increase risk of injury on land. The buoyancy of the water allows for limited or easily modified high-impact movements for most participants, reduces the risk of side-to-side movements, and supports weight for single-limb activities.

A temperature range of 80 to 86 degrees Fahrenheit (27-30 °C) is recommended for obese participants. Overheating can be an issue for obese participants, even in the water, because of increased thermal insulation provided by excess body fat. Program design should be carefully considered if water temperature exceeds 88 degrees Fahrenheit (31 °C; Yazigi et al. 2013). The exercise program should help to develop body control, promote proper posture and alignment, and maintain full range of motion; therefore, tempo is an important consideration. Music can be an excellent way to motivate participation for longer periods of exercise (Thakur and Yardi 2013).

Body Mass Index (BMI)

Body mass index (BMI) is used to assess weight in relation to height. BMI is an individual's weight in kilograms divided by the square of height in meters. The ACSM defines overweight as a BMI of ≥25, obese as a BMI of ≥30, and extremely obese as a BMI of ≥40.

Programming Considerations

Safety. Obese people require safe and comfortable access for entering and exiting the pool. Steps, ramps, and ladders in the shallow area of the pool may serve this purpose; however, some participants might require the assistance of a chair lift. Remind participants to wear shoes on the pool deck to prevent slips and falls. Clothing choices or application of lubricant to the skin may help prevent chafing where areas of the body rub together during repetitive movements.

Programming. Avoid exercises that cause discomfort or may be discouraging for participants with larger bodies. Design programming to allow success with participation while improving participants' self-efficacy and adherence. Body mass can affect range of motion, so modifications might need to be given for some exercises. Some participants, especially those with existing musculoskeletal considerations, might need alternatives for impacting in shallow-water programming. Cue for proper knee and foot position, since many participants have lower leg and ankle misalignments. The exercise program should help to develop body control, promote proper posture and alignment, and maintain full range of motion.

Leadership skills. Create an atmosphere that makes the overweight participant feel at ease. Let participants know where they can find aquatic clothing, such as bike shorts, supportive bras, and larger-sized swimsuits. Suggest the option of wearing a shirt over their swimsuits if that makes them feel more comfortable to prevent self-consciousness from becoming a deterrent or excuse for not participating in an exercise program. Additionally, make sure that you dress appropriately, keeping your larger participants in mind. Do not assume that all overweight participants are unfit; each participant will have a different fitness level. Many have never been encouraged to participate in any kind of exercise activity and will benefit from positive reinforcement and encouragement.

Equipment. Initially focus on proper body control and exercise technique before adding resistance equipment. Drag resistance may be the most suitable equipment choice when a training progression is needed. Gloves allow for changes in intensity with simple adjustments to hand position, limit joint overload, and allow greater freedom of movement with the use of hands for balance and propulsion in the water. Buoyancy resistance equipment, such as hand bars, may compromise body control because the participants will naturally be more buoyant due to higher percentages of body fat. On the other hand, the use of deep-water flotation equipment might still be necessary to help participants maintain proper alignment and form. Be sure to have belts that are large enough or can be adjusted or combined to accommodate all participants.

Musculoskeletal Considerations

Musculoskeletal considerations include a wide range of illnesses or conditions related to the muscles, bones, joints, cartilage, tendons, ligaments, and nerves. This section discusses two key musculoskeletal considerations often seen in aquatic exercise classes: rheumatic diseases and lower-back pain (figure 12.4).

Rheumatic Diseases

Rheumatic diseases are characterized by inflammation and degeneration of the body's muscles, joints, and connective tissue. More than 100 types of rheumatic diseases exist.

General Characteristics

In this section, we briefly discuss four of the common types seen in aquatic participants: osteoarthritis, rheumatoid arthritis, fibromyalgia, and osteoporosis.

Osteoarthritis (OA) is also known as degenerative joint disease because the cartilage in the joint breaks down, causing

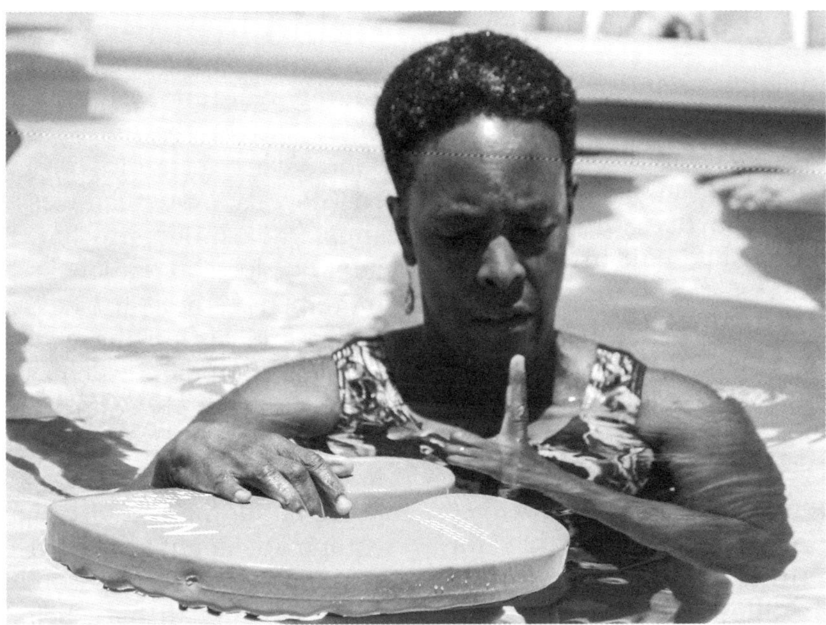

Figure 12.4 Exercising in the water provides much less impact upon the joints of those with limited mobility.

the bones to rub together. This is the most common form of arthritis, and typically begins after the age of 45. OA affects the knees, hips, hands, and spine; however, the knees are the most commonly affected weight-bearing joint (Williams and Spector 2006). OA can significantly influence quality of life due to its effect on functional activities, such as walking, going up and down stairs, and squatting (Arden and Nevitt 2006; Issa and Sharma 2006; Gabriel and Michaud 2009), and the consequent loss of independence for the individual. The causes of OA are not completely understood, but it is thought to be related to biomechanical, genetic, and environmental issues (Dieppe 1998).

Rheumatoid arthritis (RA) is an autoimmune disease where the body's immune system mistakenly attacks the joints, creating inflammation. The inflamed joint lining releases an enzyme that can damage cartilage and bone, resulting in a loss of joint stability, structure, and alignment. The chronically high levels of inflammation can create problems throughout the body, including issues of the eyes, mouth, skin, lungs, and blood vessels. RA commonly affects women between 20 and 50 years of age. The hands, feet, wrists, elbows, ankles, and knees are the most commonly affected joints, and symptoms are usually symmetrical (joints on both sides of the body are affected). Although the cause of RA is not fully understood, evidence indicates that genetics, hormones, and environmental factors are involved (Arthritis Foundation, n.d.). Research has shown that exercise is an effective and essential component in the management of arthritis (Kaptein et al. 2013; Levy et al. 2012; Wilcox et al. 2015).

Fibromyalgia syndrome is a chronic condition characterized by fatigue and widespread pain in the muscles, ligaments, and tendons. It is believed that a number of factors contribute to the development of fibromyalgia. These include chemical changes in the brain, sleep disturbances, injury, infection, abnormalities of the autonomic nervous system, and changes in muscle metabolism. Family history is also considered a risk factor. Signs and symptoms of fibromyalgia include widespread pain, fatigue and sleep disturbances, irritable bowel syndrome, chronic headaches and facial pain, heightened sensitivity, depression, numbness or tingling in the hands and feet, difficulty concentrating, mood changes, chest or pelvic pain, irritable bladder, painful menstrual periods, dizziness, a sensation of swollen hands and feet, and dry eyes, skin, and mouth. Because of the array of symptoms, many types of treatment are prescribed, including medication, relaxation techniques, and physical conditioning.

Osteoporosis (*osteo* = bone; *porosis* = porous) is a systemic skeletal disease characterized by low bone mass and deterioration of bone strength, leading to bone fragility and an increased risk of fracture. Risk factors for osteoporosis include genetics, age, lifestyle (e.g., smoking, lack of physical activity, diet), and medications. Exercise is beneficial in the management of osteoporosis and water exercise can be an integral part of a well-rounded training program. Water is a relatively safe environment that minimizes fear and injury in falls, enhances kinesthetic feedback, provides buoyancy for reduced joint stress, and offers resistance for muscular conditioning. Exercising in a safe and comfortable environment can also encourage social interaction that may decrease feelings of depression and anxiety. Aquatic exercise has been shown to be efficient in decreasing **bone resorption** (the breakdown and absorption of old bone) and enhancing bone formation (Moreira et al. 2014). Additionally, significant improvements in balance and overall health improvements suggest that aquatic exercise is a viable alternative for older women with osteoporosis (Arnold et al. 2008).

Exercise Guidelines

People with arthritis benefit from including regular exercise into their lifestyle. The ACSM recommends that flexibility exercises be performed daily, resistance training be performed two or three days per week and cardiorespiratory activities be performed three to five days per week. Aerobic exercises should both involve limited joint stress and be performed at an appropriate intensity to minimize injury and exacerbation of joint symptoms.

People with fibromyalgia should also include exercise into their lifestyle. The ACSM recommends low-impact or non-weight-bearing aerobic exercise (progressing gradually from 1 or two days per week up to 3 days per week), muscular resistance exercises (two or three days each week), and non-weight-bearing stretches (gradually progressing from one day per week up to five days per week). The ACSM also provides specific recommendations for intensity and time that can assist you with designing programs and providing self-monitoring suggestions for participants.

The ACSM recommends sessions of 30 to 60 minutes of exercise that combines both weight-bearing aerobic activities (4-5 days per week) and resistance training (2 or 3 days per week) for people with osteoporosis. Aerobic exercise should be of a moderate intensity, and resistance for muscle conditioning should allow 8 to 12 repetitions to be performed with good technique.

Programming Considerations

Safety. Shoes should be worn in the locker room, on pool decks, and in the pool to minimize the risk for slips and falls while providing support and impact absorption. Pool entry and exit areas should be carefully marked, and offer easy access for those with limited mobility. Pools should have a clear delineation of changes in water depths. When possible, submerge the moving joint under the water to help participants benefit most from the aquatic environment. This may be achieved by moving to different water depths or repositioning the body. Recommended water temperatures may vary with the population and the intensity level of the program. A temperature of 90 degrees Fahrenheit (32 °C) is suggested for people with fibromyalgia, who are generally intolerant of cold. Encourage your participants to be mindful of how their bodies feel during exercise and provide options for reduced intensity, range of motion, and impact.

Programming. Structure classes to provide a balanced workout while achieving specific goals of the population and consider the relationship between physical, psychological, and social symptoms often associated with a chronic condition.

Arthritis. The AEA Arthritis Foundation Aquatic Program (AFAP) makes the following general recommendations for aquatic classes for people with arthritis and related rheumatic diseases:

- People with arthritis need to move their joints daily.
- Exercises should be performed in a smooth and controlled manner without bouncing.
- An inflamed joint should be moved only through a pain-free range of motion.
- Exercise should be self-paced; teach and encourage self-monitoring by all participants. Participants should move to the point where they feel a gentle stretch. Move slowly and gently, allowing muscles time to relax between each repetition. Avoid overexertion.
- Follow the 2-hour pain rule. Some muscle soreness is a normal response to exercise; if you develop more joint pain that lasts for 2 hours or more after exercising, reduce exercise intensity or the duration of the next class.

Fibromyalgia. Goals for exercise programming for participants with fibromyalgia are similar to the goals for most chronic diseases: to restore and improve function and mental outlook. Like participants with arthritis, participants with fibromyalgia often find aquatic exercise to be comforting and supportive. The initial level of exercise should be determined by participant characteristics and pain tolerance. For most participants, progression should be very conservative, beginning at a low-intensity level. Light resistance training with an emphasis on proper form and technique can help build muscular endurance and increase pain tolerance. Flexibility exercises should also be included. Symptoms might worsen initially when first starting an exercise program; participants should be educated about this response. Pacing exercise sessions with daily activity obligations, coupled with the reduced impact stress and effects of water immersion on reducing pain perception, can assist people with fibromyalgia to initiate and continue an exercise program. The resistance of the water can also develop muscular strength and endurance and improve balance. Additionally, exercise in warm water has been shown to decrease pain and improve cognitive function in middle-aged women with fibromyalgia (Munguia-Izquierdo and Legaz-Arrese 2007).

Osteoporosis. A well-balanced aquatic exercise program for people with osteoporosis might include the following general concepts to provide functional improvement (Harush and Yazigi 2016):

- Include specific exercises to target posture, balance (static and dynamic), gait, coordination, hip and trunk stabilization, range of motion, and flexibility.
- Emphasize ankle-related muscles to reduce risk of falls.
- If there is no pain, 10 to 15 minutes of exercise at higher intensity is preferred over a longer duration of low to moderate intensity. For pain management, low- to moderate-intensity aerobic exercise is recommended.

Proper form and alignment are important. Cue and correct participants as necessary. Allow adequate time for participants to rest and recover between exercises as well as between sessions.

Choose exercises according to the anatomic region. Lower limb (hip) and the lumbar region of the spine have better responsiveness to the ground reaction forces, so include impact exercises. The wrist and upper limb are more responsive to strength training due to the tension that muscles exert through the tendons on the bones.

Deep-water exercise, although nonimpact, does offer benefits to people with osteoporosis, such as during pain occurrences and in cases of severe osteoporosis to improve balance, posture, and functional movements. Muscular contractions during deep-water exercise can also exert forces on the bone that stimulate bone growth.

Most exercise limitations are specific to land-based exercise due to excessive force being placed on the weakened bone structure. Since gravity is reduced in the aquatic environment, the precautions are less restrictive. Avoid spinal flexion on land to prevent vertebral fractures. In the water, some spinal flexion can be performed, including flexion in a modified supine position. Focus on bracing the core by contracting the transverse abdominis. Avoid twisting movements on land, such as a golf swing (Ekin and Sinaki 1993). In the water, a slow range of rotational motion is acceptable as an active stretch.

Leadership skills. Understanding the unique considerations of various rheumatic diseases will allow you to better provide a safe and effective class for a wide range of participants. Providing educational components to the class can assist participants in better understanding how to manage symptoms, which can improve their exercise adherence. Recognize that symptoms will vary from person to person with the same disease. Individual symptoms may also vary on a daily basis or even throughout the day. Many participants appreciate and benefit from activities that encourage socialization, both within the class and outside of the class setting (e.g., social functions for participants).

Equipment. Webbed gloves or mitts are a safe option for added resistance for arthritis programming in the pool. This type of drag resistance allows for changes in intensity with simple adjustments to hand position, limits joint overload, and allows greater freedom of movement with the use of hands for balance in the water. Drag resistance may provide the necessary overload to address bone density concerns for people with osteoporosis. For participants who have balance concerns or are not completely comfortable in the aquatic environment, buoyancy kickboards or noodles held at the surface of the water can provide stability and comfort during exercises. Buoyancy equipment is not recommended for submerged use, however, and actually decreases the already limited impact that is beneficial for people with osteoporosis. As participants progress and as body control and fitness levels improve, all varieties of equipment may become appropriate. Equipment choices should be based on the ability to control the equipment and perform the exercise with proper form. If participants are unable to achieve this, they should not use equipment until they achieve suitable strength and ability levels.

Lower-Back Pain (LBP)

It is estimated that 80 percent of adults suffer from at least one episode of lower-back pain severe enough to cause absence from work. Lower-back pain is one of the primary causes of disability in the United States and is one of the most widely experienced health-related problems in the world (Buchbinder et al. 2013).

General Characteristics

Lower-back pain can be acute or chronic in nature, and may be associated with other diseases or conditions. According to the National Institute of Health, the majority of LBP is mechanical in nature, often associated with the general degeneration of the spine from the normal wear and tear of aging ("Low back pain fact sheet" n.d.). Reduced muscular strength and endurance in the core have also been associated with LBP (Abenhaim et al. 2000). In addition, certain factors may increase the risk of developing lower-back pain, including genetics, age, fitness level, pregnancy, being overweight, and some job-related factors (NIH "Low back pain fact sheet" n.d.).

Physical activity is often recommended for both treatment and prevention of LBP. Aquatic exercise, both shallow-water and deep-water formats, may benefit participants with lower-back pain by targeting activation of the core muscles, allowing a greater pain-free range of motion, assisting with balance (dynamic and static), and enhancing coordination.

Exercise Guidelines

The ACSM (2018) recommends that people with chronic lower-back pain follow the exercise guidelines for adults, which can be found in chapter 1. Exercise programs should provide individual modifications for cardiorespiratory endurance, muscular strength and endurance, and flexibility.

Programming Considerations

Safety. Activities that increase lower-back pain should be avoided or eliminated. Shoes should be worn in the locker room, on the pool deck, and in shallow water to provide better traction and cushioning.

Programming. Although water reduces joint impact as compared to similar land-based activities, it still may be necessary to adjust the movements to reduce impact stress further (e.g., using level II, level III, or grounded exercises or deep-water formats). Research indicates that deep water substantially decreases the compressive load on the spine, making deep-water exercise a valuable tool in training progressions. Deep-water training is also very effective for training the core musculature, which is important for good posture and back health. Participants with lower-back pain might need to alter exercise positions or substitute exercises that support the lower back to avoid pain.

Generally, classes for those with lower-back pain would focus on strengthening the abdominal, gluteus maximus, hamstrings, and back extensor muscles while including flexibility exercises for the hip flexors, quadriceps, and hamstrings. Careful attention should be paid to proper posture and core stabilization.

Leadership skills. Educational information for proper posture, lifting techniques, and lower-back health are helpful. Encourage self-monitoring, provide options for reducing impact as needed, and cue to allow adequate time for safe transitions.

Equipment. Deep-water participants will need flotation equipment such as a properly fitted flotation belt or vest that helps maintain proper posture and alignment. Some participants may prefer buoyant upper-arm cuffs designed specifically for aquatic exercise. If impact is an issue during shallow-water exercise, flotation devices that are normally used for deep-water training can be employed to further reduce impact forces.

Cardiovascular Disease (CVD)

Cardiovascular disease (CVD) is the leading global cause of death for both men and women. It is a complex disease involving the heart and blood vessels. CVD can be hereditary, like congenital heart defects, but improper diet and lifestyle management are also major contributing factors.

General Characteristics

CVD encompasses a broad spectrum of health problems that include atherosclerosis, heart attack, irregular heart rhythms, heart valve dysfunction, and stroke.

- **Atherosclerosis** develops when plaque builds up in the walls of the arteries. This plaque buildup can cause narrowing in the arteries, compromising circulation that may damage the heart, brain, or other organs. If a blood clot forms, it can stop the blood flow completely, causing a heart attack or stroke.
- A **heart attack** occurs when the blood flow in the coronary arteries becomes blocked by plaque or blood clots (known as **coronary artery disease**). If the blockage cuts off the blood flow completely, the part of the heart muscle supplied by the artery begins to die.
- **Irregular heart rhythms** (too fast, too slow, extra or abnormal beats) occur when there is a disturbance to the heart's electrical system. These abnormal heartbeats and rhythms can be a contraindication to exercise. Early detection and participant education, as well as aquatic fitness instructor education, are important.
- **Heart valve dysfunction** occurs when the major valves of the heart are compro-

mised, leading to mechanical dysfunctions. This may impair the heart's ability to pump effectively, which can contribute to exercise intolerance. Heart valve dysfunction can result in inadequate blood flow or heart failure (congestive heart failure).

- A **stroke** or cerebrovascular accident is caused by a disruption of blood supply to the brain. When blood does not supply oxygen and other nutrients to the brain, the cells in the affected area cannot function properly, and might be permanently damaged.

The American Heart Association (2016) targets seven key factors contributing to heart disease and stroke:

1. Manage blood pressure (see table 12.1)
2. Control cholesterol
3. Reduce blood sugar
4. Get active
5. Eat better
6. Lose weight
7. Stop smoking

Exercise Guidelines

The ACSM recommendations for people with cardiovascular disease include both aerobic exercise and resistance exercise. Aerobic interval training offers greater long-term improvements than continuous training. Aerobic activity should begin with a short (5- to 10-minute) duration and gradually progress by 1 to 5 minutes, with intensity ranging from 40 to 80 percent of HRR depending on the individual's risk level. Similarly, resistance training is recommended at an intensity allowing for 10 to 15 repetitions without significant fatigue.

Programming Considerations

Safety. Water temperatures that are too warm or too cold may result in greater stress on the cardiovascular system. Take care to see how participants react to initial water immersion. Throughout classes, communicate about exertion as well as general physical well-being.

Programming. Continuous moderate-level aerobic conditioning is generally prescribed for participants with cardiovascular disease, although interval training has also been beneficial in some situations. With either continuous or interval formats, be sure to include warm-up, cool-down, and flexibility segments.

Leadership skills. The American Heart Association (AHA), the American Stroke Association (ASA), the American College of Sports Medicine (ACSM), and the American Association of Cardiovascular Pulmonary Rehabilitation (AACVPR) are valuable resources for fitness professionals. They provide information on CVD treatment, cardiac rehabilitation, general exercise recommendations and guidelines, and overall quality of life management for this complex disease.

Equipment. Equipment options will depend on the participant's fitness level and experience with water exercise. You may use equipment as long as you consider intensity and restrictions for your clients. Be mindful that most equipment increases effort

Table 12.1 Blood Pressure Categories

Top number (systolic)		Bottom number (diastolic)	Category
Below 120	and	Below 80	Normal blood pressure
120-139	or	80-89	Prehypertension
140-159	or	90-99	Stage 1 hypertension
160 or more	or	100 or more	Stage 2 hypertension

Source: American Heart Association.

and intensity. Additionally, if equipment causes greater amounts of concentration and effort, participants may resort to holding their breath. Breath holding during exercise exertion can be dangerous, especially in this population, and should be avoided.

Pulmonary (Lung) Disease

Lung disease is any disease or disorder stemming from improper function of the lungs. Lung disease is responsible for one in seven deaths, and is the third leading killer in the United States ("Lung Diseases" n.d.). Pulmonary diseases limit the body's ability to provide oxygen to the body's tissues.

General Characteristics

This section discusses chronic obstructive pulmonary disease and asthma. However, there are many additional lung diseases and disorders, including cystic fibrosis, lung transplant, lung cancer, mesothelioma, and tuberculosis. Note that some of these conditions may prevent participation in aquatic exercise.

Chronic obstructive pulmonary disease (COPD) is a lung disease where the lung is damaged, making it hard to breathe. Symptoms of COPD include coughing, mucus production, shortness of breath (especially with exercise), wheezing, and chest tightness. **Emphysema** is a type of COPD in which the walls between many of the air sacs (alveoli) in the lungs are damaged. The normal small air sacs are replaced with fewer, larger air sacs with less surface area. The reduced surface area of the air sacs in the lungs reduces the amount of oxygen that enters the blood (Mayo Clinic 2017). The ability to exchange oxygen and carbon dioxide is impaired, causing shortness of breath. In **chronic bronchitis**, the airways have become inflamed and thickened, and there is an increase in mucus production. This contributes to excessive coughing and difficulty getting air in and out of the lungs.

Breathing in irritants to the lungs over a long period of time causes the airways to become inflamed and narrowed and destroys the elastic fibers that allow the lungs to stretch and then return to resting shape. Cigarette smoking is the most common cause of COPD. Other factors that might contribute to COPD include the following:

- Working around certain kinds of chemicals and breathing in the fumes
- Working in a dusty area
- Heavy exposure to air pollution
- Exposure to second-hand smoke

Asthma, a chronic lung disease that inflames and narrows the airways, can be life threatening. Bronchial asthma is a syndrome characterized by reversible obstruction to airflow and increased bronchial responsiveness to a variety of allergy and environmental stimuli (Durstine and More 2002). Asthma results in wheezing, chest tightness, shortness of breath, and coughing. When symptoms become worse or more symptoms occur, it is referred to as an asthma attack.

When considering exercise, participants can be placed in one of three categories (Durstine and More 2002) that help to identify exercise intensity and duration for participants with asthma:

- Exercise-induced asthma (EIA) without any other symptoms. The causes of exercise-induced asthma are not known. EIA typically occurs 5 to 15 minutes following exercise.
- Mild asthma: Breathing limitation does not restrain submaximal exercise.
- Moderate to severe asthma: Breathing limitation restrains submaximal exercise.

Exercise Guidelines

The ACSM recommends that aerobic exercise be performed three to five days per week. Interval training may be appropriate, with the peak intensity depending on the individual's ability (anywhere from light to vigorous). People with COPD could follow the resistance and flexibility exercise guidelines provided for older adults.

The body's need for oxygen intake and carbon dioxide removal is increased during exercise, so participants with pulmonary disease must learn how to cope with diminished lung capacity and increased oxygen demands. Gas exchange impairments also create problems for the cardiovascular and muscular systems. Many people with pulmonary disease can exercise safely and benefit from a regular exercise program.

Participants with controlled EIA should see relatively normal conditioning gains (Durstine and Moore 2002). Participants with COPD might see impairments in exercise response caused by inadequate oxygen in the blood; thus, a very conservative exercise progression is key to adaptation. Adaptation capability is determined by the severity of the disease and individual characteristics.

Inactivity can lead to a vicious cycle for these participants. Shortness of breath and fatigue during exercise lead to cessation of exercise, resulting in diminished lung capacity that makes it more difficult to exercise. Pacing, both in daily activities and exercise, is an important skill for participants with diminished lung capacity. Ability will fluctuate day to day and even hour to hour.

Programming Considerations

Safety. Participants might be sensitive to chemical fumes in the aquatic environment; be aware of air quality. The warmth and humidity in the aquatic environment might assist with breathing for some participants. However, the hydrostatic pressure can make it more difficult to breathe when immersed, so participants might need to start in waist-deep water and gradually transition to chest-deep water. COPD participants might feel better exercising at certain times of the day or shortly after they have taken their medication. It is typically recommended that participants with asthma take medication 10 minutes prior to exercise and carry an inhaler at all times. Asthma symptoms might develop during prolonged exercise; the threshold for producing symptoms is typically around 75 percent of predicted maximal heart rate.

Programming. Program formats will vary depending on limitations and abilities. The ACSM recommends interval formats that combine vigorous-intensity phases with low-intensity phases. Some participants will be able to tolerate a cardiorespiratory format, and others might be capable of performing only basic toning and stretching exercises. Improved coordination, balance, form, and technique will help to conserve energy and provide more oxygen to working muscles. Choose activities that have reasonable RPE values and will improve participants' ability to perform usual activities of daily living, and that participants perceive as enjoyable.

Leadership skills. Participants with pulmonary disease can exercise more comfortably and successfully when they are desensitized to dyspnea (difficult or labored breathing), fear, and other limiting symptoms. You can play an important role in helping participants build confidence and tolerance to exercise. Instruct participants in pursed lips breathing (breathe in through the nose, keeping the lips together except at the very center; exhale by blowing the air out with a firm steady effort), which slows the breathing rate and helps with a sense of control.

Equipment. Equipment options depend on the participant's fitness level and experience with water exercise. You can use equipment as long as you consider intensity and restrictions for your clients. Be mindful that most equipment increases effort and intensity. Additionally, if equipment causes greater amounts of concentration and effort, participants may resort to holding their breath. Breath holding during exercise exertion can be dangerous, especially in this population, and should be avoided.

Diabetes

Diabetes mellitus is characterized by abnormalities in **insulin** action, insulin production by the pancreas, or both. This causes a problem with metabolism and results in glucose intolerance. Chronic **hyperglycemia**

(elevated blood sugar levels) is associated with long-term damage, dysfunction, and failure of various organs, including the eyes, kidneys, nerves, heart, and blood vessels. The classic symptoms of diabetes include intense thirst, high urine output, and unexplained weight loss.

General Characteristics

The complete lack of insulin production, in the case of type 1 diabetes, requires insulin injections or an insulin pump to sustain life. Type 1 diabetes is thought to be primarily genetically determined. Although type 1 diabetes can occur at any age, it usually occurs before the age of 30. It affects 5 to 10 percent of the 16 million people with diabetes in the United States.

The more common type 2 diabetes results from the low production of insulin and decreased cellular receptivity to insulin. Type 2 diabetes sometimes requires insulin through injection. Oral medications are available to enhance production and utilization of insulin, helping people with type 2 diabetes avoid or delay the need for insulin injections. The development of insulin sensitivity is believed to be caused by several factors, including obesity and genetics. In most cases, type 2 diabetes develops after the age of 40; however, it has become more common in children with the increasing incidence of overweight conditions and obesity. Because it is often undetected until it has been present for some time, it can cause organ damage before it is diagnosed. Gestational diabetes occurs during pregnancy. The risk factors include family history, obesity, and previous babies with large birth weight. Gestational diabetes differs from type 1 and 2 diabetes in that it resolves after pregnancy.

Exercise Guidelines

ACSM exercise guidelines recommend that people with diabetes perform aerobic exercise three to seven days per week, accumulating 150 minutes of moderate intensity exercise or 75 minutes of vigorous intensity exercise per week. Moderate intensity is the general suggestion; however, better blood sugar control may be achieved if the participant can tolerate exercise above 60 percent HRR. Resistance training guidelines are the same as those provided for older adults; flexibility guidelines are the same as for the general adult population.

Diabetes responds very well to exercise, and exercise is considered to be a cornerstone of diabetic care. Exercise provides many benefits, including the following:

- Possible improvement in blood sugar control for type 2 diabetes
- Improved glucose sensitivity and often a reduced need for insulin
- Improvements in body composition with decreases in body fat, leading to better insulin sensitivity
- Reduction in the risk of cardiovascular disease
- Stress reduction and consequent better control of diabetes
- Prevention of type 2 diabetes

Exercise has an insulin-like effect, increasing the risk of **hypoglycemia** (low blood sugar). One of the primary concerns for diabetics when exercising is to prevent a hypoglycemic event. You can share the following tips with participants to help minimize exercise-related hypoglycemic events:

- Measure blood glucose before, during, and after exercise. A participant with type 1 diabetes needs to have blood glucose reasonably controlled to exercise safely.
- Avoid exercise during periods of peak insulin activity.
- Precede unplanned exercise with extra carbohydrate and decrease postexercise insulin.
- Reduce insulin doses when exercise is planned in accordance with the intensity and duration of the exercise and personal experience.
- Consume easily accessible carbohydrate during exercise.

- Eat a carbohydrate-rich snack after exercise.
- Exercise with a partner and carry medical identification and a fast-acting carbohydrate.

Programming Considerations

Safety. Because diabetes affects peripheral circulation, especially in the feet, any type of injury or infection might be difficult to heal and may even lead to amputations. Participants should wear shoes at all times in the locker room, in the pool, and on deck to avoid cuts or abrasions. Be aware that medications such as beta-blockers might interfere with the ability to discern hypoglycemic symptoms. People with diabetes are typically at higher risk for heat-related disorders, and should avoid exercising in excessive heat. Participants should be encouraged to check their blood sugar before and after exercise to ensure safe levels and also to monitor the response to the aquatic exercise session. Quickly absorbable carbohydrate-rich foods such as orange juice or glucose tabs should be kept on deck in case participants show signs of hypoglycemia.

Programming. Continuous cardiorespiratory exercise, resistance training, and flexibility exercises through a variety of program formats are recommended. Exercise programs for diabetics should be individualized and based on medication schedule, diabetic complications, and individual characteristics.

Leadership skills. Sensation, coordination, and balance may be impaired within this special population. Incorporate exercises that challenge coordination and balance while ensuring safety with additional support, such as the use of a noodle or holding onto the wall as needed. Each participant will begin to show signs of hypoglycemia at different glucose levels. Additionally, the signs and symptoms of hypoglycemia can be different from person to person. Make sure your participants are aware of their glucose levels and their hypoglycemic symptoms. This will help you respond appropriately to changes in their health or behavior if necessary.

Equipment. Equipment options depend on the participant's fitness level and experience with water exercise. You can use equipment as long as you consider intensity and restrictions for your clients. Be mindful that most equipment increases effort and intensity. Additionally, if equipment causes greater amounts of concentration and effort, participants may resort to holding their breath. Breath holding during exercise exertion can be dangerous and should be avoided.

Multiple Sclerosis (MS)

Multiple sclerosis (MS) is a chronic, potentially debilitating disease that affects the central nervous system (brain and spinal cord). The body directs antibodies and white blood cells to break down proteins in the myelin sheaths surrounding the nerves in the brain and spinal cord. Inflammation and injury to the sheath cause scarring (sclerosis); the damage slows or blocks muscle coordination, visual sensation, and other nerve signals. The National Multiple Sclerosis Society (NMSS) estimates that 2.3 million people worldwide are affected by MS (2016).

General Characteristics

The disease, typically occurring in adults between the ages of 20 and 50, can range in severity from mild illness to permanent disability. MS symptoms are variable and unpredictable; they fluctuate over time. The NMSS website reports the following more common symptoms associated with MS:

- Fatigue
- Walking difficulties
- Numbness or tingling
- Spasticity (feeling of stiffness and involuntary muscle spasms)
- Weakness
- Vision problems
- Dizziness and vertigo

- Bladder and bowel problems
- Sexual problems
- Pain
- Cognitive and emotion changes

Women are two to three times more susceptible for developing MS, and genetic factors are thought to play a significant role in susceptibility.

Exercise Guidelines

For participants with multiple sclerosis, the ACSM recommends a combination of aerobic exercise (2-5 days per week), resistance exercise (2 days per week), and flexibility exercise (5-7 days per week). As with some other special conditions, gradual progression in exercise duration is important and based on the participant. For aerobic exercise, a minimum of 10 minutes is recommended, progressing up to 60 minutes.

Programming Considerations

Safety. Heat intolerance is a key factor. Most participants with MS are more comfortable exercising in water temperatures at or below 84 degrees Fahrenheit. The general recommendation is 80 to 84 degrees Fahrenheit (27-29 °C). Cool water is key in keeping core body temperature from rising and minimizing the risk of increasing the symptoms of MS while exercising. When developing programming for a participant with MS, remember that fatigue, sensory loss, spasticity, and impaired balance can affect exercise tolerance and performance. Discontinue exercise if there is an increase or sudden change in fatigue level, spasticity, balance, vision, or general weakness (MSAA 2013). Safe access for entering and exiting the pool is very important due to balance concerns.

Programming. Participants with MS will fatigue easily, so choose class lengths and times of day accordingly. Focus programs on maintaining or developing cardiorespiratory endurance, muscular strength and endurance, and joint flexibility to increase energy and efficiency. According to the *Aquatic Exercise & Multiple Sclerosis: A Healthcare Professional's Guide*, multiple aquatic techniques and formats are beneficial for people with MS (MSAA 2013). For example, a community-based group exercise class could include aerobic activity that is challenging but not too fatiguing to assist with daily activities; resistance training to help correct muscle weakness and improve power and endurance; stretching to help manage spasticity, maintain range of motion, and improve function; and social interaction to increase motivation, fun, and sense of support among participants.

Leadership skills. Since MS is so variable, plan to have multiple options for exercises as well as class lengths to accommodate all participants. Encourage self-monitoring and allow participants to adjust the program as needed. Open communication will help ensure safety and comfort levels.

Equipment. With gradual progression, you can include many types of equipment in aquatic programming to assist with muscular training, such as gloves or mitts and other equipment for drag resistance, buoyancy (hand bars, cuffs, noodles), and rubberized resistance. Discontinue the exercise when movement quality is reduced or when fatigue symptoms begin (MSAA 2013).

Parkinson's Disease (PD)

Parkinson's disease (PD) is a disorder that affects nerve cells in the part of the brain controlling muscle movement. The four fundamental signs are resting tremors (usually of the hands and head), muscle rigidity (hardness or stiffness of the muscles), slowness of movement, and postural instability. PD is often identified by tremors of the hands and sometimes the head and the legs.

General Characteristics

Parkinson's disease is progressive, with tremors followed by muscular rigidity, slowness of movement, and loss of facial expression. Posture and gait become problematic, but general health is not greatly affected. Many people have years of productive living with good quality of life after being diagnosed.

PD is generally associated with a reduction in the neurotransmitter dopamine. Symptoms might fluctuate from day to day, week to week, or even hour to hour. Treatment currently consists of medications and implantation of a brain stimulator (similar to a heart pacemaker) to provide deep brain stimulation to control symptoms. At this time, researchers believe that PD might result from a combination of genetic and environmental factors or from a number of drugs taken over a long period of time or in excessive doses. Unlike genetic and environmental factors, symptoms caused by drugs usually reverse when the drug is no longer taken.

Exercise Guidelines

The ACSM recommends that people with Parkinson's disease combine aerobic exercise (3 days per week), resistance exercise (2 or 3 days per week), and flexibility exercise (at least 2-3 days per week, although daily is most effective). Resistance exercises should focus on lower-body muscles, particularly the trunk and hip extensors. Slow, static stretches are best for improving flexibility. Exercise will not reverse the symptoms of PD, but it can enhance the quality of life and help maintain functional independence.

Programming Considerations

Safety. The nervous system of people with PD is more vulnerable to sudden or unexpected changes, such as cool water temperatures. Water temperature of 90 to 92 degrees Fahrenheit (32-33 °C) is often ideal for PD exercise programs (American Parkinson's Disease Association 2012). Make adjustments to the program and to participant clothing as needed for the environmental conditions. Shallow water (not greater than mid chest) is recommended, and accommodations should be made for balance concerns or freezing (a sudden, brief inability to start movement or continue with a rhythmic repeated movement). For example, standing within arm's length of the pool wall or holding a noodle for support may be beneficial for some participants. Volunteers (family members or caregivers) may be needed to provide assistance and emotional support.

Programming. The goals of an aquatic exercise program for people with PD should be to lessen the degree of disability, assist with ADLs, and promote independent living for a longer period of time. The general class format should include flexibility, aerobic training, functional training, strengthening, and neuromuscular training components. The format should also target balance, posture, and gait training. Breathing and relaxation exercises will also help with muscle rigidity.

Leadership skills. Remember that participants might be at various stages of disease progression, so you will need to modify exercises and activities. Creating a positive social environment might help with the depression and social isolation often experienced with this disease. Be aware that beginning an exercise class may be stressful (i.e., being in a new environment, meeting new people, not knowing what to expect), which could cause an acute attack of PD symptoms.

Equipment. Equipment may be an effective tool to assist with independent movement, exercise performance, and balance. Equipment options depend on the participant's fitness level and experience with water exercise. You can use equipment as long as you consider intensity and restrictions. Be mindful that most equipment increases effort and intensity. Additionally, if equipment causes greater amounts of concentration and effort, participants may resort to holding their breath. Breath holding during exercise exertion can be dangerous and should be avoided.

Cerebral Palsy (CP)

Cerebral palsy (CP) is a general term referring to abnormalities of motor control caused by damage to a child's brain early in the course of development. The damage might occur during fetal development, the birth process, or the first few months after birth.

General Characteristics

CP can take one or a combination of three major forms. Spastic individuals suffer from hypertonia (excessive muscle tensions). Athetoid individuals have involuntary, uncontrolled movements of hands or feet and often have slurred speech and defective hearing. Ataxic individuals have a disturbed sense of balance, faulty depth perception, and walk with a staggered gait.

CP is difficult to diagnose in the first six months after birth. It is usually found when the child is 1 or 2 years old. Symptoms may include delays in motor skill development, weakness in one or more limbs, standing and walking on tiptoes, one leg dragging while walking, excessive drooling or difficulties swallowing, and poor control over hand and arm movement. CP can develop after meningitis, but for most children, a specific cause is unknown.

CP is a lifelong disease that can result in difficulty with mobility and necessary maintenance of physical function. The participant with CP might have difficulty in performing skilled movements, experience muscle imbalances and poor functional strength, or have a limited range of motion attributed to very tight muscles and tendons. Strong evidence in literature exists supporting the psychological and physiological benefits of exercise for people with CP. Long-term programs have been shown to reduce muscle spasms and the need for antispasmodic medication.

Exercise Guidelines

Although some people with cerebral palsy can follow the general ACSM exercise recommendations for adults, those with more severe limitations may need to adjust some areas. For example, it may be best to perform frequent, brief bouts of exercise and then progress to 20-minute training segments. Similarly, resistance exercise might be better performed with several short sessions that are combined with stretching. To reduce spasticity, 30 minutes spent on sustained stretching may be prudent.

Programming Considerations

Safety. Participants may need a walking aid or a chairlift to enter and exit the pool. Water shoes are recommended for participants who drag their feet or need better traction on the pool bottom. Some participants report an increase in spasticity after exercise, especially strenuous exercise.

Programming. Programs should develop cardiorespiratory endurance, muscular fitness, and flexibility. Low cardiorespiratory fitness and muscular weakness and imbalances are common, and can be addressed with water exercise. Program progression should be slow and emphasize exercises for improving daily function and independence.

Leadership skills. CP symptoms vary among people. Some show only physical signs, while others have a mental impairment as well. Leadership and instruction should cater to these individual needs. Give additional emphasis to range of motion and functional mobility exercises. Devote time to walking patterns and balance skills while providing additional cues to improve form and mechanics. Consider any visual and auditory impairments that could be present. Using both auditory and visual cueing can help ensure that everyone understands your directions.

Equipment. Equipment may be an effective tool to assist with independent movement, exercise performance, and balance. Using noodles for support or ankle weights for additional grounding can be very helpful in achieving a successful exercise session. You can use equipment as long as you consider intensity and restrictions for your clients. Be mindful that most equipment increases effort and intensity. Additionally, if equipment causes greater amounts of concentration and effort, participants may resort to holding their breath. Breath holding during exercise exertion can be dangerous and should be avoided.

Cancer

Cancer is the name given to a collection of related diseases where some of the body's cells begin to divide without stopping and spread into surrounding tissue. Cancer can start almost anywhere in the human body. When cells become old, damaged, or abnormal, new cells develop to take their place. When cancer develops, the damaged cells survive even when they should die, they and continue to form new extra cells where they are not needed. These extra cells can divide without stopping and may form tumors.

Many cancers form tumors or masses of tissue, but some do not, such as leukemia. Cancer tumors can be malignant, meaning they can invade nearby tissues. As they progress, they can break off and travel to distant places throughout the body and form new tumors. Benign (non-cancerous) tumors do not spread to invade neighboring tissues. When removed, they usually do not grow back, whereas malignant tumors can reoccur.

General Characteristics

More than 100 types of cancer exist. Types of cancer are usually named for the organs or tissues where the cancer forms. Cancer is caused by changes to the genes that control how our cells function, especially as they grow and divide. These changes can be inherited, or can arise from damage to DNA caused by environmental exposures such as tobacco smoke and ultraviolet rays from the sun. The most studied, known, or suspected risk factors for cancer include age, alcohol consumption, cancer-causing substances, chronic inflammation, diet, hormones, obesity, radiation, sunlight, tobacco, and infectious agents (National Cancer Institute 2015).

Exercise Guidelines

People with cancer benefit from an exercise program that targets cardiorespiratory, muscular conditioning, and flexibility. The ACSM recommends three to five days of aerobic activity, two or three days of resistance training, and daily stretching. It may be more beneficial to include multiple, shorter bouts of aerobic exercise than a single, continuous session. One set of 8 to 12 repetitions, avoiding avoid areas involved in treatments, is recommended for resistance training.

A comprehensive review of literature in 2000 by Courneya, Mackey, and Jones indicates that exercises has a positive effect on many aspects related to quality of life for individuals who have been diagnosed with cancer. Physicians who prescribe exercise for their cancer patients see improvements in motivation and adherence. Benefits of exercise for participants with cancer include the following:

- Improved overall physical function
- Decreased depression
- Improved sleep patterns
- Decreased pain and nausea
- Improved aerobic fitness, muscular strength, and flexibility
- Improved or maintained ideal body size
- Increased bone health
- Increased energy

Lymphedema, swelling that occurs in the arms or legs, is most commonly caused by removal of or damage to the lymph nodes as part of cancer treatment, either through surgery or from radiation. Aquatic exercise appears to be a useful method to assist in controlling breast cancer lymphedema (Tidhar et al. 2004). The buoyancy effect of the water makes range of motion more comfortable and the hydrostatic pressure compresses the submerged limbs. This assists the flow of lymph and blood without stressing other body parts. Water temperatures above 94 degrees Fahrenheit (34 °C) should be avoided with this condition (no hot tubs or spas). In general, pool temperatures ranging from 72 to 92 degrees Fahrenheit (22-33 °C) are preferred, with cooler temperatures for more strenuous exercise and warmer temperatures for gentle movements to help relax the muscles and soften hardened tissues.

Programming Considerations

Safety. In some instances, exercise is contraindicated in cancer participants. You must require participants to obtain and follow guidelines from their health care provider. Pool participation during active treatment (chemotherapy, radiation, alternative therapies) may be prohibited. Those undergoing radiation should avoid pools since the chlorine may cause irritation at the treatment site. People with weak immune systems (low white blood cell counts) should avoid pools and public gyms until their immunity improves. Anyone with an open wound should also avoid the pool until the site heals.

Programming. Exercise programs must be individualized for each participant; exercise may also need to be modified according to fatigue during periods of treatment. Goals of exercise might be altered depending on whether the participant is under active treatment or in remission. Program objectives should include returning the participant to former levels of physical and psychological function prior to diagnosis and preserving or enhancing function. General exercise guidelines suggest moderate- to vigorous-intensity cardiorespiratory exercise three to five days a week for 20 to 30 minutes per session. Resistance training and flexibility exercises are also recommended.

Leadership skills. Work hand in hand with the participant's medical team (e.g., oncologist, radiologist, and surgeon) to provide safe and effective care. Understand that people with cancer, specifically those undergoing treatment, will experience energy fluctuations from day to day and even hour to hour. Be prepared to increase or decrease intensity according to the energy level of the participants. Pay special attention to gentle, broad movements that promote circulation, range of motion, and lymph massage. Adding relaxation components into the class may also be of benefit to assist in reduction of stress and anxiety associated with the diagnosis of cancer.

Equipment. You can use equipment as long as you consider intensity and restrictions for your clients. Be mindful that most equipment increases effort and intensity. Additionally, if equipment causes greater amounts of concentration and effort, participants may resort to holding their breath. Breath holding during exercise exertion can be dangerous and should be avoided.

Summary

Special populations are groups of people with similar characteristics, health conditions, or common age range. Some special populations may find the water a more manageable, comfortable, and enjoyable environment in which to exercise, thus promoting better health and overall wellness.

Many participants will need a medical evaluation prior to initiating an exercise program. They may receive specific guidelines to follow in terms of frequency, intensity, time, and type of exercise. You can assist participants by encouraging self-monitoring and providing exercise modifications, but know your professional limitations and refer participants to a more qualified instructor, trainer, or health professional when necessary.

Knowing the basic information regarding the general characteristics, exercise guidelines, and programming considerations of special populations will allow you to better accommodate these people into your classes.

Review Questions

1. List four sensory changes associated with aging.
2. Heart rate and respiration rate are both higher in younger children and gradually decrease or normalize with age.
   a. True
   b. False
3. Due to the enlarging abdomen women experience during pregnancy, aquatic programming should consider the degree of ________________ with sagittal-plane lower-body movements.
   a. knee flexion
   b. knee extension
   c. hip flexion
   d. All of the above
4. For a general weight loss program, the ACSM recommends a reduction of ______________ initial weight over 3 to 6 months by an intervention of moderate to vigorous aerobic exercise, resistance training, and behavior intervention.
   a. 1-5%
   b. 3-10%
   c. 10-15%
   d. 15-20%
5. Define the 2-hour pain rule:
6. ________________________ is a chronic condition characterized by fatigue and widespread pain in the muscles, ligaments, and tendons.
   a. Osteoarthritis
   b. Osteoporosis
   c. Rheumatoid arthritis
   d. Fibromyalgia syndrome
7. People with CVD should exercise to the point of chest pain or angina.
   a. True
   b. False

8. For people with pulmonary disease, the hydrostatic pressure can make it more difficult to breathe when immersed. What programming consideration may be helpful to participants?

   a. Exercise only in water that is hip deep.
   b. Start in neck-deep water and gradually transition to chest-deep water.
   c. Start in waist-deep water and gradually transition to chest-deep water.
   d. Do not participate in water exercise; it is too risky.

9. For people with diabetes, exercise can help improve body composition by decreasing body fat, leading to better insulin sensitivity.

   a. True
   b. False

10. Heat intolerance is a key factor for _______________, who are more comfortable exercising in water temperatures at or below 84 degrees Fahrenheit (29 °C).

    a. participants with Parkinson's disease
    b. participants with multiple sclerosis
    c. older adults
    d. children

See appendix D for answers to review questions.

References and Resources

Abenhaim, L., M. Rossignol, J. Valat, M. Nordin, B. Avouac, F. Blotman, J. Charlot, et al. 2000. The role of activity in the therapeutic management of back pain. Report of the International Paris Task Force on Back Pain. *Spine* 25(4):1S-33S.

Alderman, B., R. Olson, et al. 2016. MAP training: Combining meditation and aerobic exercise reduces depression and rumination while enhancing synchronized brain activity. *Translational Psychiatry* 6:e726.

Altman, R., D. Block, et al. 1990. Osteoarthritis: Definitions and criteria. *Annals of the Rheumatic Diseases* 49(3):201.

American College of Sports Medicine. 2008. *ACSM Fit Society® page: The heart* www.acsm.org/docs/fit-society-page/2008-summer-fspn_the-heart.pdf?sfvrsn=0.

———. 2018. Guidelines for exercise testing and prescription. 10th edition. Baltimore: Lippincott, Williams & Wilkins.

American Congress of Obstetricians and Gynecologists. 2016. *Exercise During Pregnancy. FAQ119.* www.acog.org/Patients/FAQs/Exercise-During-Pregnancy.

American Heart Association. 2016. My life check—Life's simple 7.www.heart.org/HEARTORG/Conditions/My-Life-Check---Lifes-Simple-7_UCM_471453_Article.jsp#.V6JhWo52n7g.

American Parkinson's Disease Association. 2008. *Aquatic Exercise An Exercise Program for People with Parkinson's Disease*. Staten Island, NY: APDA, Inc.

Arden, N., and M. Nevitt. 2006. Osteoarthritis: Epidemiology. *Best Practice & Research: Clinical Rheumatology* 20(1):3-25.

Arnold, C. M., A.J. Busch, C.L. Schachter, E.L. Harrison, and W.P. Olszynski. 2008. A randomized clinical trial of aquatic versus land exercise to improve balance, function, and quality of life in older women with osteoporosis. *Physiotherapy Canada* 60(4): 296-306.

Arthritis Foundation. n.d. Rheumatoid Arthritis. www.arthritis.org/about-arthritis/types/rheumatoid-arthritis/

Barbosa, T., M. Garrido, and J. Bragada. 2007. Physiological adaptations to head-out aquatic exercises with different levels of body immersion. *Journal of Strength & Conditioning Research* 21(4):1255-1259.

Baste, V., and J. Gadkari. 2014. Study of stress, self-esteem and depression in medical students and effect of music on perceived stress. *Indian Journal of Physiology and Pharmacology* 58(3):298-301.

Becker, B. 2009. Aquatic therapy: Scientific foundations and clinical rehabilitation applications. *PM&R* 1(9):859-872.

Buchbinder, R., F. Blyth, L. March, P. Brooks, A. Woolf, and D. Hoy. 2013. Placing the global burden of low back pain in context. *Best Practice & Research: Clinical Rheumatology* 27(5):575-589.

Cavalcante, S., J. Cecatti, R.I. Pereira, E.P. Baciuk, A.L. Bernardo, and C. Silveira. 2009. Water aerobics II: Maternal body composition and perinatal outcomes after a program for low risk pregnant women. *Reproductive Health* 6:1.

Centers for Disease Control and Prevention. Adult obesity causes and consequences. www.cdc.gov/obesity/adult/causes.html. Last reviewed June 16, 2015. Last updated August 15, 2016. Accessed June 10, 2017.

Cooper, C., S. Snow, et al. 2000. Risk factors for the incidence and progression of radiographic knee osteoarthritis. *Arthritis & Rheumatology* 43(5):995-1000.

Courneya, K.S., J.R. Mackey, and L.W. Jones. 2000. Coping with cancer: can exercise help? *Physicians and Sports Medicine* 28(5): 49-73.

Creamer, P., M. Lethbridge-Cejku, et al. 2000. Factors associated with functional impairment in symptomatic knee osteoarthritis. *Rheumatology (Oxford)* 39(5):490-496.

de Brito Fontana, H., A. Haupenthal, C. Ruschel, M. Hubert, C. Ridehalgh, and H. Roesler. 2012. Effect of gender, cadence, and water immersion on ground reaction forces during stationary running. *Journal of Orthopedic & Sports Physical Therapy* 42(5): 437-443.

Dieppe, P. 1998. Osteoarthritis. *Acta Orthopaedic Scandinavica. Supplementum* 281:2-5.

Durstine, J. and G Moore. 2002. *ACSM's exercise management for person with chronic disease and disabilities, 2nd edition*. Champaign, IL: Human Kinetics Publishers.

Ekin, J.A., and S. Mehrsheed. 1993. Vertebral compression fractures sustained during golfing: report of three cases. *Mayo Clinic Proceedings* 68(6).

Englund, M. 2010. The role of biomechanics in the initiation and progression of OA of the knee. *Best Practice & Research: Clinical Rheumatology* 24(1):39-46.

Gabriel, S., and K. Michaud. 2009. Epidemiological studies in incidence, prevalence, mortality, and comorbidity of the rheumatic diseases. *Arthritis Research & Therapy* 11(3):229.

Gill, T., L. DiPietro, et al. 2000. Role of exercise stress testing and safety monitoring for older persons starting an exercise program. *JAMA* 284(3):342-349.

Granath, A., M. Hellgren, and R.K. Gunnarsson. 2006. Water aerobics reduces sick leave due to low back pain during pregnancy. *Journal of Obstetric, Gynecologic, & Neonatal Nursing* 35(4):465-471.

Haffner, S.M., L. Ruilope, B. Dahlof, E. Abadie, S. Kupfer, and F. Zannad. 2006. Metabolic syndrome, new onset diabetes, and new end points in cardiovascular trials. *Journal of Cardiovascular Pharmacology* 47(3):469-75.

Hartmann, S., and R. Huch. 2005. Response of pregnancy leg edema to a single immersion exercise session. *Acta Obstetricia et Gynecologica Scandinavica* 84(12):1150-1153.

Harush, M. and F. Yazigi. 2016. Osteoporosis & aquatic exercise. *Akwa* 29(6): 6.

Himes, C., and S. Reynolds. 2011. Effect of obesity on falls, injury and disability. *Journal of American Geriatrics Society* 60(1):124-129.

Holmes M., W. Chen, D. Feskanich, C. Kroenke, and G. Colditz. 2005. Physical activity and survival after breast cancer diagnosis. *Journal of the American Medical Association* 293(20):2479-2486.

Issa, S., and L. Sharma. 2006. Epidemiology of osteoarthritis: An update. *Current Rheumatology Reports* 8(1):7-15.

Kaptein, S., C. Backman, E. Badley, D. Lacaille, D. Beaton, C. Hofstetter, and M. Gignac. 2013.

Choosing where to put your energy: A qualitative analysis of the role of physical activity in the lives of working adults with arthritis. *Arthritis Care & Research* 65: 1070–1076.

Karsdal, M., D. Leeming, et al. 2008. Should subchondral bone turnover be targeted when treating osteoarthritis? *Osteoarthritis and Cartilage* 16(6):638-646.

Kent, T., J. Gregor, L. Deardorff, and V. Katz. 1999. Edema of pregnancy: A comparison of water aerobics and static immersion. *Obstetrics & Gynecology* 94(5 Pt 1):726-729.

Levy, S., C. Macera, J. Hootman, K. Coleman, R. Lopez, J. Nichols, and S. Marshall. 2012. Evaluation of a multi-component group exercise program for adults with arthritis: Fitness and Exercise for People with Arthritis (FEPA)." *Disability and Health Journal* 5(4): 305-311.

Martin, K., D. Kuh, et al. 2013. Body mass index, occupational activity, and leisure-time physical activity: An exploration of risk factors and modifiers for knee osteoarthritis in the 1946 British birth cohort. *BMC Musculoskeletal Disorders* 14:219.

Mayo Clinic. 2017. Emphysema. www.mayoclinic.org/diseases-conditions/emphysema/home/ovc-20317003

McTiernan, A. 2006. *Cancer prevention and management through exercise and weight control.* Boca Raton, FL: Taylor and Francis.

Messier, S. 2008. Obesity and osteoarthritis: Disease genesis and nonpharmacologic weight management. *Rheumatic Disease Clinics of North America* 34(3):713-729.

Messier, S., D. Gutekunst, C. Davis, and P. DeVita. 2005. Weight loss reduces knee-joint loads in overweight and obese older adults with knee osteoarthritis. *Arthritis & Rheumatology* 52(7):2026-2032.

Moreira, L.D., M.L. Oliveira, A.P. Lirani-Galvao, R.V. Marin-Mio, R.N. Santos, and M. Lazaretti-Castro. 2014. Physical exercise and osteoporosis: effects of different types of exercises on bone and physical function of postmenopausal women. *Arquivos Brasileiros de Endocrinologia & Metabologia* 58(5): 514-522.

Multiple Sclerosis Association of America. 2013. *Aquatic exercise & multiple sclerosis: A healthcare professional's guide.* Cherry Hill, NJ: Multiple Sclerosis Association of America.

Munguía-Izquierdo, D., and A. Legaz-Arrese. 2007. Exercise in warm water decreases pain and improves cognitive function in middle-aged women with fibromyalgia. *Clinical & Experimental Rheumatology* 25(6): 823.

Muthuri, S., M. Hui, et al. 2011. What if we prevent obesity? Risk reduction in knee osteoarthritis estimated through a meta-analysis of observational studies. *Arthritis Care & Research (Hoboken)* 63(7):982-990.

National Cancer Institute. 2015. What is cancer? www.cancer.gov/about-cancer/understanding/what-is-cancer#related-diseases. Updated February 9, 2015. Accessed June 10, 2017.

National Institutes of Health. National Institute of Neurological Disorders and Stroke. n.d. Low back pain fact sheet. Accessed August 2, 2016. www.ninds.nih.gov/disorders/backpain/detail_backpain.htm.

National Institute of Mental Health. 2016. Depression. www.nimh.nih.gov/health/topics/depression/index.shtml.

National Multiple Sclerosis Society. 2016. Who gets MS? Epidemiology. www.nationalmssociety.org/What-is-MS/Who-Gets-MS.

Pinto, B., G. Frierson, C. Rabin, J. Trunzo, and B. Marcus. 2005. Home based physical activity intervention for breast cancer patients. *Journal of Clinical Oncology* 23(15):1377-3587.

Polman, R., M. Kaiseler, and E. Borkoles. 2007. Effect of a single bout of exercise on the mood of pregnant women. *Journal of Sports Medicine and Physical Fitness* 47(1):103-111.

Rahmann, A. 2010. Exercise for people with hip or knee osteoarthritis: A comparison of land-based and aquatic interventions. *Open Access Journal of Sports Medicine* 1:123-135.

Rai, M., and L. Sandell 2011. Inflammatory mediators: Tracing links between obesity and osteoarthritis. *Critical Reviews in Eukaryotic Gene Expression* 21(2):131-142.

Reginster, J., O. Bruyere, et al. 2003. New perspectives in the management of osteoarthritis. Structure modification: Facts or fantasy? *Journal of Rheumatology Supplement* 67: 14-20.

Repka, C. 2015. Physiological benefits of exercise in cancer patients. *ACSM's Certified News* 3(25):8, 14-15.

Riebe, D., B. Franklin, et al. 2015. Updating ACSM's recommendations for exercise preparticipation health screening. *Medicine & Science in Sports & Exercise* 47(11):2473-2479.

Scopaz, K., S. Piva, et al. 2009. Relationships of fear, anxiety, and depression with physical function in patients with knee osteoarthritis. *Archives of Physical Medicine and Rehabilitation* 90(11):1866-1873.

Silveira, C., B. Pereira, J.G. Cecatti, S.R. Cavalcante, and R.I. Pereira. 2010. Fetal cardiotocography before and after water aerobics during pregnancy. *Reproductive Health* 7: 23.

Smith, S., and Y. Michel 2006. A pilot study on the effects of aquatic exercises on discomforts of pregnancy. *Journal of Obstetric, Gynecologic, & Neonatal Nursing* 35(3):315-323.

Sturmer, T., K. Gunther, et al. 2000. Obesity, overweight and patterns of osteoarthritis: The Ulm Osteoarthritis Study. *Journal of Clinical Epidemiology* 53(3):307-313.

Tanamas, S., F. Hanna, et al. 2009. Does knee malalignment increase the risk of development and progression of knee osteoarthritis? A systematic review. *Arthritis & Rheumatology* 61(4):459-467.

Thakur, A., and S. Yardi 2013. Effect of different types of music on exercise performance in normal individuals. *Indian Journal of Physiology and Pharmacology* 57(4):448-451.

Tidhar, D., A. Shimony, and J. Drouin. 2004. Aqua lymphatic therapy for postsurgical breast cancer lymphedema. *Rehabilitation Oncology* 22(3): 6-14.

van der Kraan, P. 2012. Osteoarthritis year 2012 in review: Biology. *Osteoarthritis and Cartilage* 20(12):1447-1450.

Wadden, T., M. Butryn, and K. Byrne. 2004. Efficacy of lifestyle modification for long-term weight control. *Obesity Research & Clinical Practice* 12 Suppl:151S-162S.

Waller, B., J. Lambeck, and D. Daly. 2009. Therapeutic aquatic exercise in the treatment of low back pain: A systematic review. *Clinical Rehabilitation* 23(1):3-14.

Wang, T., B. Belza, E.F. Thompson, J.D. Whitney, and K. Bennett. 2007. Effects of aquatic exercise on flexibility, strength and aerobic fitness in adults with osteoarthritis of the hip or knee. *Journal of Advanced Nursing* 57(2):141-152.

Wieland, H., M. Michaelis, et al. 2005. Osteoarthritis—an untreatable disease? *Nature Reviews Drug Discovovery* 4(4):331-344.

Williams, F., and T. Spector. 2006. Osteoarthritis. *Medicine* 34(9):364-368.

Williams, M., W. Haskell, P. Ades, E. Amsterdam, V. Bittner, B. Franklin, M. Gulanick, et al. 2007. Resistance exercise in individuals with and without cardiovascular disease: 2007 update: a scientific statement from the American Heart Association Council on Clinical Cardiology and Council on Nutrition, Physical and Metabolism. *Circulation* 116(5):572-584.

Wilcox, S., B. McClenaghan, P.A. Sharpe, M. Baruth, J.M. Hootman, K. Leith, and M Dowda. 2014. The steps to health randomized trial for arthritis: a self-directed exercise versus nutrition control program. *American Journal of Preventive Medicine*. 48(1): 1-12.

World Health Organization. 2003. The burden of musculoskeletal conditions at the start of the new millennium. *World Health Organization Technical Report Series* 919:i-x, 1-218, back cover.

———. 2012. Depression in Europe. www.euro.who.int/en/health-topics/noncommunicable-diseases/pages/news/news/2012/10/depression-in-europe.

Yazigi, F., S. Pinto, J. Colado, Y. Escalante, P.A. Armada-da-Silva, R. Brasil, and F. Alves. 2013. The cadence and water temperature effect on physiological responses during water cycling. *European Journal of Sport Science* 13(6):659-665.

Zhang, W., D. McWilliams, et al. 2011. Nottingham knee osteoarthritis risk prediction models. *Annals of the Rheumatic Diseases* 70(9):1599-1604.

Part IV

Safety, Scope of Practice, and Legal

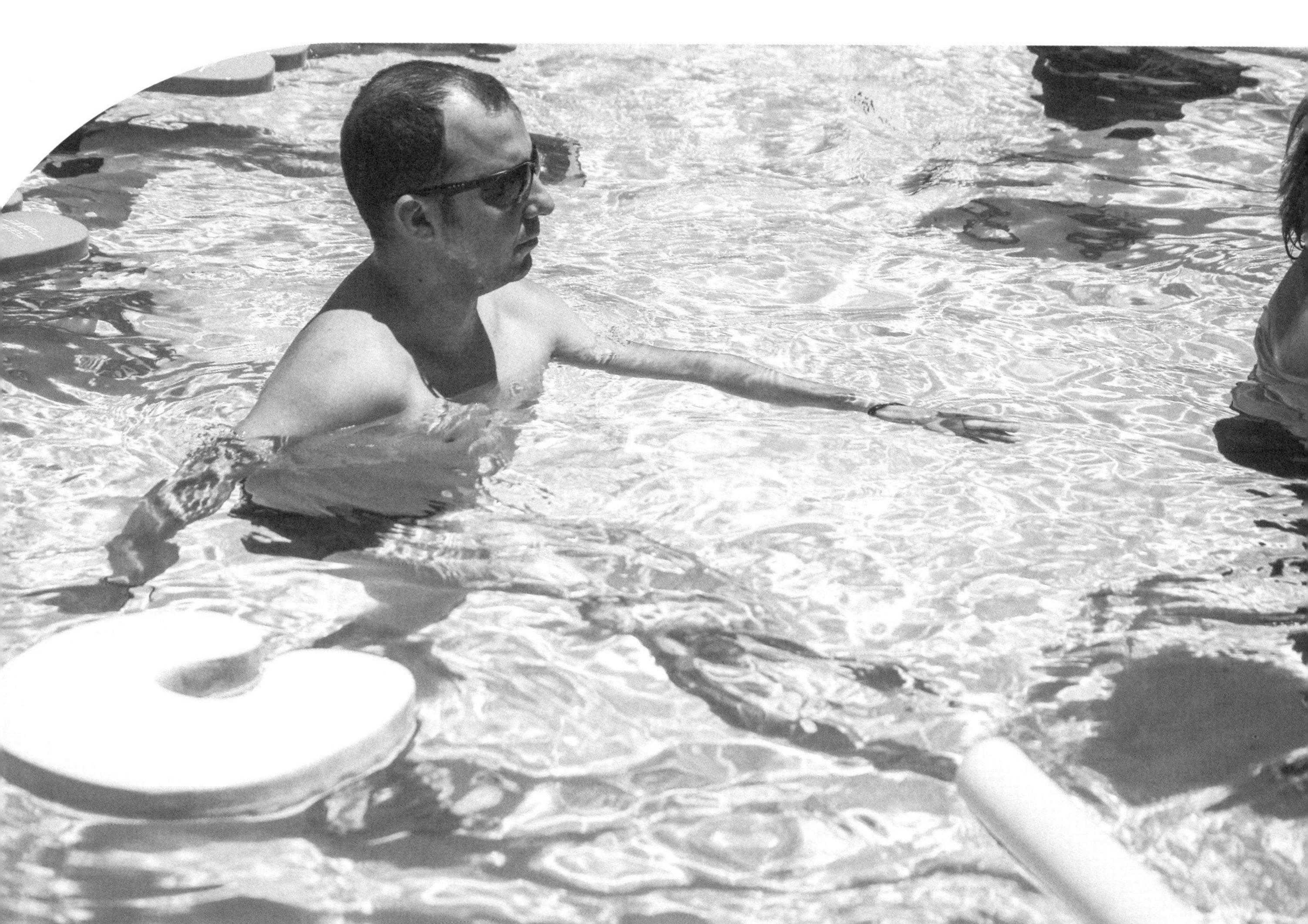

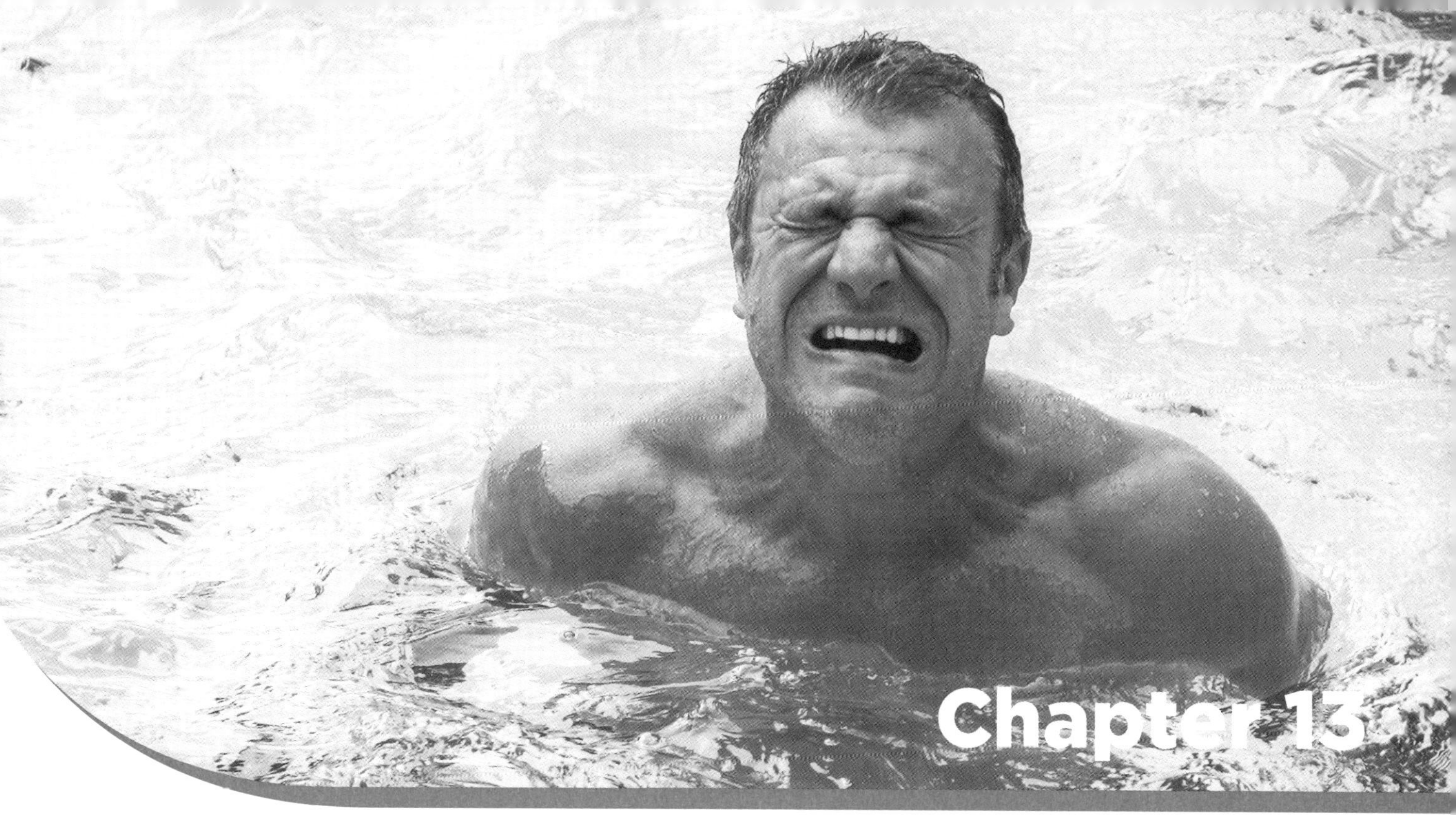

Safety, Emergencies, Injuries, and Instructor Health

Introduction

This chapter presents information intended to help you appreciate general water safety and risk management concepts and the various emergencies and injuries that can occur, as well as learn about your health as a fitness professional. In your position as an aquatic fitness professional, you might be required to provide initial first aid, initiate CPR, or use an AED. However, the information in this chapter is neither intended to be a replacement for training courses on water safety, first aid, CPR, or AED, nor is this information meant to eliminate the need for hiring properly trained and certified lifeguarding staff at pool facilities. Rather, the information reviews the basics that you need to know as an aquatic fitness professional.

Key Chapter Concepts

- Know the required and recommended safety training for aquatic fitness professionals.
- Understand risk management strategies to reduce the occurrence of injury, illness, or drowning in your aquatic programs.
- Define emergency action plan (EAP) and assessment procedures for responsive and unresponsive people.
- Recognize the difference between a distressed person and a drowning situation, and understand how to make a safe assist based on your level of training.
- Understand the emergency first aid procedures for sudden illnesses common to aquatic fitness classes.
- Differentiate between acute and chronic injuries; know basic first aid for acute injuries and aquatic program strategies to help prevent chronic injuries.
- Recognize both the potential danger of electrical shock in the aquatic environment and how to minimize its risk.
- Be aware of health considerations relevant to aquatic fitness professionals.

As aquatic fitness professionals, we hope never to experience an emergency situation in our classes, training sessions, pool decks, or locker rooms. However, it is prudent to always be prepared because emergencies do happen—and they happen quickly.

Instructors and personal trainers working in and around the pool must maintain certification or training in **cardiopulmonary resuscitation (CPR)**, including the use of an **automated external defibrillator (AED)**. Additional training in general water safety and basic first aid is also highly recommended. The more knowledge and practice you have in these areas, the more confident you will be should an emergency situation arise. You will improve your response, as well as the outcome of emergencies, with a well-considered and practiced emergency action plan for each facility where you work or train.

Safety and Risk Management

Safety should always be a primary consideration in and around the pool. **Risk management** is the process of measuring or assessing potential risk and developing strategies to manage the risk. You should be prepared to recognize potential risk, adhere to policies to reduce risk, and react to emergency situations that may arise when conducting exercise programs in an aquatic environment.

The following is a sample of emergency scenarios that participants might experience:

- Lose footing or unexpectedly find themselves in deep water and unable to stand up.
- Slip off unattached flotation equipment and panic.
- Begin the drowning process if submerged under water.
- Have a heart attack, sudden cardiac arrest, stroke, seizure, or other sudden illness.
- Become injured due to a fall on the pool deck or locker room.

In addition, the environment may create potentially harmful conditions:

- Approaching severe weather or lightning

- Chemical reaction, leak, or spill
- Exposure to bloodborne, waterborne, or airborne pathogens
- Slippery deck surfaces
- Broken ladders, loose rails on steps, loose tiles on the pool bottom, chipped gutters
- Improperly grounded electrical outlets
- Improper drain covers (as per the Virginia Graeme Baker Pool and Spa Safety Act of 2007)

The foundation of safety is to understand the foreseeable risks and then take steps to reduce the risk, when possible, through prevention strategies. Risk can never be completely eliminated, so emergencies can and will occur. In these situations, being prepared is the next level of safe practices. See chapter 15 for additional information and policies on risk management.

There are several things described in other areas of this text that will help you reduce the risk of injury, illness, or drowning. Understand how movement in water differs from movement on land and how different types of aquatic equipment influence the muscle actions (see chapter 4). Conduct programs only when water quality, air quality, temperatures, and humidity are within recommended ranges (see chapter 7). Evaluate each new participant in deep-water exercise for comfort and ability, and follow recommendations for choosing proper flotation equipment (see chapter 9). When teaching from the pool deck, follow AEA Standards and Guidelines for Deck Instruction to ensure your personal safety (see chapter 10). Realize that special populations and participants with health conditions will require program modifications (see chapter 12). Be aware of prevention strategies to decrease the risk of common chronic injuries (discussed later in this chapter).

In addition, consider these risk management strategies:

- Conduct a preclass safety inspection.
    - Pause before you approach. Ask yourself, "Does everything seem okay on first glance?" Generally, your first impression is correct.
    - Observe your surroundings. Are there any obvious potential safety hazards? What is there about the deck, water quality, or other conditions that could cause injury or harm?
    - Ask yourself about people traffic. Will the number of participants coming into the area cause a safety hazard or concern?
    - Protect yourself! Are you wearing the appropriate footwear? Should you be wearing sunscreen and sunglasses? Are bodily fluids present? If so, do you have personal protective equipment?
    - Consider the unknown. What is unique about the situation that could cause concern?

Information provided courtesy of the Park District Risk Management Agency (www.pdrma.org).

- Know the emergency action plan at each facility where you work and the responses expected of you.
- Be trained in the proper use of emergency response and rescue equipment (first aid supplies, personal protective equipment, rescue tube, ring buoy, AED, and telephone) and make sure that the equipment is available.
- Follow facility procedures in the event of fecal or vomit contamination of the pool water or surrounding deck areas to prevent recreational water illness (described later in this chapter).
- Scan (look at) every participant about every 10 seconds and be able to recognize signs and symptoms of illness, distress, or drowning.

Having a lifeguard on duty provides an important prevention strategy because distress or drowning can happen quickly and the lifeguard's primary focus will be looking for signs of distress or drowning. Many locations have a regulatory requirement that a lifeguard be on duty during hours of operation, but some do not. As an instructor, your

AEA Standards and Guidelines for Aquatic Fitness Programming

Lifeguard

Country, state, county, and local codes relating to lifeguard regulations should always be followed. For maximal safety of participants and limited liability for the Aquatic Fitness Professional and facility, AEA recommends that a certified lifeguard, in addition to the Aquatic Fitness Professional leading the class or session, should be on duty at the pool facility when aquatic fitness classes are being held.

If an additional certified lifeguard is not present during the aquatic fitness class or session, AEA recommends:

- The Aquatic Fitness Professional to be certified in water safety and basic water rescue techniques.
- The Aquatic Fitness Professional to remain on deck while leading the class or session unless it is a one-on-one session or small group training (2-5 participants) that requires in-water assistance or guidance.
- The Aquatic Fitness Professional to be fully aware of the facility's emergency action plan (EAP) and the professional's role in this plan.

focus is on leading activities and looking to see if participants are performing them correctly. However, if there is not a lifeguard on duty during your class, you have added responsibilities of ensuring the safety of participants. See the sidebar for standards and guidelines for aquatic fitness programming.

Emergency Procedures

Your role during an emergency situation will vary, depending on whether or not a lifeguard is on duty. You should know what to do when you are the closest person to the scene of an emergency situation or if an injury occurs during a class or training session.

Emergency Action Plans

An **emergency action plan (EAP)** is a preconceived plan of action for emergency situations. Its purpose is to prepare the staff to deal with emergencies in a coordinated effort. Each facility should be prepared for emergencies and each staff member should be well trained in the procedures. Emergency action plans should include the following information:

- Course of action for all staff on duty at the time (who does what and when)
- Instructions about how to call **emergency medical services** (EMS) or other agencies that would respond to your specific location
- List of people to be notified of an emergency and the contact numbers (this information should also be posted near the phones)

An EAP should be created for each type of emergency that requires different procedures. For example, a facility might have one plan for a non-life-threatening event, another for a drowning, and even another for a weather or environmental emergency. Each EAP should be practiced by the included staff and evaluated for effectiveness on a regular basis. Should an actual emergency occur, the facility should also have follow-up procedures to evaluate the event and determine if the EAP or prevention strategies need to be revised. Additionally, it is important to document details of the situation by completing appropriate incident or injury report forms (see chapter 15 for more information).

Assessment

Quick action during an emergency is often important, but first you need to assess the situation to determine your course of action. Depending on the agency through which you obtained first aid training, you may know these steps as Check–Call–Care (American Red Cross), Assess–Alert–Attend (Health and Safety Institute), Chain of Survival (American Heart Association), or something similar.

- **For a person who appears to be unresponsive**, check the scene and approach if it is safe. Shake the person and loudly ask, "Are you OK?" If there is no response, quickly check for normal, easy, rhythmic breathing. Occasional gasps are not normal breathing. If there is no response and the person is not breathing normally, signal for help to activate the EAP so that EMS is called. Begin CPR.
- **For a person who is responsive**, check the scene and approach if it is safe. Ask the person if it is OK to help. Determine if there are any life-threatening problems by checking for an altered mental status, signs of stroke, or serious bleeding or injury. If the person appears to be weak, confused, seriously ill, or injured, activate the EAP so that EMS is called. Begin first aid care and continue until EMS arrives. For non-life-threatening conditions, provide first aid care as needed.

Distress and Drowning

The aquatic environment adds a safety concern not found in land-based fitness programs—the potential for drowning. People in **distress** can swim or float, and are still breathing but having difficulty remaining on the surface to breathe. They might have lost footing on the bottom, developed a cramp, or swallowed water. Or they may be fatigued or experiencing a sudden illness. These people have some water skills and may or may not be able to wave, signal, or call out for help. This condition can quickly deteriorate if fear takes hold or if the person is unable to keep the mouth or nose above the surface and the drowning process begins.

Drowning is a process that begins when the mouth and nose are covered with water, preventing the person from taking a breath. The process continues until the person gets a breath, either spontaneously (if still conscious when lifted above the surface) or through rescue breathing (if the person has gone unresponsive due to lack of oxygen). Drowning does not always result in death. It can result in one of three outcomes, primarily depending on how quickly the drowning process is interrupted.

1. The person may live and be fine.
2. The person may live but experience lifelong mild to severe neurological problems (brain damage).
3. The person may die.

Drowning is not a lung problem; it is a brain problem. Very little water enters the lungs during drowning. During drowning, the heart stops because of lack of oxygen to the brain. Brain damage can begin after just a few minutes without oxygen. The heart will not continue to beat when oxygen levels drop past a certain point.

Drowning is silent and quick. A person who is drowning is actually being suffocated by the water and thus cannot call out for help. Drowning symptoms may be difficult to detect; a person may appear to be bobbing up and down, which gives the illusion of being in control or playing. People, even those nearby, are often unaware that the person is struggling and that a drowning is taking place. Often, the person slips quietly below the surface or is unresponsive and floating at the surface with no visible struggle. This is particularly true with children or when a person suffers a sudden illness while in the water.

Making an Assist

If you are in the position to assist a distressed person, a **reaching** or **throwing assist** is the safest way to help that person. Another type of assist is a **wading assist**.

If you are not trained, attempting a swimming rescue is *not* recommended. It might create a double drowning situation. A safety slogan to keep in mind if you are not trained for swimming assists is, "Reach, throw, but never go!"

Reaching Assist

- Be sure you are not in danger of being pulled into the water yourself.
- Keep your center of gravity low to the ground and extend a rescue tube, pole or shepherd's crook, your arm, leg, towel, pool noodle, or shirt.
- When extending a pole, place it on the edge of the pool and slide it out and under the victim's outstretched arms. *Do not aim for the face or chest area.*
- If you extend a shepherd's crook, turn the crook away from the victim as you extend it. Once alongside the victim, turn the pole and rotate the crook and hook it around the victim's waist. Slide it up to the armpits and pull the victim in slowly.

Throwing Assist

- Any item that floats and that can be thrown can be used in a throwing assist.
- When throwing a ring buoy or other flotation device with a rope attached, attempt to throw it just past the person and instruct the person to grab hold. Do not throw the device with the entire rope; stand on the end of rope or have it attached to your wrist. You can pull the device and person to safety.
- When throwing a device without a rope, attempt to have it land just in front of the person so that it will drift under their arms. If you are unsuccessful and you can safely swim, push the device to the person, avoiding body-to-body contact. You can tow the device and person to safety.

Wading Assist

- Lean your body toward safety (e.g., side of pool) before making contact with the person.
- When possible, take a rescue tube or other flotation device with you to extend to the victim. Keep the flotation device between you and the person, avoiding any body-to-body contact.

Sudden Illness

Sudden illness can occur to anyone, anywhere. You might not know what the illness is, but you can still provide care. If you think something is wrong or if the participant looks or feels ill, check for a medical alert tag. Don't be afraid to ask questions to gain insight as to what is wrong; their condition can deteriorate very quickly. Keep in mind that you are not required to perform any skills beyond your level of training. The following are some sudden illness situations that you might experience in an aquatic class.

Hypoglycemia is not a disease, but rather an indicator of a health problem. It is a condition characterized by an abnormally low level of blood sugar (glucose), which is the body's main energy source. Low levels of blood sugar can cause lethargy, weakness, dizziness, and, in severe cases, fainting.

Often associated with diabetes, hypoglycemia can result from a variety of conditions. Participants who have not eaten for several hours and come to exercise may suffer low-level hypoglycemia symptoms. You might want to encourage participants to eat breakfast before morning classes or consume a healthy snack before afternoon or evening classes. Immediate treatment of hypoglycemia requires a return of blood sugar levels to the normal range, either with high-sugar foods, glucose tablets, or medications. Because treatment should occur immediately, items such as glucose tabs, juice, or sugar (cubes or gels) should be kept on the pool deck in the first aid kit. Participants subject to becoming hypoglycemic should have some type of food with them when they come to class in case of an emergency.

Early Signs and Symptoms of Hypoglycemia

Early signs and symptoms of diabetic hypoglycemia include the following:

- Shakiness
- Nervousness or anxiety
- Sweating, chills, and clamminess
- Irritability or impatience
- Confusion, including delirium
- Rapid heartbeat
- Lightheadedness or dizziness
- Hunger and nausea
- Sleepiness
- Blurred or impaired vision
- Tingling or numbness in the lips or tongue
- Headaches
- Weakness or fatigue
- Anger, stubbornness, or sadness
- Lack of coordination
- Nightmares or crying out during sleep
- Seizures
- Unconsciousness

Source: American Diabetes Association, www.diabetes.org.

A **heart attack**, also called a myocardial infarction, occurs when blood flow to the heart is blocked, causing damage to part of the heart muscle. Some heart attacks are obvious—sudden and intense. However, most heart attacks start with mild discomfort and pain, leaving the affected person confused about what is wrong and waiting too long to get help. Recognition of the symptoms of a heart attack is important, and immediate action is critical. If you suspect someone is having a heart attack, call emergency medical services immediately. Have the person lie down and monitor them closely. If the person has been prescribed nitroglycerin and has it available, encourage them to take the

Heart Attack Warning Signs

Heart attack warning signs include the following:

- **Chest discomfort.** Most heart attacks involve discomfort in the center of the chest that lasts more than a few minutes or that goes away and comes back. It can feel like uncomfortable pressure, squeezing, fullness, or pain.
- **Discomfort in other areas of the upper body.** Symptoms can include pain or discomfort in one or both arms, the back, neck, jaw, or stomach.
- **Shortness of breath** with or without chest discomfort.
- **Other signs** may include breaking out in a cold sweat, nausea, or lightheadedness.
- As with men, women's most common heart attack symptom is chest pain or discomfort. But women are somewhat more likely than men to experience some of the other common symptoms, particularly shortness of breath, nausea or vomiting, and back or jaw pain.

Source: American Heart Association, www.heart.org.

Cardiac Arrest Symptoms

Sudden cardiac arrest symptoms are immediate and drastic and include the following:

- Sudden collapse
- No pulse
- No breathing
- Loss of consciousness

Sometimes other signs and symptoms precede sudden cardiac arrest. These may include fatigue, fainting, blackouts, dizziness, chest pain, shortness of breath, weakness, palpitations, or vomiting. But sudden cardiac arrest often occurs with no warning.

Source: Mayo Clinic, www.mayoclinic.org.

medication. Have the facility's AED available and begin CPR if necessary.

Cardiac arrest is caused when the heart's electrical system malfunctions. Death results when the heart suddenly stops working properly. A heart attack may cause cardiac arrest and sudden death; however, a heart attack is not the same as cardiac arrest. If cardiac arrest occurs, call emergency medical care immediately and begin CPR. When the AED becomes available, power it on, attach the chest pads, and follow the prompts. Early administration of both CPR (a combination of chest compressions and rescue breathing) and defibrillation (the process of delivering electrical shock to allow the heart to spontaneously develop an effective rhythm) increases the chance for survival.

For chest compressions to be effective in CPR, the person should be placed on their back on a flat, firm surface. It is not possible to perform effective chest compression in the water, so the individual must be removed from the water before CPR can be initiated. Removing an unresponsive person from the pool involves skills that must be practiced. Attend a water safety or rescue course to learn and perform the removal skills and practice the methods used at your facility with others who would respond to an emergency. Additionally, certain precautions must be taken when operating an AED to ensure the safety of the person, the rescuers, and bystanders. An AED is safe to use if a person has been completely removed from the water, and is not lying in a puddle of standing water. The person's chest must be dry for the AED pads to adhere correctly.

A **stroke** is a "brain attack." A stroke occurs when blood flow to an area of the brain is cut off; brain cells are deprived of oxygen and begin to die and abilities controlled by that area of the brain are lost. Prompt response and care for stroke victims is imperative for survival and effective treatment. In the case of a stroke, the fight is to save brain tissue and avoid permanent loss of function. If a stroke is suspected, call emergency medical care immediately, lay the person down, and monitor them carefully. Use the American Heart Association's FAST acronym to quickly determine the presence of a stroke if you should suspect one:

Face. Ask the person to smile. Does one side of the face droop?

Arms. Ask the person to raise both arms. Does one arm drift downward?

Speech. Ask the person to repeat a simple phrase. Is their speech blurred?

Time. If you observe any of these signs, call EMS immediately.

Sudden Signs of Stroke

Beyond FAST, other symptoms of stroke include the following:

- Sudden **numbness** or weakness of face, arm, or leg, especially on one side of the body
- Sudden **confusion**, trouble speaking or understanding speech
- Sudden **trouble seeing** in one or both eyes
- Sudden **trouble walking**, dizziness, loss of balance or coordination
- Sudden **severe headache** with no known cause

Source: American Stroke Association, www.strokeassociation.org.

A **seizure** occurs when there is abnormal electrical activity in the brain. Seizures may go virtually unnoticed or may produce loss of consciousness and convulsions. Seizures usually come on suddenly and vary in duration and severity. Recurrent seizures are known as epilepsy, or a seizure disorder. In the event that a seizure takes place in the water, the steps taken vary from those followed on land. Your primary concern is to keep the person's head above the water and the airway open. Do *not* attempt to remove the person from the pool during a seizure. As soon as the seizure is over, check for normal breathing and an obvious pulse. Provide rescue breathing or CPR as indicated. The potential for aspiration of pool water during a seizure can lead to a severe lung infection. Call EMS in the event of a seizure that takes place in the water or recommend that the person immediately obtain evaluation by a health care professional.

Hyperthermia is elevated body temperature that occurs when a body produces or absorbs more heat than it dissipates. Everyone is susceptible to heat-related illness, although the very young and very old are at greater risk. Heat-related illnesses can become serious or even deadly if unattended. The key to avoiding these conditions is prevention. Prevention of hyperthermia in exercise includes acclimatization, identification of susceptible people, unrestricted fluid replacement (avoiding alcohol and caffeine), and a well-balanced diet.

As an aquatic fitness professional, be aware of your local weather forecasts and your exercise environment (refer to chapter 7 to review recommendations for air and water temperatures). Dress appropriately for the environment. For example, when instructing at outdoor pools in hot weather, wear loose-fitting, lightweight, light-colored clothing and a hat. Stay hydrated, and encourage your participants to stay hydrated, by drinking plenty of fluids even if you do not feel thirsty. Schedule classes at outdoor pools to avoid exercising during the hottest part of the day.

It is important to recognize signs and understand care for heat-related illness, including heat cramps, heat exhaustion, and heat stroke (American Red Cross 2016):

- **Heat cramps.** Heat cramps represent the least severe stage of heat-related illness. The muscle pains and spasms, usually occurring in the legs or abdomen, are often the first signals that the body is having difficulty with heat. Caused by exposure to high heat and humidity along with the loss of fluids and electrolytes, heat cramps should be considered a warning of a potential heat-related emergency. A person with heat cramps should move to a cooler location, drink cool water, and gently stretch the muscles affected by the cramps.
- **Heat exhaustion.** More severe than heat cramps, heat exhaustion is usually a consequence of losing body fluids through heavy sweating without proper rehydration. Signs of heat exhaustion include headache,

nausea, dizziness, weakness or exhaustion, heavy sweating, and skin that is cool, moist, pale, ashen, or flushed. After moving the individual to a cooler location, give cool water and observe for changes in condition. If the person refuses water, vomits, or begins to lose consciousness, call EMS.

- **Heat stroke.** Although the least common, heat stroke is the most serious of the three conditions. It can be life-threatening. The person loses the ability to sweat and cool the body because the temperature control system stops functioning. The body temperature can elevate dangerously, resulting in brain damage and death if the body is not cooled quickly. Signs of heat stroke include red skin that may either be dry or moist; changes in consciousness; rapid, weak pulse; and rapid, shallow breathing. Call EMS and move the person to a cooler location and apply cold towels or ice packs. Give small amounts of cool water every 15 minutes.

Hypothermia occurs when heat loss exceeds heat production; signs include shivering, numbness, glassy stare, impaired judgment, and loss of consciousness. Hypothermia could be a risk in some environmental situations, such as outdoor pools during cold weather or indoor pools with cooler water. Water can cool the body rapidly, and some participants might become chilled to the point of discomfort and shivering. Hypothermia can be a health hazard equally as dangerous as hyperthermia. Once again, dressing for the environment is helpful in prevention. Participants in the pool might consider full-length tights and long-sleeved jackets designed for aquatic exercise; wearing a hat can also help to reduce heat loss.

Injuries

The responsibility of an aquatic fitness professional is to offer a safe and effective class or training session. Even with effective program design, proper cueing, and maintaining a safe environment, accidents and injuries may happen.

Acute Injuries

An **acute injury** is defined as one with a sudden onset and short duration. An example of an acute injury is a participant who slips on the pool deck and sprains their ankle. The onset is sudden and the length of time to full recovery can vary, depending on the severity. Basic first aid for soft-tissue injuries, such as sprains or strains, focuses on reducing swelling and pain while aiding the healing process.

Various acronyms have been used to summarize first aid for acute injuries. For example, RICE indicates rest, ice, compression, and elevation. Another version (PRICE) includes protection of the injured area with a sling, brace, or other immobilization technique or device. Although applying ice has been a long-recommended treatment for acute injuries, some recent studies indicate that ice may not be the best option (Tseng et al. 2013). A newer acronym (MCE) reflects this change and encourages movement (when possible) rather than rest.

Move (exercise) safely when you can do so without pain.

Compress soft tissues (with items such as clothing or elastic bandage).

Elevate when possible.

Should the need arise to provide first aid to an acute injury, follow the protocol in your facility's EAP, including the completion of required injury or incident reports.

However, some injuries that could occur at the pool are more serious than bumps, bruises, strains, or sprains. Fractures, dislocations, and neck or head injuries require emergency help.

Chronic Injuries

Chronic injuries are injuries that have a long onset and long duration. Although there is a wide variety of chronic injuries, the primary underlying causes are very similar. Chronic injuries can result from repetitive movement, poor alignment (posture or a single joint), muscle imbalances, muscle fatigue, using equipment incorrectly or for too long, exercising on uneven surfaces, exercising in water that is too shallow or too deep, improper exercise progression (adding too much too soon), or not providing the support a body part may need (either muscular or external, such as shoes).

Chronic injuries related to extended participation in aquatic fitness classes include the following:

- **Anterior shin splints**: Characterized by pain in the front of the lower leg along the tibia.
- **Plantar fasciitis**: Characterized by pain on the bottom of the foot or around the heel.
- **Tendonitis** and **bursitis**: Characterized by pain in or around the affected tendon or bursa that can occur anywhere in the body, but most commonly in the shoulder, elbow, hip, knee, and Achilles tendon.
- **Back pain:** Characterized by pain in any portion of the back (cervical, thoracic, or lumbar).
- **Carpal tunnel syndrome**: Characterized by pain, numbness, or tingling in the wrist, hand, or fingers.

Although these chronic injuries are very different from one another, the prevention strategies that you can employ as an instructor have many commonalities:

- Maintain proper alignment—postural and joint alignment.
- Allow for breaks during exercise to reduce muscle fatigue and overuse. This is particularly important if you begin to see that the participants' form is breaking down or if you are using equipment. Encourage participants to rest if alignment becomes compromised due to fatigue.
- Provide exercises that promote muscle balance—the anterior and posterior as well as lateral muscles.
- If exercising on sloped surfaces, change footing to reduce overuse at one specific angle.
- Utilize proper water depth for the designated type of activities.
- Promote wearing aquatic footwear that provides appropriate support, mobility, and shock absorption.
- Plan a balanced exercise program that does not overemphasize one joint or one repetitive movement.
- Apply the concept of progressive overload to your class planning.
- Include exercises that reduce the risk of chronic injuries—mobility, strengthening, and muscle endurance exercises.

If the symptoms of chronic injury arise, you should recommend that the participant seek medical attention for proper diagnosis and treatment.

Electrical Shock

Electricity and pool water can be a deadly mix, resulting in injury from electrical shock. Many instructors use boom boxes, microphones, pace clocks, and other electrical devices to teach aquatic fitness programs. Keep electrical appliances away from the pool unless they are approved for poolside use and labeled as safe to use around water with a sticker from NSF International, Underwriters Laboratories, or a similar company. Electrical outlets, lights, or other electrical fixtures must be properly installed and grounded according to code. Do not take any chances with faulty or damaged outlets. Dry off before touching electrical appliances, cords, or outlets. Wear rubber-soled shoes to prevent tissue burns or disruption in electrical heart signals if shocked. Refer to the National Electrical Code published by the National Fire Protection Association for additional information and safety tips.

Another potential risk associated with electrical shock involves lightning. Swimming pools are connected to a much larger surface area through underground water pipes, gas lines, and electric and telephone wiring. According to the National Lightning Safety Institute (NLSI), lightning that strikes anywhere on this metallic network could result in electrical shocks elsewhere. Keep in mind the NLSI safety slogan: "If you see it, flee it. If you hear it, clear it."

The National Swimming Pool Foundation *Pool and Spa Operator Handbook* (NSPF 2014) follows the American Red Cross guidelines pertaining to outdoor swimming pools. Clear everyone from the outdoor pool and the surrounding deck area at the first sound of thunder or first sighting of lightning. When possible, move everyone inside and away from the water. Most organizations also recommend clearing indoor swimming pools during a thunderstorm. Some policies suggest clearing the indoor pool when lightning is within 8 miles (13 km) or when thunder is heard within 30 seconds of a lightning flash. Other policies recommend clearing indoor pools at the first sign of either thunder or lightning, regardless of the storm's distance. It is generally recommended to wait 30 minutes after the last observed lightning or thunder before resuming activities in or around the pool.

Ultimately, you must comply with state, county, and local safety codes. In an electrical storm, adhere to safety policies and know your role in the emergency action plans for all pools where you work or train.

Fitness Professional Health

Just as it is important for you to be proactive in the safety and health of your class participants, you must monitor your personal health. In addition to a personal exercise program, you will want to maintain a healthy eating plan, stay hydrated (especially when teaching your classes), manage your stress levels, and get adequate sleep. It is impossible to provide the highest level of performance without good health, and you must set a good example for your participants. The following are some specific health considerations that are of concern for aquatic fitness professionals.

Recreational Water Illness

A growing concern in the aquatic environment worthy of mention is **recreational water illness**. You need to be aware of the risk of illness caused by fecal contamination of pool water, improperly sanitized water, and poor indoor air quality in swimming venues. This risk affects you as well as your participants. Mild to life-threating gastrointestinal symptoms of diarrhea and vomiting can be caused by pathogens such as *Giardia*, *Cryptosporidium*, and *E. coli* that enter the water through fecal contamination. Additionally, skin and respiratory conditions can develop as a result of poor water or air quality.

The U.S. Centers for Disease Control and Prevention (CDC) is an excellent reference for the most up-to-date, evidence-based prevention and response protocols. You can access this information at www.CDC.gov.

Overtraining

More is not always better in terms of exercise. Inappropriate levels of training can lead to a potentially serious condition called **overtraining**. Overtraining occurs when someone trains too hard, too often, or too long. Many overtraining syndromes are a function of the rate of progression—in other words, doing too much too quickly. The body reacts negatively to excessive exercise, leading to decreased performance, extreme soreness, and fatigue.

Prevention includes varying program components, practicing periodization (see chapter 11 for more information), and incorporating appropriate rest. There is no accurate measurement for the onset of overtraining. Once symptoms occur, the most effective treatment is rest. The participant should cut back on frequency, duration, and intensity of exercise sessions. Overtraining can often be avoided by changing the type or mode of exercise.

The causes of overtraining are multifaceted, and include physiological as well as psychological factors. It is important to understand that overall health is made up of many different things; exercise is only one component. There is a fine line between abusive exercise (or exercise addiction) and healthy exercise. Healthy exercise leaves a person feeling refreshed, rejuvenated, mentally alert, and productive.

Anyone from athletes to fitness professionals to participants in exercise classes can be at risk for overtraining. Some participants become overenthusiastic and participate in too many classes or complete too many training sessions, resulting in symptoms of overtraining. Likewise, some instructors teach multiple classes in addition to continuing their own workout routines and experience symptoms of overtraining.

The following list includes some of the signs and symptoms of overtraining. If you or your participants exhibit any of the symptoms listed, consider re-evaluating current exercise behavior and programming.

Symptoms of overtraining include but are not limited to the following:

Extended muscle soreness
Elevated resting heart rate
Insomnia or chronic fatigue
Decreased appetite
Persistent flu-like symptoms
Increase in injuries
Loss of concentration
Feelings of depression or anxiety
Decrease in motivation
Decreased performance

Vocal Use and Abuse

Vocal injury is recognized as any alteration in your normal manner of speaking. Vocal abuse afflicts singers, actors, ministers, classroom teachers, and anyone who has an occupation that requires excessive talking. Fitness professionals are often at risk, and should learn the warning signs and symptoms of vocal abuse and take proper care of their voice to prevent injury. Voice problems in fitness professionals are often related to speaking over music (without a microphone), shouting during class (either out of necessity to be heard or a means of motivation), and working in settings with poor acoustics, as often experienced in pool environments.

A variety of early symptoms might indicate vocal misuse, abuse, or injury. The progression of symptoms is very gradual.

Symptoms or warning signs of vocal abuse include the following:

Harsh, gravelly, rough voice
Habitual use of lower pitch
Pain when swallowing
Feeling of something in your throat
Difficulty swallowing
Dry mouth
Clearing throat frequently (more than two times an hour)
Frequent hoarseness, voice loss
Pitch breaks, voice cracking
Reduced range for the singing voice
Voice not heard clearly (muffled)
Frequently asked if you have a cold or to repeat a sentence
Comments on how sexy your voice sounds
Vocal fatigue (worse at night)
Voice tired after talking a lot

If you think you might be experiencing a voice injury, seek a professional opinion from an otolaryngologist (ear, nose, and throat specialist). The earlier vocal abuse is detected, the easier it is to treat. You may also find it necessary to work with a speech therapist. However, prevention of voice injury is your first line of defense. To reduce your risk of vocal abuse, try the following:

- Keep your throat moist and your vocal cords lubricated. Drink plenty of water throughout the day.
- Avoid overuse. Limit the number of classes you teach and minimize the use of loud vocal cues. Include more body language and nonverbal cues.
- Maintain proper breathing.

- Use a microphone.
- If using music, keep it at a moderate level. Consider speaker placement and the location from which you project your voice.
- Check ventilation and chemical fume levels in the pool area.
- Project your voice with proper posture and body alignment. Maintain the neck in neutral alignment.
- Minimize background noise as much as possible.
- Limit talking when you have an upper respiratory infection. The vocal folds are already swollen and inflamed.
- Substitute a swallow for excessive throat clearing. Try to cough quietly to bring the vocal folds together gently.

Summary

Instructors and personal trainers working in and around the pool must maintain certification or training in cardiopulmonary resuscitation (CPR), including the use of an automated external defibrillator (AED). Additional training in general water safety and basic first aid is also highly recommended.

The foundation to safety, a primary consideration in and around the pool, is to understand foreseeable risks and reduce the risk through prevention strategies.

An emergency action plan (EAP) should be created for each type of emergency that requires different procedures. Although quick action is important, you first need to assess the situation to determine your course of action during an emergency.

A person in distress is still breathing but is having difficulty remaining on the surface of the water to breathe. If you are in the position to assist a distressed person, a reaching or throwing assist is the safest way to help.

The drowning process begins when the mouth and nose are covered with water and the person is prevented from taking a breath. Drowning can result in one of three outcomes, primarily depending on how quickly the drowning process is interrupted.

Sudden illness can occur to anyone, anywhere. You can provide care in many situations; however, you are not required to perform any skills beyond your level of training. Similarly, you may need to provide, or assist with, first aid of acute injuries that occur in or around the pool.

Prevention strategies for chronic injuries that you can employ as an aquatic fitness professional include programming and teaching techniques. However, if the symptoms of chronic injury arise, you should recommend that the participant seek medical attention for proper diagnosis and treatment.

Electricity creates a potential risk when working in and around the aquatic environment. Injury from electrical shock can result from the use of electrical equipment as well from lightning strikes.

Just as it is important for you to be proactive in the safety and health of your class participants, you must also monitor your personal health.

Review Questions

1. An ______________________________ is a preconceived plan of action designed to prepare staff to deal with emergencies in a coordinated effort.

   a. assessment
   b. evacuation action plan
   c. emergency action plan
   d. risk strategy

2. For a person who ____________________, check the scene and approach if it is safe.

   a. appears to be unresponsive
   b. is responsive
   c. both A and B
   d. None of these.

3. The drowning process continues until the person gets a breath, either spontaneously or through rescue breathing.

   a. True
   b. False

4. You should always remove a victim from the water before administering CPR.

   a. True
   b. False

5. ________________ occurs when blood flow to the heart is blocked, causing damage to part of the heart muscle.

   a. A stroke
   b. Cardiac arrest
   c. A seizure
   d. A heart attack

6. List three tips to avoid vocal abuse and injury.

7. An AED is safe to use if the person has been removed completely from the water and is not lying in a puddle.

   a. True
   b. False

8. An acute injury is defined as an injury with a long onset and long duration.
   a. True
   b. False
9. Define the American Heart Association's FAST acronym, which is used to quickly determine whether someone has experienced a stroke.
10. ________________is a condition characterized by an abnormally low level of blood sugar (glucose).
   a. Hypothermia
   b. Hypoglycemia
   c. Hyperglycemia
   d. Hyperthermia

See appendix D for answers to review questions.

References and Resources

American Diabetes Association. www.diabetes.org.

American Diabetes Association. n.d. Hypoglycemia (low blood glucose). Accessed June 27, 2016. www.diabetes.org/living-with-diabetes/treatment-and-care/blood-glucose-control/hypoglycemia-low-blood.html.

American Heart Association. www.americanheart.org.

American Heart Association. 2014. Chain of survival. www.heart.org/HEARTORG/CPRAndECC/WhatisCPR/EC%C2%ACCIntro/Chain-of-Survival_UCM_307516_Article.jsp#.V3wTrvkrJaQ.

American Lifeguard Association. www.americanlifeguard.com.

American Red Cross. www.redcross.org.

American Red Cross. n.d. Heat Wave Safety. Accessed June 30, 2016. www.redcross.org/get-help/prepare-for-emergencies/types-of-emergencies/heat-wave-safety#/About.

———. 2006. *First Aid/CPR/AED for schools and the community, participant's manual.* 3rd edition. Yardley, PA: StayWell.

———. 2012. *Lifeguarding manual.* Yardley, PA: StayWell.

———. 2016. Learn how to stay safe during a heat wave. www.redcross.org/images/MEDIA_CustomProductCatalog/m4340158_HeatWave.pdf.

American Stroke Association. www.strokeassociation.com.

Arnheim, D. 1989. *Modern principles of athletic training.* 7th edition. St. Louis: Times Mirror/Mosby College.

Cailliet, R. 1983. *Knee pain and disability.* 2nd edition. Philadelphia: F.A. Davis.

Ekstrom, M. 1987. Lower leg pain can stop athletes in their tracks. *The First Aider 56*(5):1.

Howley, E.T., and D.L. Thompson. 2012. *Fitness professional's handbook.* 6th edition. Champaign, IL: Human Kinetics.

Mayo Clinic. 2016. Plantar fasciitis. www.mayoclinic.org/diseases-conditions/plantar-fasciitis/home/ovc-20268392. Accessed June 11, 2017.

Mayo Clinic. 2015. Diseases and conditions—Hypoglycemia. www.mayoclinic.org/diseases-conditions/hypoglycemia/basics/definition/CON-20021103.

Nachemson, A.L. 1985. Advances in low back pain. *Clinical Orthopedics and Related Research* 200:266-278.

National Lightning Safety Institute. n.d. Lightning and aquatics safety: A cautionary perspective for indoor pools. Accessed July 14, 2016. www.lightningsafety.com/nlsi_pls/indoor_pools.html.

National Swimming Pool Foundation. www.nspf.org.

National Swimming Pool Foundation. 2014. *Pool and spa operator handbook*. Colorado Springs: Author.

Pia, F. 1971. *On drowning*. 2nd edition. Larchmont, NY: Water Safety Films.

———. 1974. Observations on the drowning of nonswimmers. Warsaw, IN: The YMCA Society of North America.

Prentice, W. 2001. *Rehabilitation techniques in sport medicine with PowerWeb: Health and human performance*. 3rd edition. New York: McGraw-Hill.

Tseng, C.-Y., J.-P. Lee, Y.-S. Tsai, S.-D. Lee, C.-L. Kao, T.-C. Liu, C.-H. Lai, M.B. Harris, and C.-H. Kuo. 2013. Topical cooling (icing) delays recovery from eccentric exercise–induced muscle damage. *Journal of Strength and Conditioning Research* 27(5):1354-1361.

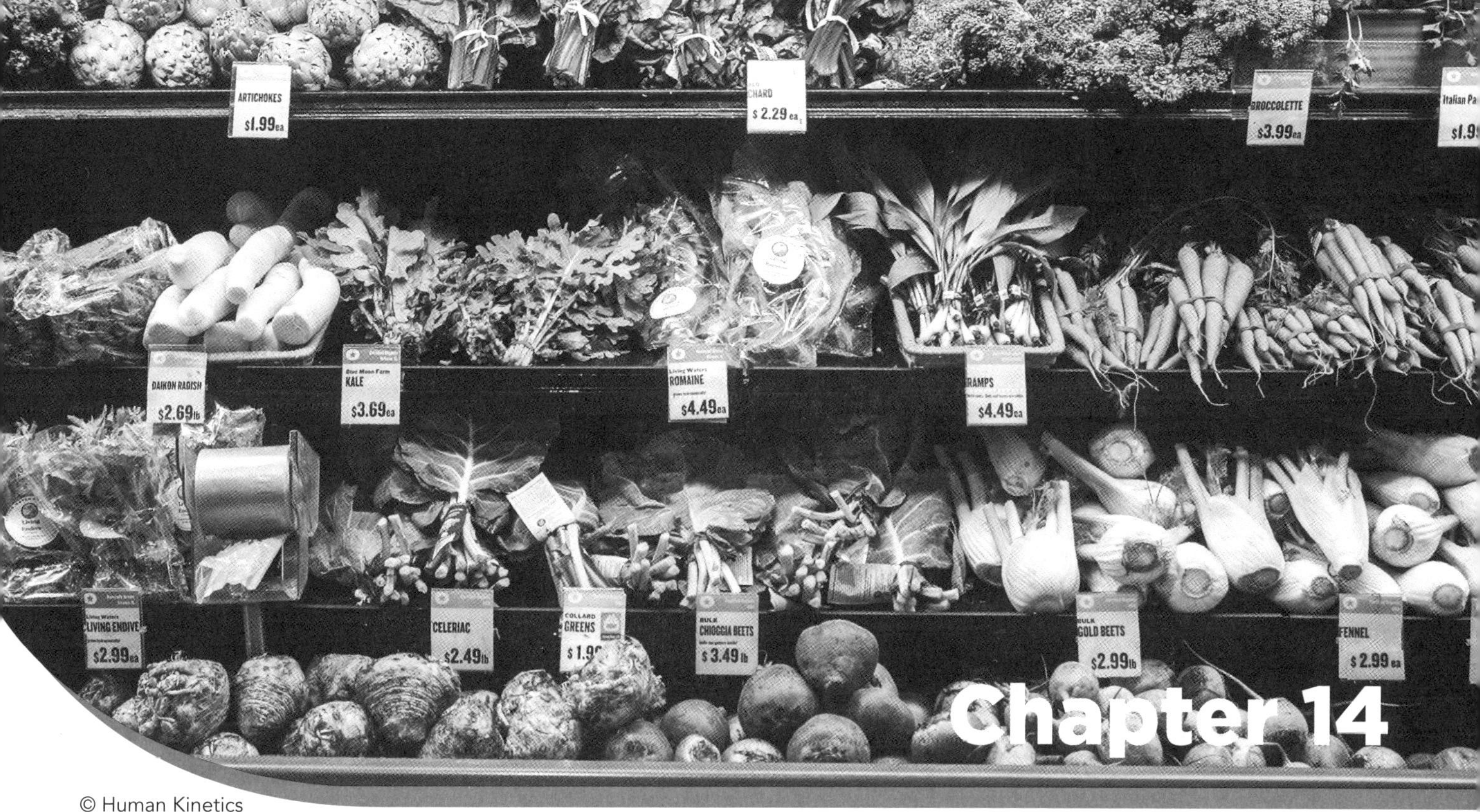

Chapter 14

Basic Nutrition and Weight Management

Introduction

Nutrition and exercise go hand in hand. You must have a basic understanding of nutrition in order to guide your aquatic exercise participants to healthier eating habits. However, it is important to stress that, as a fitness professional, you are not trained as a registered dietitian and therefore are not qualified to write or disseminate specific dietary information (such as a written diet plan) outside of what is provided by the United States Department of Agriculture (USDA) and the Department of Health and Human Services (HHS). Your limitation with dietary advice is necessary because every participant has their own unique dietary needs that can positively and negatively affect their health.

Americans spend billions of dollars annually on weight control. Weight management resources and products represent a never-ending supply of opinions, so it is important to be able to sort fact from fiction when helping a participant understand nutrition information. Since weight loss is a goal for many fitness enthusiasts, basic nutrition knowledge and an understanding of behavior modification techniques will allow you to assist participants in altering their eating habits to maximize progress. Your job is to guide clients and participants in the right direction. It may be that *Dietary Guidelines for Americans* are enough to help your participants reach their goals, or you may need to assist them in finding a licensed professional who can customize a food plan to enhance their health and well-being.

Key Chapter Concepts

- Understand the six essential nutrients required for normal growth and function and differentiate between macronutrients and micronutrients.
- Define simple and complex carbohydrates, soluble and insoluble fiber, essential and nonessential amino acids, complete and incomplete proteins, water-soluble and fat-soluble vitamins, and unsaturated, saturated, and trans fat.
- Explain how carbohydrates, fat, and protein work together to provide energy for the body's needs, including resting metabolic rate (RMR), activities of daily living, and exercise.
- Recognize how the information provided on packaged food nutrition labels is one way to better understand food quality and make healthier choices.
- Learn how the *Dietary Guidelines for Americans* offer science-based advice to promote health and reduce risk for major chronic diseases through diet and physical activity.
- Explain the three ways that the body burns calories—thermic effect of food, thermic effect of physical activity, and resting metabolic rate—and how they can be manipulated to assist in weight management.
- Understand the signs of common eating disorders so that you can identify participants who may be at risk of developing these conditions and provide professional referrals as needed.

General Nutrition

Nutrition is the process of fueling the body with food to provide **nutrients** for the growth, function, and rebuilding or replacement of tissue. Proper nutrition can help your participants achieve many goals by supplying the body with the nutrients needed to grow, perform, and recover. Food provides the energy that the body needs to function every day, and these needs increase with physical activity. For the majority of your participants, you will find that eating in accordance with the *U.S. 2015-2020 Dietary Guidelines for Americans* and USDA ChooseMyPlate.gov guidelines will provide an adequate diet for healthy people.

Information on caloric consumption (calories in) and caloric expenditure (calories out) often interchange the word *calorie* with the term *kilocalorie*. Within this chapter, we refer to the energy derived from food as a calorie. A **calorie** is the amount of heat energy required to raise the temperature of 1 gram of water 1 degree Celsius. Although consuming 1 calorie will not change your weight, consuming an abundance of calories in your food or using an excessive number of calories during exercise will change your weight.

Nutrients

The human body requires six nutrients to ensure normal growth and function. These nutrients are classified as either macronutrients or micronutrients.

Macronutrients are needed in large amounts every day while **micronutrients** are needed in smaller amounts every day. Macronutrients that contain calories and supply the body with energy include carbohydrates, protein, and fat. They each serve different purposes in the functioning of the body, as outlined in table 14.1. Water is the only noncaloric macronutrient. We need water in large amounts every day, but water does not supply the body with any fuel in the form of calories. The micronutrients, vitamins and minerals, are also free of calories but vital to disease prevention and overall well-being.

What follows is a simplified explanation of these six essential nutrients.

Carbohydrates. **Carbohydrates** are the primary source of energy for the skeletal muscles and the exclusive source of energy for the brain and nervous system. It is recommended that adults (19 years and older) obtain 45 to 65 percent of daily calories from carbohydrates (U.S. Department of Health and Human Services and U.S. Department of Agriculture 2015). Both healthy and unhealthy carbohydrate-rich foods exist. Carbohydrate-rich foods that are high in vitamins, minerals, and fiber provide greater nutritional value to your diet.

Carbohydrates are classified into two specific subgroups: simple and complex. Regardless of the type of carbohydrate, the ultimate breakdown is **glucose**, which is used either immediately for energy, stored in the liver and muscles as **glycogen**, or (if consumed in excess) stored as fat in the adipose tissue.

Simple carbohydrates are easily digested and absorbed into the blood stream from the digestive tract. Because they are easily broken down and digested, simple sugars provide a rapid source of energy for the muscles, brain, and nervous system. Simple carbohydrates are sugars. Sugar occurs naturally in nutrient-rich foods such as fruit and milk; other foods (e.g., cookies, cakes, and non-diet carbonated beverages) have added sugars. **Complex carbohydrates** involve a more complicated digestive process and provide a steady stream of

Healthy Carbohydrate Choices

- Beans
- Legumes
- Fruits
- Vegetables
- Whole grains (unprocessed or minimally processed)

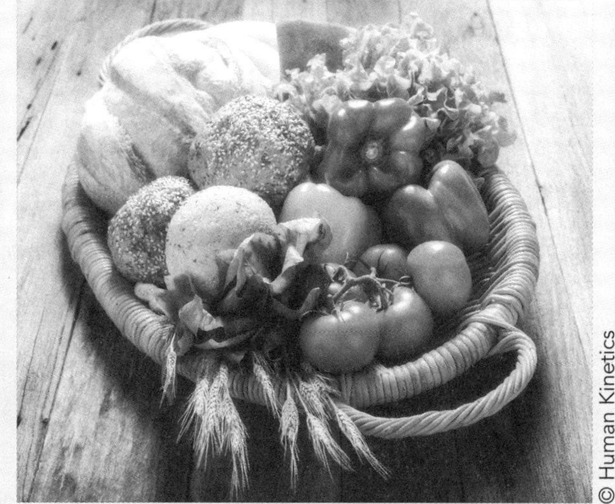

© Human Kinetics

Whole grain versions of baked goods can be part of a healthy diet.

glucose in the blood. Complex carbohydrates include vegetables and whole-grain products, such as brown rice and wheat bread, that contain **dietary fiber** and glucose.

There are two forms of dietary fiber. **Soluble fiber** dissolves in water to form a gel while **insoluble fiber** does not break down. Soluble fiber is found in barley, legumes, oats, and some fruits and vegetables. It assists in lowering blood cholesterol levels and slows the process of digestion, allowing for greater absorption of nutrients. Insoluble fiber sources include some fruits, seeds, some vegetables, and whole grains. These fibers provide roughage, for example, the string of celery, the skins of corn kernels and legumes, and the outer layer of brown rice. Insoluble fibers soften stools, regulate bowel movements, and speed transit of fecal matter through the colon; improve the body's handling of glucose (especially helpful for people with diabetes); and reduce the risk of diverticulosis, cancer, and appendicitis.

Proteins. **Proteins** are considered the building blocks of the human body. Every cell in the body contains protein. Proteins are long chains of **amino acids** that play a role in the growth, repair, and maintenance of all bodily tissues. Eighty amino acids occur in nature, but only 20 are found in the human body. The amino acids that are synthesized in the body are considered **nonessential amino acids**; those that must be consumed in the diet because the body cannot make them are known as **essential amino acids**.

If a protein-rich food contains all nine essential amino acids in the ratio required by the body, the protein is considered **complete**. Complete proteins usually come from animal food products, but some plant products contain all 9 essential amino acids, such as soy, quinoa, and buckwheat. If a protein is lacking in one or more essential amino acids, it is considered **incomplete**. Even though most plant proteins are incomplete proteins, it is possible to consume complete proteins by combining certain foods. For example, legumes are high in the amino acid lysine but lack methionine. Whole grains are extremely high in methionine but lack lysine. If a meal is composed of whole-grain bread and natural peanut butter (legume), then all essential amino acids are consumed.

The recommended dietary allowance (RDA) for men and women is 0.8 grams of

Healthy Protein Choices

- Plant-based proteins (nuts, seeds, beans, lentils, soy, quinoa, buckwheat)
- Fish and seafood
- Poultry (including eggs)
- Dairy products (low-fat milk, cheese, cottage cheese, yogurt)

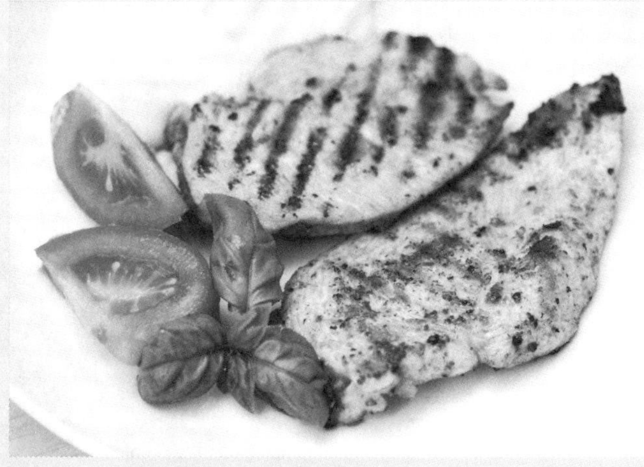

Protein is an important part of everyone's diet and additional protein may be necessary for those who are physically active.

high-quality protein per kilogram of body weight per day. To determine the amount of protein needed in a diet, multiply a person's weight in kilograms by 0.8.

$$\text{Weight in pounds} \div 2.2 = \text{Weight in kilograms}$$

$$\text{Weight in kilograms} \times 0.8 = \text{Estimated dietary protein need}$$

Proteins contain 4 calories per gram. It is recommended that 10 to 35 percent of our daily calories come from low-fat protein sources such as lean meats, beans, vegetables, and whole grains (U.S. Department of Health and Human Services and U.S. Department of Agriculture 2015). Keep in mind that as we become more physically active, we may need to consume a slightly greater amount of protein because the amino acids help repair any damage done to the muscle cells.

Fat. **Fat** is an energy-rich macronutrient with 9 calories in each gram. The role of fat in the diet is to provide energy, protect vital organs, insulate, and transport fat-soluble vitamins. Fats store easily and are a good source of energy for long-duration, low-intensity exercise. Fats contribute to the taste, texture, and smell of foods that stimulate appetite and assist in providing satiety (feeling full). It is recommended that fats make up 20 to 35 percent of our daily calories (U.S. Department of Health and Human Services and U.S. Department of Agriculture 2015).

Two main types of dietary fat naturally occur: saturated and unsaturated. **Saturated fats** are derived mostly from animal sources and contain an excess of cholesterol, which can contribute to cardiovascular diseases. Saturated fat intake should remain under 10 percent of total calories; the American Heart Association (2016) recommends making dietary choices that limit saturated fats to 5 to 6 percent.

Unsaturated fats (monounsaturated and **polyunsaturated)** do not increase the risk of heart disease. Examples include olive oil, canola oil, most types of nuts, and fatty fish oils, such as salmon, herring, and tuna. Unsaturated fats may help raise the healthy HDL cholesterol in our bodies. All fatty acids are a combination of saturated and unsaturated

Healthy Fat Choices

Monounsaturated fats (avocados, olives, nuts and natural nut butters from almonds, peanuts, pecans, cashews, hazelnuts, and macadamia nuts)

Polyunsaturated fats (walnuts, seeds [sunflower, sesame, pumpkin], flaxseed, fatty fish [salmon, tuna, mackerel, herring, trout, sardines], soymilk, and tofu)

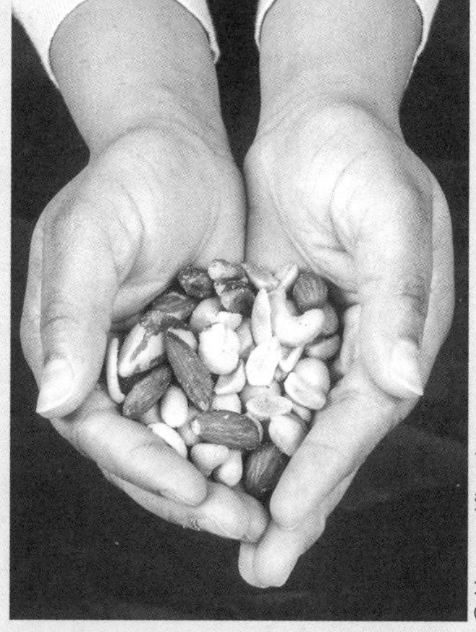

Everyone needs fat in their daily diet, preferably derived from healthy sources.

fats. Foods are classified by the type of fat that is most dominant. The less saturated the fat, the more liquid it is at room temperature. Conversely, the more saturated a fat, the more solid it is at room temperature.

Trans fats, hydrogenated unsaturated fats with physical properties similar to saturated fats, are typically found in man-made food products. They were developed to increase the food's shelf life as well as improve texture and mimic characteristics of frying. They are found mainly in chips, crackers, cookies, cakes, pies, and frozen processed foods. Trans fats provide a much greater risk to heart health because they raise LDL (unhealthy cholesterol) levels while also lowering HDL.

Water. **Water** is the only non-caloric macronutrient, but it plays an irreplaceable role in the body. It is the major element for all of the workings of the human body and the single most important nutrient during exercise. A decrease in water leads to dehydration, which can cause fatigue, muscle breakdown, and even death in extreme situations. As the demand for water increases through exercise, heat, and general exertion, the consumption of water must also increase.

Relationship Between Cardiovascular Disease, Fat, and Cholesterol

The risk for a myocardial infarction (heart attack), atherosclerosis (process in which plaque builds up on artery walls), and heart disease increases as cholesterol reaches unhealthy levels. A total cholesterol level less than 200 milligrams per deciliter is recommended by most health care organizations.

Total cholesterol levels are determined based on a ratio of LDL, HDL, and triglycerides.

- **Low-density lipoproteins (LDL)** can cause buildup of plaque on the walls of arteries. The more LDL in the blood, the greater the risk of heart disease.
- **High-density lipoproteins (HDL)** help the body get rid of LDL cholesterol in the blood. The higher the level of HDL cholesterol, the better. If your levels of HDL are low, your risk of heart disease increases.
- **Triglycerides** are another type of fat carried in the blood. They represent the major form of fat stored by the body. They are produced by the body and also derived from the food we eat. Excess calories are converted into triglycerides and stored in fat cells throughout the body. High levels of triglycerides in the blood increase the risk of heart disease.

Cholesterol and triglyceride levels can be linked to both heredity (family history) and behavior (diet, exercise, weight management). Foods high in saturated fat or cholesterol can increase your LDL and triglycerides. Losing weight, participating in regular physical activity, increasing fiber and water, and substituting unsaturated fats for saturated fats can reduce triglycerides and LDL and increase HDL.

Omega-3 fatty acids found in certain cold-water fish have also been associated with a decreased risk of cardiovascular disease. Omega-3 fatty acids seem to help control blood platelets so they don't form as many clots. Fish rich in omega-3 fatty acids include European anchovy, blue fish, Atlantic and Pacific herring, mackerel, mullet, sablefish, salmon, Atlantic and common sturgeon, lake trout, white albacore or bluefin tuna, and lake whitefish.

Table 14.1 Basic Functions of Carbohydrates, Protein, and Fat

Carbohydrate	
4 calories per gram	Energy and muscular fuel Cholesterol and fat control Digestion assistance Nutrient and water absorption
Protein	
4 calories per gram	Energy source (if carbohydrates are depleted) Delivery of essential amino acids Essential for developing new tissue Essential for maintaining existing tissue Substances for manufacturing enzymes, antibodies, and hormones Fluid balance Carriers of substances in the blood
Fat	
9 calories per gram	Delivery of fat-soluble vitamins Delivery of essential fatty acids Energy and muscular fuel for low-intensity activities Satiety control Substance in many hormones

Water is in every cell and tissue of the body and is the primary carrier for all nutrients. It is responsible for the removal of metabolic by-products and wastes in the body. Water works with the liver to metabolize fat efficiently through cardiorespiratory training and works directly in the muscle to assist muscular contraction for strength gains.

A general fluid intake guideline for the average exercise enthusiast is five to eight 8-ounce (240 ml) glasses per day, adjusting the intake if thirst arises or if in hot and humid conditions. The goal is to keep a consistent level of fluids coming into the system to prevent thirst. When the body lacks water, it sends out the feeling of thirst; if thirst is not addressed, the next alarm is hunger. You should replenish whenever you are thirsty, but note that thirst is not a reliable indicator of when to drink. When the sensation of thirst ensues, you are already partially dehydrated. The thirst response is further reduced during exercise in water. Studies show that people exercising in water do not elicit strong thirst responses and thus are not driven to hydrate while performing aquatic exercise (Sagawa et al. 1992). Promoting water breaks during your class is highly recommended; even though your participants may not feel thirsty, they should be encouraged to drink water during aquatic exercise.

The American College of Sports Medicine 2007 Position Stand on Exercise and Fluid Replacement emphasizes individualized hydration considerations and provides details on hydration before, during, and after exercise. The official ACSM pronouncement was published in the February 2007 issue of *Medicine and Science in Sports and Exercise*, and includes the following key points:

- Variability in fluid requirements during exercise will exist among individuals and different physical activities, as well as under different environmental conditions. The sweat rate and loss of fluids will vary based on individual characteristics, including but not limited to body weight, genetic predisposition, and metabolism.
- Fluid replacement before exercise is for the purpose of initiating physical activity at normal levels of water and electrolytes. Fluid should be consumed several hours before exercise, which enables absorption and allows urine output to return to normal levels.
- During exercise, fluid replacement prevents excessive dehydration (>2% reduction from baseline body weight) and helps avoid excessive changes in electrolyte balance, which may compromise performance. The rate of consumption and the amount of fluids will depend on the individual and the activity, including opportunities to drink. Most people will benefit from drinking water during a 60-minute exercise class; however, participants in longer duration exercise programs or athletes may benefit from beverages containing electrolytes and carbohydrates.

- Fluid replacement after exercise is needed to fully replace any fluid and electrolyte losses. Regular meals and beverages will restore normal hydration levels, when time permits. The speed at which rehydration is needed and the level of electrolyte loss will determine if a more specific rehydration program is necessary.

Caffeine, alcohol, and certain medications contribute to dehydration. These should be kept to a minimum, but extra amounts of water help to counterbalance the effects if they are consumed. Note that the constant use of your voice can contribute to dehydration. Be sure to drink before, during, and after a class and to maintain adequate amounts of hydration throughout the day. For those teaching outside, the hydration process should begin well before the class and continue throughout the class to maintain an adequate hydration level.

Micronutrients are nutrients needed in small amounts every day. Vitamins and minerals are the two classes of micronutrients. Thirteen known vitamins and 17 minerals are found in the human body. This section focuses on the major vitamins and minerals that are important in the metabolism of energy in the body. Continuing education courses may provide additional information on vitamins and minerals. However, always make sure you stay within your scope of practice when discussing nutrition issues with participants and refer them to registered dietitians when appropriate.

Vitamins. **Vitamins** are the body's regulators that perform every internal action necessary for maintaining life. They are non-caloric, organic nutrients that can be classified as water soluble or fat soluble. Water-soluble vitamins are generally absorbed directly into the bloodstream. Because they are not stored in the tissues to any great degree, excesses are excreted in the urine, reducing the potential for toxicity. Fat-soluble vitamins follow the same absorption pathway as fat, and are stored in the body's fatty tissues. Excess amounts can lead to toxic concentrations accompanied by detrimental effects.

Fat-Soluble Vitamins

The fat-soluble vitamins include vitamins A, D, E, and K. Although each plays various roles in the body, the main functions are listed as follows.

Vitamin A: Maintains the skin and mucous membrane and plays an integral part in the health of the eyes.

Vitamin D: Assists the body in the absorption of calcium for optimal bone health.

Vitamin E: Assists the body in tissue repair, and is an **antioxidant** to terminate the chain reaction of free radicals in the body.

Vitamin K: Plays an integral part in blood clotting.

Water-Soluble Vitamins

The water-soluble vitamins include the vitamin B complexes and vitamin C.

Vitamin B: Maintains energy metabolism of all macronutrients.

Vitamin C: A primary antioxidant, involved in most bodily functions; assists in cartilage and tendon health and in immune function.

Minerals. **Minerals** are naturally occurring substances that work as regulators of body processes and are components of various body cells (e.g., iron in red blood cells) or are components of various structures (e.g., bone). As is true of vitamins, oversupplementation of minerals can upset the normal balance of body processes. Some of the minerals the human body needs to function properly include the following:

Iron: Involved in the manufacturing of hemoglobin, a major component of red blood cells, it also assists in the delivery of oxygen to the cells and protects the body from infection. This mineral is the most common deficiency in physically active women.

Magnesium: Involved in every facet of the internal system of the body, such as protein synthesis, energy production, nervous function, and muscle contraction. A deficiency has been linked to muscle cramping.

Selenium: An antioxidant that helps protect cells against damage by free oxygen particles and assists in normal heart function.

Calcium: Helps to maintain strong bones and teeth, and has been shown to assist the body in combating high blood pressure and certain forms of cancer. This mineral is also very important in muscle contraction.

Potassium: A major component in maintaining proper heart rhythm, muscle contraction, and regulation of blood pressure. From a fitness standpoint, a deficiency of potassium has been linked to muscle cramping and fluid imbalance.

Sodium: Assists in fluid balance and muscle contraction, and is essential to replenish after long, strenuous exercise bouts, especially in humid or high-temperature environments.

The recommended amounts for each vitamin and mineral are listed at the USDA National Agricultural Library website at www.nal.usda.gov.

Alcohol. We do not consider **alcohol** as a nutrient, but it does contain calories. Alcohol has 7 calories per gram (more than protein or carbohydrates), but these calories provide no benefit as an energy substrate. Alcohol contributes to dehydration, can decrease performance, and lengthens the time needed for recovery. It directly interferes with the body's absorption, storage, and use of other nutrients.

Putting It All Together

Macro- and micronutrients are absorbed into the body through the digestive process, and are responsible for all human function. The process begins the moment we put foods or liquids into our mouths. Digestive enzymes begin to break the food into components, which are distributed throughout the body. The absorption of nutrients gives us the energy to exercise and the strength to maintain healthy bodies free from illness and disease. Our food choices determine the nutrients that our bodies have available for recovery, growth, and energy sources. Every nutrition choice that we make has consequences, some positive and some negative. As a society, we have been programmed to eat for comfort, for social occasions, or simply for fun. We need to train ourselves to eat for nutrition so that our bodies will function and perform at optimal levels.

Carbohydrates, fat, and protein all work together to provide the energy that our bodies use on a daily basis. The calories needed to maintain the processes of life constitute **resting metabolic rate (RMR)**, which in a clinical setting is referred to as **basal metabolic rate**. Activities of daily life, as well as exercise, require additional calories that are derived from a mixture of these three macronutrients. We are continually using carbohydrates, fat, and protein as fuel regardless of the activity we are performing. Our metabolism functions on a mixture of the fuels, although one is usually dominant.

How many calories people should consume in a day depends on many factors, including their height, weight, age, gender, body composition, and activity level. In general, a person who wants to lose weight must produce a negative energy balance through a combination of exercise (burning of calories) and reducing the amount of food calories consumed. However, it is important not to restrict calorie intake below one's RMR. Doing so causes fatigue and decreases performance. This also makes it harder to lose weight. In fact, weight gain may occur because the body recognizes that it is not being fueled, so it begins to conserve energy. Fitness professionals can provide participants with basic nutrition information and encourage them to make healthier nutrition choices, but they should leave creating a specific caloric game plan to licensed professionals.

Food Nutrition Labels

Food quality should be one of the primary components of healthy nutrition. Encourage your participants to look for nutritionally fulfilling foods that promote good physical health and optimal performance, and you should do the same. Nutritionally, 200 calories of fries are not equal to 200 calories of sautéed vegetables and fish. You might be providing your body with its caloric energy needs, but the lack of nutrients makes the body desire more food until its nutrition needs are met. Once your body's needs are fulfilled with high-quality foods, it can function properly.

Using the information provided on packaged food nutrition labels is one way to better understand food quality and make healthier choices. The American Heart Association (AHA) (2014) provides the following tips for understanding food nutrition labels:

- The serving information will tell you the size of a single serving and how many servings are in the package.
- Pay attention to calories per serving. If you consume more than one serving, the calories and nutrients increase accordingly.
- Notice the amounts of specific nutrients of the food. The AHA recommends limiting certain nutrients (e.g., saturated fat, trans fat, sodium) while making sure to get adequate amounts of others (e.g., dietary fiber, protein, calcium, iron).
- The % Daily Value explains the percentage of each nutrient in a single serving as it relates to the daily recommendations.
- Keep in mind that the % Daily Value is based on a diet of 2,000 calories per day, so this may need to be adjusted based on your required caloric intake.
- If a food contains "0 g" of trans fat, but includes "partially hydrogenated oil" in the ingredient list, it does contain trans fat—but less than .5 grams per serving. However, this adds up if you eat more than one serving or multiple foods that have a similar trans fat content.

In May of 2016, the Food and Drug Administration (FDA) announced a new Nutrition Facts label for packaged foods, which is intended to assist consumers in making better-informed food choices (see figure 14.4). This label reflects new scientific information, including the link between diet and chronic conditions. The compliance date is 2018 for food manufacturers and 2019 for smaller companies. Read more information on the new food labels at the FDA website, www.fda.gov.

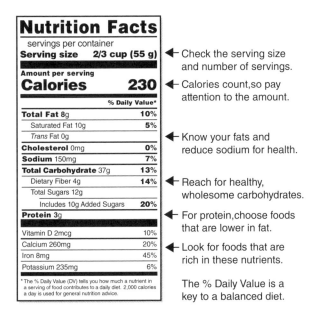

Figure 14.4 New Nutrition Facts food label.

Dietary Guidelines for Americans

The ***Dietary Guidelines for Americans*** offer science-based advice for promoting health and reducing risk for major chronic diseases through diet and physical activity. Specific diseases linked to poor diet and physical inactivity include, but are not limited to, cardiovascular disease, type 2 diabetes, hypertension, osteoporosis, and certain cancers. Additionally, poor diet and physical inactivity represent the most important factors contributing to the increase in overweight and obese individuals in the United States.

The *Dietary Guidelines for Americans* were first published in 1980 and are reviewed and updated every five years. Published by the Department of Health and Human Services (HHS) and the USDA, the 2015 guidelines provide five general recommendations to encourage overall healthy eating.

1. Follow a healthy eating pattern all your life. This includes both food and beverage choices. The chosen eating pattern should include the number of calories that will help you maintain or achieve a healthy body composition, support nutrient adequacy, and reduce the risk of chronic disease.
2. Focus on variety, nutrient density, and amount. All food groups should be included in the daily diet, with an emphasis on foods that contain more nutrients and fewer calories (nutrient-dense foods). For example, fruits and vegetables contain more vitamins and minerals at a lower caloric value than processed toaster pastries.
3. Limit calories from added sugars and saturated fats and reduce sodium intake. Sugar, saturated fats, and sodium should be limited to help ensure healthy eating patterns. They do not need to be removed entirely because small amounts do have a place in a healthy eating plan.
4. Shift to healthier food and beverage choices. Again, choose nutrient-dense foods and beverages that are lower in calories in place of less healthy choices. Americans often consume excess sugar calories in soft drinks.
5. Support healthy eating patterns in all aspects of the community. Community design and philosophy can influence healthy eating and active living from school lunch programs to worksite nutrition polices.

The *Dietary Guidelines for Americans* (2015) contain additional recommendations for specific populations. The entire publication can be downloaded free of charge at www.health.gov/DietaryGuidelines.

Another excellent tool to help your participants can be found at www.choosemyplate.gov. The USDA introduced **MyPlate** in 2011 to replace the previously standard food pyramid, providing a more individualized approach to an overall food guidance system for improving diet and lifestyle. MyPlate represents the recommended portions of foods from each food group and focuses on making smart food choices in every food group, every day. It incorporates recommendations from the *Dietary Guidelines for Americans* and uses an interactive format to assist people in determining their personal daily calorie needs based on age, gender, and physical activity. ChooseMyPlate.gov offers a variety of other features that make this food guidance system accessible to all ages. The online SuperTracker can help people plan, analyze, and track diet and physical activity. The **body mass index (BMI)** calculator has options, both for adults and for children and teens, for calculating current weight status.

Weight Management

Many of your class participants or personal training clients will have some type of weight loss goals in mind. You must be able to provide quality information to your participants while staying within your scope of practice. Both overweight and obesity are conditions related to a higher body weight. Body mass index, or BMI, is commonly used to classify these disorders and further define the level of severity (CDC 2008, ACSM 2018).BMI equal to or greater than 25 is considered overweight, equal to or greater than 30 is considered obese, and equal to or greater than 40 is extremely obese. BMI works as a weight-estimating tool for the majority of people; however, it does not take into account lean body mass, and therefore may not be appropriate for athletes. More information on BMI can be found in chapter 12.

The body burns calories in three ways. The **thermic effect of food (TEF)**, which accounts for calories that are burned during digestion; the **thermic effect of physical activity (TEPA)**, which accounts for calories that are burned during physical activity or exercise; and the resting metabolic rate (RMR), which accounts for calories burned to sustain everyday bodily functions such as heartbeat, respiration, and thermal regulation. Physical activity might help to maintain RMR during weight loss, but it is unsure whether exercise training can increase the RMR if muscle mass is not increased. However, metabolic demands can increase during and after exercise. These increases result in greater caloric expenditure both during and following exercise and are dependent primarily on the exercises intensity and duration.

Thermic Effect of Food (TEF)

- Digestion increases oxygen consumption after a meal.
- Can account for 10 to 15 percent of our total energy expenditure.
- The energy cost of meals is highest for protein, lower for carbohydrates, and lowest for fat.

Thermic Effect of Physical Activity (TEPA)

- Exercise is the most variable side of energy expenditure equation (5-40 % of daily energy expenditure).
- Exercise might decrease appetite slightly.
- Dieting appears to reduce lean tissue as well as fat tissue, however, exercise can assist in limiting the amount of lean tissue loss.

Resting (Basal) Metabolic Rate (RMR)

- Energy is expended by the body to sustain living processes.
- Represents 60 to 75 percent of total energy expenditure in the average sedentary person.
- Proportional to fat-free mass (muscle, bone, organs).

These methods of caloric expenditure (burning calories) can be manipulated to assist in weight management. If a person increases energy intake without adjusting energy expenditure, weight is gained. On the other hand, if a person decreases energy intake and increases energy expenditure, weight is lost.

3,000-calorie intake – 3,000-calorie expenditure = Energy balance

3,000-calorie intake – 2,000-calorie expenditure = Energy imbalance (weight gain)

2,000-calorie intake – 3,000-calorie expenditure = Energy imbalance (weight loss)

Finding the appropriate energy balance equation is not an easy task. It often takes time and multiple manipulations to achieve the goals that your participants seek. Food logs that include activity trackers can assist participants in finding the perfect mix of caloric intake and caloric expenditure (physical activity). You can recommend that your participants use the SuperTracker at ChooseMyPlate.gov or refer them to a registered dietitian for assistance with tracking caloric intake and expenditure.

When someone goes on a weight loss diet without exercise, the body uses more protein for energy than with diets that include exercise. The protein may be broken down from muscle cells. When the person goes off the diet-only weight loss plan and regains body weight, the regained weight is typically from a greater percentage of fat than muscle. Dieting plus exercise protects muscle tissue because the muscle is continually used during exercise. Eating an appropriate amount of carbohydrates, protein, and fat will allow the body to burn calories during exercise and use appropriate nutrients for recovery, resulting in weight loss.

Research clearly indicates that you can effectively burn calories in a vertical aquatic workout (Colado et al. 2009; Gaspard et al. 1995; Nagle et al. 2003). It appears that the water's resistance makes up for the reduced workload associated with reduced weight bearing in the buoyant environment. Several variables affect caloric expenditure during vertical water exercise:

- Water depth, which affects weight bearing, control of movement, and the amount of resistance
- Speed of movement, which affects the amount of drag and resistance
- Amount of force applied against the water's resistance (The harder you work, the more calories you burn.)

Aquatic Exercise and Weight Loss

Although some aquatic studies have not resulted in weight loss, those using proper frequency, duration, intensity, and study length have clearly indicated weight loss with aquatic exercise. A study by Gappmaier et al. in 2016 summed up the prevailing attitude on aquatic exercise and weight loss with this conclusion: "Results indicate that there are no differences in the effect of aerobic activities in the water versus weight-bearing aerobic exercise on land on body composition components as long as similar intensity, duration, and frequency are used" (564). In other words, if proper intensity is reached in aquatic exercise, oxygen consumption and caloric expenditure occur at the same rate even if the water suppresses heart rate. Carefully applying a proper heart rate deduction and diligently monitoring intensity, duration, and frequency in aquatic exercise can successfully lead to weight loss and improvements in body composition for most participants.

- Length of the person's limbs, which affects the amount of resistance encountered when moving against the water
- Environmental factors (water temperature, air temperature, humidity, chemicals, and so on)

Eating Disorders

Eating disorders are complex, life-threatening diseases that revolve around an unhealthy relationship with food, weight, and body image. The cause of eating disorders is unknown, but research shows a link to psychological factors. People with eating disorders might believe that they would be happier and more successful if they were thin. They often have a need to be perfect and are consumed with the pressures that society places on body shape and size. They allow stress, overcommitment, and the urge to be in control to dictate their feelings about themselves.

Most often, eating disorders are found in teenage girls and young women, but they can also occur in teenage boys and young men. Eating disorders are commonly thought of as being primarily concerned with weight loss, but weight gain is another area where an eating disorder can develop. Treatment often includes medical intervention, counseling or therapy, and, in some cases, hospitalization.

Because eating disorders are psychological disorders, the role of a fitness professional is to refer the participant to a trained specialist. Identification of participants is your primary role in the treatment process. Provide professional referrals (registered dietitian or behavior specialist, such as a psychologist) to those whom you suspect have an eating disorder.

Medical and psychological complications associated with eating disorders include the following:

- Gastrointestinal (digestive) problems
- Cardiac arrhythmia (irregular heart beat)
- Hypotension (low blood pressure)
- Hypothermia (cold intolerance)
- Dehydration
- Amenorrhea
- Osteoporosis
- Sleep disorders
- Excessively dry skin
- Low self-esteem
- Depression, anger, anxiety
- Low frustration tolerance
- High need for approval

Anorexia

Anorexia is a condition in which a person is obsessed with being thin. People with anorexia attempt to lose a great amount of weight, and are terrified of gaining it back. They don't want to eat and might constantly worry about how many calories they consume or how much fat is in their food. They often use diet pills, laxatives, and water pills to lose weight. They are often obsessed with exercising. The warning signs of anorexia include the following:

- Deliberate semi-self-starvation with weight loss
- Fear of gaining weight
- Refusal to eat
- Denial of hunger
- Constant exercising
- Greater amounts of hair on the body or the face (lanugo)
- Sensitivity to cold temperatures
- Absent or irregular periods (amenorrhea)
- Loss of scalp hair
- A self-perception of being fat when they are actually too thin

Anorexia Athletica

A disorder that is most commonly seen in competitive athletes, **anorexia athletica** can occur in the general population as well. An individual with anorexia athletica has a preoccupation with diet and weight loss and thus compulsively and excessively exercises. Excessive exercise interferes with the person's daily function, often leads to isolation, and consumes all their thoughts. Someone with this disorder uses exercise to try to remedy the distorted perception of their body.

People with anorexia athletica meet five criteria:

- Excessive fear of becoming obese
- Restriction of calorie intake
- Weight loss
- No medical disorder to explain leanness
- Gastrointestinal complaints

In addition, they meet one or more of these related criteria:

- Disturbance in body image
- Compulsive exercising
- Binge eating
- Use of purging methods
- Delayed puberty
- Menstrual dysfunction

Bulimia

Bulimia is an eating disorder characterized by recurrent binge eating followed by compensatory behaviors—called purging—such as self-induced vomiting, fasting, exercising excessively, or using laxatives, enemas, or diuretics. Typically, people with bulimia are of normal weight or overweight with mild fluctuations. The warning signs of bulimia include the following:

- Preoccupation with food (binges on carbohydrates, high fluid intake, fast eating in large bites, refusal to waste food, awareness of calories)
- Relentless pursuit of thinness; significant body dissatisfaction
- Bitter or sour breath (halitosis)
- Unusual eating habits and behaviors
- Menstrual irregularities
- Dental and gum disease
- Permanently swollen salivary glands from repetitive vomiting (chipmunk cheeks)
- Gastrointestinal problems
- Dehydration
- Complications associated with diuretic and laxative use, such as bloating, diarrhea, constipation, fatigue, muscle cramps, and decreased bone density

Binge Eating Disorder

Also referred to as compulsive overeating, **binge eating disorder** is characterized by eating unusually large amounts of food and, often, feeling guilty or secretive. People with a binge eating disorder have different relationships with food. At first, food might provide sustenance or comfort, but eventually it might become the focus of guilt or distress. People with this condition eat large amounts of food quickly and feel completely out of control as they are binging. It is different from occasionally eating too much.

This disorder differs from anorexia and bulimia because people with binge eating disorder are usually overweight. The most common health risks are the same as those that accompany obesity. The causes are unknown, but many people who binge eat say that it is triggered by feelings of anger, sadness, boredom, depression, or anxiety. The warning signs of binge eating disorder include the following:

- Eating a lot of food quickly
- A pattern of eating in response to emotional stress, such as family conflict, peer rejection, and poor academic performance
- Feeling ashamed or disgusted by the amount of food eaten
- Finding food containers hidden in the person's room or house
- Possessing an increasingly irregular eating pattern, such as skipping meals, eating lots of junk food, and eating at unusual times (like late at night)

Body Dysmorphic Disorder

Body dysmorphic disorder (BDD), or **dysmorphophobia**, is a mental disorder where the person cannot stop thinking about one or more perceived defects or flaws in their appearance. From excessive exercise to plastic surgery, people with BDD become fixated on making a change. As a fitness professional, you need to be able to communicate realistic goals and encourage positive self-esteem.

Other Specified Feeding and Eating Disorder

Other specified feeding and eating disorder (OSFED) is an eating disorder that does not meet the exact criterion for a specific, defined eating disorder, such as anorexia, anorexia athletica, bulimia, binge eating disorder, or body dysmorphic disorder. It also includes eating disorders that have a mixture of the various conditions (NEDA 2016). The significance of this classification is that professionals can identify and help people who do not quite fit into the profile.

You are faced with a wide array of participants on a day-to-day basis; they trust you to help them reach their physical goals. If you think your participants have one of the preceding issues with food, guide them to a medical professional as quickly as possible. These disorders can have detrimental effects on the body and the participant's health. You are placed in an uncomfortable position, but your inspiration and guidance can make a positive difference in the person's health and well-being. Some confrontations with participants who have eating or self-image disorders are well received, and others are not; your job is to guide these people as best you can for the betterment of their health.

Nutrition References

A referral system is the best way to provide class participants or personal training clients with a customized food plan to meet specific needs. An effective referral system provides mutual benefits to all involved. You must understand the qualifications of each kind of nutrition professional in order to guide your participants in the right direction. A **registered dietitian (RD)** is an expert on food and nutrition who has credentials from academic and professional study. A **nutritionist** is a person who advises people on dietary matters relating to health, well-being, and optimal nutrition. Unfortunately, no legal definition exists for nutritionists, so educational levels for nutritionists can vary from a simple continuing education course all the way to a master's degree in chemistry. When working with nutritionists, investigate their background to fully understand their level of education and expertise.

Searching the Internet is a common practice for people looking to lose weight or increase physical activity. With so many confusing and misleading websites, your participants might look to you for good, useful information. The following are science-based websites that you and your participants can consult with confidence:

www.eatright.org (Academy of Nutrition and Dietetics)

www.fda.gov (U.S. Food and Drug Administration)

www.nationaldairycouncil.org (National Dairy Council)

www.nutrition.gov (Nutrition.gov)

www.fruitsandveggiesmorematters.org (Fruits and Veggies—More Matters)

www.cspinet.org (Center for Science in the Public Interest)

www.cancer.org (American Cancer Society)

www.mayoclinic.org (Mayo Clinic)

www.hhs.gov (U.S. Department of Health and Human Services)

www.usda.gov (U.S. Department of Agriculture)

www.choosemyplate.gov (USDA Center for Nutrition Policy and Promotion)

www.health.gov (Office of Disease Prevention and Health Promotion)

www.nih.gov (National Institutes of Health)

www.cdc.gov (Centers for Disease Control and Prevention)

Summary

Nutrition is the process of fueling the body with food to provide nutrients for the growth, function, and the rebuilding or replacement of tissue. For the majority of your participants, eating in accordance with the *U.S. 2015-2020 Dietary Guidelines for Americans* and USDA ChooseMyPlate.gov guidelines will provide an adequate diet for health.

The human body requires six nutrients to ensure normal growth and function. These nutrients, classified as either macronutrients (carbohydrates, protein, fat, and water) or micronutrients (vitamins and minerals), are absorbed into the body through the digestive process. They are responsible for all human function, including the energy to exercise and the strength to maintain healthy bodies free from illness and disease. Our food choices determine the nutrients that are available to our bodies for recovery, growth, and energy sources.

The *Dietary Guidelines for Americans* offer science-based advice for promoting health and reducing risk for major chronic diseases through diet and physical activity. They provide five general recommendations for encouraging overall healthy eating. The USDA MyPlate incorporates recommendations from the *Dietary Guidelines for Americans* with an individualized and interactive approach to determine daily calorie needs based on age, gender, and physical activity.

You must be able to provide participants with quality information regarding weight management while staying within your scope of practice. You can recommend that your participants use the SuperTracker at ChooseMyPlate.gov or refer them to a registered dietitian for assistance with tracking caloric intake and expenditure. You can also assist participants through appropriate exercise programming.

Because eating disorders are psychological disorders, your role as a fitness professional is to recognize participants who may have an eating disorder and refer them to a trained specialist (to a registered dietitian or behavior specialist, such as a psychologist).

A referral system is the best way to provide class participants or personal training clients with a customized food plan to meet specific needs. You may also gain knowledge from science-based websites that you and your participants can consult with confidence.

Review Questions

1. Which of the following is a non-caloric (calorie-free) micronutrient?
   a. Water
   b. Vitamins
   c. Minerals
   d. All of these
   e. B and C only
2. ________________ are the primary source of energy for the skeletal muscles and the exclusive source of energy for the brain and nervous system.
   a. Carbohydrates
   b. Fats
   c. Proteins
   d. Vitamins and minerals
3. ______________________ found in barley, legumes, oats, and some fruits and vegetables assists in lowering blood cholesterol levels and slows the process of digestion, allowing for greater absorption of nutrients.
   a. Complete fiber
   b. Essential fiber
   c. Soluble fiber
   d. Insoluble fiber
4. The amino acids that must be consumed in the diet, because the body cannot make them, are known as _________________.
   a. complete proteins
   b. incomplete proteins
   c. nonessential amino acids
   d. essential amino acids
5. The recommended dietary allowance (RDA) for men and women is 0.8 grams of high-quality protein per kilogram of body weight per day.
   a. True
   b. False

6. ________________ provide a much greater risk to heart health because they raise LDL (unhealthy cholesterol) levels while also lowering HDL.

   a. Saturated fats
   b. Monounsaturated fats
   c. Polyunsaturated fats
   d. Trans fats

7. Total cholesterol levels are determined based on a ratio of low-density lipoproteins, high-density lipoproteins, and________________.

   a. triglycerides
   b. omega-3 fatty acids
   c. mid-density lipoproteins
   d. saturated fats

8. The % Daily Value listed on prepackaged food labels is based on a diet of __________ per day, so this may need to be adjusted based on your required caloric intake.

   a. 1,200 calories
   b. 1,500 calories
   c. 2,000 calories
   d. 2,200 calories

9. Specific diseases are linked to poor diet and physical inactivity, including cardiovascular disease, type 2 diabetes, hypertension, osteoporosis, and certain cancers.

   a. True
   b. False

10. Which of the following is true regarding BMI?

    a. BMI ≥ 25 is considered overweight.
    b. BMI ≥ 30 is considered obese.
    c. BMI ≥ 40 is considered extremely obese.
    d. All of these
    e. None of the above

See appendix D for answers to review questions.

References and Resources

American College of Sports Medicine. 2016. *Resources for the personal trainer.* 4th edition. Baltimore: Lippincott, Williams and Wilkins.

American Heart Association. 2014. Understanding food nutrition labels. www.heart.org/HEARTORG/HealthyLiving/HealthyEating/Nutrition/Understanding-Food-Nutrition-Labels_UCM_300132_Article.jsp#.V6nU-wI52n7g.

———. 2016. Saturated fats. www.heart.org/HEARTORG/HealthyLiving/HealthyEating/Nutrition/Saturated-Fats_UCM_301110_Article.jsp#.V6itrI52n7g.

Bernardot, D. 1992. *Sports nutrition—A guide for the professional working with active people*. 2nd edition. Chicago: American Dietetic Association.

Centers for Disease Control and Prevention (CDC). 2008. Prevalence of overweight, obesity and extreme obesity among adults: United States, trends 1960-62 through 2005-2006. www.cdc.gov/nchs/data/hestat/overweight/overweight_adult.pdf.

Chewning, J. 2002. *How many calories? AEA Research Council.* Nokomis: FL: Aquatic Exercise Association.

Coburn, J.W., and M.H. Malek. 2012. *NSCA's essentials of personal training*. 2nd edition. Champaign, IL. Human Kinetics.

Colado, J.C., V. Tella, N.T. Triplett, and L.M. González. 2009. Effects of a short-term aquatic resistance program on strength and body composition in fit young men. *Journal of Strength and Conditioning Research* 23(2):549-559.

Colgan, M. 1982. *Your personal vitamin profile.* New York: Quill.

Dietary Guidelines Advisory Committee. 2015. *Dietary guidelines for Americans*. Washington, D.C.: U.S.

Freeman, V., and L. Kravitz. 2004. Women and weight loss: Practical applications for water fitness instructors. *AKWA* 18(3):26-30.

Gappmaier, E., W. Lake, A.G. Nelson, and A. Fisher. 2006. Aerobic exercise in water versus walking on land: Effects on indices of fat reduction and weight loss of obese women. *Journal of Sports Medicine and Physical Fitness* 46(4):564-569.

Gaspard, G., J. Schmal, J. Porcari, N. Butts, A. Simpson, and G. Brice. 1995. Effects of a seven-week aqua step training program on aerobic capacity and body composition of college-aged women. *Medicine and Science in Sports and Exercise* 27:1003-1011.

Mayo Clinic. 2016. Body dysmorphic disorder. www.mayoclinic.org/diseases-conditions/body-dysmorphic-disorder/home/ovc-20200935.

Moore, G.E., J.L. Durstine, and P.L. Durstine. 2016. *ACSM's exercise management for persons with chronic diseases and disabilities*. 4th edition. Champaign, IL: Human Kinetics.

Nagle, E.F., A.D. Otto, J.M. Jakicic, R.J. Robertson, F.L. Goss, and J.L. Ranalli. 2003. Effects of aquatic plus walking exercise on weight loss and function in sedentary obese females. *Medicine and Science in Sport and Exercise* 35(5):S136.

National Eating Disorder Association. 2016. Other specified feeding or eating disorder. www.nationaleatingdisorders.org/other-specified-feeding-or-eating-disorder

National Heart, Blood and Lung Institute. 2005. *High blood cholesterol, what you need to know.* Washington, DC: Department of Health and Human Services. www.nhlbi.nih.gov/health/public/heart/chol/wyntk.htm.

Oz, M., and M. Roizen. 2006. *You on a diet.* New York: Simon and Schuster.

Sagawa, S., K. Miki, F. Tajima, H. Tanaka, J.K. Choi, L.C. Keil, K. Shiralei, and J.E. Greenleaf. 1992. Effect of dehydration on thirst and drinking during immersion in men. *Journal of Applied Physiology* 72:128-134.

Sawka, M.N., L.M. Burke, E.R. Eichner, R.J. Maughan, S.J. Montain, and N.S. Stachenfeld. 2007. American College of Sports Medicine position stand: Exercise and fluid replacement. *Medicine and Science in Sport and Exercise* 39:377-390.

U.S. Department of Health and Human Services and U.S. Department of Agriculture. 2015. *2015–2020 Dietary Guidelines for Americans.* 8th edition. http://health.gov/dietaryguidelines/2015/guidelines.

U.S. Food and Drug Administration. 2016. Changes to the Nutrition Facts. www.fda.gov/Food/GuidanceRegulation/GuidanceDocumentsRegulatoryInformation/LabelingNutrition/ucm385663.htm.

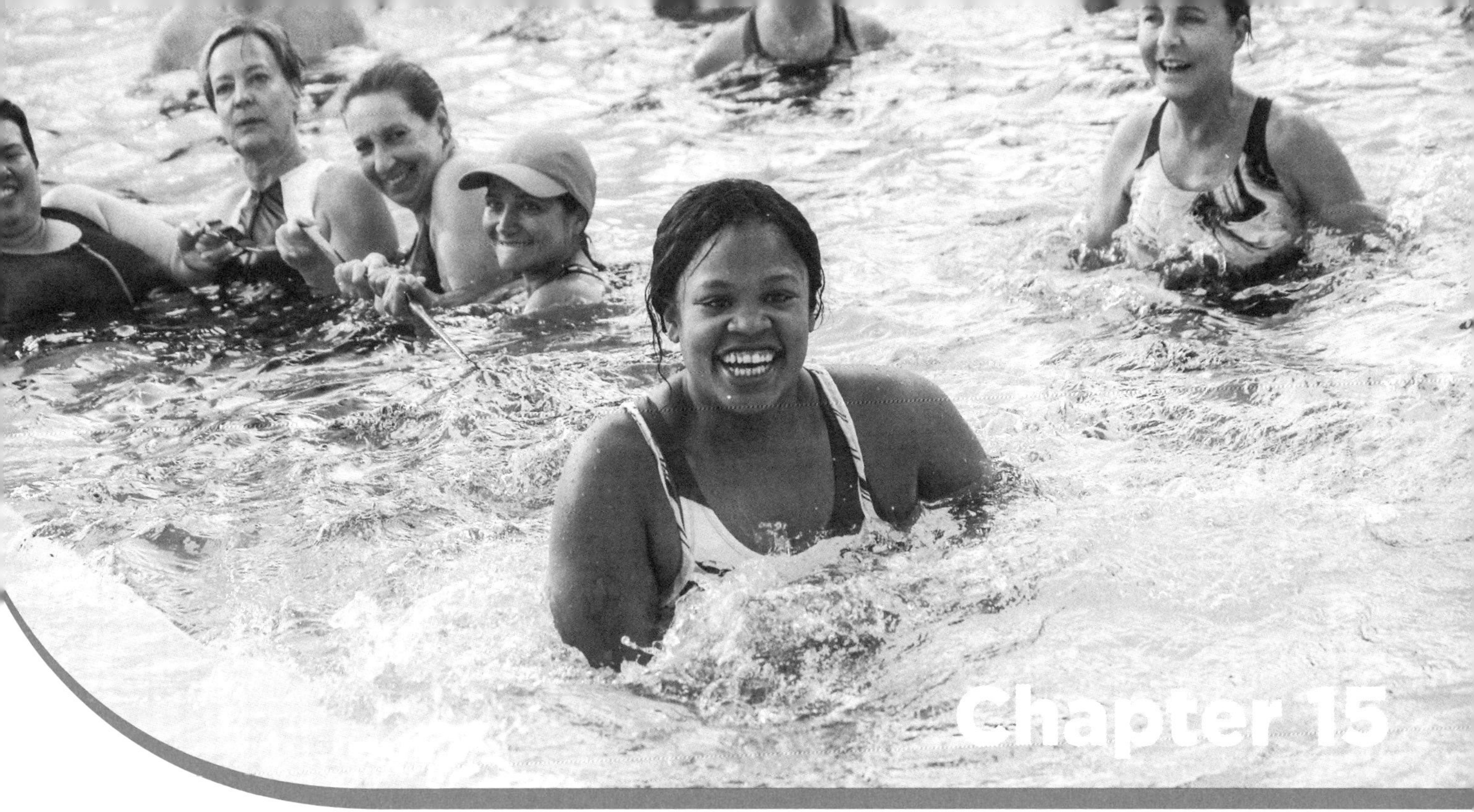

Business Issues and Legal Considerations

Introduction

The purpose of this chapter is to provide an overview of good practices with regard to business issues, considerations, and responsibilities within the fitness industry. More important, it shares key knowledge to help you keep your classes and students as safe as possible within the scope of a certified fitness professional. The information provides a clear understanding of your leadership responsibilities as a fitness professional, as well as basic knowledge of business and legal issues. This chapter also discusses the Americans with Disability Act (ADA) regulations and amendments involving group fitness and swimming pool issues. Legal considerations regarding the use of music are also discussed in this chapter.

This chapter should be considered a supplemental resource for legal and business issues in the fitness industry relating to group exercise programming and leadership. All terms and definitions are based on U.S. practices; terms and definitions may vary in other countries. The AEA recommends that all aquatic fitness professionals retain appropriate legal and business counsel for individual needs or concerns. Legal considerations include federal, state, and local levels and vary considerably across the United States and abroad. Business considerations may also vary, since fitness professionals may have more than one labor status qualification (such as employee and business partnership). It would be best to consult with an attorney, accountant, and the Department of State to ensure all requirements are met.

Key Chapter Concepts

- Recognize the difference in employment status for employees and independent contractors and understand various options for setting up your own fitness business.
- Define the most common types of insurance applicable to fitness professionals.
- Understand the concept of risk management and specific examples of risks associated with the aquatic environment.
- Define standard of care and be aware of two key sets of standards provided by the AEA: *AEA's Certified Aquatic Fitness Professional Code of Ethics and Conduct* and *AEA's Standards and Guidelines for Aquatic Fitness Programming.*
- Recognize the five general factors that influence liability and the four factors that must be present in order to demonstrate professional negligence.
- Understand the importance of proper documentation within the legal aspect of the fitness industry, including informed consent, waiver or liability, injury reports, and recommendations for identifying clients who would benefit from obtaining medical clearance prior to initiating an exercise program.
- Understand the legalities of music use within the fitness industry and how you can remain in compliance.
- Be aware of the responsibilities of fitness facilities and swimming pools under the Americans with Disabilities Act (ADA).

Employee Versus Independent Contractor

In the fitness industry, two common terms are associated with instructors, group exercise leaders, and personal trainers: employee and independent contractor (also referred to as a subcontractor). Each has a unique definition, and the responsibilities and liabilities vary between the two. It is possible that you are an employee at one location but an independent contractor at another facility, or that you provide services in both capacities in the same location.

The Internal Revenue Service (IRS) provides simple common law rules to determine the differences between an employee and an independent contractor. The three factors they use are behavioral (Does someone control how you do your job?), financial (Does someone control the business aspects of your job?), and type of relationship (Are there written contracts, employee benefits, insurances, vacation pay, and so on?). These and other factors must be considered when determining the status of your relationship with the organization as an employee or independent contractor. It's important to look at the entire relationship, including duties performed and expectations. How a fitness facility hires instructors often depends on their corporate structure.

Employee

As an **employee**, you are hired to provide services to a company on a regular basis in exchange for wages. Your employer (company) is responsible for deducting federal and state required taxes from your payroll and reporting all taxes to the appropriate agencies. You would be covered by your company's professional and general liability insurance when teaching in the company's facilities, or any time you represent the company and are receiving wages for your services. You would be hired to perform certain tasks (e.g., to teach group fitness, aquatic classes, personal training), and your employer would specify your job description, duties, and benefits. Policies and procedures should be reviewed and should be found in your employee handbook or benefits package.

Independent Contractor (Self-Employed)

If you are self-employed, you are more than likely teaching classes as an **independent contractor** (also referred to as a subcontractor). You may teach classes or provide personal training for a facility, but you are not considered an employee. You would follow guidelines specified in a contract or agreement, but you would provide services based on your schedule, expertise, and preferences. Unlike an employee, an independent contractor does not necessarily work on a regular basis for one facility and may work for more than one facility. As an independent contractor, you assume all liability, financial obligation, debt, claim, or potential loss. It would be prudent to seek the advice of business advisors, lawyers, and insurance agents to adequately protect your own future and financial stability.

As an independent contractor, you are responsible for filing all federal and state taxes based on the compensation you receive for services provided (e.g., teaching classes, personal training). You are also responsible for having proper insurance. You may need to provide proof of coverage to each contracted company (e.g., fitness facility, hotel, or private condominium). (Note: Definitions of various types of insurance are discussed later in this chapter.) You would need to maintain professional liability insurance in the event of a lawsuit and you would need general liability insurance, especially if you own or rent a facility or provide services in your home or pool. If you work on the premises, the company's general liability insurance may assume some of the legal responsibility in the event of loss or injury. Additionally, it is recommended that you consider options for health and disability insurance since you are not an employee and will not be offered health benefits from the company. You also cannot sue an employer for a wrongful act or injury suffered on the job because you are not an employee.

Independent Contractor—IRS Definition

"The general rule is that an individual is an independent contractor if the payer has the right to control or direct only the result of the work and not what will be done and how it will be done."

"You are not an independent contractor if you perform services that can be controlled by an employer (what will be done and how it will be done). This applies even if you are given freedom of action. What matters is that the employer has the legal right to control the details of how the services are performed" (IRS 2016b).

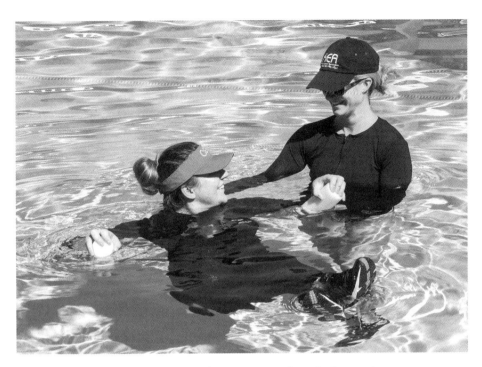

Aquatic personal trainers may choose to work as independent contractors or as employees.

Setting Up Your Own Business

As the fitness industry continues to grow and evolve, some professionals will choose to set up a business or structured company due to legal or financial considerations. If you are providing services, such as offering in-home personal training or fitness classes, or providing aquatic fitness programs at a condominium, residential community pools, or hotels, it might be in your best interest to speak to a lawyer or business advisor regarding setting up a formal company. It may be beneficial for you to consider setting up one of the business models discussed in the following sections.

Sole Proprietorship

A **sole proprietorship** is a business structure in which an individual and the company are considered a single entity for tax and liability purposes. A sole proprietorship is a company that is not registered with the state as a limited liability company or corporation.

Partnership

Partnerships are also common in the fitness industry. This type of business is composed of two or more people who control the business, and are personally liable for the partnership's debts. Partners are not considered employees. Profits and losses are split between the parties and the income or losses are split between all parties on their individual or personal income tax returns.

Limited Liability Company (LLC)

A limited liability company (LLC) is a business structure allowed by state statute that is common in the fitness industry. Owners of an LLC are called members; some states do allow a single owner of LLCs. The IRS may treat the LLC like a partnership or a corporation, depending on how many members are involved. It is best to check your state's requirements and the IRS website for more detailed information if you are considering forming an LLC.

Corporations

Corporations in the fitness profession are generally registered businesses organized for the purpose of providing professional services as defined by the specific state laws. There are several types of corporations with different shareholders and tax configurations. Your business advisors can help you choose the type of corporation that is most beneficial for your business structure.

Insurance

Carrying liability insurance creates a sense of professionalism and credibility and protects you from potential loss. The most common types of insurance associated with the fitness profession include, but are not limited to, those listed here.

General liability insurance protects you or your company in the event that a participant is injured on your premises, or if you or one of your employees injures someone or damages property at a participant's location.

Professional liability insurance provides protection when you are held legally liable for how you rendered or failed to render professional services.

Umbrella liability is sometimes referred to as a bridge or additional coverage to your professional liability coverage. It can supply additional coverage if your professional liability isn't enough to cover all expenses for damages resulting from litigation.

Property insurance protects business property and inventory (assets) against physical loss or damage by theft, accident, or other means, even if that property is removed from your place of business when it is lost or damaged.

Sexual abuse liability insurance provides coverage in the event you are accused or sued for sexual harassment by a class participant or client. Some professional liability insurance policies include this type of coverage, and it is best to check with your insurance provider.

Service interruption or business interruption insurance is a special type of insurance that covers indirect losses that occur when a direct loss (that results from a covered peril, such as a fire) forces a temporary interruption of business. Depending on policy structure, business interruption insurance reimburses policyholders for the difference between normal income and the income earned during the enforced shutdown period.

Worker's compensation insurance provides wage replacement and medical coverage for employees who sustain job-related injuries. Generally, these worker's compensation insurance policies cover employees' medical expenses and reimburse them for some percentage of lost wages. Some states have a mandatory worker's compensation program that you must participate in, whereas other states require you to have coverage through a private broker.

If you are working at a club or a private or public pool facility, you may be required to provide a certificate of insurance listing the facility as an **additional insured**. This means a business added to your liability insurance policy for purposes of protecting them against your negligence. Some insurance companies may charge a fee for this service.

As you can see, there are several types of insurance policies, and it is best to consult your insurance agent to determine insurance requirements based on your professional needs, business structure, and services provided. It is also important to look at the amount of coverage recommended or, in some instances, mandated by the state.

Risk Management and Standard of Care

Risk management is the process of measuring or assessing potential risk and developing strategies to manage that risk. Risk management includes regulating and enforcing conduct and safety guidelines to ensure the safety of participants. The management of fitness and aquatic facilities should identify both potential health and safety risks and establish specific policies and guidelines to reduce the risk of injuries and accidents. Rules, guidelines, and potential risks should be posted for all exercise activities and areas. The rules should be visible to all participants and clients and strictly enforced by the staff. Lack of appropriate risk-management practices can lead to potential damages or injuries.

Examples of potential risks for aquatic fitness participants include the following:

- Slippery deck surface
- Broken ladders, loose rails on steps into pool
- Chipped gutters
- Loose or chipped floor tiles (e.g., lap lane tiles) on pool bottom
- Improperly grounded electrical outlets
- Pool chemical and sanitation problems
- Improper drain covers (as per the Virginia Graeme Baker Pool and Spa Safety Act of 2007)

The ability to identify existing and potential risk is important for fitness professionals. All fitness professionals and facilities should create and implement policies with clear guidelines. The guidelines should be evaluated regularly to continually ensure the welfare of all of the participants.

Standard of care is defined as the degree of care a reasonable person would take to prevent an injury to another. You should know your limitations and boundaries as a fitness professional and develop a comfortable standard of care based on personal knowledge and skill. Always act within those boundaries and limitations. An example of this is CPR certification. Your CPR training certifies you to perform choking victim care, rescue breathing, and CPR. A reasonable person with a CPR certification would provide rescue breathing to a person who is not breathing but has a pulse. This would be the standard of care for this specific situation. You can see how certifications and education would alter your personal standard of care. Fitness professionals are responsible for keeping all certifications current and attending continuing education courses. Ongoing education is critical for remaining up to

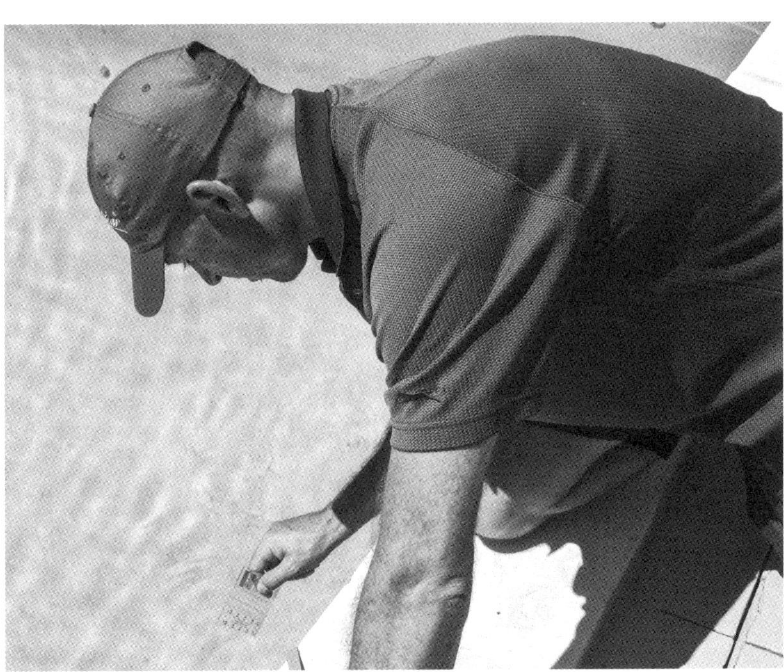

Regular testing will help maintain proper water quality.

date with the latest knowledge and changes in the fitness industry. Reading professional journals and researching reputable sources and organizations on the Internet will help you grow and gain fresh ideas for safe and effective programming.

The AEA provides two sets of standards. The first is ***AEA's Certified Aquatic Fitness Professional Code of Ethics and Conduct***, which defines baseline standards that AEA-certified fitness professionals are expected to follow.

The second standard is the AEA published ***Standards and Guidelines for Aquatic Fitness Programming***, which provides important information for professional leadership and application, environmental concerns, facility recommendations, and instructional issues for the overall safety of the participants serviced. Several of the standards and

Aquatic Exercise Association Certified Aquatic Fitness Professional Code of Ethics and Conduct

- I will maintain high standards of professional conduct at all times.
- I will remain aware of current AEA Standards and Guidelines for Aquatic Fitness Programming. I will not knowingly contradict current accepted industry standards.
- I shall maintain my AEA certification through continuing education to stay abreast of the industry. I recognize that a minimum of 15 hours of continuing education is recommended for each 2-year renewal period of my AEA certification.
- I will maintain training and certification in cardiopulmonary resuscitation (CPR) and will obtain training in the use of an automatic external defibrillator (AED).
- I will maintain recommended levels of training in first aid and water safety.
- I will acknowledge my skills and limitations as an aquatic fitness professional. I will practice ethically and properly represent my qualifications.
- I shall maintain clear and honest communications with my clients and students and uphold confidentiality at all times.
- I shall respect and cooperate with all health care and fitness professionals to promote the betterment of the aquatic fitness industry.
- I will contribute to the health, safety, and welfare of my clients and students to gain continued respect for the aquatic industry.
- I shall uphold the standards, policies, and procedures as outlined by the aquatic facility for which I work.
- I shall dress in a professional and appropriate manner when representing the aquatic fitness industry.
- I shall refrain from using any mind-altering drugs, alcohol, or intoxicants when conducting classes or instructing clients.
- I shall provide the highest quality of service possible to my clients and students in conjunction with the standards, guidelines, and objectives of the Aquatic Exercise Association.

guidelines have been included in various places in this manual. The complete standards and guidelines document is available at the AEA website and is updated regularly.

Liability

Rules and regulations will be designated by the facility where you teach or train clients in addition to industry standards and guidelines. However, there is always a possibility of injury or damage when participating in fitness programs. **Liability** is an obligation, debt, or responsibility owed to someone. As an aquatic fitness instructor, you have the legal obligation and responsibility to ensure the safety of all participants. Making sure you understand and follow industry standards and the facilities' guidelines, policies, and procedures will minimize liability and ensure both your safety and the safety of the class participants before, during, and after the class.

Five general factors influence liability:

1. Ignorance of the law: not knowing the law.
2. Ignoring the law: doing something that you know is contrary to the law.
3. Failure to act: you know that you should do something but you fail to do it.
4. Failure to warn: not making participants or supervisors sufficiently aware of inherent dangers.
5. Expense: failing to budget or spend money to further safety objectives.

The following points can help reduce liability within the fitness setting:

- Every participant should read, understand, and sign an informed consent and waiver of liability that is professionally drafted by the facility's attorney. This is further discussed later in this chapter.
- All participants should complete appropriate health screening forms and obtain medical clearance to exercise when necessary.
- Encourage participants to participate in fitness testing to identify initial fitness levels and abilities.
- Follow recommended procedures for paperwork and policies for class participants and personal training clients. Policies and procedures may vary due to the type of services being provided.
- Follow facility procedures with regard to incident reports and injury reports. Properly document all incidents and injuries immediately following the incident.
- Avoid high-risk exercises. Teach safe exercises with proper form and technique. Recommend that participants maintain appropriate exercise intensities for their fitness level, existing medical conditions, and age.
- Remain certified, educated, and up to date with industry practices, including but not limited to CPR, AED, first aid, and water safety skills.
- Check and ensure that the environment pool area, locker room, and any other area used by participants or clients are safe and free of hazards.
- Determine that all equipment is in good working order.
- Maintain adequate personal and professional insurance protection.

Duty of Care

Duty of care refers to the level of responsibility that one has to protect another from harm under the circumstances (ASCM 2013). You have the responsibility and moral obligation as an aquatic fitness professional to perform services following industry standards and guidelines.

In a potential lawsuit or trial, the judge and jury would examine whether the individual (defendant) acted in accordance with industry standards to avoid damage or acted in any way to promote damage. An instructor may be held liable for doing something incorrectly or for failing to act in a preventive way. The following is a list of factors that must be present in order for an instructor to be considered responsible for the damage or injury; if any one of these factors is missing, liability or damage cannot be charged.

- Presence of the duty: was it your responsibility to provide the duty in question to the participant?
- Breach of duty: was that duty breached or compromised? Did you act inappropriately or fail to act to prevent damage?
- Cause of the injury: was your breach of duty the direct cause of the injury?
- Extent of the injury: what was the actual extent of the injury?

Negligence

Negligence is simply defined as failure to use reasonable care that a reasonably prudent person would use in a similar situation, resulting in injury or damages. Two concepts determine negligence:

- Did you have a duty?
- Did you breach that duty?

Four factors must be present in order to demonstrate professional negligence or malpractice:

- Proximate cause: were your actions the cause of the injury?
- Damages: the injured party must show damages.
- Duty: did you have a duty?
- Breach of duty: did you breach (fail to do) that duty?

A fitness professional can be considered negligent if a client or class participant is injured as a result of the instructor or trainer not acting in a manner consistent with the industry standard, or if they did something that was outside their scope of practice.

Informed Consent

By legal definition, consent is a person's agreement to allow something to happen. You should inform all fitness participants of the risks and potential injury inherent in participation in exercise programming. An **informed consent** explains the risks of participating in physical activity and shows that the participant or client understands these risks and voluntarily assumes responsibility for taking the risks. An informed consent is often included in the initial contract or binding agreement of a participant for professional services provided.

Liability Release (Waiver of Liability)

A **liability release** or **waiver of liability** is commonly used in the fitness industry to protect the facility or fitness professional from damages and potential lawsuits. Participants agree that they are willingly using the facility and participating in the activity and waive all rights to assign damage or negligence. Essentially, participants waive their rights for future lawsuits and damages that could result from participation.

In the United States, wavier law varies from state to state. Some states have very lenient enforcement requirements, others are very strict, and a few states currently disallow waivers. Regardless, it is recommended to use a well-written waiver. It is also suggested to work with a lawyer who has experience in the liability waiver laws of your state when developing your forms (Lowe 2015). The language utilized in the form must be very clear and explicit; some states even require that a waiver contain specific words (Cotton 2006). Additionally, some legal considerations cannot be waived. In most states, courts will not enforce a waiver designed to protect against reckless conduct, gross negligence, or intentional acts (Lowe 2015).

In many cases, the informed consent and waiver of liability are combined into one form that must be signed by all participants. Signing this form should be mandatory before joining the program. For most facilities, members sign these forms in their initial agreement with the facility. If you have a guest or one-day participant, be sure to have a version of a waiver of liability and informed consent available and policies in place to have these participants sign the form. If you are a subcontractor, be sure to have an informed consent and waiver of liability form drafted by an attorney in your area to follow state or area guidelines. Periodically have your form reviewed and updated by your attorney. Be sure to have all participants sign the form before participating. Figure 15.1 is a sample of an informed consent or waiver of liability form. However, as mentioned, you will want to work with a lawyer who is experienced in the specific liability waiver laws of your state when developing a form for your facility or your class sessions.

Injury Report Form

Although fitness professionals use a variety of risk management techniques to prevent injuries, injuries still occur. **Injury reports** are essential, and should be properly filled out and documented for all accidents or injuries sustained by any participant or guest. You should properly document and record all events immediately after an incident. It is very difficult and considered irresponsible to try to rely on memory when completing an injury report, even the day

Figure 15.1 Sample Informed Consent, Waiver of Liability, and Release of Liability.

Name of facility or logo

I, ______________________________ , have enrolled in a program of strenuous physical activity, including (but not limited to) aerobic training, resistance training, deep- and shallow-water exercise, interval training, circuit training, and the use of various aerobic and conditioning machinery and free weights offered by [name of facility or business] and/or exercise equipment owned by ______________________ (participant, homeowner).

I hereby affirm that I am in good physical condition and do not suffer from any disability that would prevent or limit my participation in this exercise program.

In consideration of my participation in the [name of facility or business] program, I, ______________________________ , for myself, my heirs and assigns, hereby release [name of facility or business], its employees, owners, and subcontractors from any claims, demands, and causes of action arising from my participation in the exercise program.

I fully understand that I might injure myself as a result of my participation in the [name of facility or business] exercise program and I, _________________________, hereby release [name of facility or business] exercise program and I, ____________________________ __, hereby release [name of facility or business], its employees, and owners, from any liability now or in the future, including (but not limited to) heart attacks, muscle strains, pulls or tears, broken bones, shin splints, heat prostration, knee, lower back, or foot injuries, and any other illness, soreness, or injury, however caused, occurring during or after my participation in this exercise program.

I acknowledge that I have carefully read this waiver and release of liability. I understand that I am waiving a legal right to bring a legal action and to assert a claim against the trainer, instructor, or facility for negligence.

Signature: ______________________________________ Date: ___________________

Printed name: ____

From Aquatic Exercise Association, 2018, *Aquatic Fitness Professional Manual, Seventh Edition* (Champaign, IL: Human Kinetics).

after the event. It may take several years for reports of injuries to result in lawsuits; therefore, proper documentation is critical. An injury report should be completed for any situation that has the possibility of damage regardless of your labor status (e.g., independent contractor, employee). Figure 15.2 is a sample of an injury report. Most facilities will have some type of injury report form for their employees or contractors. Some insurance companies may provide fitness professionals with a specific, recommended injury report form.

Figure 15.2 Sample Injury Report.

Facility name: ______________________________

Date of incident: ______________________________

Name of injured or involved: ______________________________

Address: ______________________________

Phone: ______________________________

Detailed description of incident (use back of paper if necessary): ______________________________

____

____

____

____

Signature of injured/involved: ______________________________

Date: ______________________________

Name of witness: ______________________________

Phone: ______________________________

Name of witness: ______________________________

Phone: ______________________________

Name of witness: ______________________________

Phone: ______________________________

Name of employee present: ______________________________

Name of employee present: ______________________________

Name of person filling out this report: ______________________________

Signature of person filling out this report: ______________________________

Date: ______________________________

Additional information: ______________________________

____

____

____

From Aquatic Exercise Association, 2018, *Aquatic Fitness Professional Manual, Seventh Edition* (Champaign, IL: Human Kinetics).

Music Use in Fitness

The **Copyright Act of 1976** explains the rights of copyright holders, including musical works, which affects fitness classes, personal training, and small group training, whether conducted in person or through online methods. Music played during fitness classes (even as background music) is considered a public performance, and thus requires permission by the copyright owner. This permission is generally obtained by paying music licensing fees to a performing rights organization (Yoga Alliance 2015). In the United States and abroad, fees must be paid to appropriate performing rights companies by profit and nonprofit organizations, health clubs, studios, churches, schools, and other entities or professionals who use music in their fitness programs or throughout their facilities.

Most fitness professionals want to abide by the copyright law, but may not be aware of, or not fully understand, the application to the fitness industry. ASCAP (American Society of Composers, Authors, and Publishers), BMI (Broadcast Music, Incorporated), and SESAC (Society of European Stage Authors and Composers) are the three largest performing rights organizations representing the writers and composers of songs (musical compositions). These organizations also help anyone using music for purposes other than personal enjoyment to comply with the United States copyright laws by issuing the required clearance (for a fee) to publicly use copyrighted music. Under the law, when a business or individual wishes to play music publicly, meaning outside a normal circle of friends or family, they must first obtain permission from the music's copyright owners. ASCAP, BMI, and SESAC services enable you to access and use music through agreements, licensing procedures, and the payment of fees without needing to contact each song composer individually.

Record companies own copyrights for the recordings of musical compositions performed by the original artists or bands. However, record companies traditionally don't license their recordings for the fitness industry. Therefore, fitness music companies and other businesses create or produce CDs, DVDs, music downloads, and other products specifically for various fitness applications. Producers and performers are hired to create or recreate the music and the song tracks compiled for specific programming requirements, such as an aquatic, step, cycling, walking, or interval format. These music products have appropriate counts, phrasing, adjusted beats per minutes, tempo range, rhythms, and transitions that aid in teaching an effective fitness program. The fitness music companies pay appropriate reproduction and mechanical fees for the right to produce, reproduce, sell, or duplicate these products.

When purchasing music from fitness music companies, remember that public performance fees are not covered. Thus, when using music—whether background music in the gym or locker room, for group exercise in the studio, or for aquatic programs in the pool—facilities must pay appropriate public performance rights licensing fees. It is the responsibility of the facility (employer) or independent contractor to make sure that ASCAP, BMI, SESAC, or other publisher fees are paid to ensure compliance with the copyright law. Typically, these fees are based on the average number of participants in class. In addition, fees are assessed for music played over a speaker in the general facility, even if the music is from a local radio station. These fees are typically based on the number of speakers but may also factor in the size of the club and even membership numbers.

Finally, it is not legal for you to copy or download and compile music from several original sources (e.g., albums, CDs, digital or electronic services, websites) onto a device for use in your class, because your class is a public performance. Though you may have purchased the songs, you did so for your personal enjoyment, not for commercial use. If you want to compile, sell, or distribute music programs, you must comply with all of the same regulations as the music production companies. This would require that you seek permission from the owners of all copyrights (record companies that own the recordings and music publishing companies that own or represent the musical composition). You would be required to pay advances or royalties for selling and distribution purposes, even if you gave the product away for free.

The law is simple: you play, you pay. Unless music is original and in original format or is unprotected, or if you have received written permission from the artists and writers to use the music, it is illegal to play music for classes or exercise sessions until you pay the public performance fees.

The following websites will provide additional information on music use and your responsibilities as a fitness professional.

ASCAP: www.ascap.com

BMI: www.bmi.com

SESAC: www.sesac.com

Americans With Disabilities Act (ADA)

The **Americans with Disabilities Act (ADA)** was initiated and approved in 1990. The purpose of this act was to set guidelines preventing discrimination and ensuring equal opportunities for individuals with disabilities. The ADA is a federal civil rights law that prohibits the exclusion of people with disabilities from everyday activities, such as buying an item at the store, watching a movie in a theater, enjoying a meal at a local restaurant, exercising at the local health club, or having a car serviced at a local garage. To meet the goals of the ADA, the law established requirements for private businesses of all sizes. These requirements first went into effect on January 26, 1992, and remain in effect for both profit and nonprofit businesses or organizations.

Private businesses that provide goods or services to the public are called public accommodations in the ADA. The ADA establishes requirements for 12 categories of public accommodations, including stores and shops, restaurants and bars, service establishments, theaters, hotels, recreation facilities, private museums, and schools. Almost all private businesses that serve the public are included in the categories, regardless of size. If you own, operate, or lease to a business that serves the public, then you have obligations to abide by the ADA for existing facilities, altered facilities, and new facilities. Existing facilities are typically not exempt by the "grandfather provisions" of building codes.

For small businesses, compliance with the ADA is not difficult. To help businesses with their compliance efforts, the United States Congress established a technical assistance program to answer questions about the ADA. Answers to questions about the ADA are a phone call away. The Department of Justice operates a toll-free ADA information line (800-514-0301 voice and 800-514-0383 TDD). In addition, tax credits and deductions are established that can be used annually to offset many of the costs of providing access to people with disabilities. For more information, see the Department of Justice website, www.usdoj.gov.

Summary

According to the Internal Revenue Service (IRS), employment status is based on three factors: behavior, financial, and type of relationship. Employees and independent contractors each have specific responsibilities and liabilities. It is possible to be an employee at one location and an independent contractor at another facility, or even provide your services in both capacities in the same location.

Should you choose to set up your own fitness business, the structure would depend on legal or financial considerations for the type of services you wish to provide, as well as locations where you plan to work. It would be prudent to speak to a lawyer or business advisor for guidance.

Risk management determines potential risk and develops strategies to manage that risk through regulation and enforcement of conduct and safety guidelines. Fitness and aquatic facilities should identify potential health and safety risks and establish specific policies and guidelines to reduce the risk of injuries and accidents.

Standard of care is the degree of care a reasonable person would take to prevent an injury to another. You need to know your limitations and boundaries as a fitness professional and develop a comfortable standard of care based on personal knowledge and skill. You must also act within those boundaries and limitations.

As an aquatic fitness instructor you have the liability—a legal obligation and responsibility—to ensure the safety of all participants. Understanding and following industry standards and the facilities' guidelines, policies, and procedures will minimize your liability. Duty of care refers to your level of responsibility to protect class participants and clients from harm while participating in exercise. Should injury or damage occur, negligence will be determined if you failed to provide the care that a reasonably prudent person would have used in a similar situation.

Managing risk and limiting liability within the fitness industry also requires providing proper documentation, such as informed consent and waiver of liability and injury reports, as well as recommending participants or clients obtain medical clearance when necessary.

Regulations for legal music use in the fitness industry can be found in the U.S. 1976 Copyright Act. Music played for group exercise classes and as background music within a fitness facility is subject to usage fees. ASCAP, BMI, and SESAC services enable you to access and use music through agreements, licensing procedures, and the payment of fees without needing to contact each song composer individually.

The Americans with Disabilities Act is a federal civil rights law that prohibits the exclusion of people with disabilities from everyday activities, including access to fitness facilities and swimming pools.

Review Questions

1. As a(n) ______________________, your employer (company) is responsible for deducting federal and state required taxes from your payroll and reporting all taxes to the appropriate agencies.

   a. subcontractor
   b. independent contractor
   c. employee
   d. self-employed instructor

2. ______________________________ provides protection when you are held legally liable for how you rendered or failed to render professional services.

   a. General liability insurance
   b. Professional liability insurance
   c. Property insurance
   d. Additional insured

3. Liability is the process of measuring or assessing potential risk and developing strategies to manage that risk.

   a. True
   b. False

4. What are the two sets of standards provided by the AEA?

5. As an aquatic fitness instructor, you have the liability (legal obligation and responsibility) to ensure the safety of all participants.

   a. True
   b. False

6. ___________________________ refers to the level of responsibility that one has to protect another from harm under the circumstances.

   a. Risk management
   b. Duty of care
   c. Negligence
   d. Breach of duty

7. A _______________________is commonly used in the fitness industry to protect the facility or fitness professional from damages and potential lawsuits.

8. Injury reports should be properly filled out and documented for all accidents or injuries sustained by any participant or guest ______________________________.
   a. within 1 month of an incident
   b. within 1 week of an incident
   c. within 3 days of an incident
   d. immediately after an incident
9. When using music purchased from fitness music companies, fitness facilities must still pay appropriate public performance rights licensing fees.
   a. True
   b. False
10. The ___________________________ is a federal civil rights law that prohibits the exclusion of people with disabilities from everyday activities.

See appendix D for answers to review questions.

References and Resources

Acton, M., L. Denomme, and J. Powers. 2005. *Aquatic after care manual.* 2nd edition. Venice, FL: Personal Health Trac.

American College of Sports Medicine. 2013. *ACSM's resources for the personal trainer.* 4th edition. Baltimore: Lippincott Williams and Wilkins.

American Society of Composers, Authors and Publishers. 2005. *Legislative history.* New York: Author.

———. 2008. *Music copyright in the digital age: A position paper. https://www.ascap.com/~/media/Files/Pdf/bill-of-rights/ASCAP_BillOfRights_Position.pdf.*

Broadcast Music. 2016. Common questions. www.bmi.com/licensing/entry/fitness_clubs.

Cotton, D. 2006. The ABCs of Liability Waivers. Guest Column at Recreation Management website. http://recmanagement.com/feature/200611gc03/2. Accessed June 12, 2017.

Employment Law Information Network. 2010. Liability: Workplace wellness. www.elinfonet.com/human-resources/Liability%3A-Workplace-Wellness.

Internal Revenue Service. 2016a. *Businesses—Tax information for businesses.* Washington, D.C.: Author.

———. 2016b. Independent contractor defined. www.irs.gov/businesses/small-businesses-self-employed/independent-contractor-defined.

Lowe, J.U. 2015. Why health club liability waivers are worth the cost. www.clubindustry.com/resourcebeat/why-health-club-liability-waiver-are-worth-cost. Accessed June 13, 2017.

U.S. Department of Justice. Civil Rights Division. 2011a. *ADA update: A primer for small business.* www.ada.gov/regs2010/smallbusiness/smallbusprimer2010.htm.

———. 2011b. Information and technical assistance on the Americans with Disabilities Act. www.ada.gov/2010_regs.htm.

U.S. Small Business Administration & U.S. Department of Justice. 1999. *ADA guide for small business.* 4th printing. www.ada.gov/smbusgd.pdf.

U.S. Legal. 2015. Waiver and release from liability law and legal definition. https://definitions.uslegal.com/w/waiver-and-release-from-liability.

Yoga Alliance. A crash course in yoga music licensing in the United States. https://www.yogaalliance.org/Learn/Article_Archive/A_Crash_Course_in_Yoga_Music_Licensing_in_the_United_States. Accessed June 13, 2017.

Appendix A

Shallow-Water Exercise

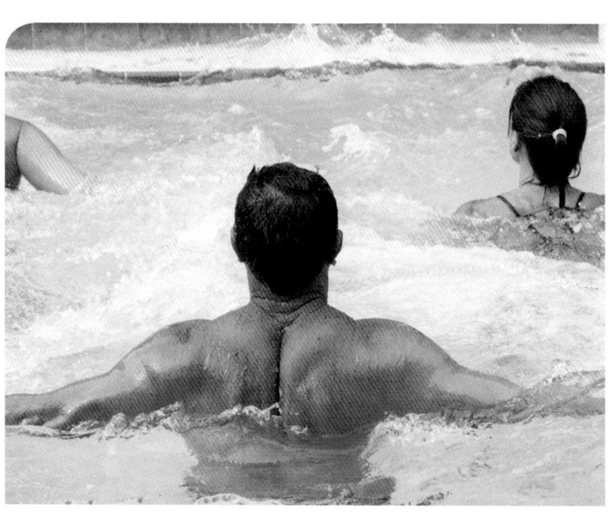

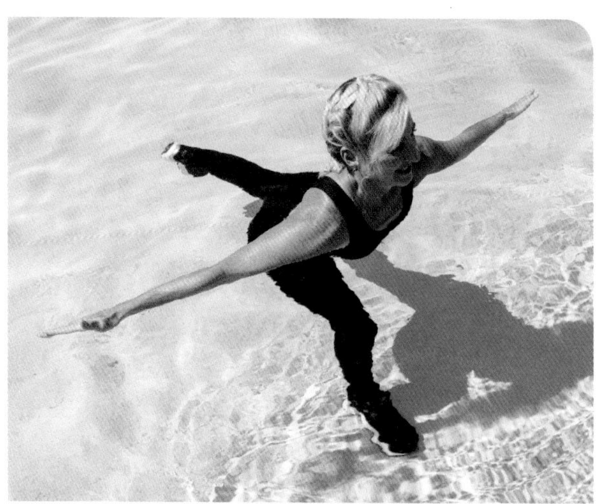

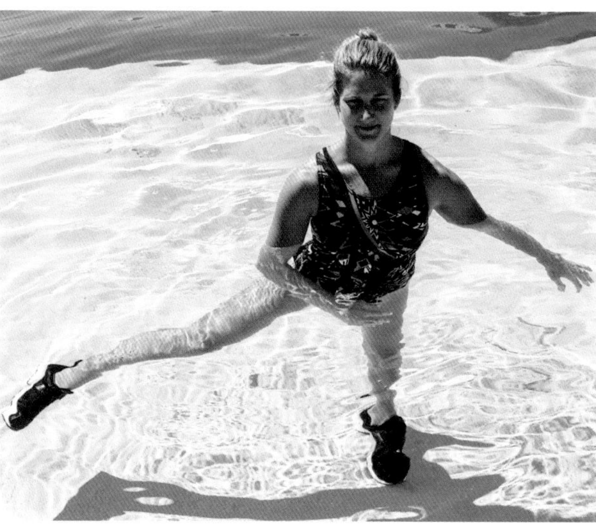

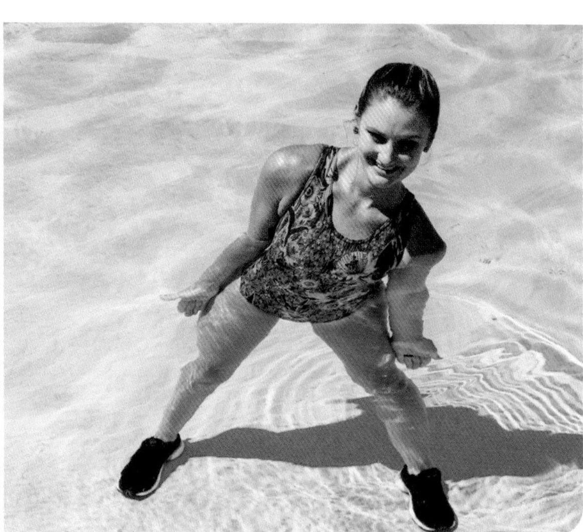

The exercises shown in this appendix represent techniques designed for the average healthy adult. Special populations or medical conditions might warrant exercise modifications. Some techniques are advanced and should be practiced with caution.

Shallow-Water Impact Levels—Jumping Jack

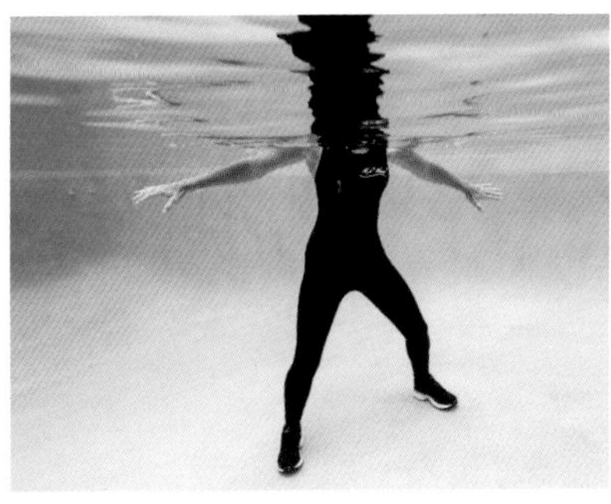

Level I: Level I movements are performed in an upright position with water level at waist to armpit depth. The degree of rebound (impact) can be altered with various methods.

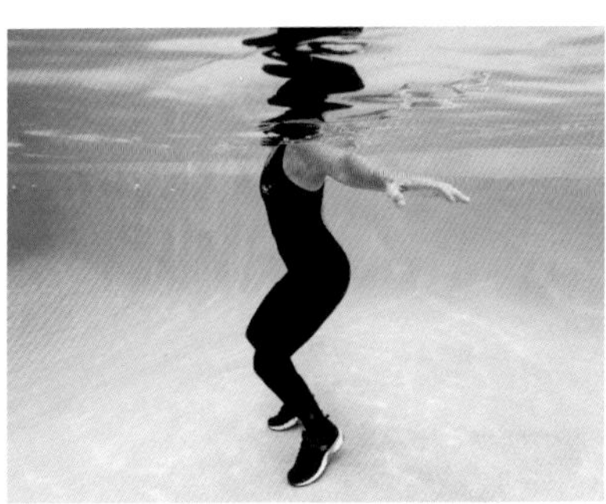

Level II: Level II movements are performed by flexing at the hips and knees to submerge the body to shoulder depth while executing the move. This is a low-impact option.

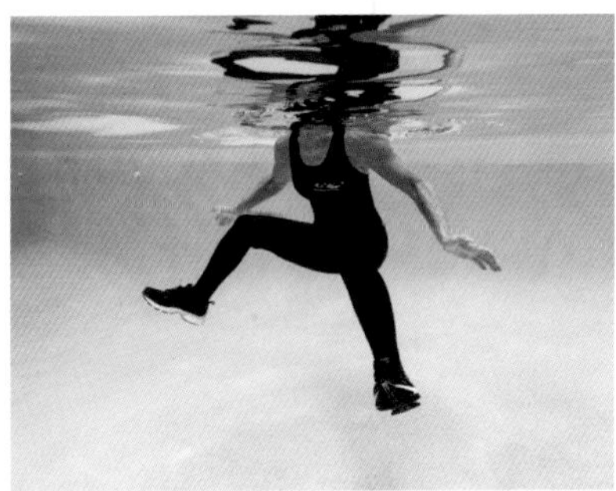

Level III: Level III movements are performed without touching the pool bottom (suspended). This is a nonimpact option.

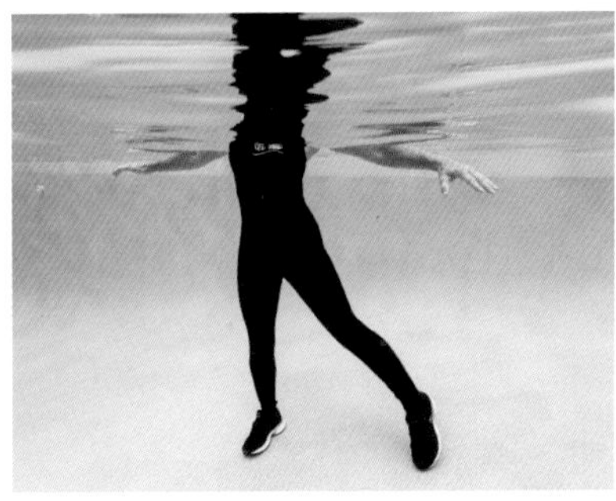

Grounded or anchored: Grounded moves are performed with one foot in contact with the pool bottom at all times. The variation pictured is a side tap, a low-impact option.

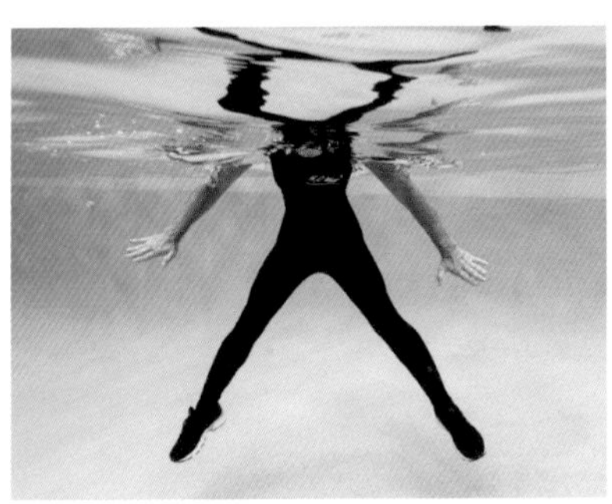

Propelled: A movement propelled up and out of the water. This is plyometric-type training, a higher impact option.

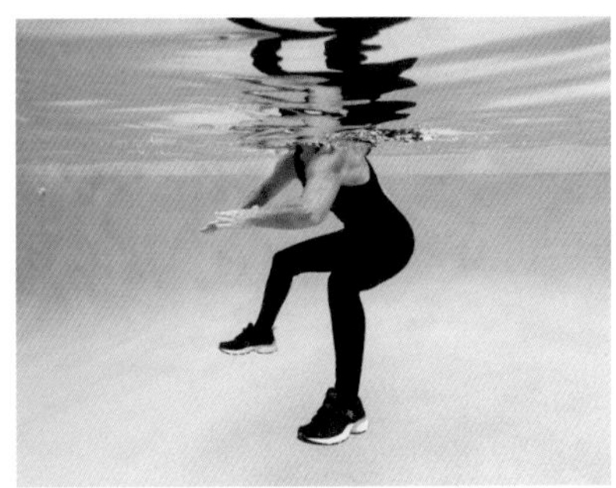

Power tuck: Variations of movements performed in level I, II and III to increase intensity and add variety. The knees pull forcefully toward the chest (tucking the knees toward the body) and then the legs push forcefully away and toward the pool bottom. In level I, power tucks increase impact, but in levels II and III, the impact is not altered.

Shallow-Water Impact Levels—Cross-Country Ski

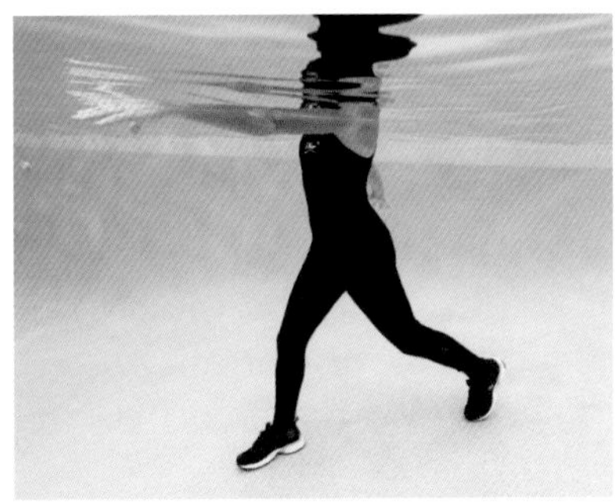

Level I: Level I movements are performed in an upright position with water level at waist to armpit depth. The degree of rebound (impact) can be altered with various methods.

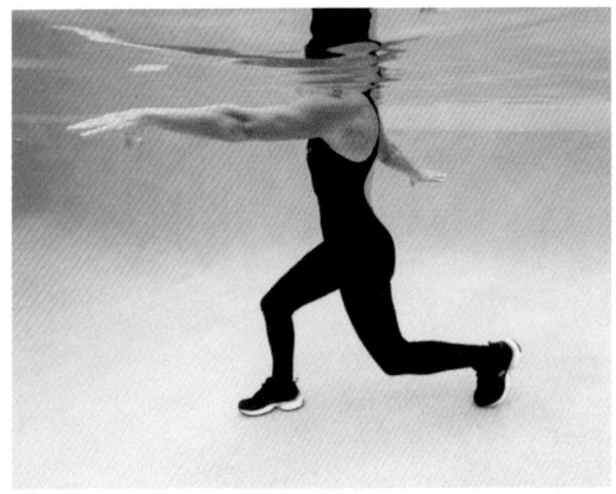

Level II: Level II movements are performed by flexing at the hips and knees to submerge the body to shoulder depth while executing the move, which is a low-impact option.

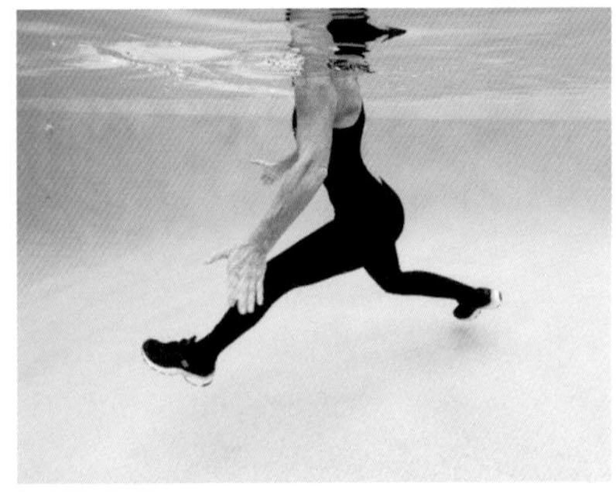

Level III: Level III movements are performed without touching the pool bottom (suspended).This is a nonimpact option.

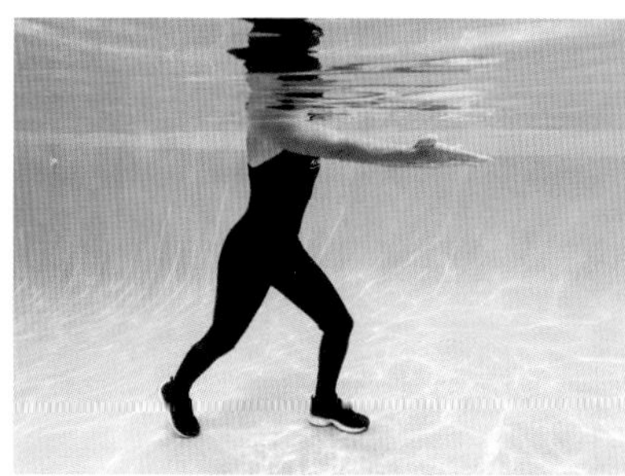

Grounded or anchored: Grounded moves are performed with one foot in contact with the pool bottom at all times. The variation pictured is a tap behind, a low-impact option.

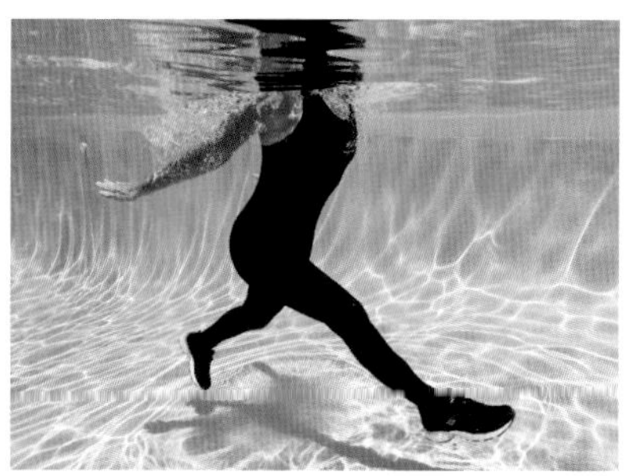

Propelled: A movement propelled up and out of the water. This is plyometric-type training, a higher impact option.

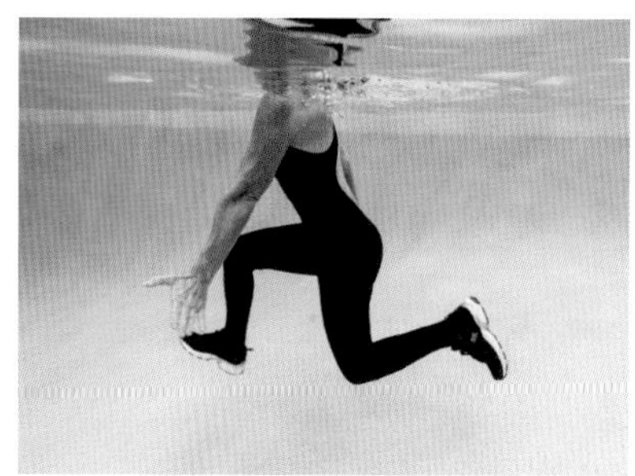

Power tuck: Variations of movements are performed in levels I, II and III to increase intensity and add variety. The knees pull forcefully toward the chest (tucking the knees toward the body) and then the legs push forcefully away and toward the pool bottom. In level I, power tucks increase impact, but in levels II and III, the impact is not altered.

Shallow-Water Cardiorespiratory Exercises (Shown at Level I)

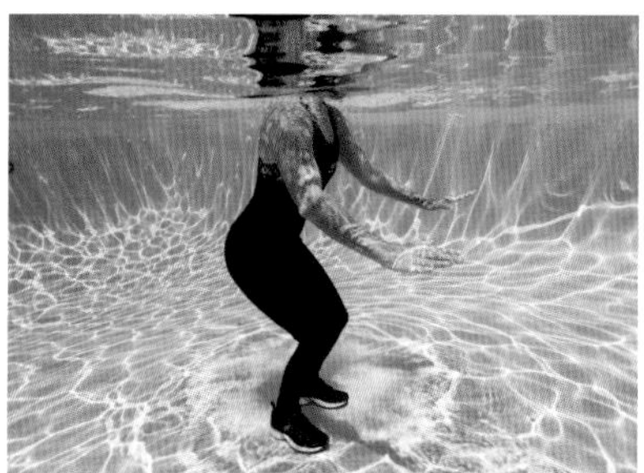

Bounce: Jumping with both feet. A common transitional move, the bounce can be performed in place or traveling, alternating front to back or side to side, or with many variations, such as a twist (rotating the body from side to side) or a tuck (pulling knees toward the chest).

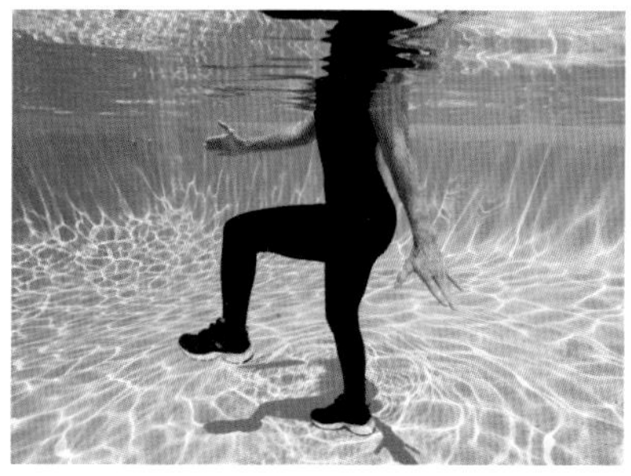

Knee lift or knee-high jog: Alternately lift the knees in front of the body while shifting the weight from one foot to the other. A low-impact alternative is a march in which the body does not rebound off the pool bottom.

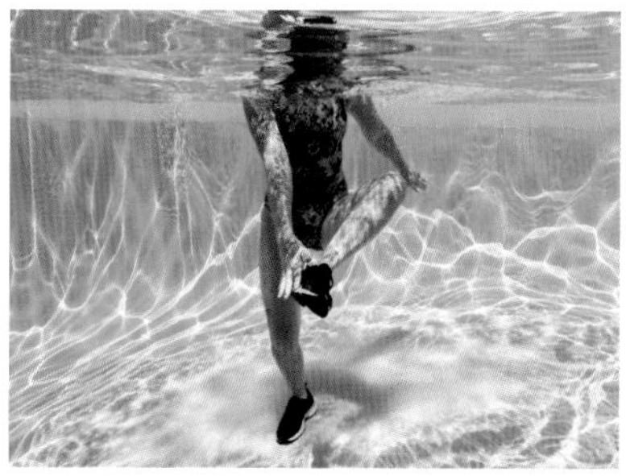

Ankle reach front: Variation of the knee lift or knee-high jog in which the hip externally rotates as the knee lifts; the opposite hand reaches toward the ankle.

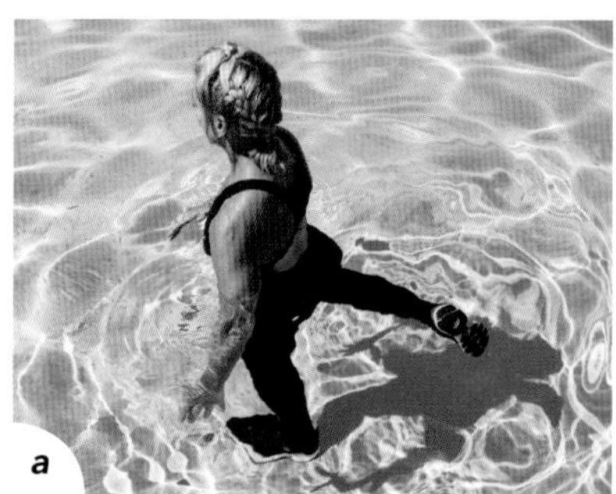

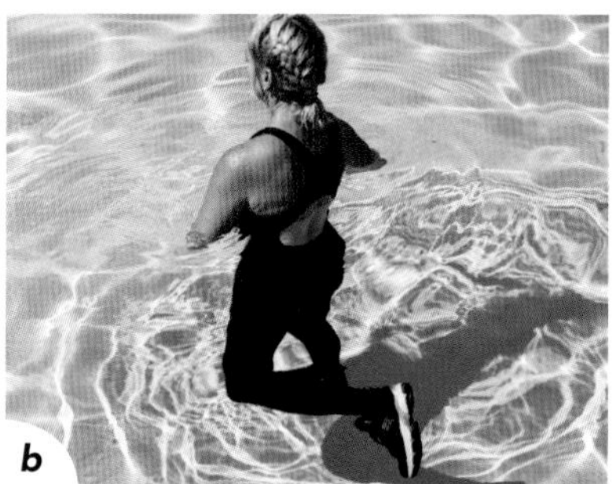

Leg curl or heel-high jog: *(a)* Alternately lift the heels behind the body while shifting the weight from one foot to the other. *(b)* Lift heels behind to about knee height; bringing heels up to the buttocks might cause stress to the knees. Compared to the knee lift or knee-high jog, this move focuses more on the posterior leg muscles.

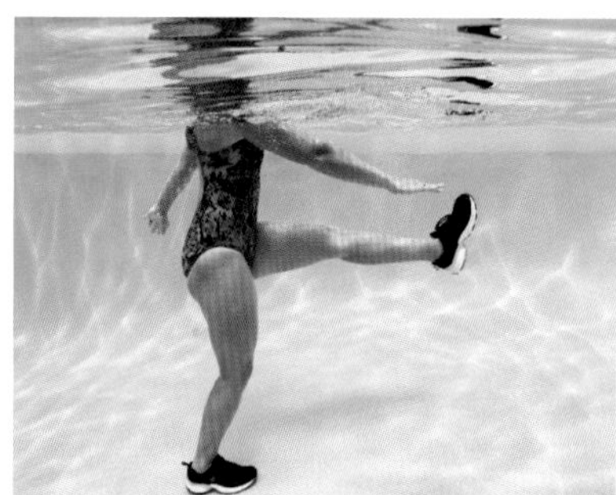

Kick front (straight leg): Kick forward of the body by flexing at the hip; the knee is extended but not locked. Focusing on the pull downward (hip extension) places more emphasis on the gluteals and hamstrings. Perform alternating between sides or with several reps on one leg before changing sides.

(continued)

Shallow-Water Cardiorespiratory Exercises (Shown at Level I) *(continued)*

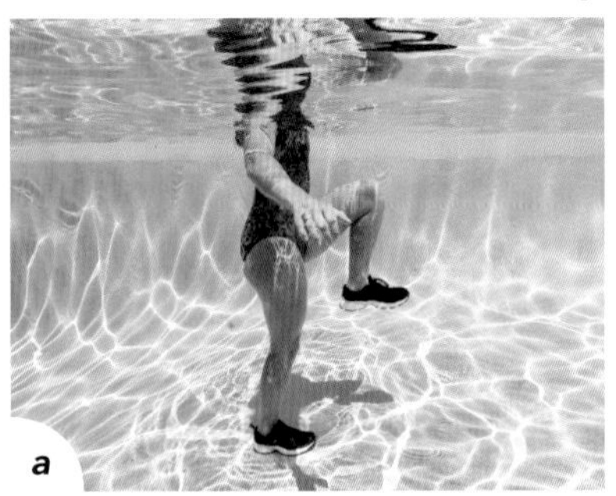
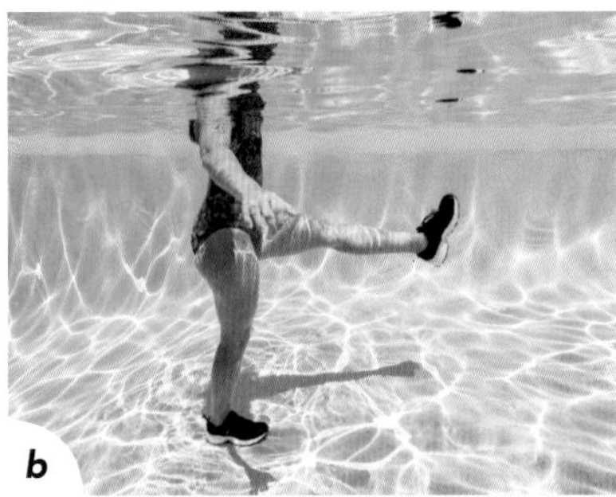
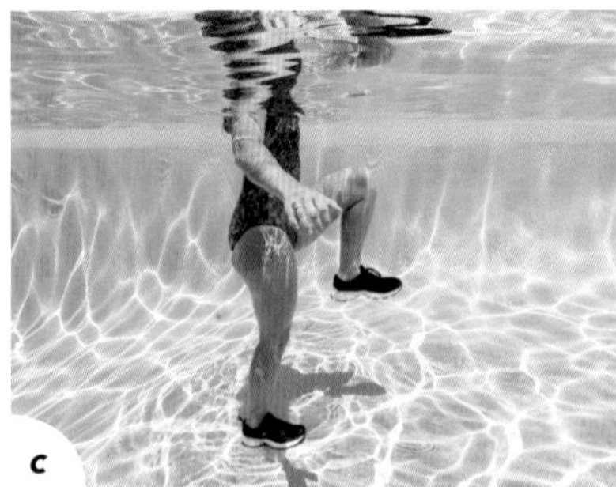

Kick front (karate): This move differs from the kick front (straight leg) by involving movement at the knee *and* the hip joint. The leg has for positions: *(a)* knee and hip flexion, *(b)* knee extension, *(c)* knee flexion, and return to start. Perform alternating between sides or with several reps on one leg before changing sides.

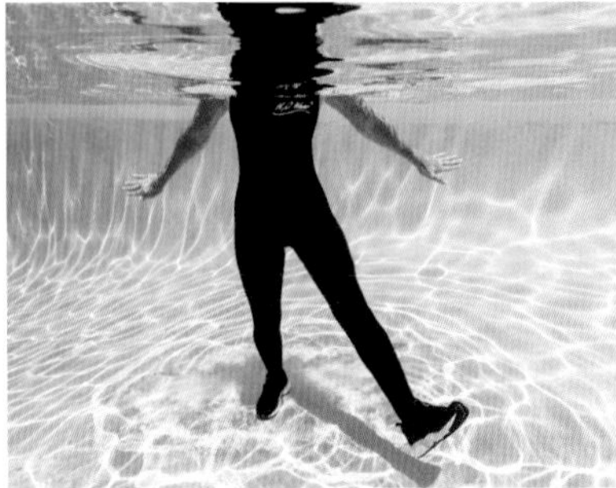

Kick corner: This move is a variation of the kick front (straight leg); here, the leg kicks toward the outside corner rather than forward. Perform alternating between sides or with several reps on one leg before changing sides.

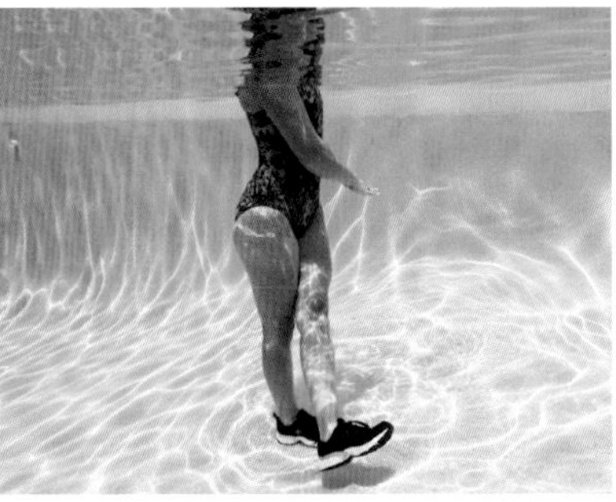

Kick across: This move is a variation of the kick front (straight leg); here, the leg kicks across the front of the body rather than straight ahead. Because this move crosses the body's midline with the legs, it may not be appropriate for all participants. Perform alternating between sides or with several reps on one leg before changing sides.

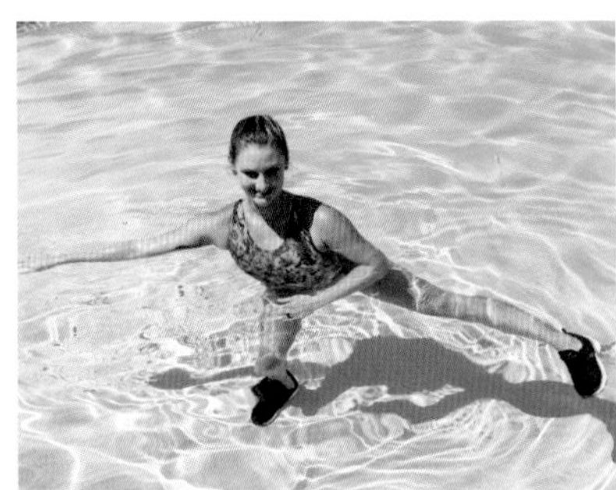

Kick side: Kick laterally by abducting at the hip; the knee is extended but not locked. Avoid rotation of the hip; the toes should face forward, not up toward the pool's surface. Variation: kick side (karate). Perform alternating between sides or with several reps on one leg before changing sides.

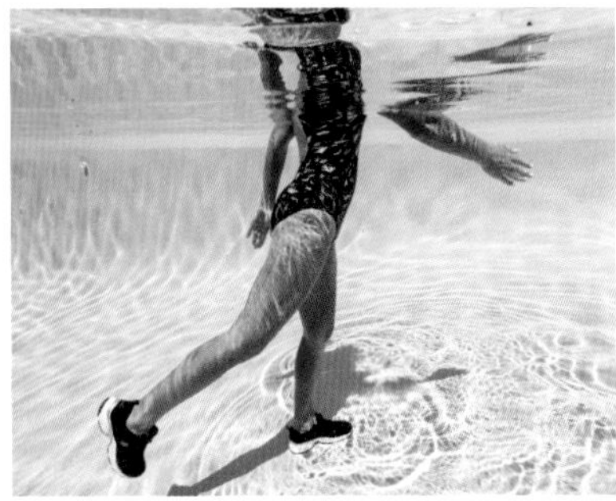

Kick back: Kick behind the body. Keep kick low enough that lower back (lumbar) does not hyperextend during the move; movement is at the hip joint. Bringing one or both arms forward also assists in maintaining spinal alignment. Variation: back kick (karate). Perform alternating between sides or with several reps on one leg before changing sides.

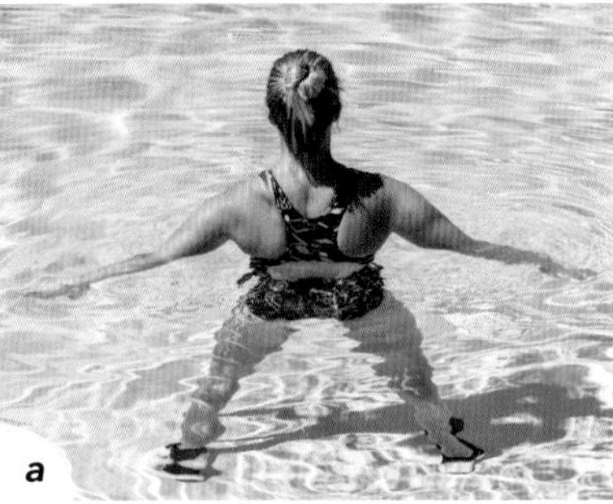
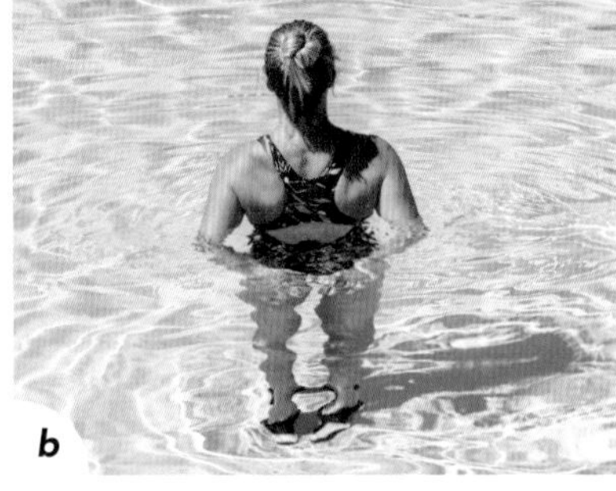

Jumping jack: *(a)* Jump with feet apart into straddle position and then *(b)* jump bringing the feet together. There are many variations of this movement including jumping jack with ankle crossovers (alternately crossing one foot in front of the other) and other variations using tempo, impact, and arm patterns (such as the arm adducting behind the body as show in photo *b*).

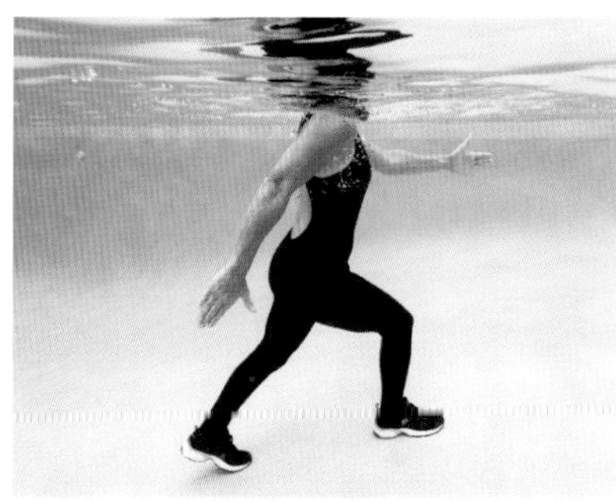

Cross-country ski: Jump with feet apart into a stride position (one leg forward, the other leg behind) and then jump to switch leg positions. There are many variations of this movement using different tempo, impact, and arm patterns.

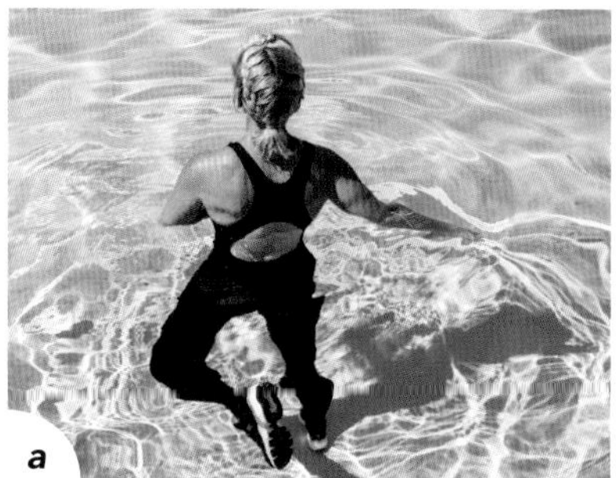

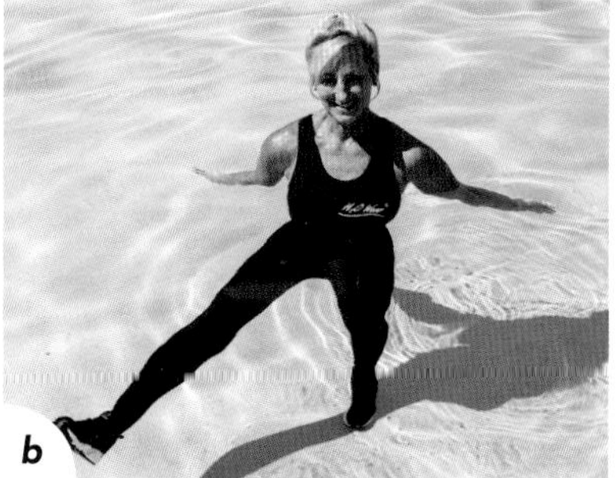

Jazz kick corner: *(a)* Lift one heel behind the body toward opposite buttock (back view). *(b)* Swing that leg diagonally (to the outside corner) forward (hip flexion) and extend the leg at the knee. Alternate legs, avoiding hyperextending the lower back (lumbar) and overextending the knees.

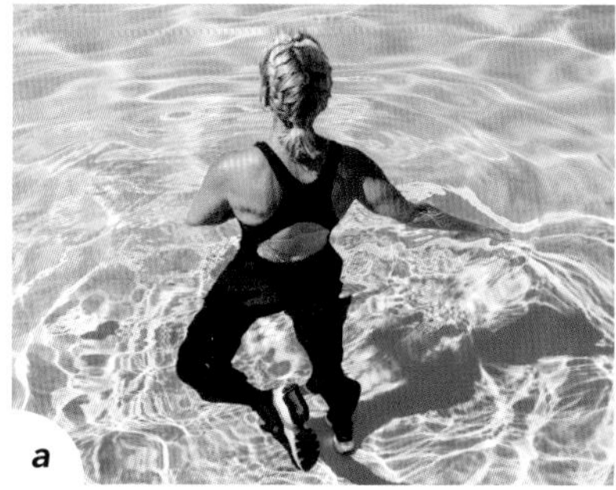

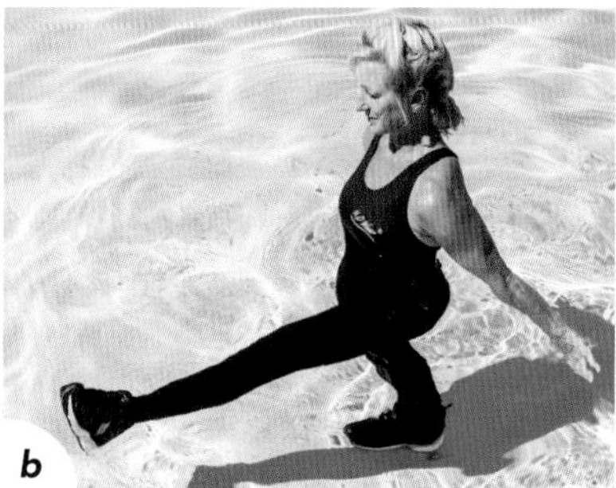

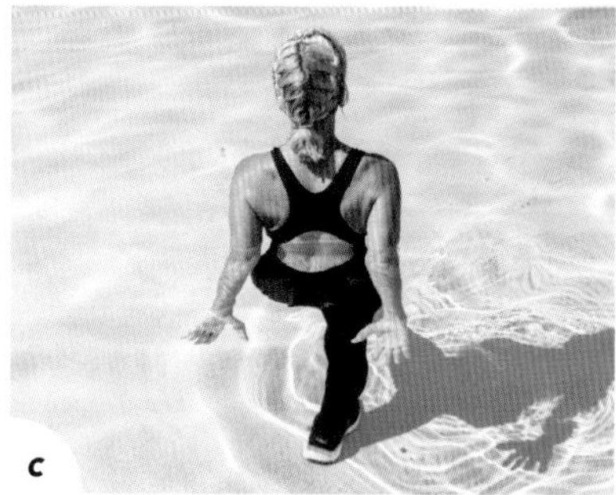

Jazz kick front: *(a)* Lift one heel behind the body. *(b)* Swing the leg forward (hip flexion) and extend the leg at the knee. Alternate legs, avoiding hyperextending the lower back (lumbar) and overextending the knees. *(c)* Arms can both press behind at the same time as the kicks forward; this can assist with balance and coordination, and add emphasis to the posterior muscles of the upper body.

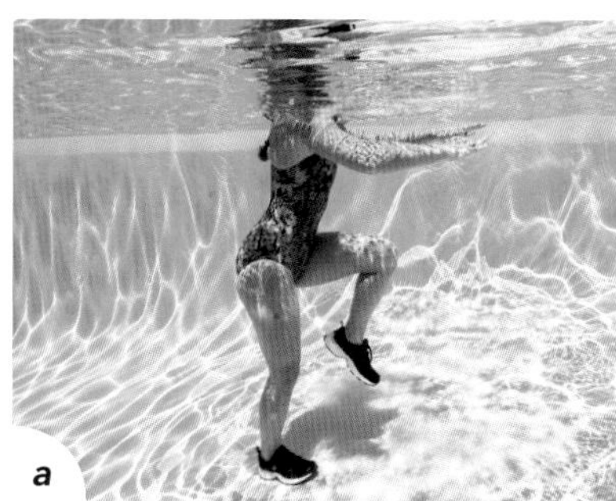

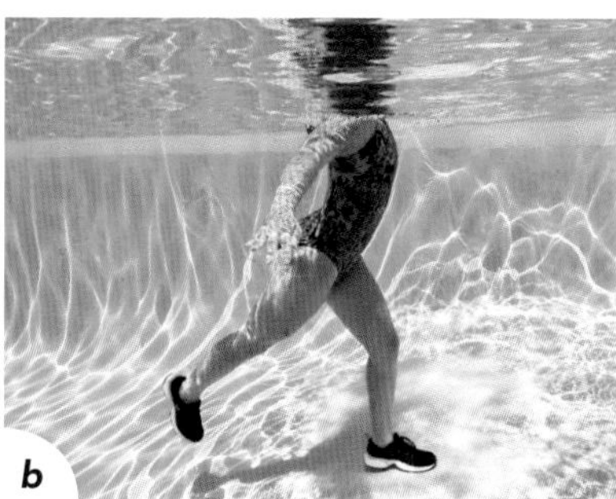

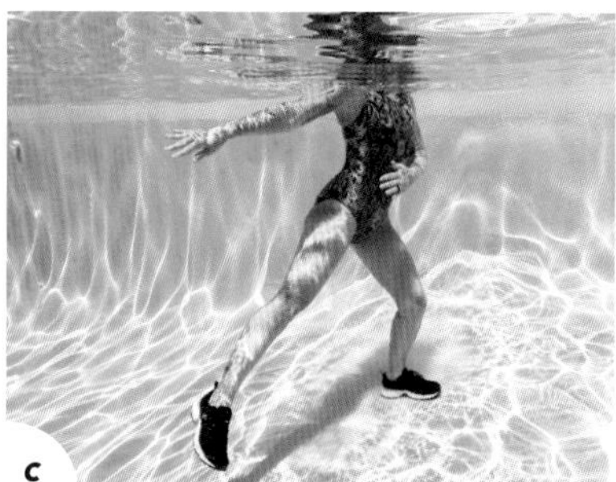

Leap: *(a)* Push off the right leg to travel forward; *(b)* land on the left leg. Step the right foot forward to meet the left; by shifting the weight to the right foot, the movement is ready to repeat. *(c)* Variation: perform the leap laterally. Repeat with the opposite leg pattern.

(continued)

Shallow-Water Cardiorespiratory Exercises (Shown at Level I) *(continued)*

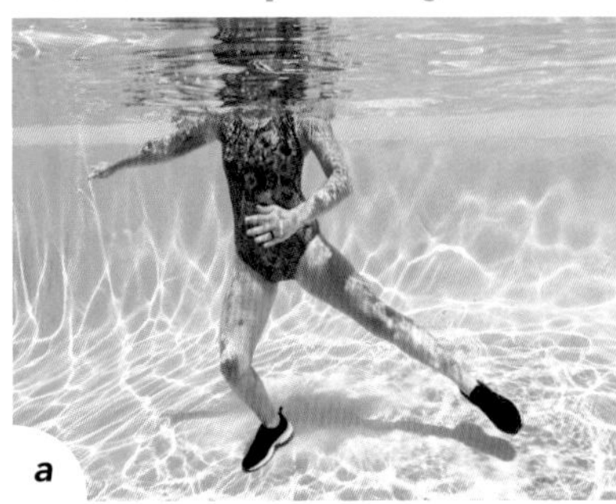
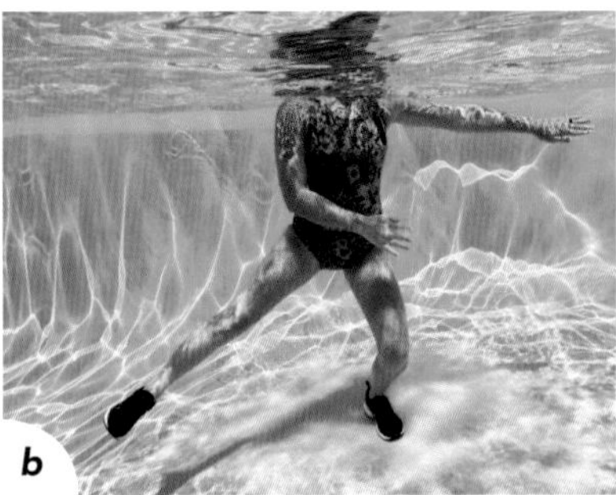

Pendulum: *(a)* Bounce on the right foot and lift the left leg laterally (hip abduction). *(b)* Pull the left leg toward the midline (hip adduction) and bounce on the left foot while lifting the right leg laterally. Shift weight from side to side like a pendulum.

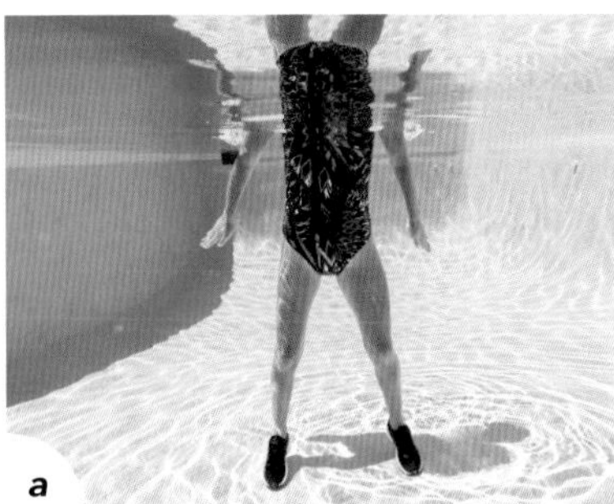
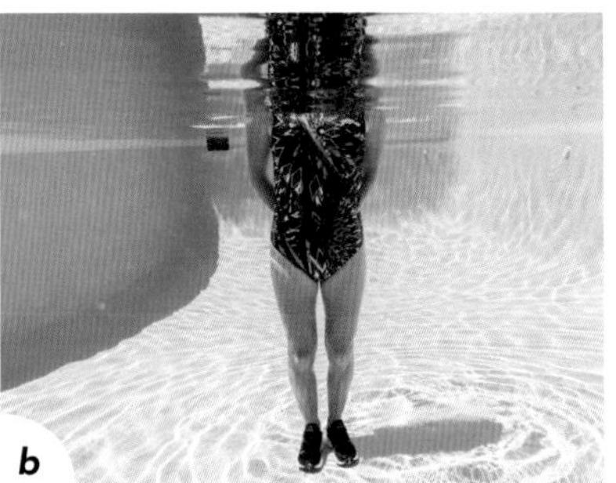

Side step: *(a)* Step right leg out to side. *(b)* Pull left leg in to meet the right. Step out with right leg again and continue to travel laterally the desired distance. Repeat with opposite lead.

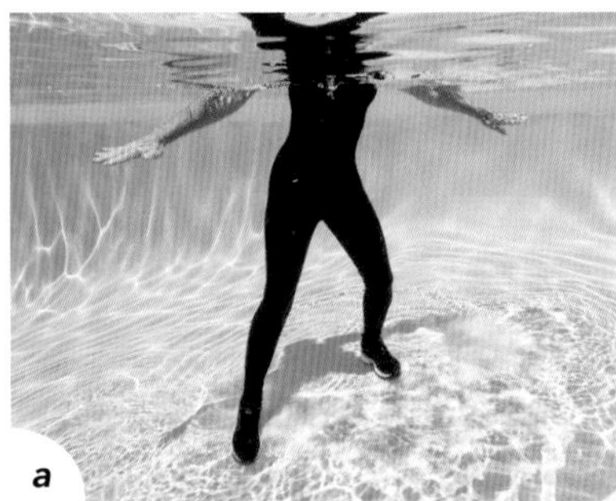
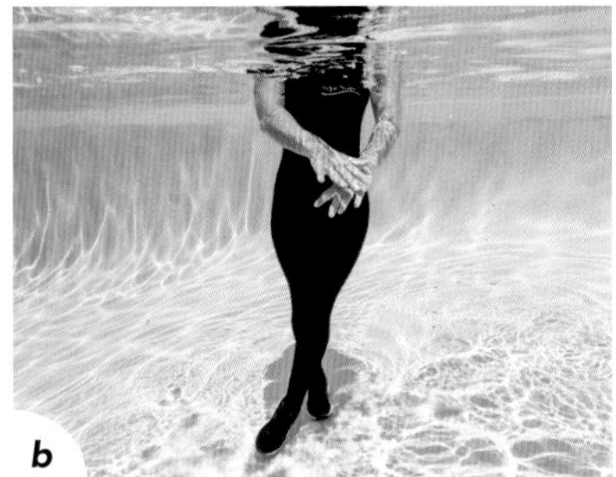

Step and cross: *(a)* Step right leg out to side. *(b)* Step left leg across the right; alternate crossing in front and behind. Repeat with opposite lead. Because this move crosses the body's midline with the legs, it may not be appropriate for all participants.

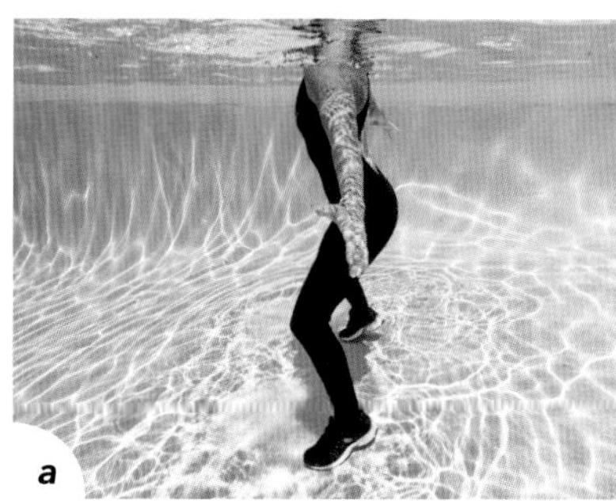
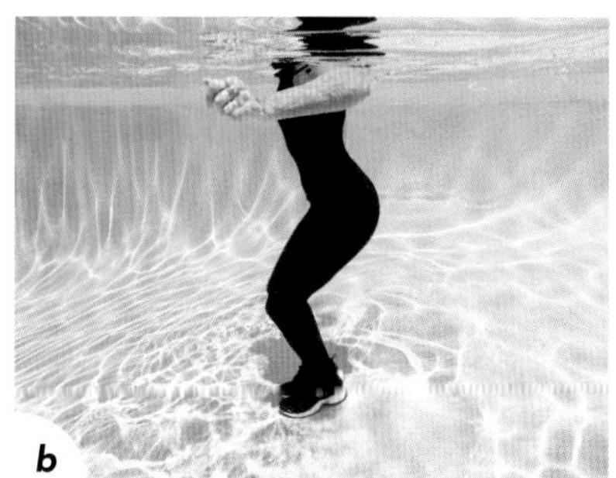
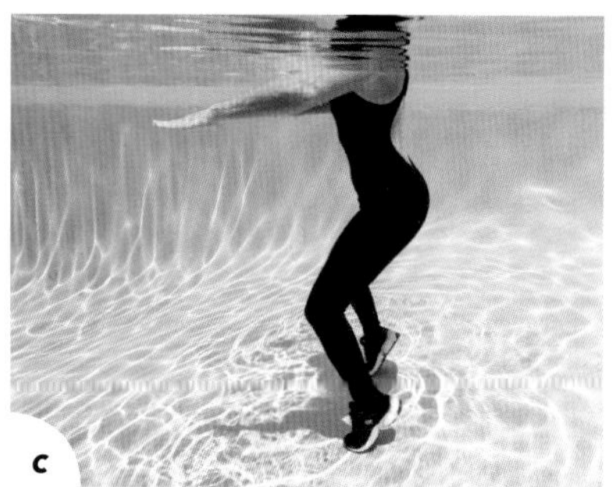

Slide: Similar to the side step but involves a rebounding action and the rhythm is syncopated. *(a)* More emphasis is placed on the lead leg and *(b)* dragging (sliding) the trailing leg in to meet the lead leg. *(c)* **Glide:** Level II variation on the toes with hips externally rotated.

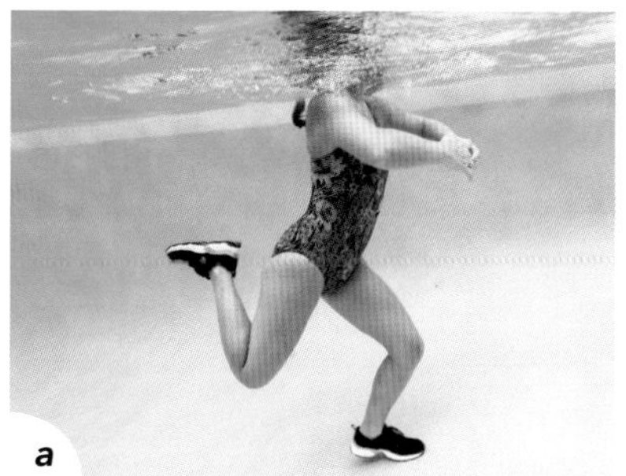
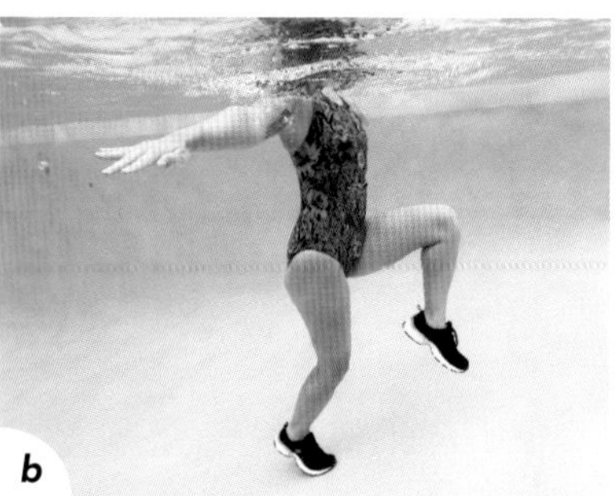

Rocking horse: *(a)* Rock the weight forward onto the left leg while lifting the right heel up behind the body. *(b)* Rock backward onto the right leg while lifting the left knee up in front of the body. Alternate the rocking motion several repetitions before switching to the opposite side.

Shallow-Water Toning Exercises (Muscle Conditioning)

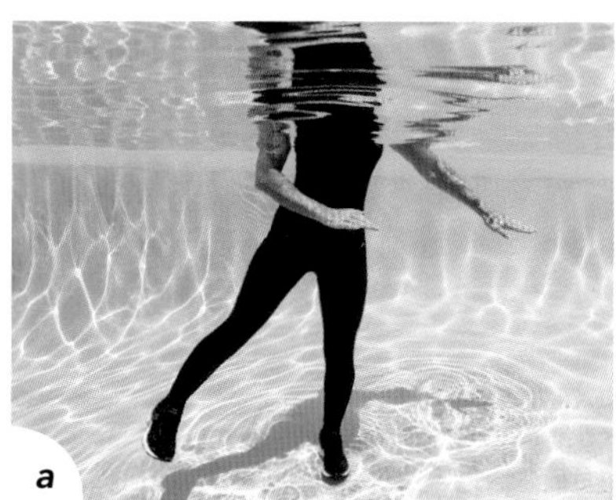
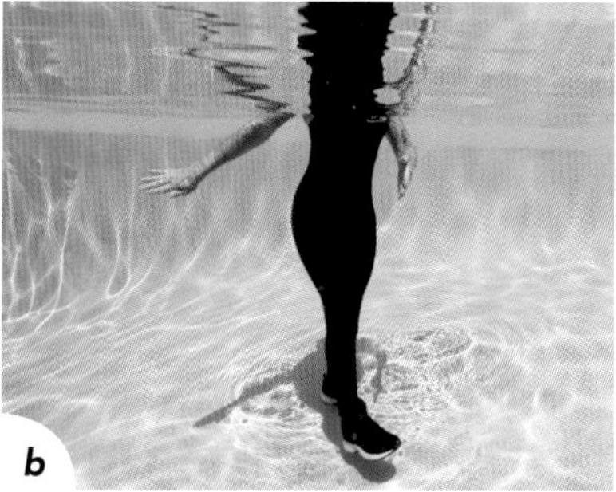
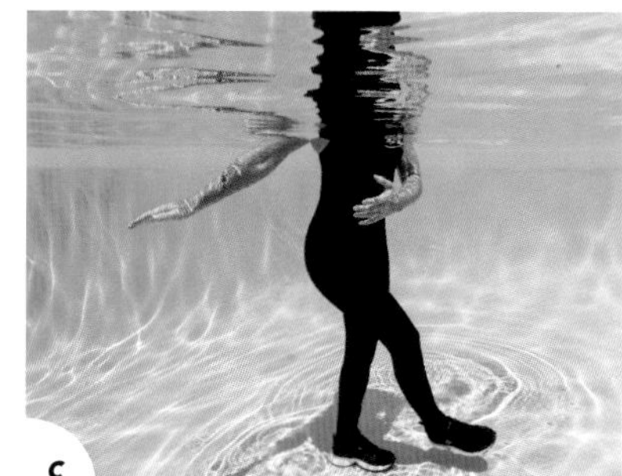

Hip abduction and adduction (hip abductors and adductors): *(a)* Lift the leg to the side with toes facing forward and *(b)* pull back down to center. *(c)* Crossing the midline is a variation of the move, but it may not be appropriate for all participants. Repeat on both legs.

(continued)

Shallow-Water Toning Exercises (Muscle Conditioning) *(continued)*

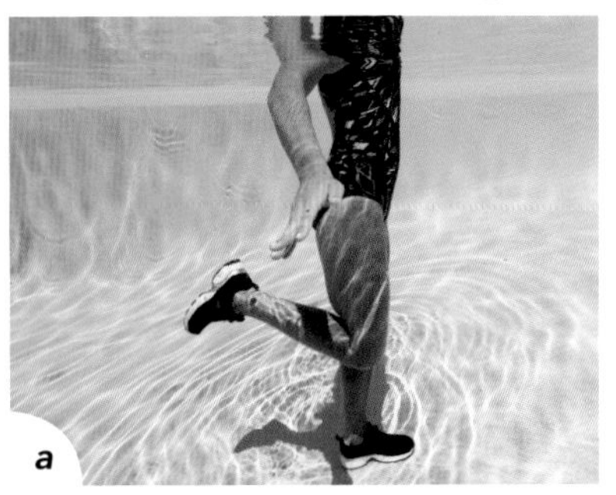
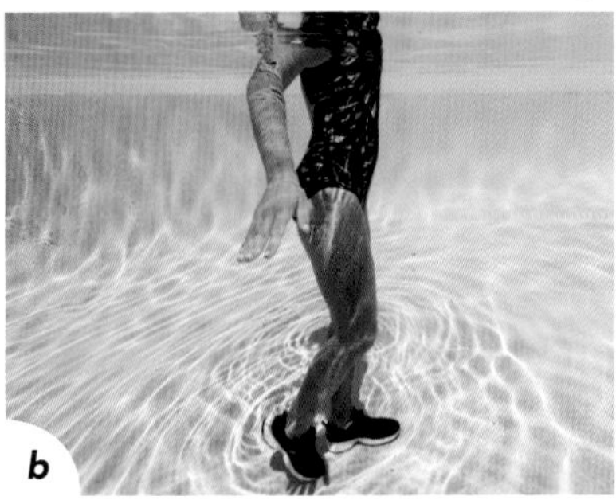
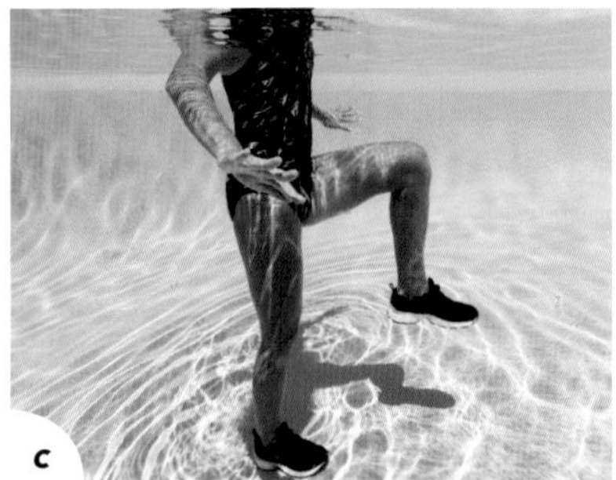

Knee flexion and extension (hamstrings and quadriceps): *(a)* Lift the heel toward the buttocks and *(b)* then return to the extended position. Variation: Begin with hip flexed (leg lifted in front of body), *(c)* bend the knee, and then straighten the leg. Repeat on both legs.

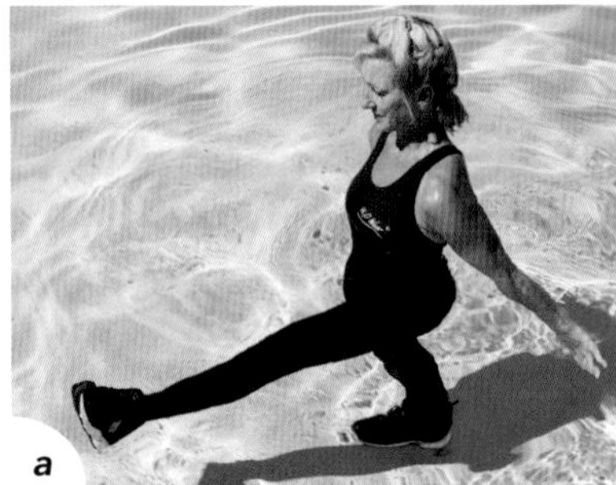
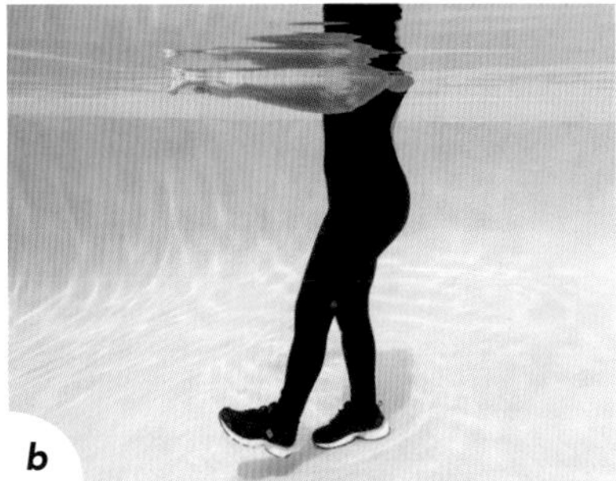
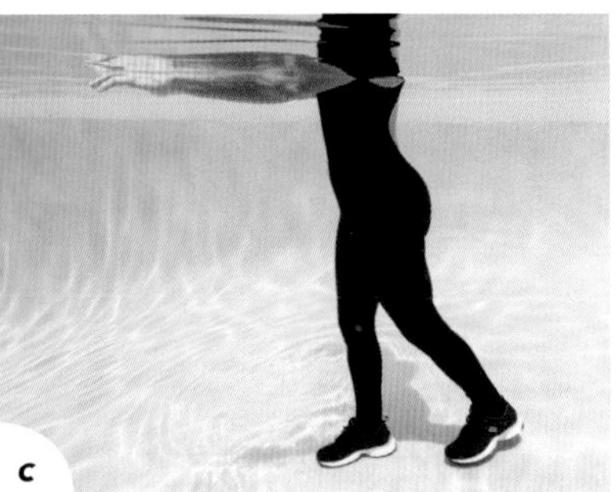

Hip flexion, extension, and hyperextension (iliopsoas and gluteals): *(a)* Flex leg at the hip. *(b)* Extend at the hip by pulling the leg down and *(c)* then slightly to the back of the body into hyperextension. Repeat on both legs.

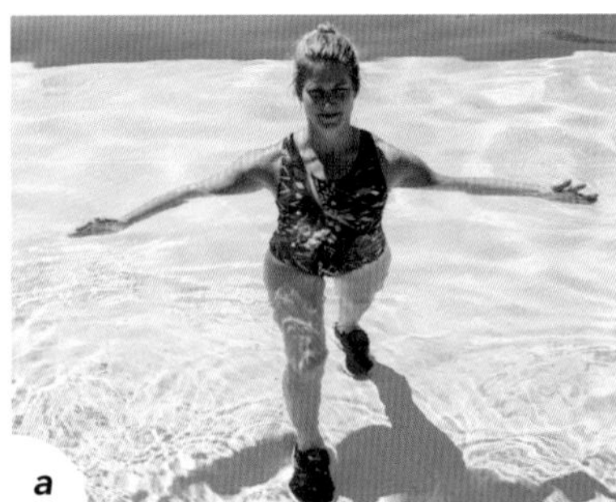
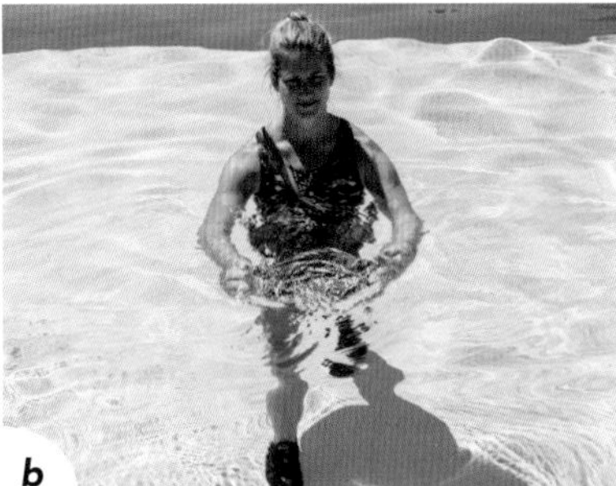
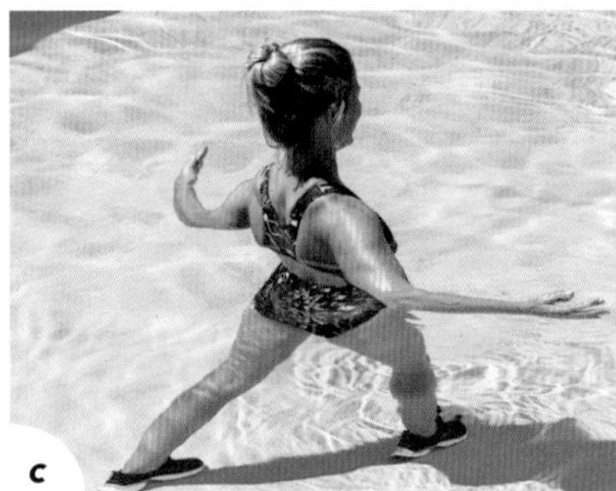

Transverse shoulder abduction and adduction (pectoralis, anterior deltoid, and posterior deltoid): *(a)* Begin with shoulders abducted. *(b)* The arms pull forward, parallel to the pool bottom (transverse adduction), and then return to the *(a)* start position (transverse abduction). *(c)* Retracting the scapulae by squeezing the shoulder blades together will target the middle trapezius.

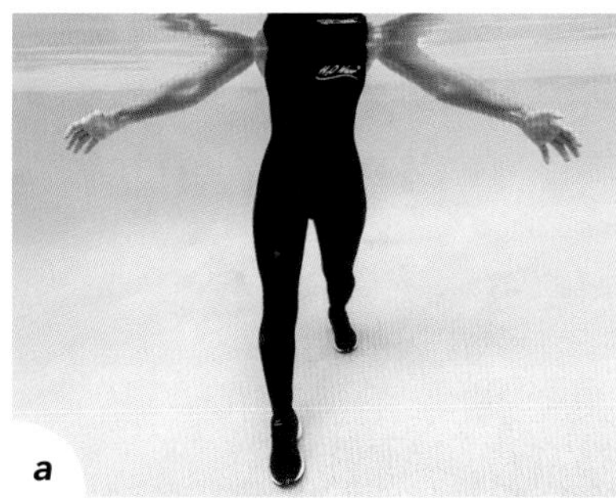
a

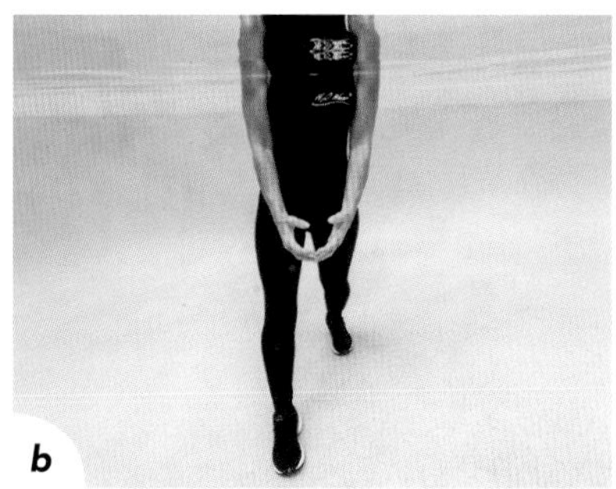
b

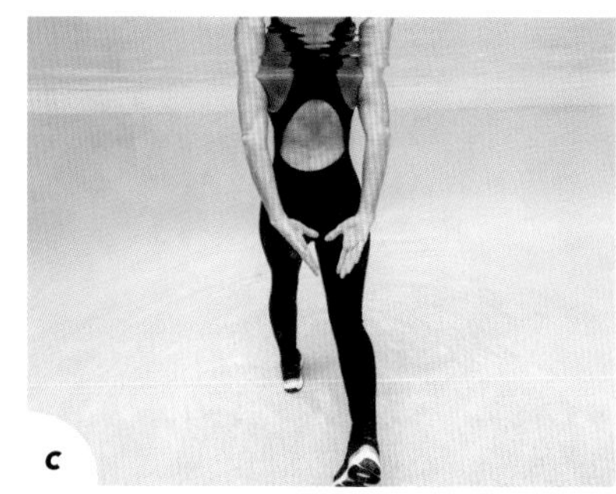
c

Shoulder abduction and adduction (deltoids and latissimus dorsi): *(a)* Lift arms laterally (abduction) and *(b)* pull the hands down to return to the sides in front of the body (adduction). Avoid lifting above shoulder height. Variation: Pull the hands down behind the body as shown in *(c)*.

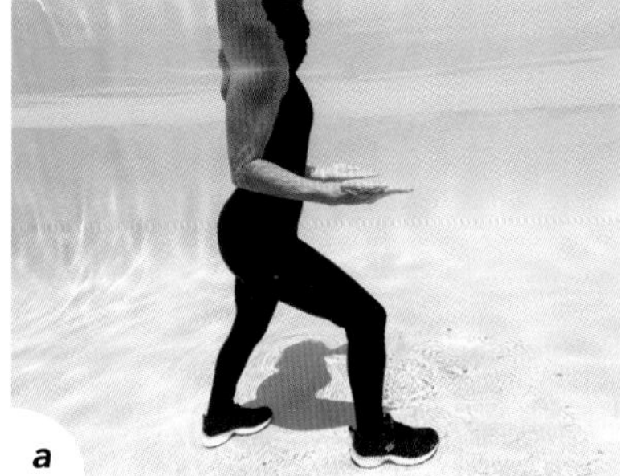
a

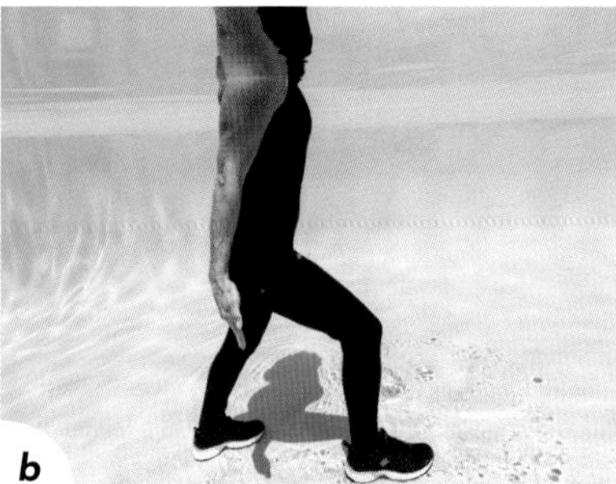
b

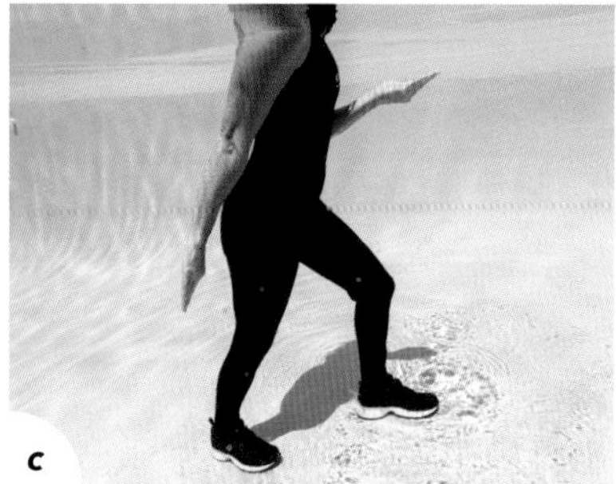
c

Elbow flexion and extension (biceps and triceps): *(a)* Bend or flex at the elbow with hands pulling forward. *(b)* Then straighten or extend the elbow with hands pressing down and back. *(c)* Variation: alternate arms.

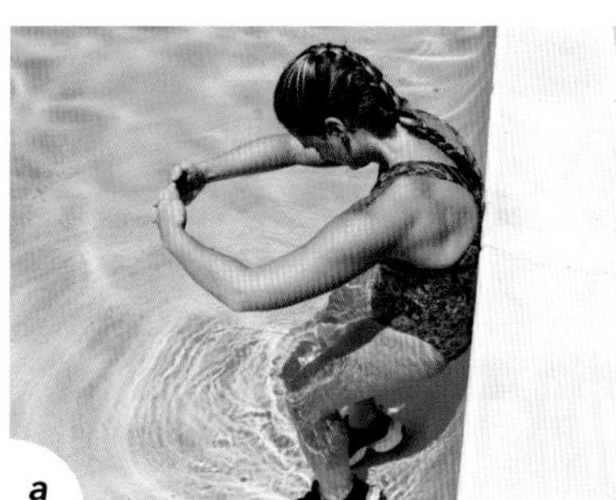
a

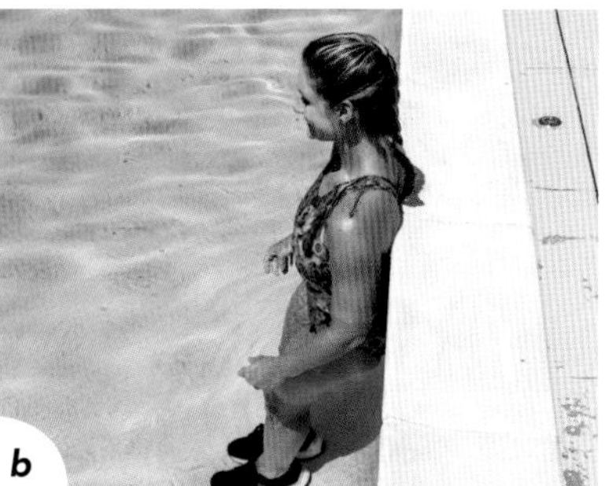
b

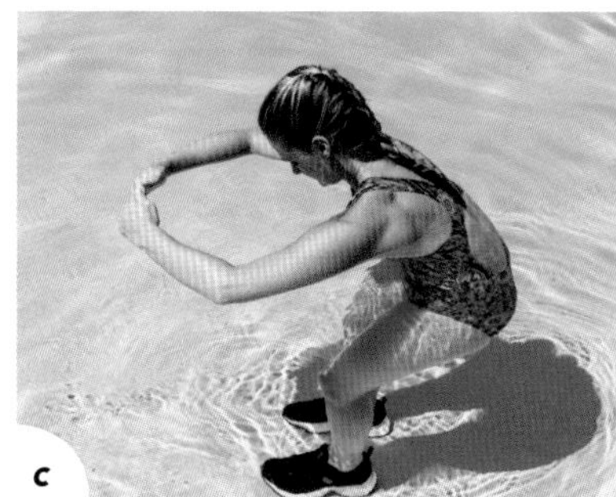
c

Standing spinal flexion and extension (rectus abdominis and erector spinae): *(a)* Flex the spine forward, bringing rib cage toward the pelvis; movement is along the spine, not at the hips. *(b)* Extend the spine, returning to upright position. Note: although the wall is a good reference point for learning this exercise *(c)*, this exercise can also be performed midpool.

(continued)

Shallow-Water Toning Exercises (Muscle Conditioning) *(continued)*

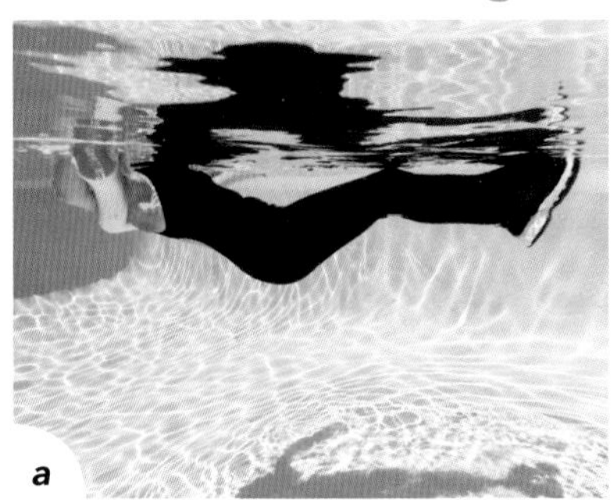
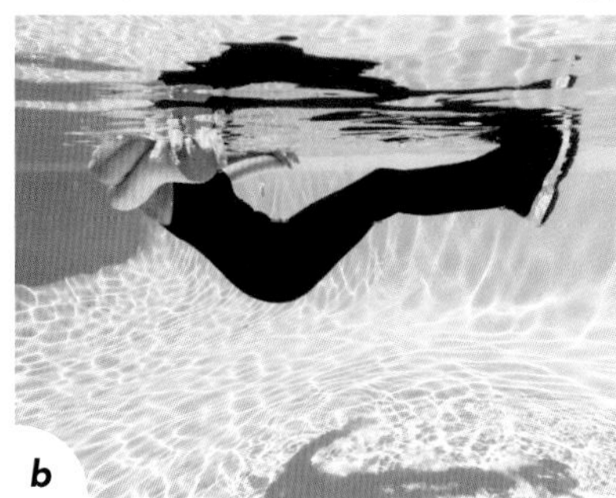
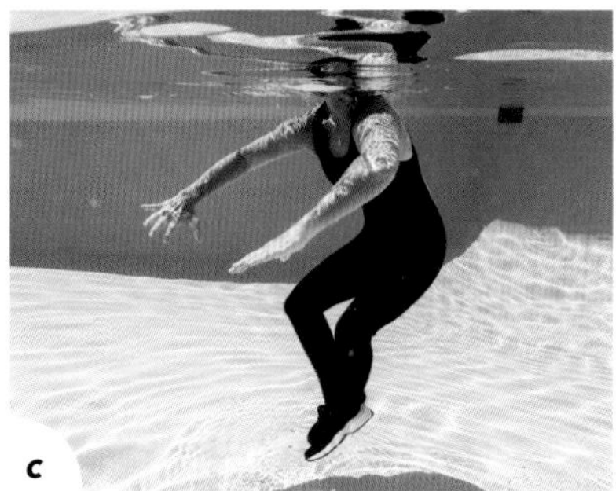

Supine spinal flexion and extension (rectus abdominis and erector spinae): *(a)* Begin suspended in a modified supine position. *(b)* Flex the spine forward, bringing rib cage toward the pelvis. *(c)* Variation: Perform suspended but in vertical position rather than supine.

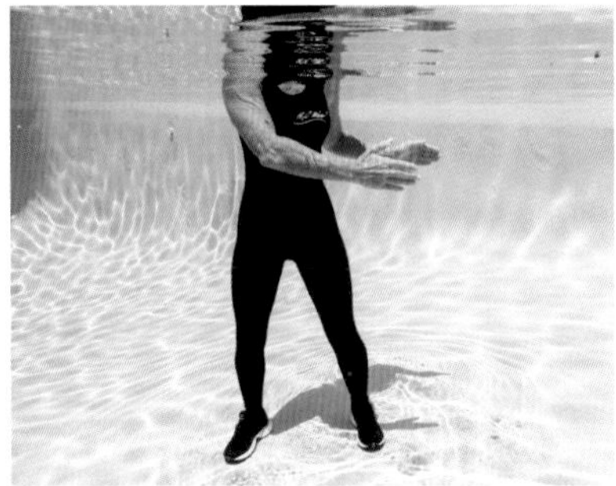

Spinal rotation (internal and external obliques): Perform rotational movement from the spine, making certain the hips remain forward. Repeat on the opposite side.

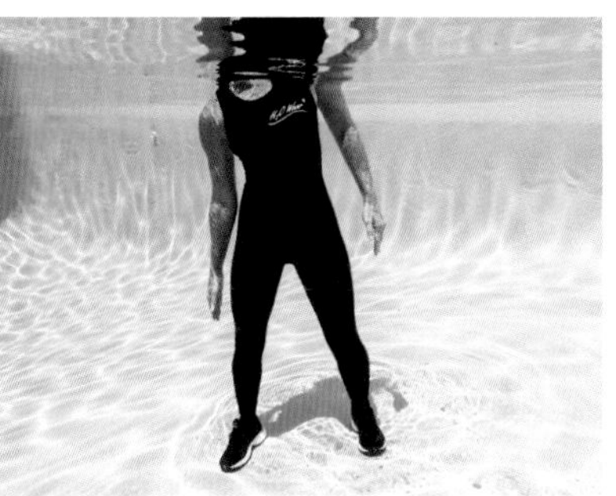

Spinal lateral flexion (quadratus lumborum and rectus abdominis): Lean the body to one side, remaining in the frontal plane (i.e., do not lean to the front or to the back). Repeat on the opposite side. Visualization cue: slide hand down side of leg.

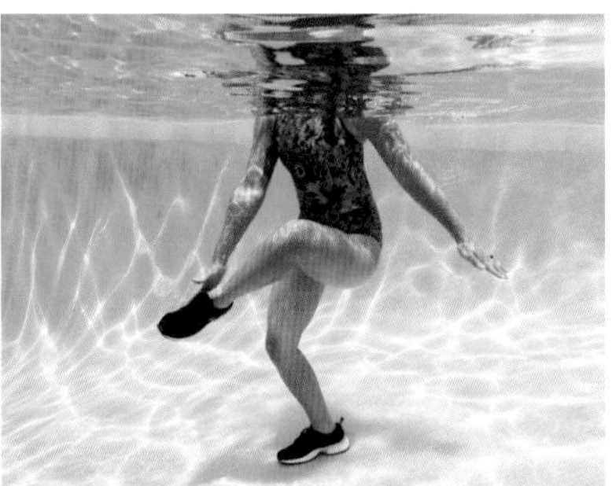

Spinal rotation and flexion (obliques, rectus abdominis, and erector spinae): Combine forward flexion with rotation by moving the shoulder toward the opposite hip. Return to the starting position and repeat on the opposite side. This combination of spinal functions may not be appropriate for all individuals.

Shallow-Water Stretches

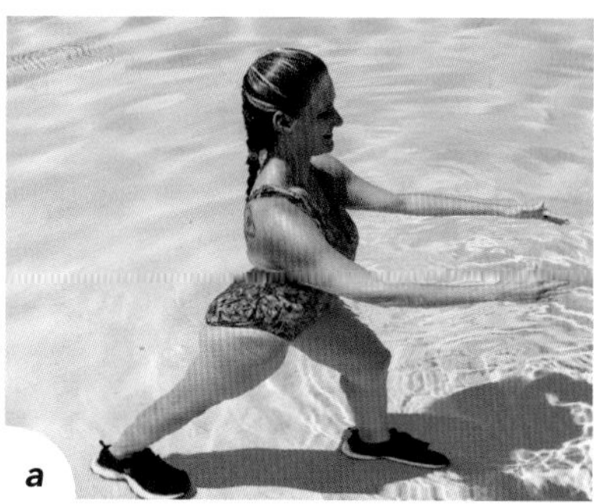

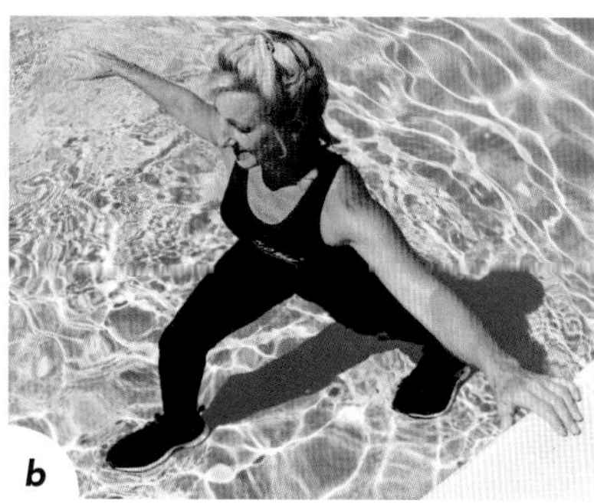

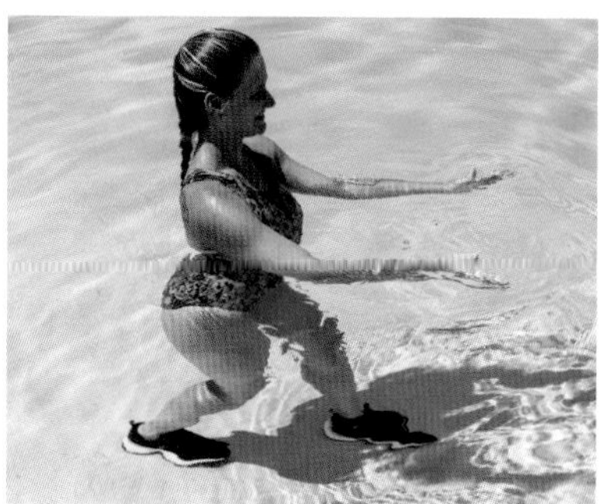

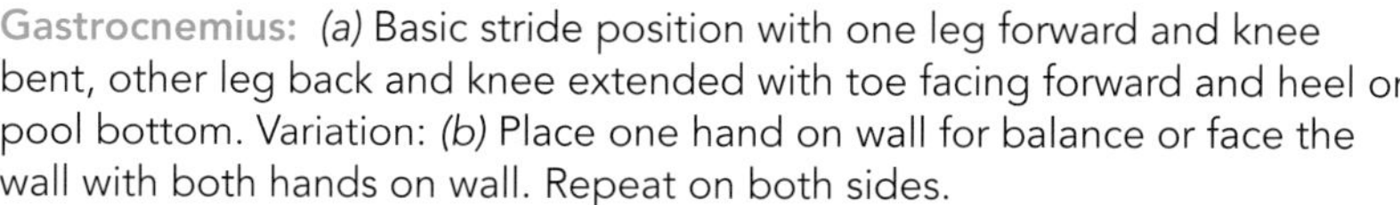

Gastrocnemius: *(a)* Basic stride position with one leg forward and knee bent, other leg back and knee extended with toe facing forward and heel on pool bottom. Variation: *(b)* Place one hand on wall for balance or face the wall with both hands on wall. Repeat on both sides.

Soleus: Beginning from the gastrocnemius stretch, slightly bend the back leg while keeping the heel down to stretch the soleus. Repeat on both sides.

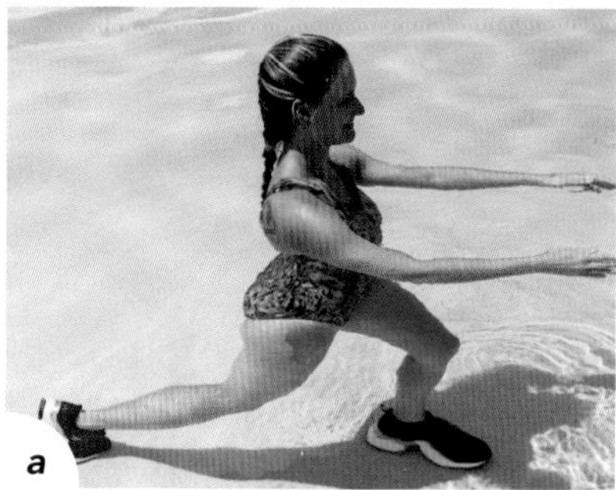

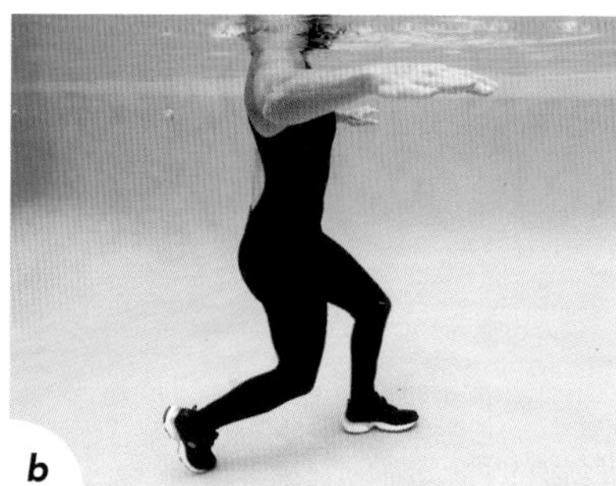

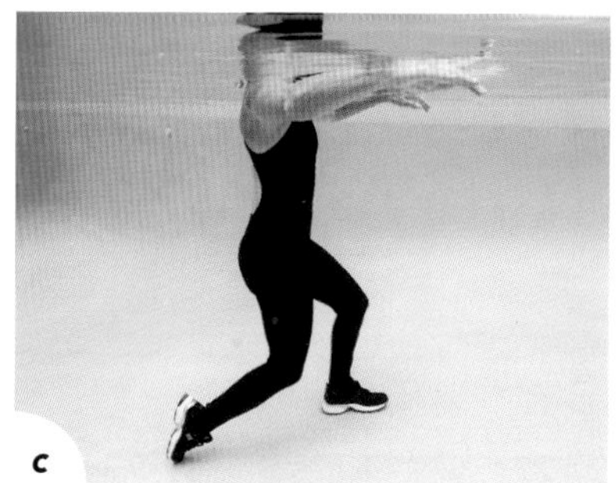

Quadriceps and iliopsoas, stride position: From a stride position, *(a)* lower the back knee and allow heel to lift; *(b)* tilt the pelvis (posterior tilt). Variation: *(c)* The top of the foot (dorsal surface) can be positioned toward pool bottom to incorporate a stretch for the tibialis anterior. Repeat on both sides.

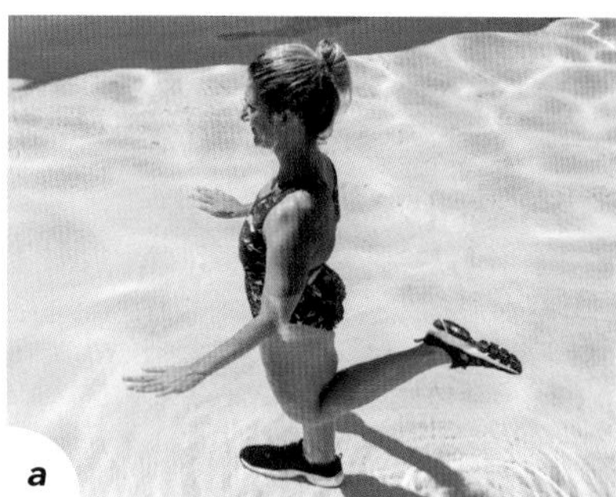

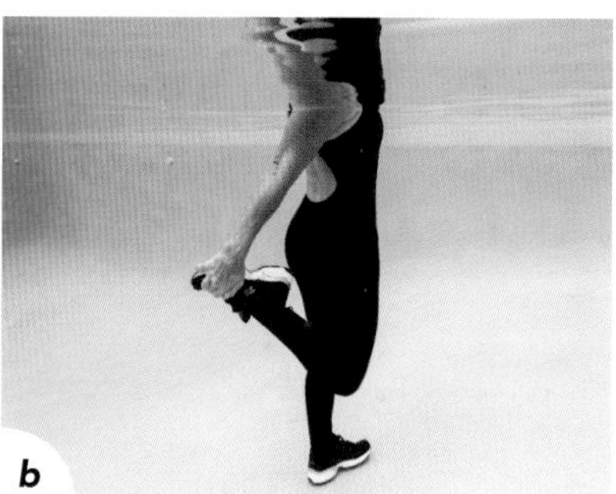

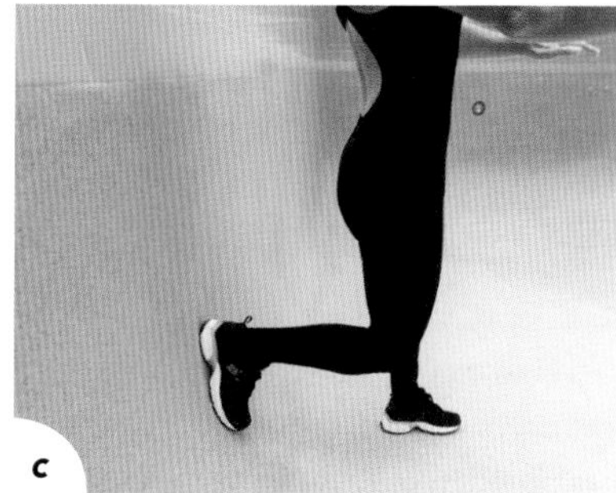

Quadriceps and iliopsoas, elevated foot position: *(a)* Lift one foot up behind the body with the knee pointed down and the pelvis tilted (posterior tilt). *(b)* If range of motion allows, the foot can be held with the hand. Option: *(c)* Foot can be placed on the pool wall. Repeat on both sides.

(continued)

Shallow-Water Stretches *(continued)*

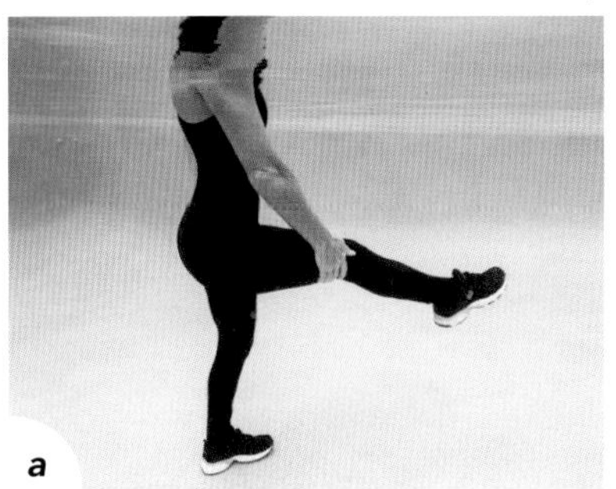
a

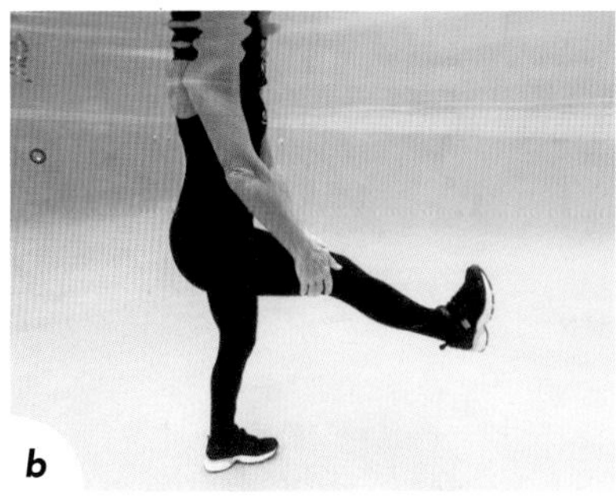
b

Hamstrings and gluteus maximus: Lift one leg up in front of the body (hip flexion with knee extension). Hold under the thigh for support if range of motion allows *(a)*. Dorsiflexing the ankle increases the stretch through the gastrocnemius *(b)*. Repeat on both sides.

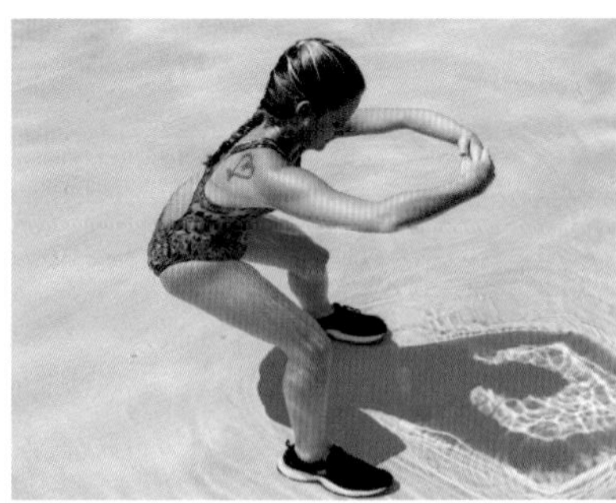

Lower back: Stand with knees soft and arms forward. Tilt the pelvis (posterior tilt) and tuck the tail bone to round the lower back.

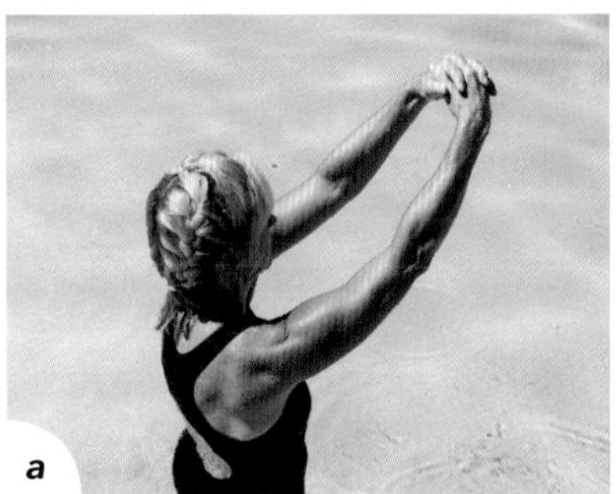
a

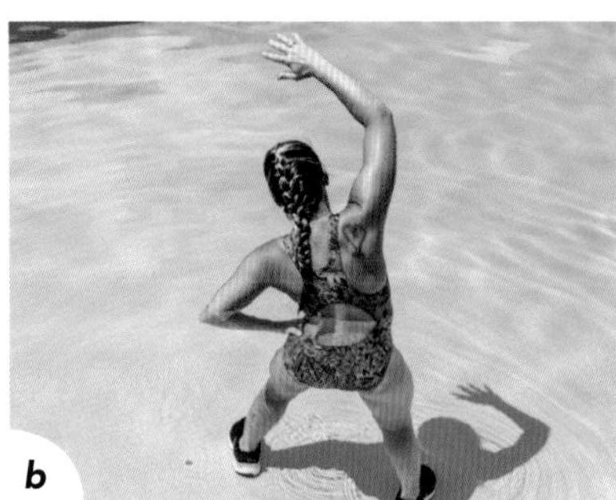
b

Latissimus dorsi: Raise both arms overhead and lift the rib cage upward. Remind participants to *(a)* keep arms slightly forward of the head to maintain proper alignment. Fingers can be interlocked or hands apart. *(b)* Variation: One-arm stretch.

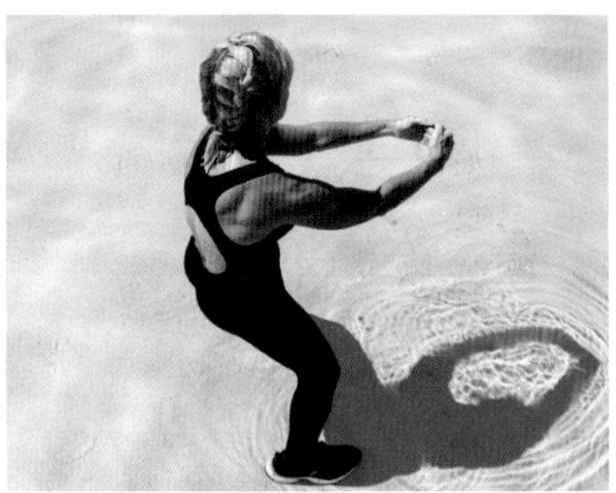

Middle trapezius: Press both arms forward, opening (protracting) the shoulder blades and rounding the upper back. The stretch can be intensified slightly by lowering the chin toward the chest.

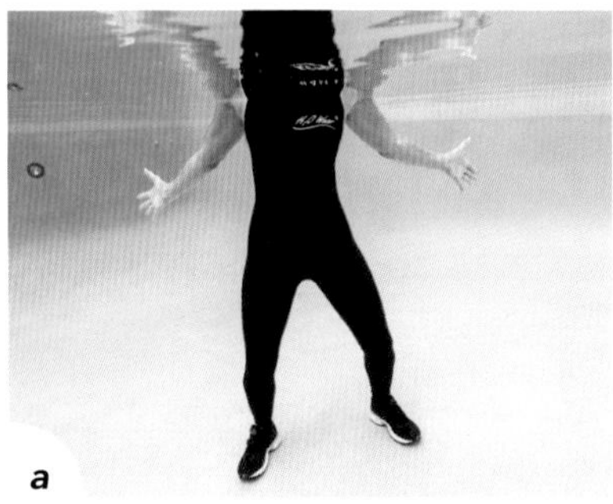
a

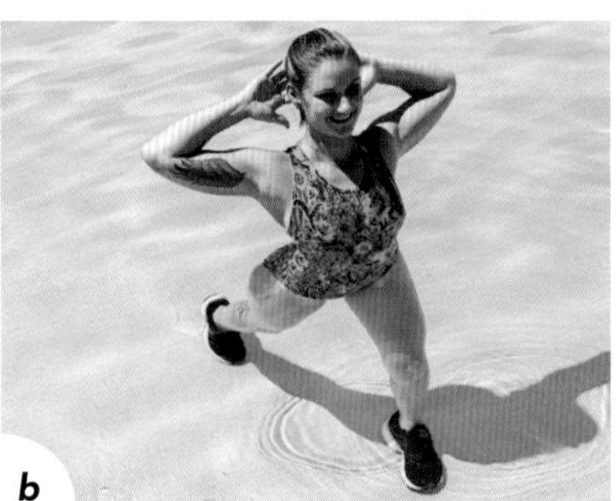
b

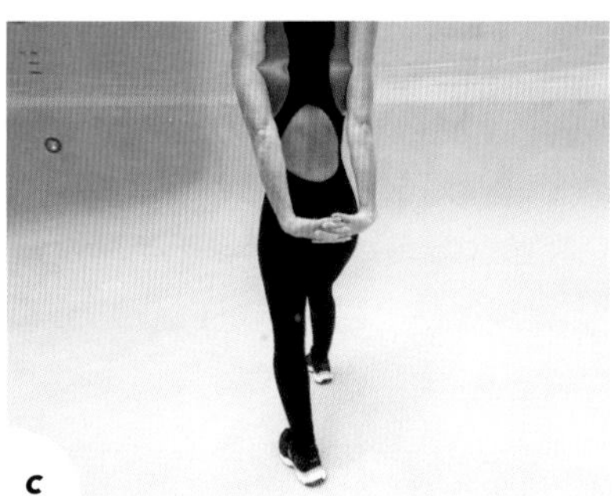
c

Pectoralis and anterior deltoid: *(a)* Abduct shoulders in transverse plane with thumbs turned up. Variations: *(b)* Place the hands behind the head and open the elbows wide, and *(c)* grasp the hands behind the back with the shoulders pulled down and back.

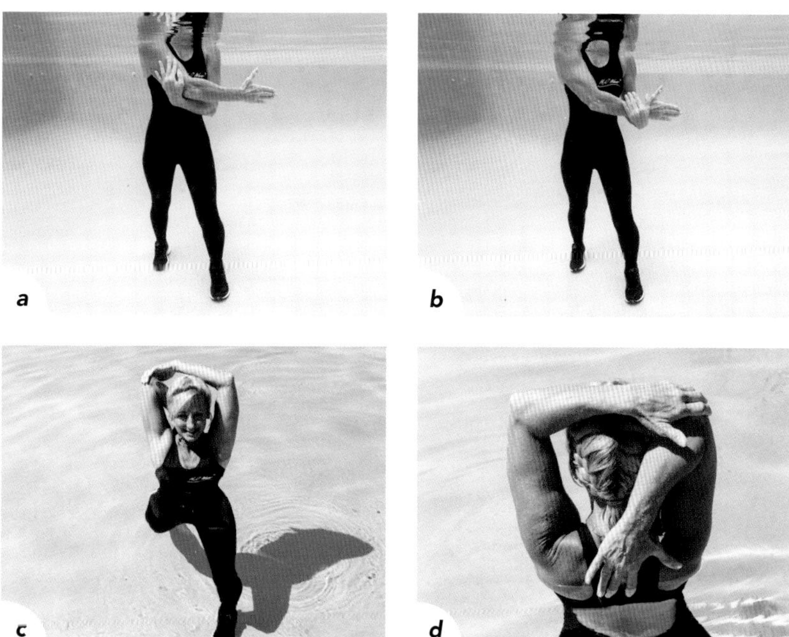

Triceps and posterior deltoid: Bring one arm across toward the opposite shoulder at midchest. *(a)* Gently pull with the other hand above the elbow or *(b)* at the forearm. Variation: *(c)* Drop one hand behind the head and push gently with the other hand above the elbow; *(d)* shows the back view. Repeat on both sides.

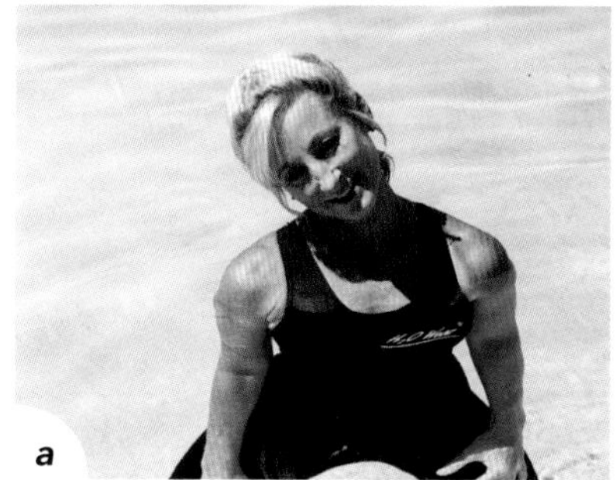

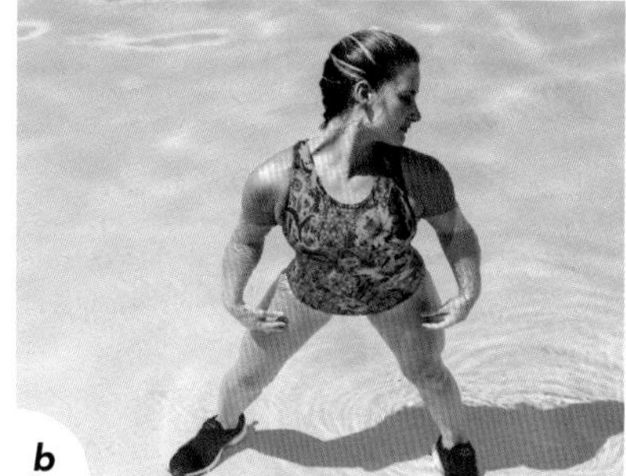

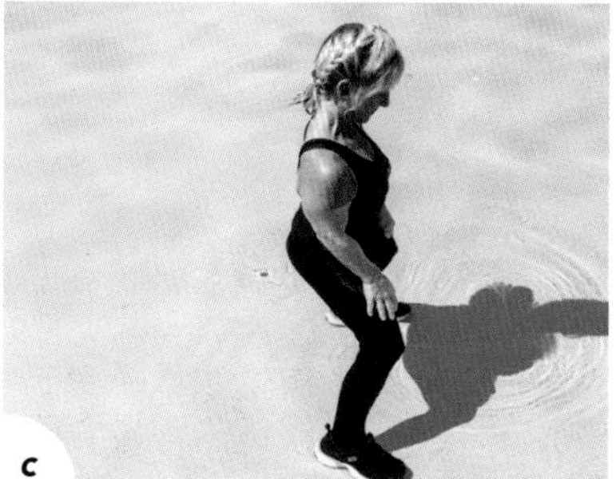

Upper trapezius and neck: *(a)* Tilt the head laterally to the right and left. *(b)* Rotate the head to look to the right and left. *(c)* Flex the neck forward and extend the neck to look up. Limit range of motion to comfortable position.

Appendix B

Deep-Water Exercise

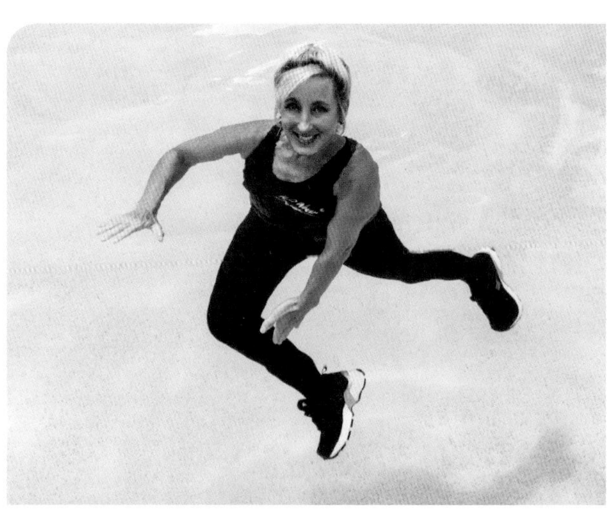

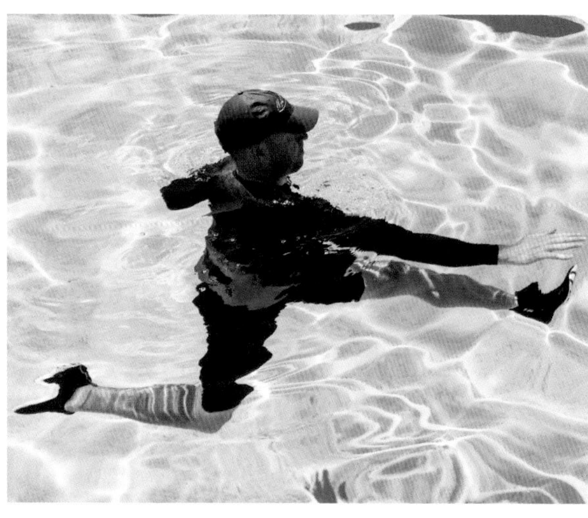

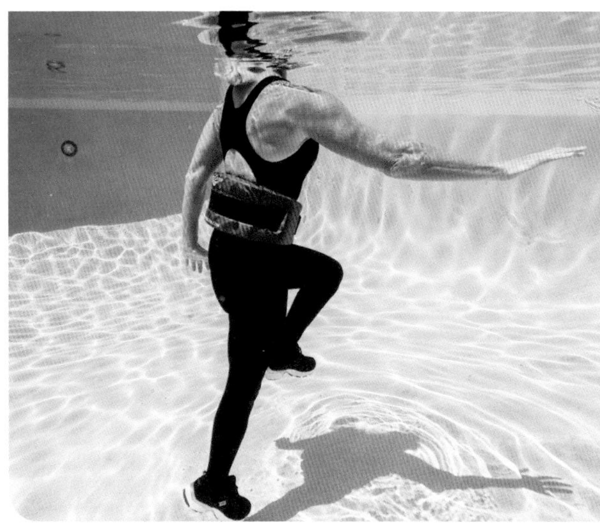

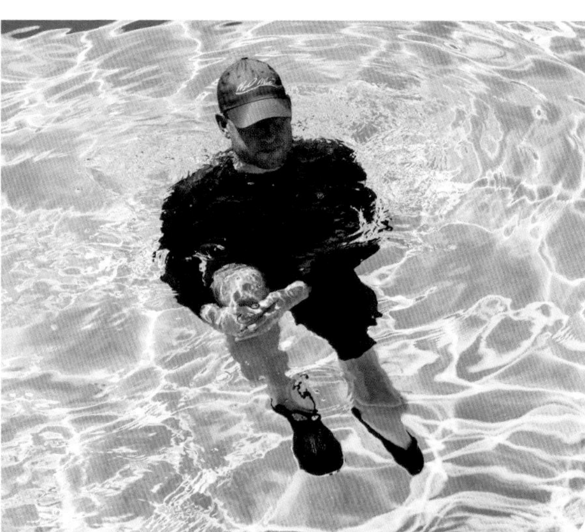

The exercises shown in this appendix are techniques designed for the average healthy adult. Special populations or medical conditions might warrant exercise modifications. Some techniques are advanced and should be practiced with caution.

Deep-Water Alignment

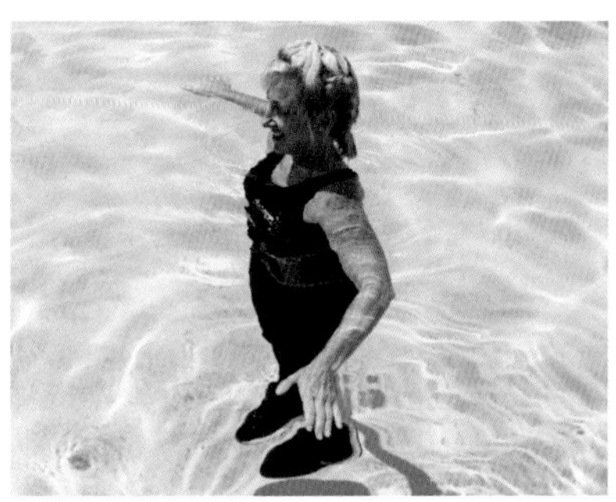

Proper alignment: This is the correct vertical position with the proper amount of flotation and belt positioning.

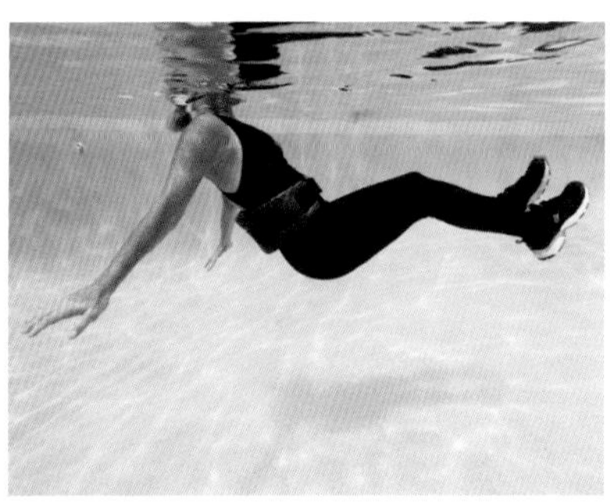

Incorrect alignment: The legs are flexed at the hips (seated position), rather than the hips being extended with the feet under the hips as in proper vertical position.

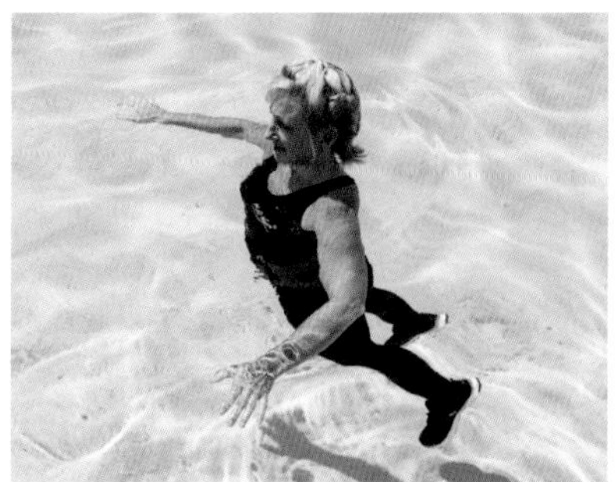

Incorrect alignment: Inability to maintain upright vertical alignment might be caused by improper placement of flotation; adjust the position of the floatation device or the amount of buoyancy as needed.

Deep-Water Cardiorespiratory Exercises

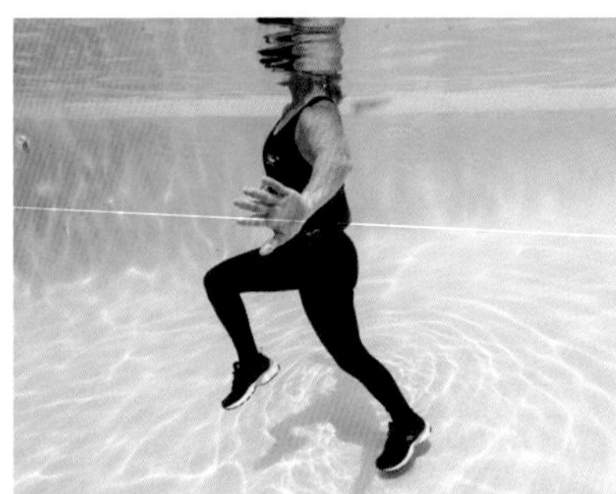

Knee-high jog, stationary: As the hip is flexed, the knee is flexed with the foot positioned slightly posterior to the knee (side view). Emphasize the flat foot pressing down as the hip and knee extend. Legs alternate from side to side but this is *not* a bicycling motion.

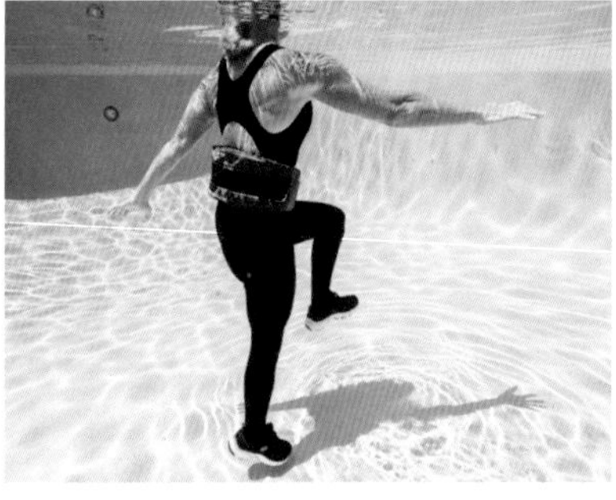

Knee lifts: This exercise differs from the stationary knee-high jog in that the move is more like a march, with the foot directly under the knee (from a side view) when the hip and knee flex. Perform on both sides.

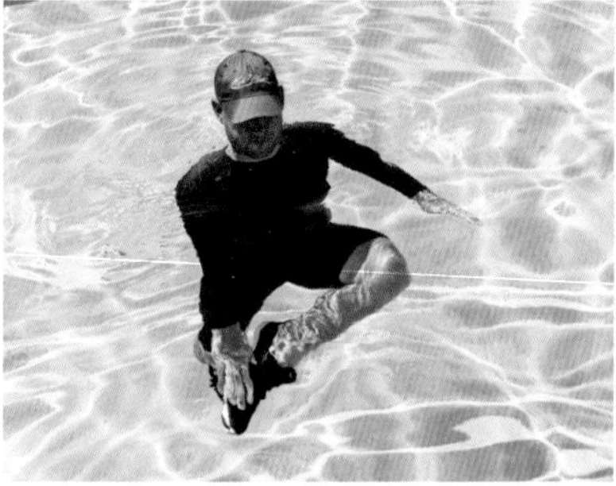

Inner thigh lift or ankle reach front: Variation of the knee-high jog; here, the hip rotates externally as the knee lifts; the opposite hand reaches toward the ankle. Alternate side to side.

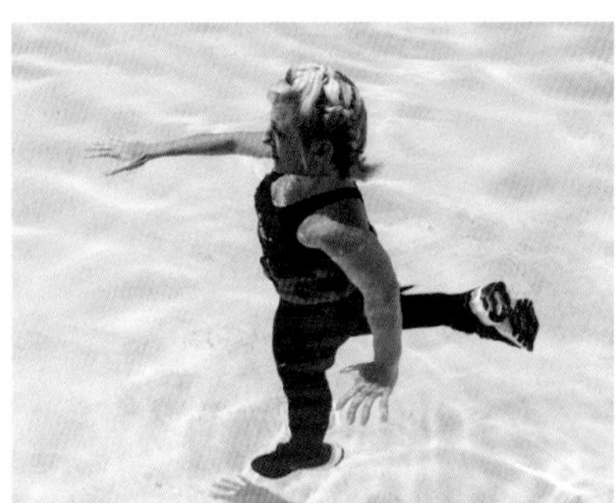

Leg curl or heel-high jog: Alternating knee flexion. Lift heels behind to about knee height. Compared to the knee-high jog or knee lift, this move focuses more on the posterior leg muscles.

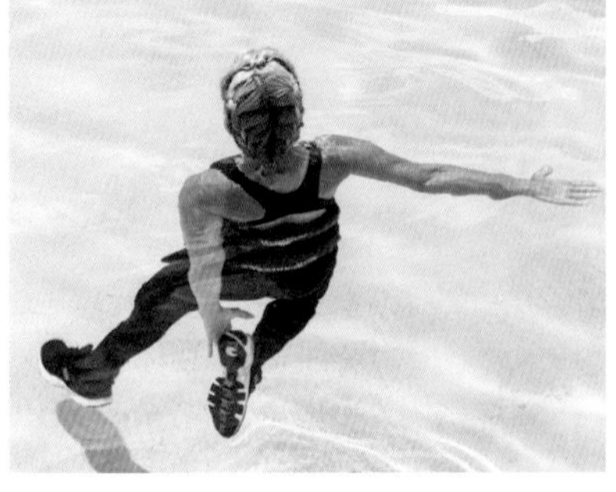

Heel reach behind (opposite hand toward heel): This move is a variation of the leg curl; here, the hip rotates externally as the knee flexes. The opposite hand reaches toward the heel behind the body. Alternate side to side.

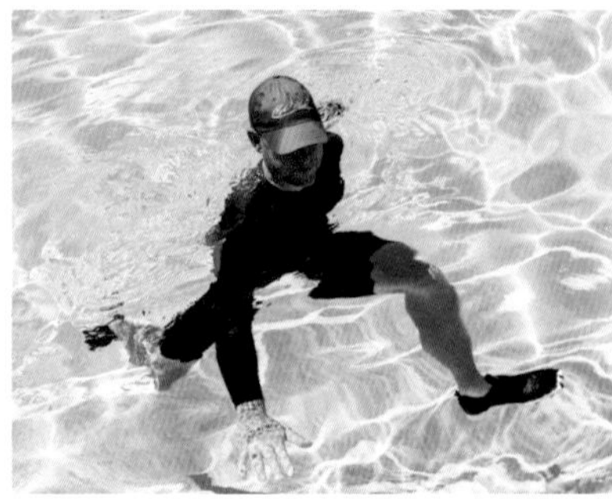

Wide jog or straddle jog: Jog with the legs in a slightly abducted position (legs apart); this may be done with knees high or heels high.

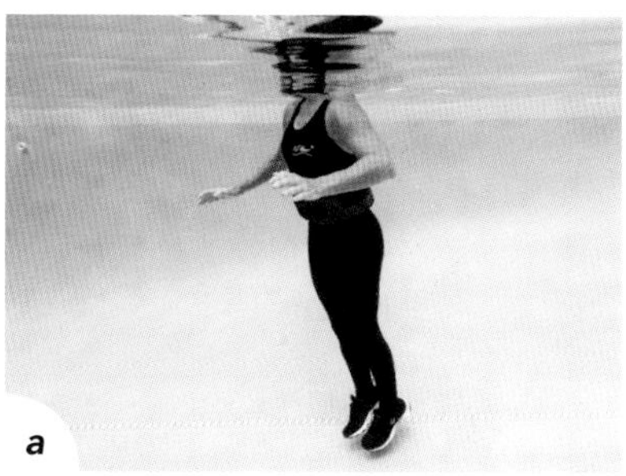

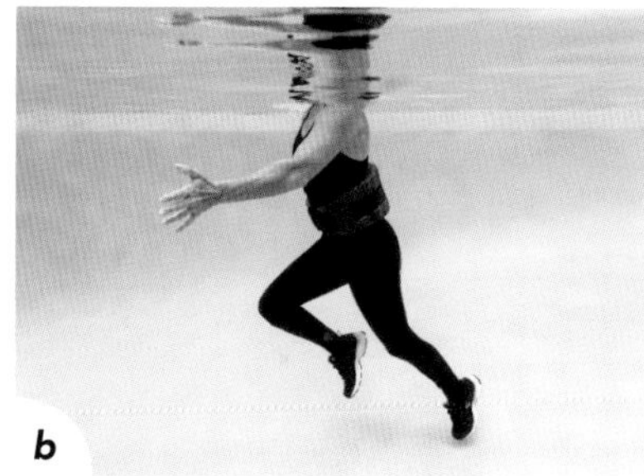

Deep-water running: This is a traveling movement. *(a)* Lean the body forward 5 to 10 degrees from vertical. *(b)* The leg action drives down and slightly diagonally backward to achieve the forward run.

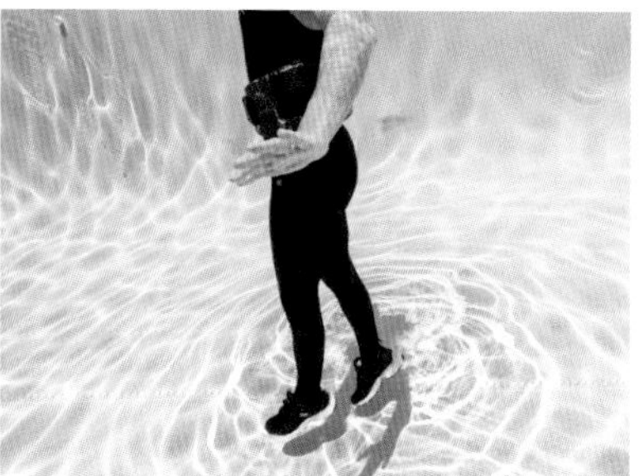

Vertical flutter kicks: Maintain correct vertical alignment and contract the core muscles. The legs perform alternating, small ROM hip flexion and extension with the knees soft. Pointing the toes (plantar flexion) lengthens the lever.

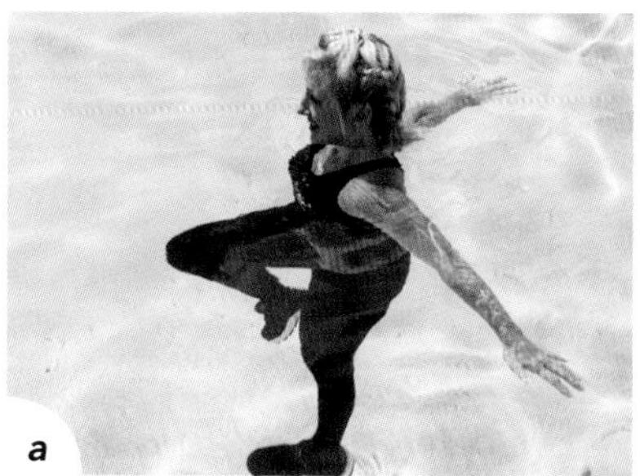

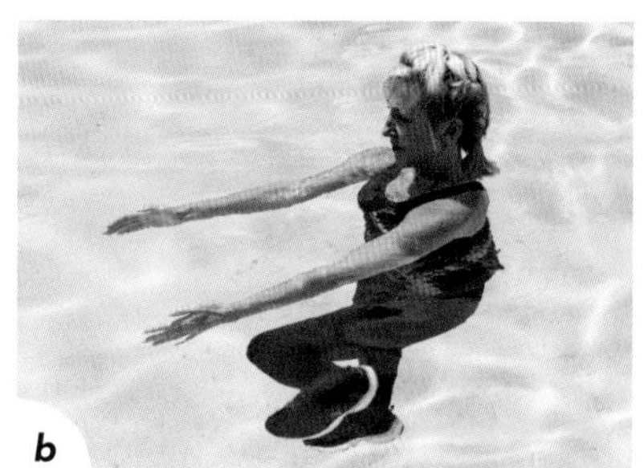

Backward jog: The leg movement is similar to riding a bicycle backward, but the body remains vertical. *(a)* The feet pedal down and back, scooping the water forward with the front of the leg and foot. *(b)* Assist by adding a symmetrical arm action, such as reverse breaststroke.

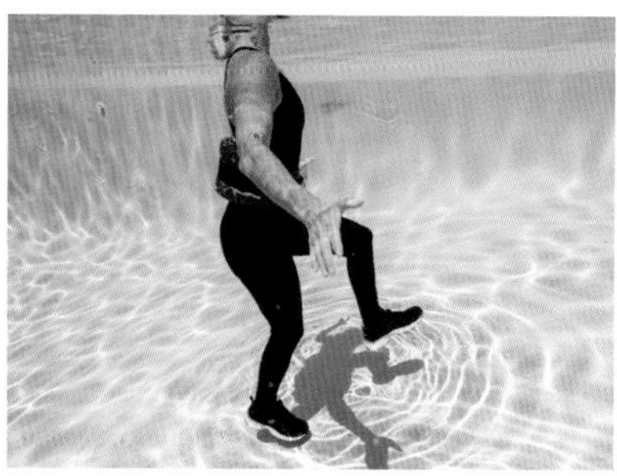

Biking: The body is positioned as if seated on a bicycle with some flexion at the hips. The legs perform a pedaling motion slightly in front of the body. Travel can be forward or backward by changing the focus of the pull with the legs.

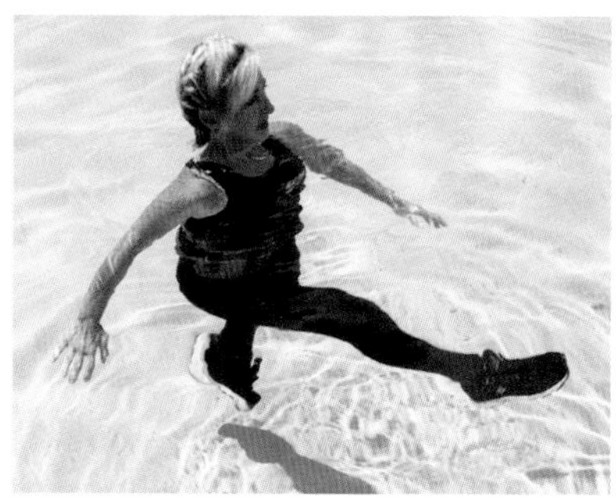

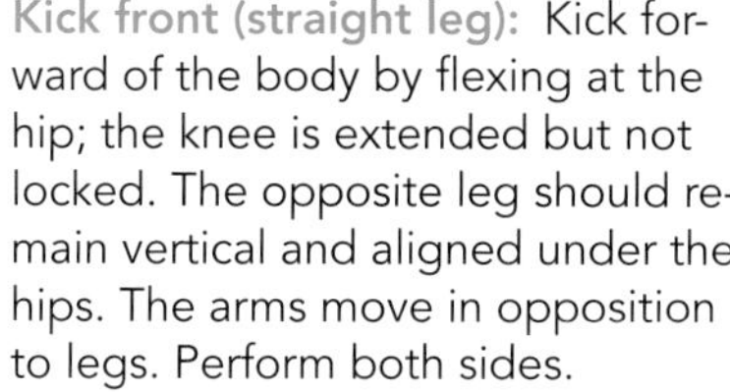

Kick front (straight leg): Kick forward of the body by flexing at the hip; the knee is extended but not locked. The opposite leg should remain vertical and aligned under the hips. The arms move in opposition to legs. Perform both sides.

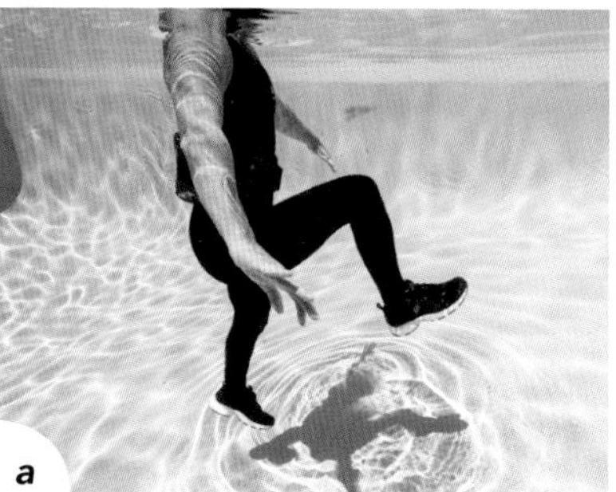

Kick front (karate): This move differs from the front kick with a straight leg by involving movement at the knee and the hip joint. The leg has four positions: *(a)* knee and hip flexion, *(b)* knee extension, knee flexion, and return to start. Perform both sides.

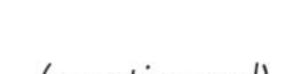

(continued)

Deep-Water Cardiorespiratory Exercises *(continued)*

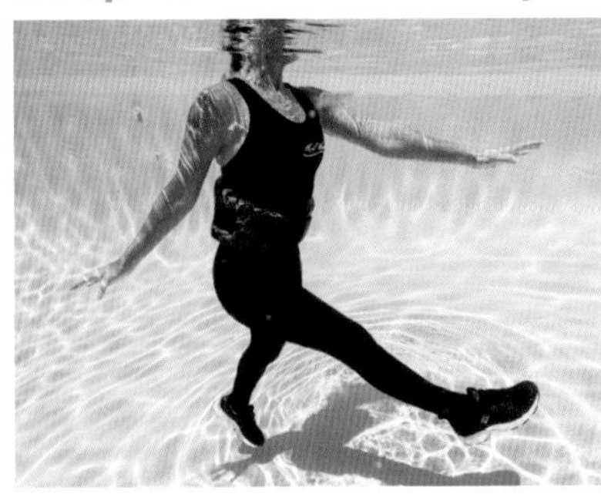

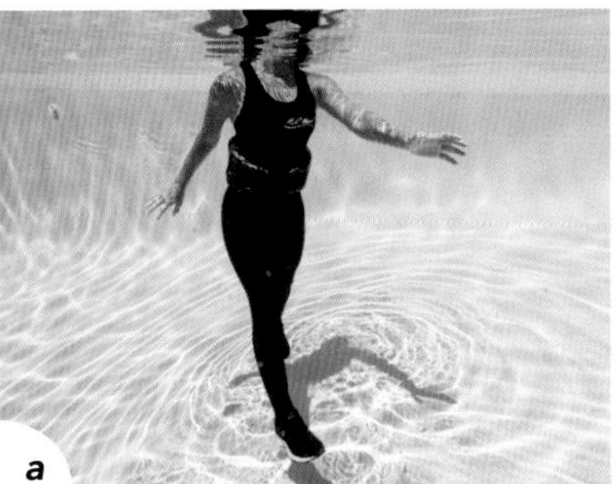

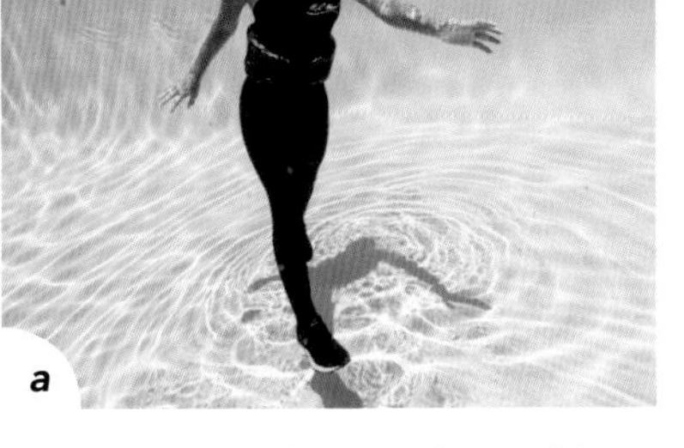

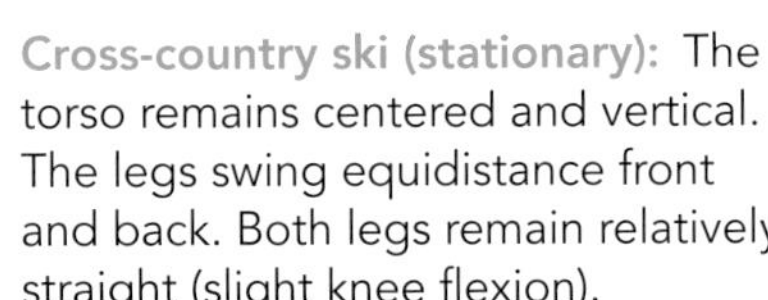

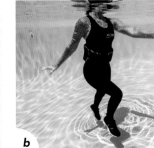

Cross-country ski (stationary): The torso remains centered and vertical. The legs swing equidistance front and back. Both legs remain relatively straight (slight knee flexion).

Cross-country ski (traveling): *(a)* Lean the body slightly forward. *(b)* The knee is slightly flexed while swinging forward and then straightens as the leg moves backward into hip hyperextension to propel the body forward.

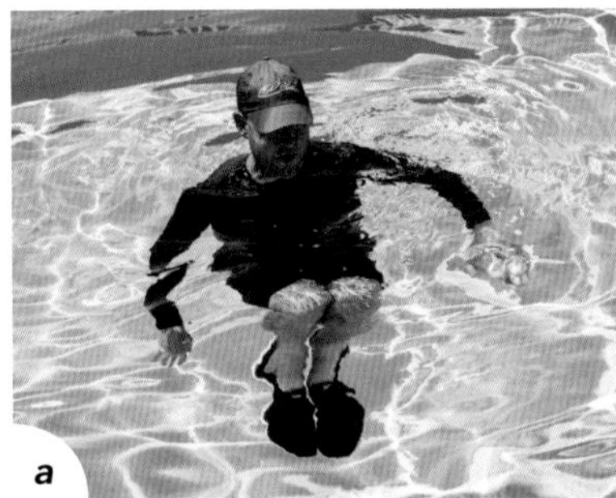

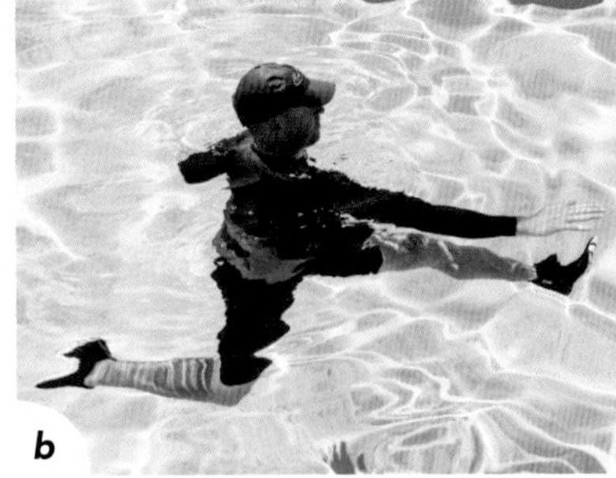

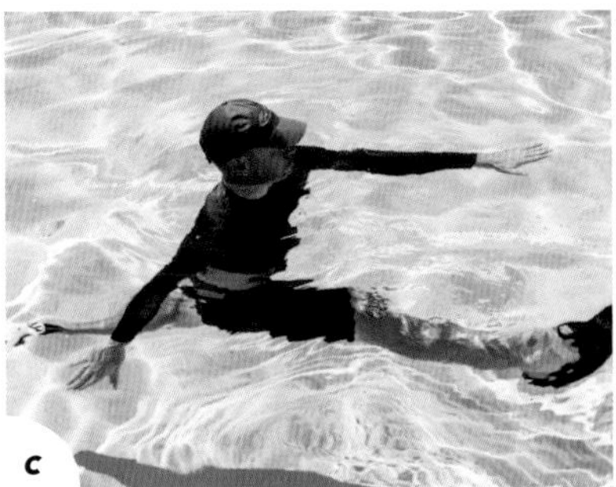

Modified hurdle: This move initiates from *(a)* a tuck position. *(b)* One leg shoots forward and straightens at the knee (without locking) while the opposite leg pushes behind and the knee remains bent. *(c)* The back leg does *not* externally rotate as in a true hurdle motion on land.

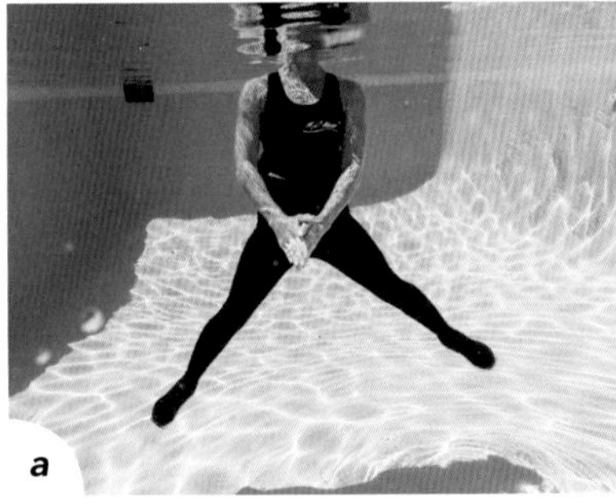

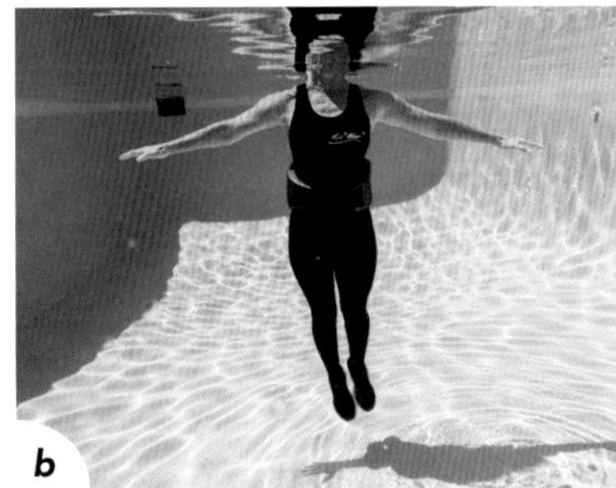

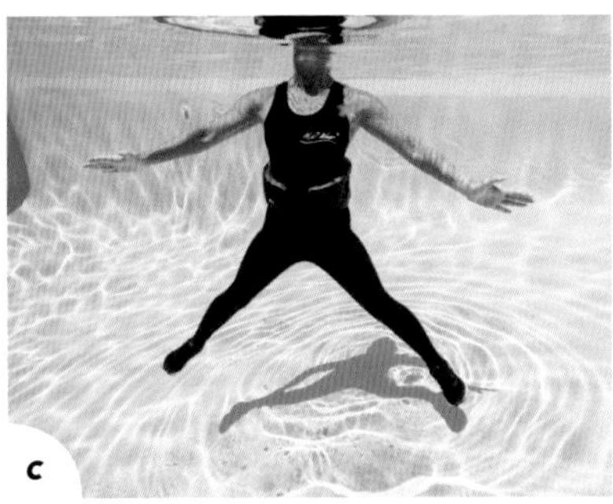

Deep-water jack: *(a)* Hip abduction and *(b)* adduction. To keep from bobbing in the water, move the arms in opposition to the legs as shown in *(a)* and *(b)*. *(c)* Arms can also move in synchrony with legs. Many variations are available; options include tempo, knee tuck, and arm patterns.

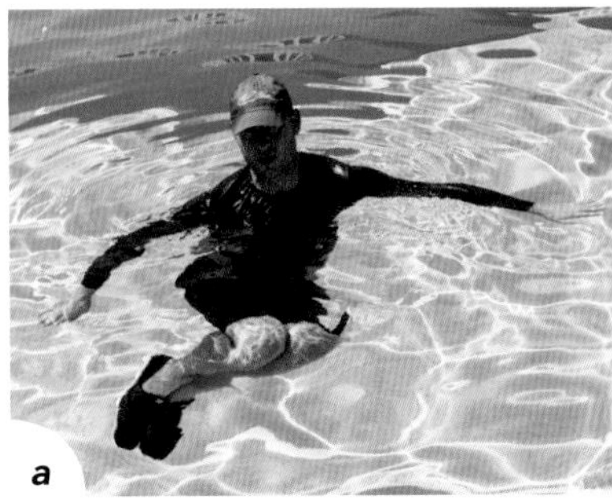

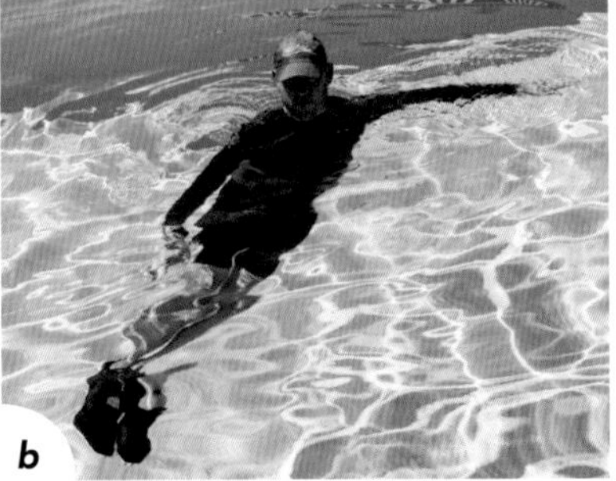

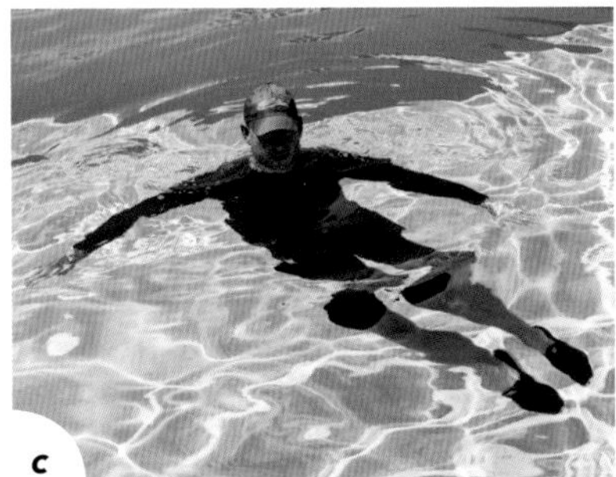

Moguls or small ROM side-to-side tuck: *(a)* Tuck the knees, then *(b)* shoot both legs to one side of the body, diagonally downward, while maintaining spinal alignment. *(c)* Tuck and repeat to opposite side. Use arms as needed for balance and stabilization.

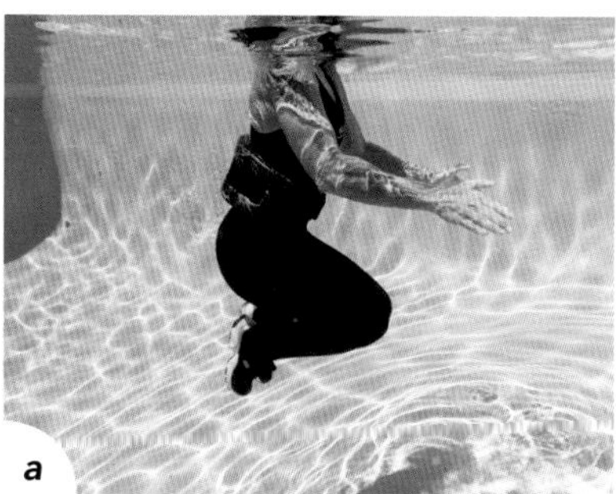

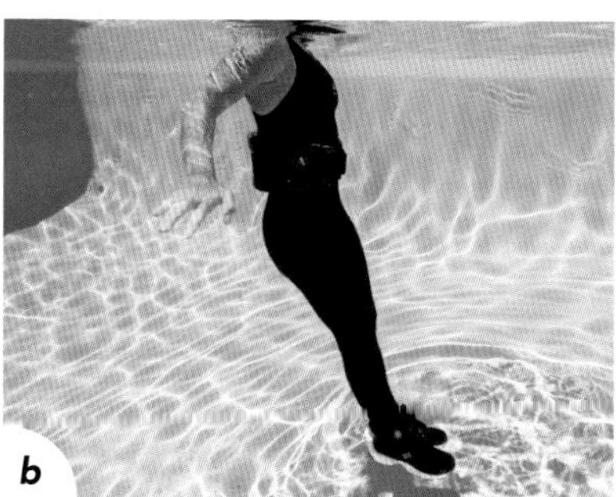

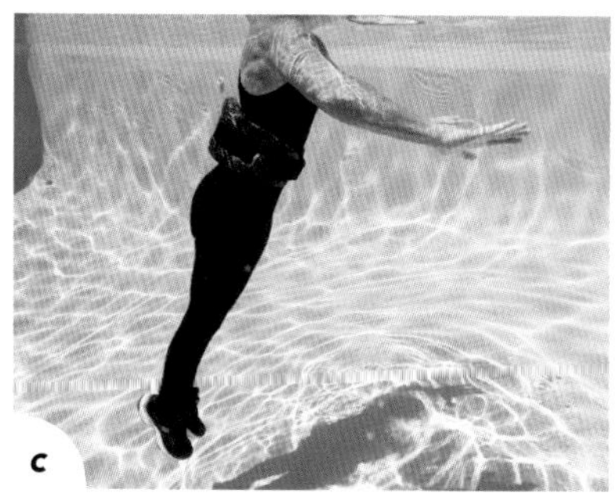

Log jump or small ROM forward and backward tuck: *(a)* Tuck knees, then *(b)* shoot both legs forward of the body, diagonally and downward, while maintaining spinal alignment. *(c)* Tuck and repeat behind the body. Use arms as needed for balance and stabilization; arms in opposition to the legs is often best.

Deep-Water Suspended Stretches

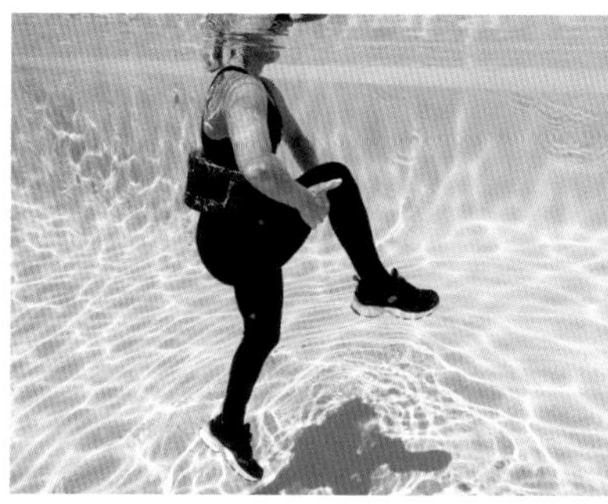

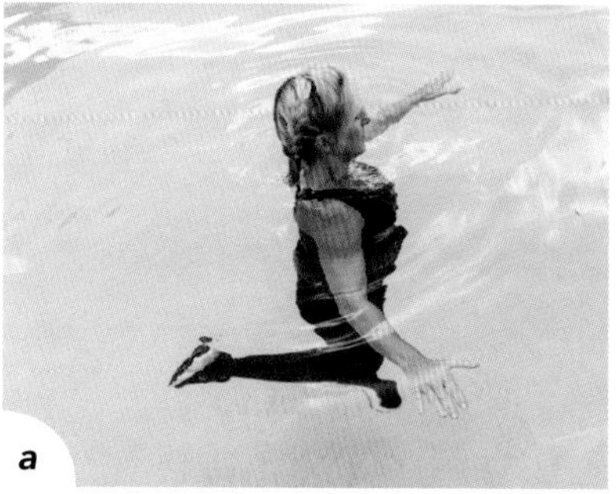

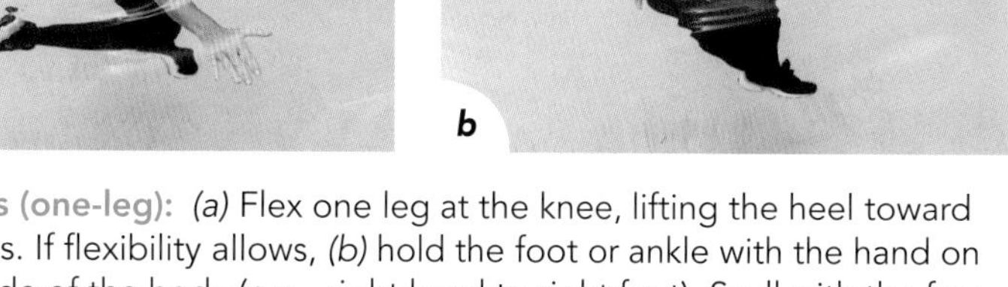

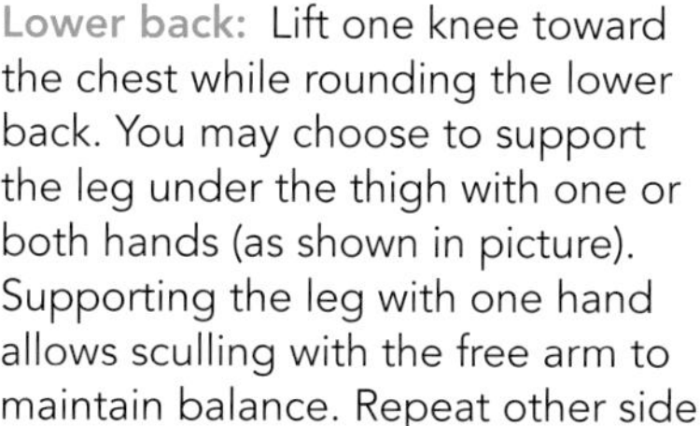

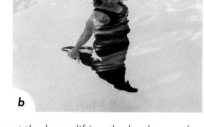

Lower back: Lift one knee toward the chest while rounding the lower back. You may choose to support the leg under the thigh with one or both hands (as shown in picture). Supporting the leg with one hand allows sculling with the free arm to maintain balance. Repeat other side.

Quadriceps (one-leg): *(a)* Flex one leg at the knee, lifting the heel toward the buttocks. If flexibility allows, *(b)* hold the foot or ankle with the hand on the same side of the body (e.g., right hand to right foot). Scull with the free arm to maintain balance. Repeat on other side.

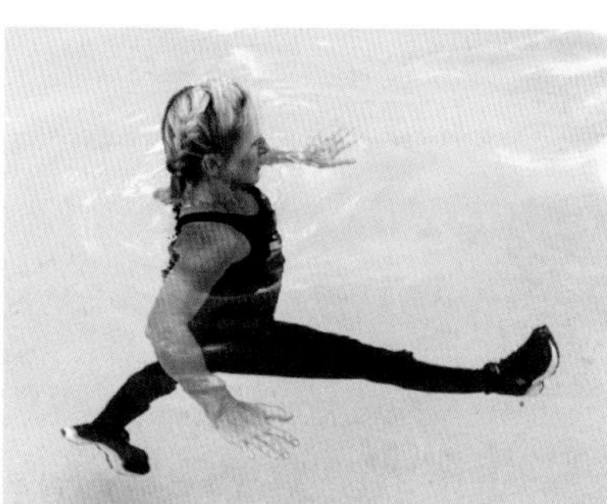

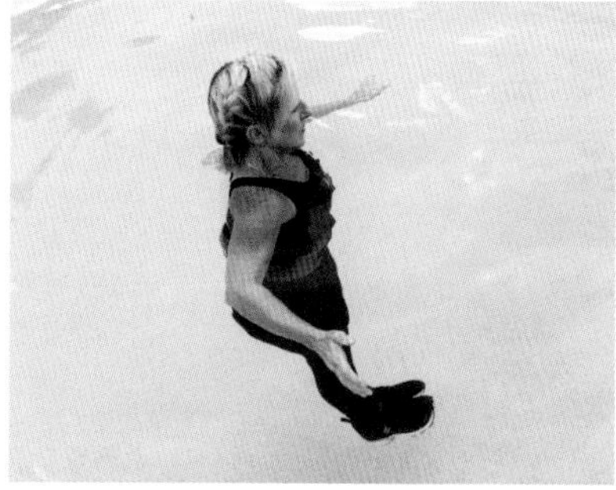

Gastrocnemius (rhythmical option): Perform a slow cross-country ski, emphasizing the forward leg movement and dorsiflexing the ankle as the leg swings forward. Repeat on the other side.

Gastrocnemius (stationary): Dorsiflex ankles with extended knees and hips while vertically suspended; arms sculling to maintain balance.

(continued)

Deep-Water Suspended Stretches *(continued)*

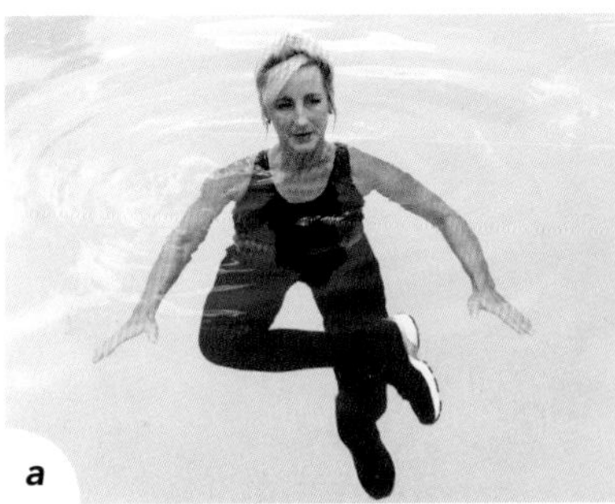

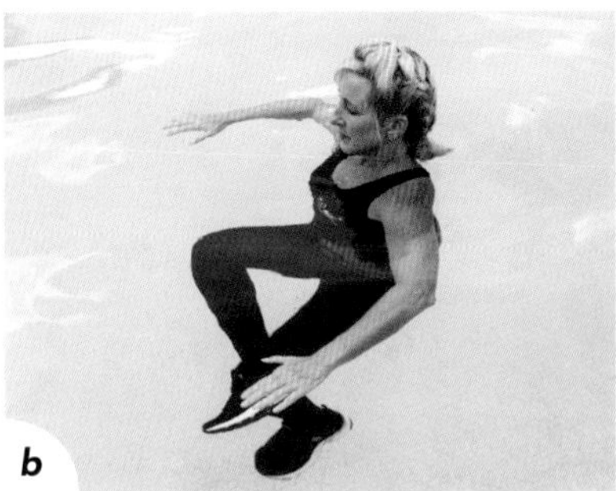

Outer thigh: *(a)* Cross ankle over opposite knee with arms sculling to maintain balance. *(b)* Maintain vertical alignment of the spine. Repeat on the other side.

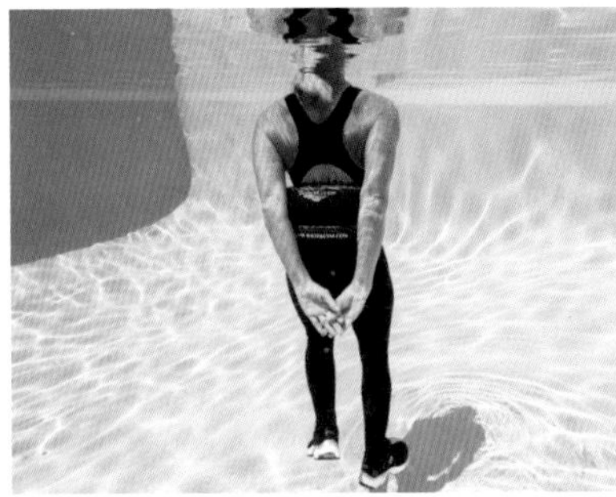

Pectoralis or anterior deltoid (stationary): Hands grasp behind the back with shoulders pulled down and back to open the chest. Perform a slow jog or biking action to maintain vertical body position.

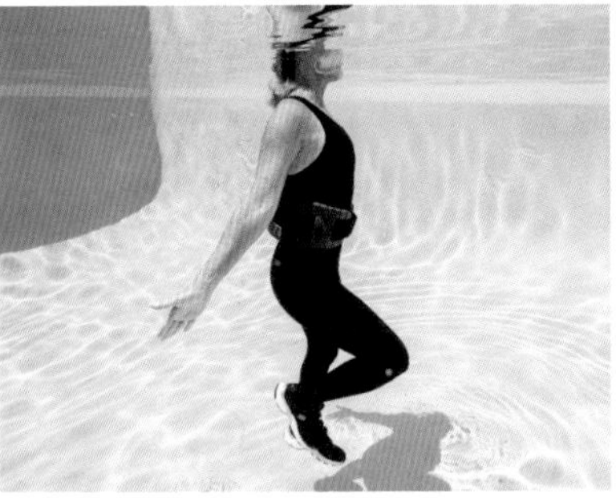

Pectoralis or anterior deltoid (traveling): Both arms abducted, shoulders rotated with thumbs up, and scapula retracted. Travel forward with a deep-water run to enhance the stretch.

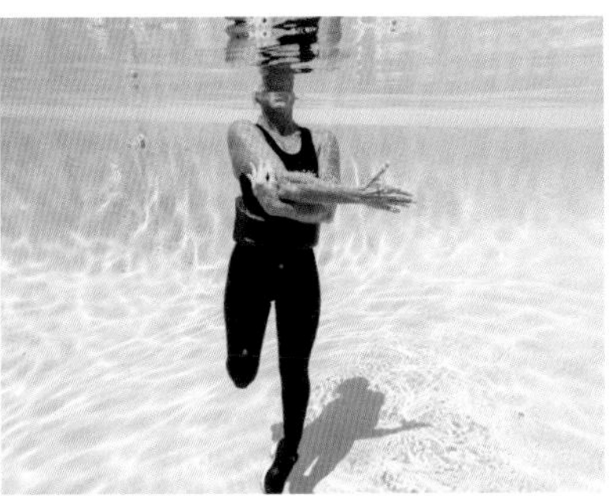

Triceps or posterior deltoids: Bring one arm across the body at midchest; assist the stretch by gently pulling with the opposite hand above or below the elbow. Keep the shoulders pressed down and back. Perform a slow jog to maintain vertical body position.

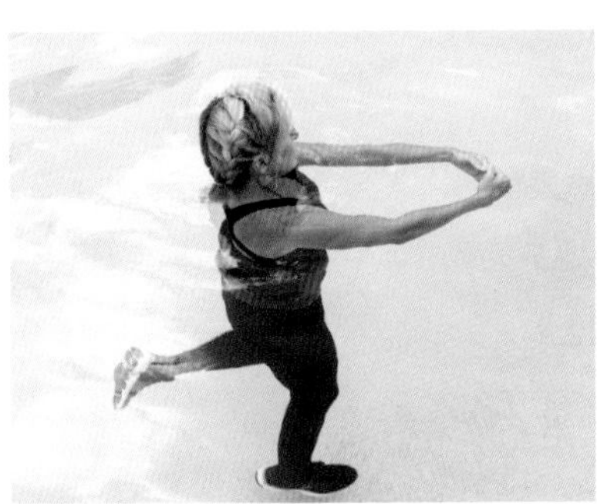

Middle trapezius: Press both arms forward, opening (protracting) the shoulder blades and rounding the upper back. Perform a slow jog or biking action to maintain vertical body position.

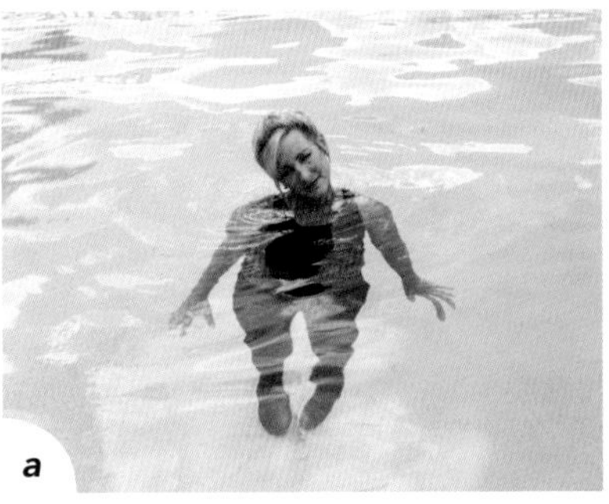

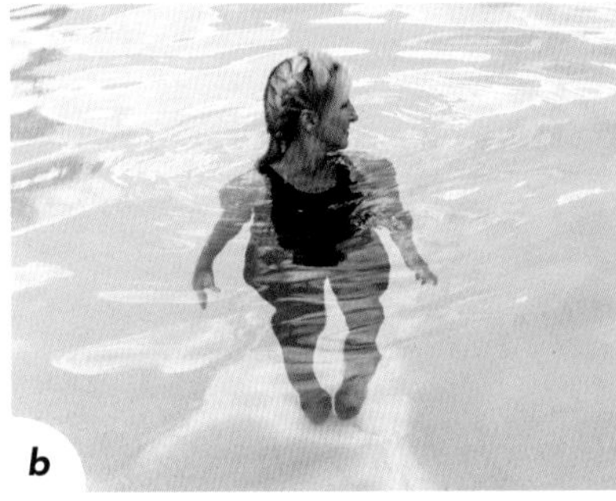

Upper trapezius and neck: *(a)* Tilt the head laterally to the right and left. *(b)* Rotate the head to look right and left. Perform a slow jog or biking action to maintain vertical body position.

Deep-Water Wall Stretches

Wall stretches might not be appropriate for all individuals.

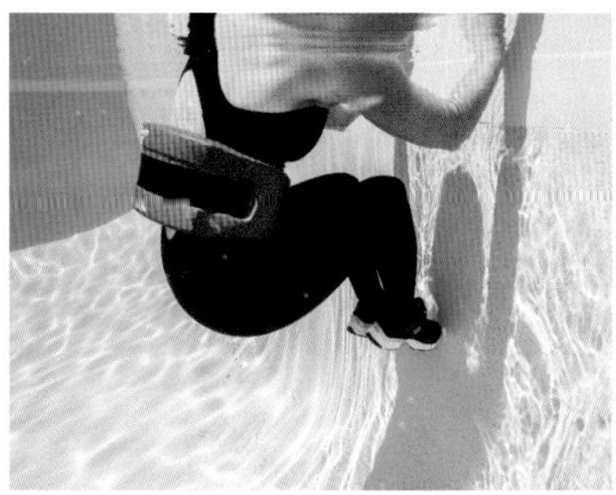

Lower back: Face the wall with both hands holding the pool edge. Place feet close together on the wall with knees bent. Keeping knees bent, round the spine forward.

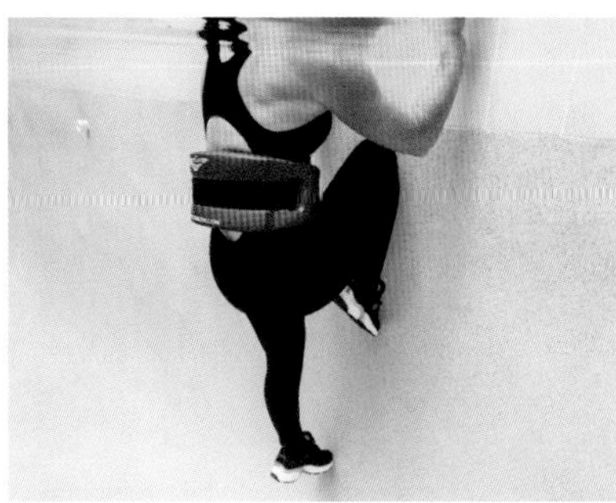

Single-leg lower back: Face the wall, place the shin of one on the wall and allow opposite leg to remain long. Both hands stay on the pool edge. Repeat on both sides.

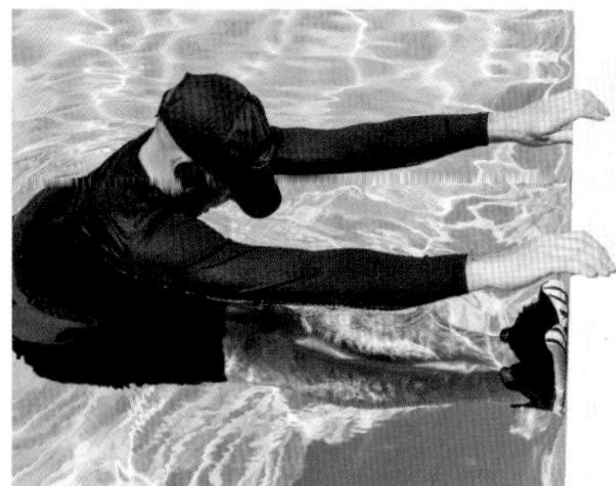

Hamstrings: Begin in the lower back wall stretch and slowly extend the knees. (Do not hyperextend or lock the knee joint.)

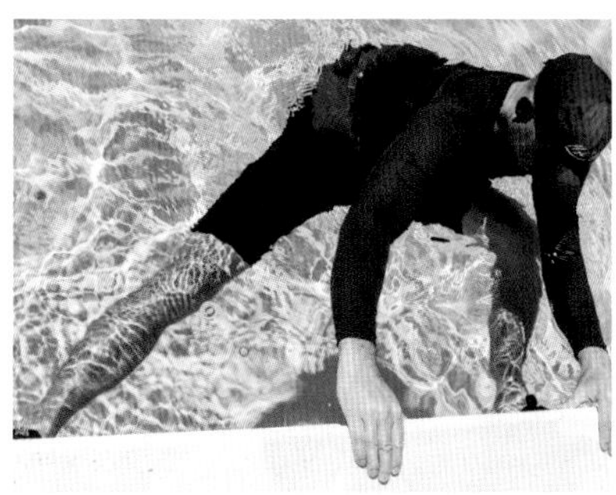

Inner thigh: Begin in the hamstrings wall stretch and move legs to a straddle position. Lean to the right side by bending the right knee; focus on pressing the left inner thigh toward the pool wall. Repeat on the other side.

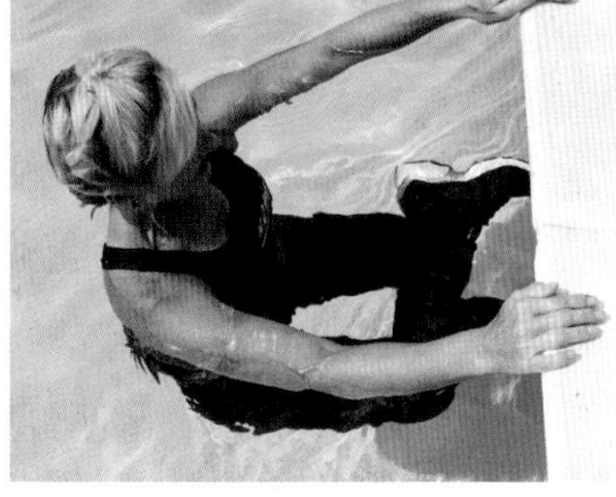

Outer thigh: Face the wall and hold the wall with both hands. Cross the right ankle above the left knee and place left foot on the wall, with knee bent. Visualize sitting in a chair with leg crossed. Repeat on the other side.

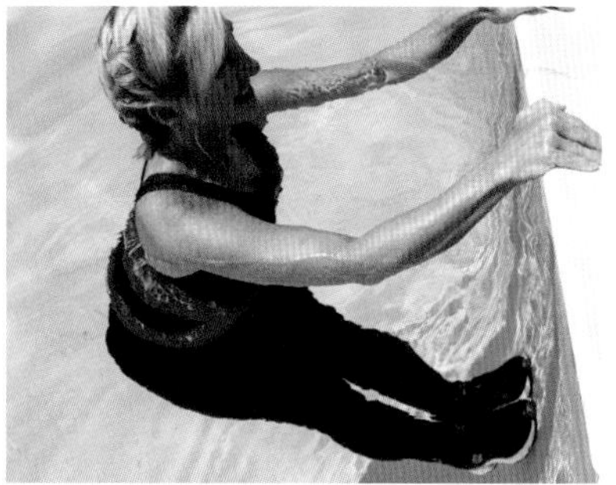

Gastrocnemius: Face the wall with the body long and vertical. Both hands hold the pool edge; the balls of the feet rest against the wall. Press the heels toward the pool bottom (dorsiflex ankles).

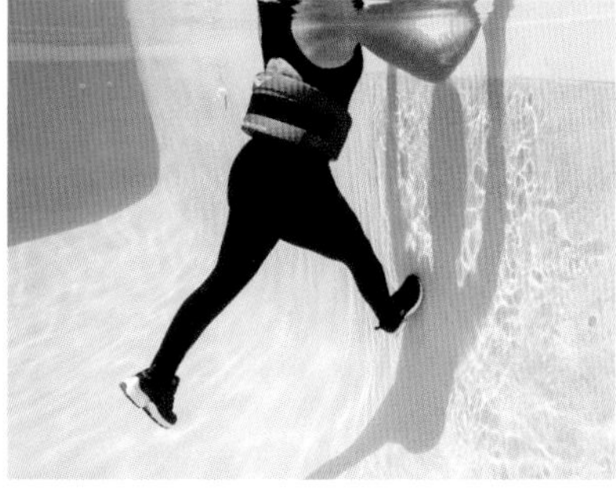

Iliopsoas: Face the wall with the body long and vertical. Both hands hold the pool edge; the balls of the feet rest against the wall. Extend one leg behind the body to stretch the iliopsoas and rectus femoris of the quadriceps. Repeat on the other side.

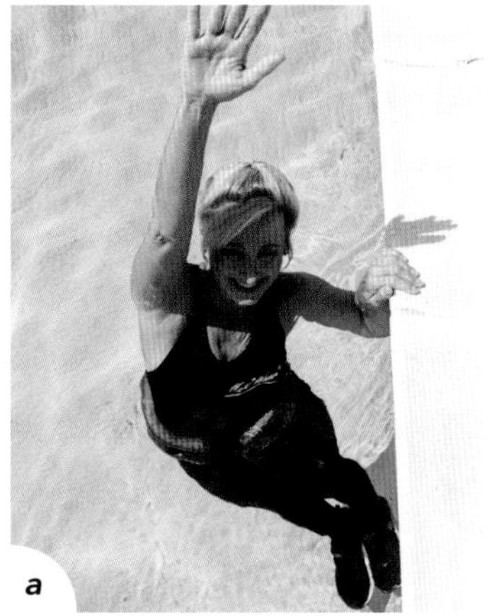

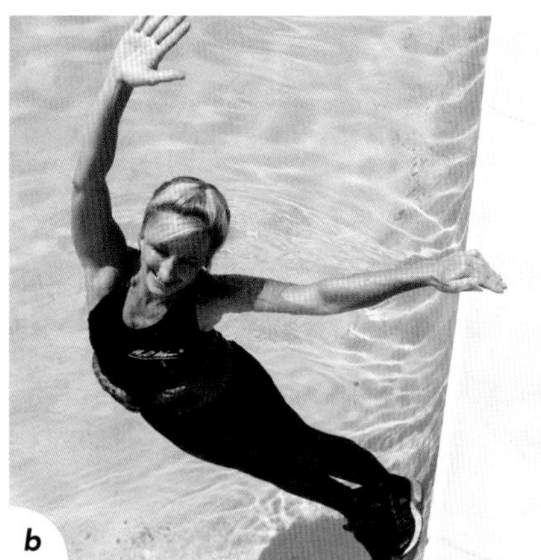

Latissimus dorsi: *(a)* Position right side toward wall with right arm holding pool edge. With the feet braced against the wall, extend left arm above head with the arm close to the ear, and then stretch toward the right upper corner. *(b)* Option: Allow the body to lean away from the wall to intensify the stretch. Repeat on the opposite side.

(continued)

Deep-Water Wall Stretches *(continued)*

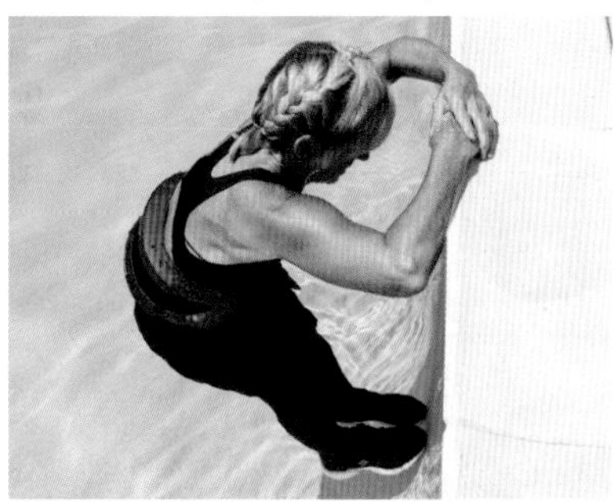

Middle trapezius: Face the wall with the body long and vertical. Both hands hold the pool edge; the balls of the feet rest against the wall. Open (protract) the scapulae. To intensify, lower the chin toward the chest.

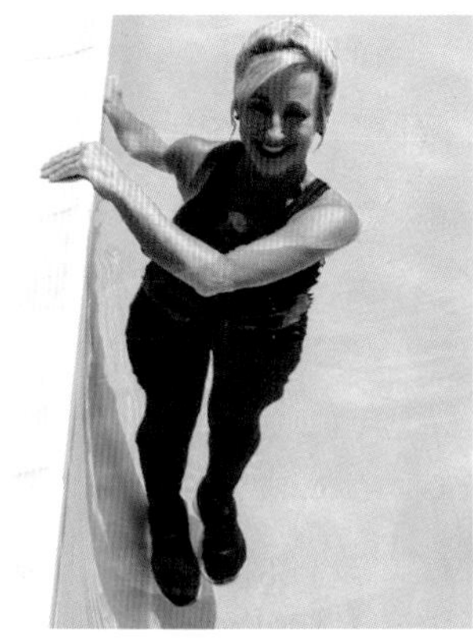

Pectoralis or biceps (single arm): Position left side toward pool wall with left hand touching the pool wall behind the body, under the water's surface. Brace with the right hand in front of the body, holding the pool wall. Repeat on the other side.

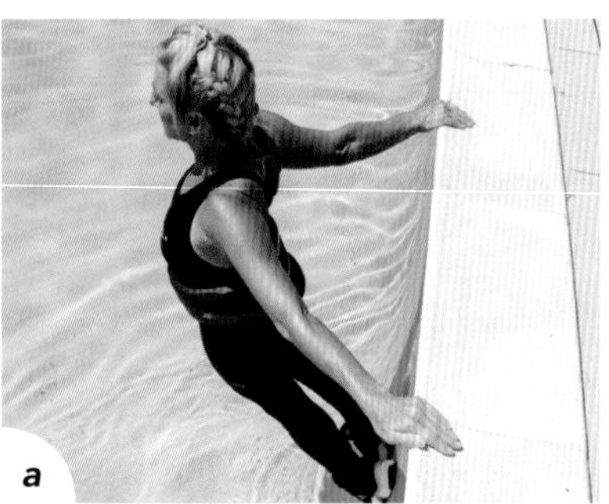

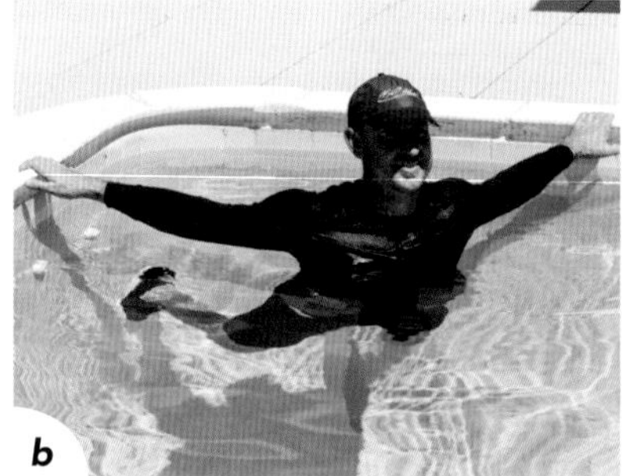

Pectoralis or biceps (double arms): Face away from the wall with feet resting on the pool wall for support. *(a)* Hold the pool edge with both arms behind the body. Lean the body away from the wall, or move arms closer together to enhance the stretch. Visualization cue: "Bust on a boat." *(b)* An option for the stretch at the corner of the pool. This stretch may not be appropriate for all populations.

Appendix C
Aquatic Fitness Equipment

As you become more familiar with the aquatic environment, you will undoubtedly learn to appreciate the versatility available in water fitness programming. Aquatic exercise equipment increases your programming potential by adding deep-water options, resistance training, fun, and variety. A wide range of fitness equipment designed specifically for the aquatic environment is available; however, some land-based equipment can also be incorporated safely and effectively.

Before choosing equipment for your aquatic programs, you must first understand how equipment choices affect program safety and training results. Chapter 4 will help you to understand how movement in water differs from movement on land and how different types of aquatic equipment influence the muscle actions. Proper use of equipment involves understanding the function, purpose, limitations, properties, safety factors, and biomechanics of the equipment.

Aquatic equipment falls into six general categories:

- *Buoyant equipment* is specific to the aquatic environment. This equipment is composed of a material such as dense closed-cell or soft-cell foam that floats in the water or is filled with air, such as a beach ball. Although lightweight, buoyant equipment can create a great deal of resistance in the water.
- *Drag equipment* usually increases the surface area or turbulence to create additional resistance for muscle movement in an aquatic environment.
- *Rubberized equipment* is usually composed of bands or tubes, and the position of the anchor point determines the muscle group being worked. Rubberized equipment is reasonably priced, compact, and easy to transport. Over time, this type of equipment will break down from exposure to pool chemicals and sunlight, so it must be inspected frequently to ensure safety.
- *Weighted equipment* in the water is very similar to land-based weight options. Weighted equipment sinks in the water and is influenced by the forces of gravity.
- *Flotation equipment* is primarily used to create neutral buoyancy. Although buoyant, it is utilized to create or maintain correct body positioning for specific exercises and class formats rather than to provide added resistance.
- *Specialized equipment* is equipment that does not fall into any of the previous individual categories. Examples include bikes, treadmills, boxing bags, poles, trampolines, and wall stations designed for use in the pool.

The following are the most common options within each equipment category.

Buoyant Equipment

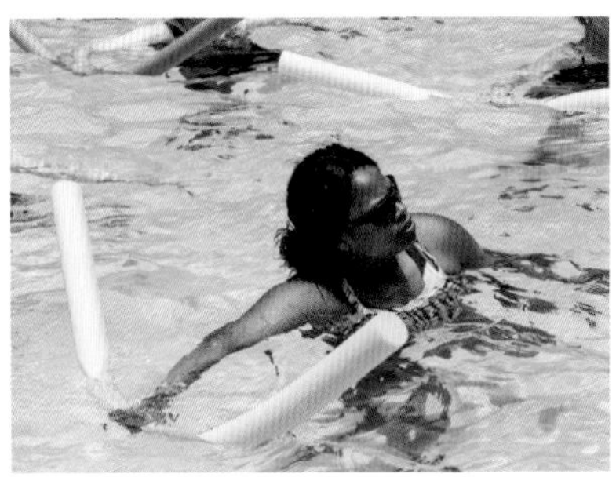

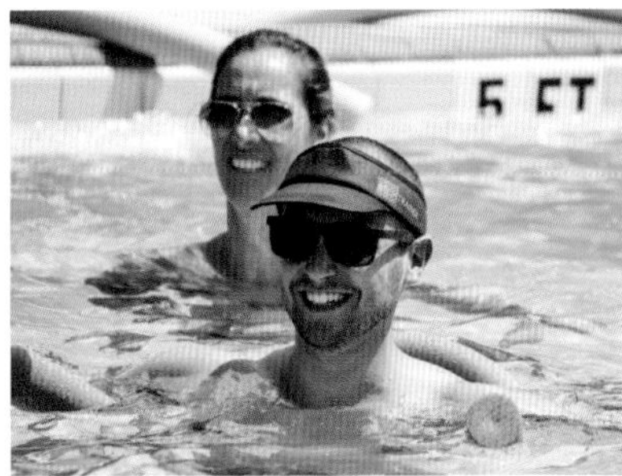

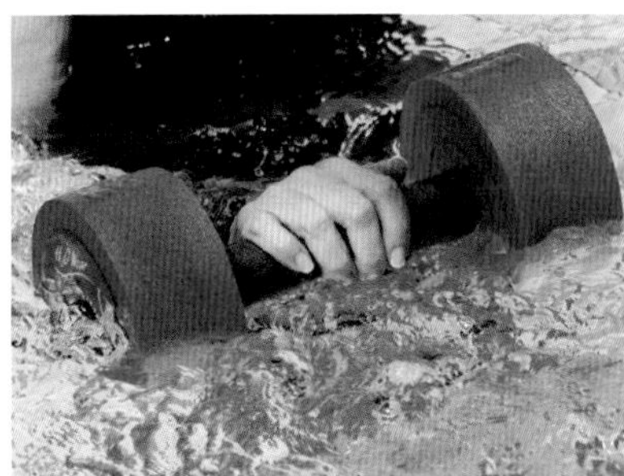

Noodles: The most widely used equipment choice in aquatic exercise classes, noodles can be utilized for unique upper- and lower-body resistance exercises, balance drills, core challenges, and fun. Noodles are not recommended as the primary flotation device during deep-water training due to the potential drowning risk should the participant lose grip or fall off the equipment. This type of training would only be appropriate for individuals with strong swim skills who are comfortable in water depths over their head.

Handheld buoyancy: Often referred to as *hand bars*, *hand buoys*, or *foam bells*, this equipment is very popular for aquatic fitness programming. Numerous options are available based on size, shape, density, and hand grip. One of the most versatile types of equipment, handheld buoyancy assists in stabilization and alignment, creates resistance when utilized underwater, and may provide an increased sense of security for some individuals.

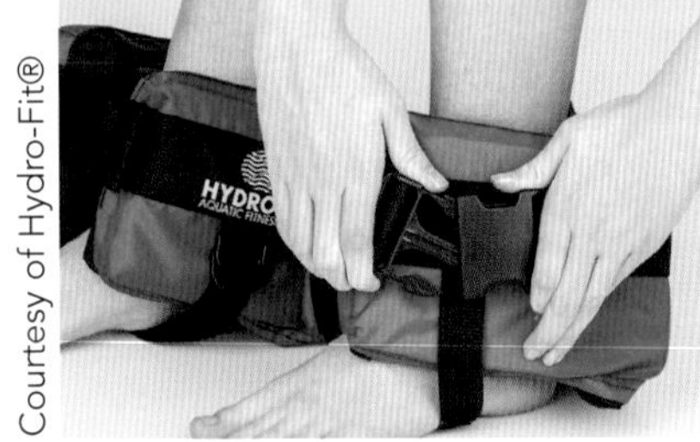

Courtesy of Hydro-Fit®

Buoyant cuffs for the ankle or arm: Soft foam cuffs are attached to the ankle or lower leg to provide buoyant resistance for shallow- and deep-water exercises or to aid in flotation if using for deep-water training. When using ankle cuffs without an additional flotation belt in deep water, the participant must have adequate core strength and proficient swim skills. Cuffs can also be attached to the upper arm to offer additional flotation and postural alignment during deep-water training.

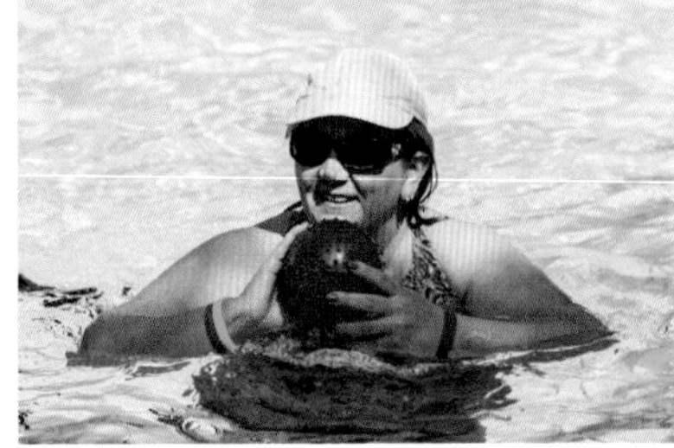

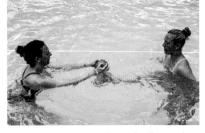

Air-filled balls: Various types of balls—e.g., beach balls, rubber balls, and Pilates balls—are used in the aquatic fitness environment. Beach balls offer options for above-water activities (passing and catching skills) or at the water's surface to assist with stabilization, coordination, and skills. Beach balls are typically not recommended for submerged exercises, because they are difficult to grip and hard to control. Smaller air-filled rubber balls, especially those with textured surfaces to provide a better grip, can be submerged for buoyancy resistance; these provide options for balance and functional training.

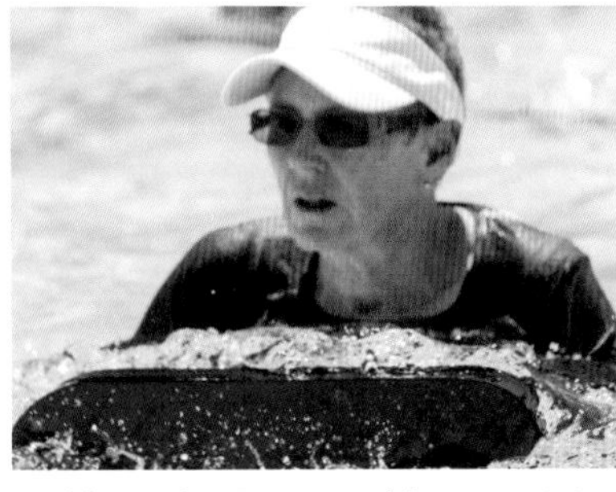

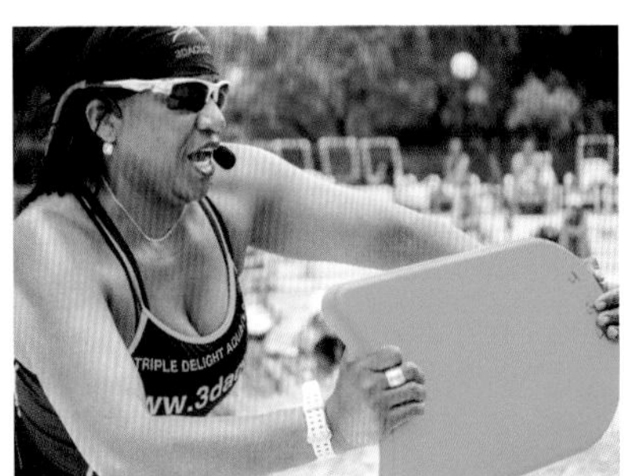

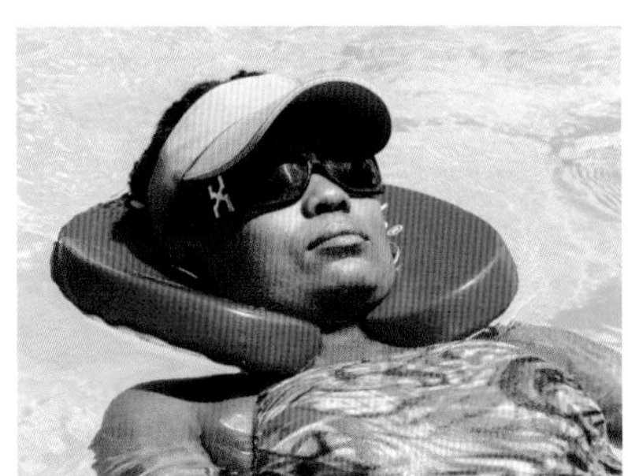

Kickboards: Designed for practicing swim skills, kickboards are a commonly found poolside tool and have multiple uses in aquatic fitness programming. They can be used in balance exercises, resistance training, and functional training, as well as sport-specific activities, such as serving as a target in aquatic kickboxing.

Nekdoodle®: This polyvinyl-coated flotation device was designed to support the head and neck while allowing the individual to float hands-free. It can also be utilized for suspension training and be used in a fashion similar to the kickboard.

Drag Equipment

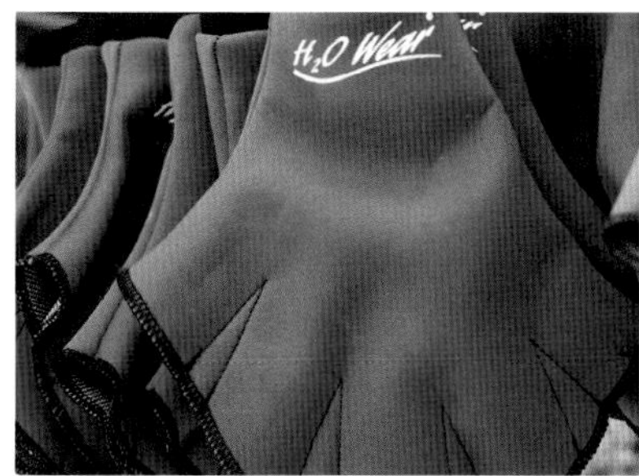

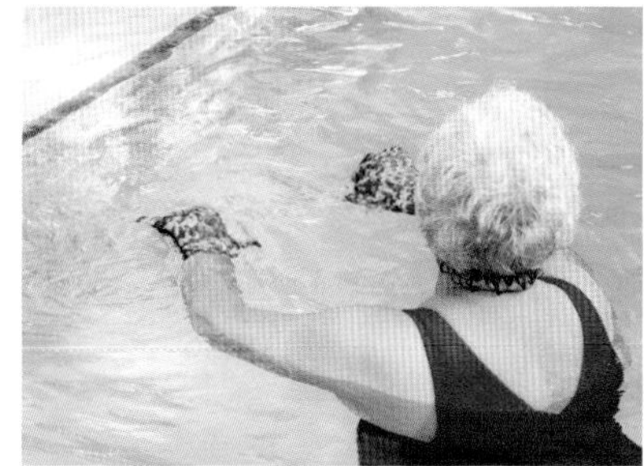

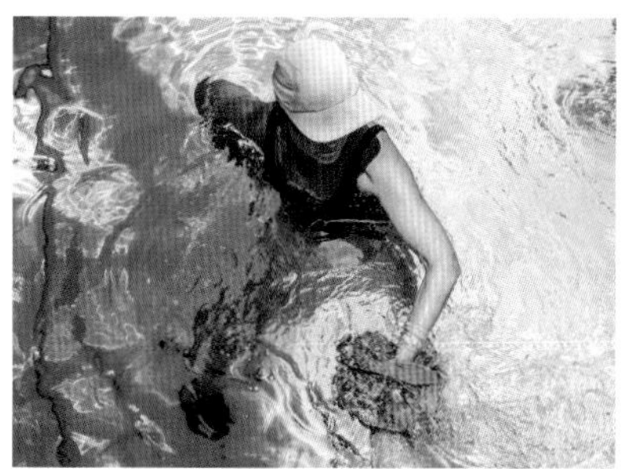

Gloves and mitts: Gloves and mitts provide additional resistance for upper-body movement and assist in balance and coordination for shallow- and deep-water programming. All fitness levels can safely use these, because hand positions can vary to alter frontal surface area and resistance levels. Gloves have individual openings for each finger, whereas mitts have a separate opening for the thumb only (like a mitten), making the mitts easier to put on, especially for individuals with arthritis or other issues with the hands and fingers.

Upper-body drag resistance: Molded rubber or plastic drag equipment for the upper body includes both handheld options and options that are attached at the wrist. Designed to increase the resistance for all submerged movement, this equipment targets upper-body muscles and the core stabilizers. Proper form, alignment, and tempo are imperative for safety and effective results.

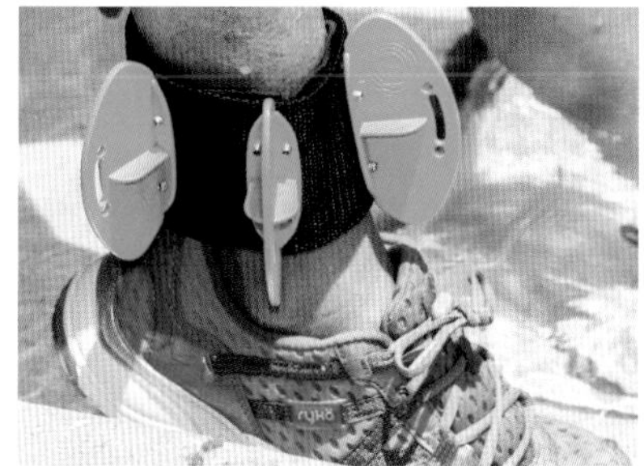

Lower-body drag resistance: Molded rubber or plastic drag equipment for lower-body drag is generally attached just above the ankle, providing a higher-intensity workout by targeting the lower body and core during all submerged movement. Proper form, alignment, and tempo are imperative for safety and effective results.

Rubberized Equipment

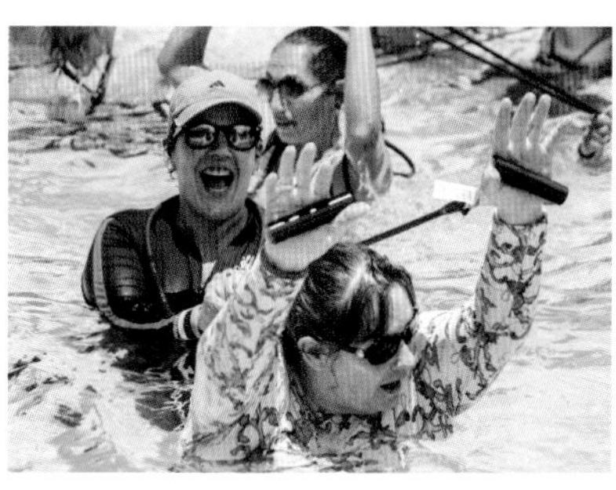

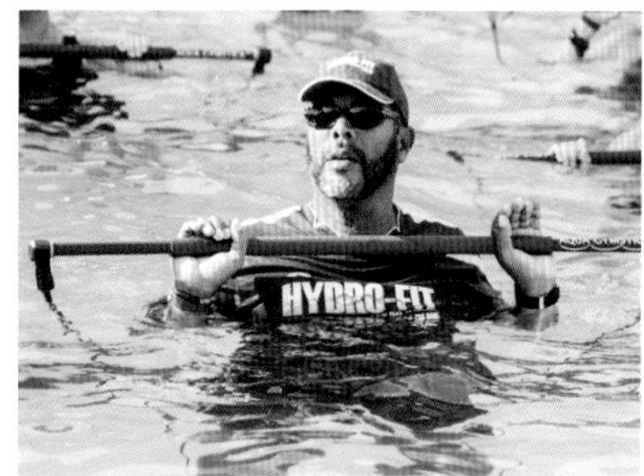

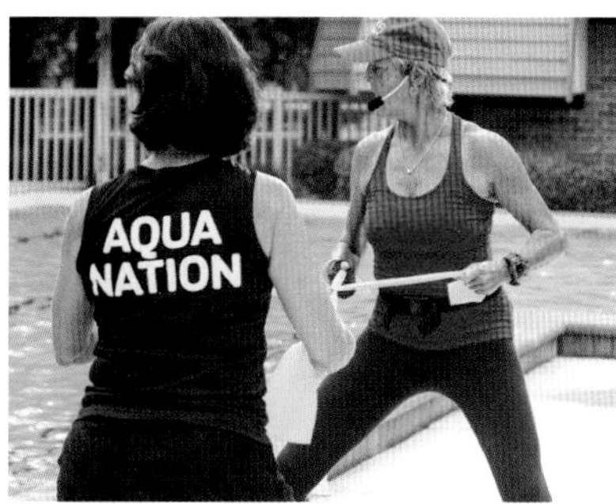

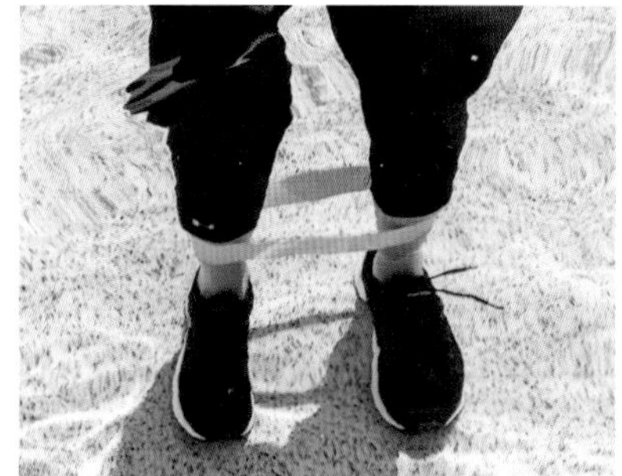

Tubing, bands, and loops: Rubberized equipment is available in different materials (e.g., tubing and flat bands) and configurations (e.g., straight, loops, figure 8), and various grips or anchors may be included. Some types of rubberized equipment also incorporate training tools or attachments, such as bars, to offer more exercise options. Similar applications and training benefits are seen on land and in the water with this versatile, inexpensive equipment option.

Weighted Equipment

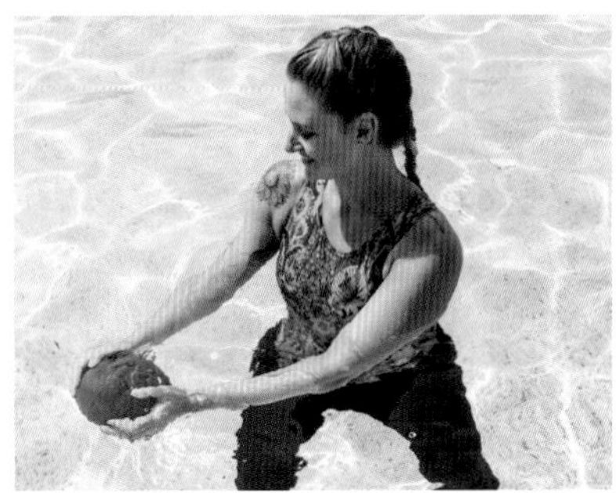

Weighted balls: One of the more common types of balls used in aquatic programming, weighted balls are used in a manner similar to land-based exercises. Weighted balls provided added resistance and are used for functional training that targets stability, endurance, coordination, and balance.

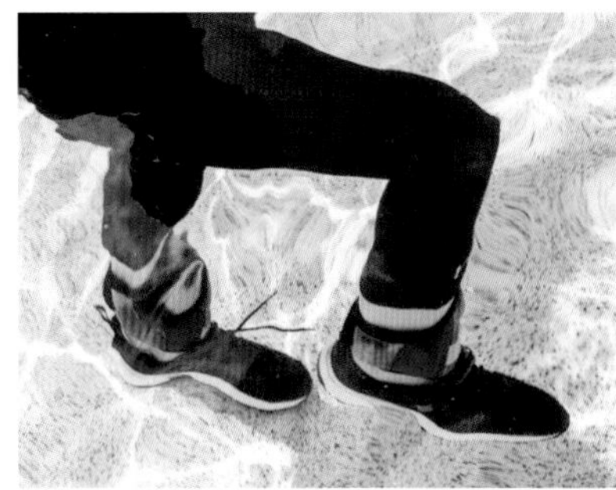

Ankle weights: Weighted equipment attached to the ankles can be utilized in water, as on land, to add resistance to specific movements of the lower body. Weights attached at the ankles can also be used for stabilization, balance activities, and gait training. In some therapeutic situations, ankle weights can also be used in vertical, suspended spinal traction. The use of ankle weights during cardiorespiratory training that involves impact is generally not recommended.

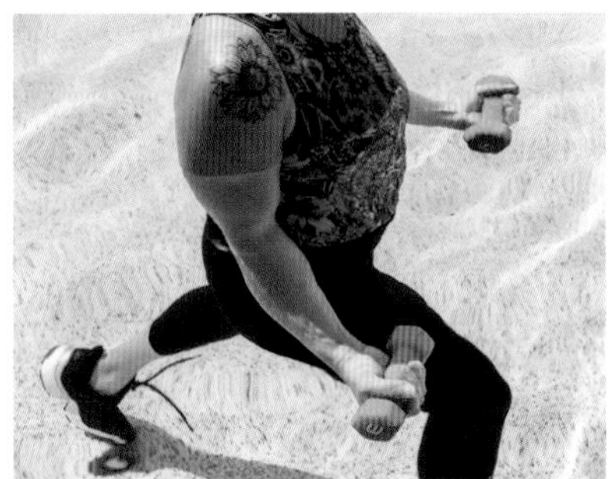

Handheld weights: Vinyl-coated weighted dumbbells can be utilized in the water to target specific muscle groups, in a similar manner to land applications. These weights are predominantly used in aquatic exercise for resistance training (e.g., to complement handheld buoyancy exercises for a balanced workout), and rehab- or therapy-type training. As with weights used on land, if the water dumbbell is dropped, it could injure the foot or toes. The dumbbell is also difficult to retrieve from the pool bottom.

Flotation Equipment

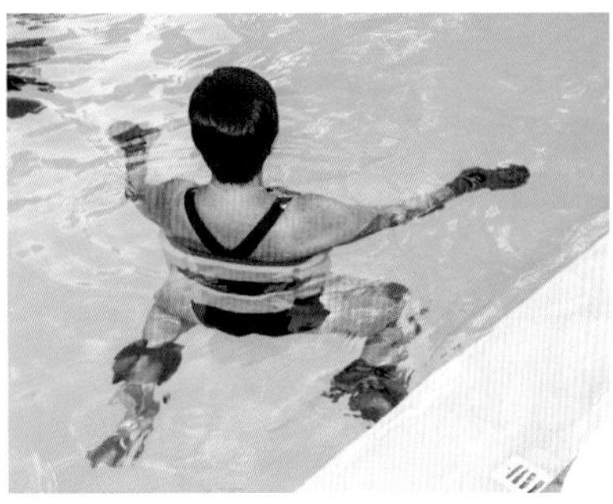

Flotation belts: Affixed at the waist, flotation belts provide stability and support for deep-water exercises, allowing the participant to maintain proper vertical alignment while performing a variety of exercises and stretches. Flotation belts may also be used in shallow water for stability training, for body awareness, or to assist specific needs. There are variations of belts available for all body types and fitness levels.

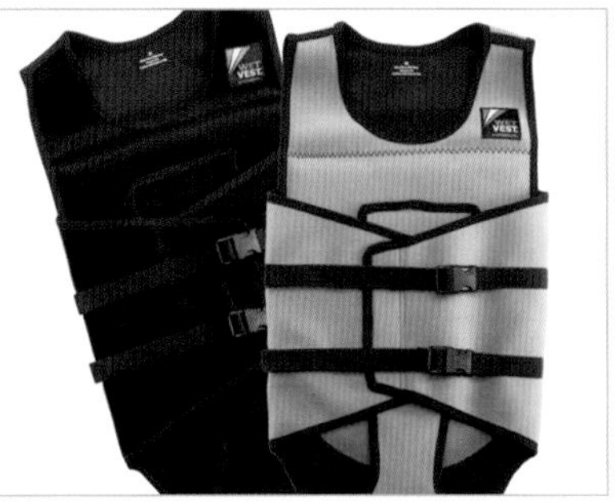

Courtesy of Hydro-Fit®

Flotation vests: Designed to provide proper alignment during deep-water exercise, these vests are worn on the upper body with zippers or straps to provide a secure fit. Some include a lower strap (positioned anterior to posterior between the legs) to secure the vest and keep it from sliding up the body.

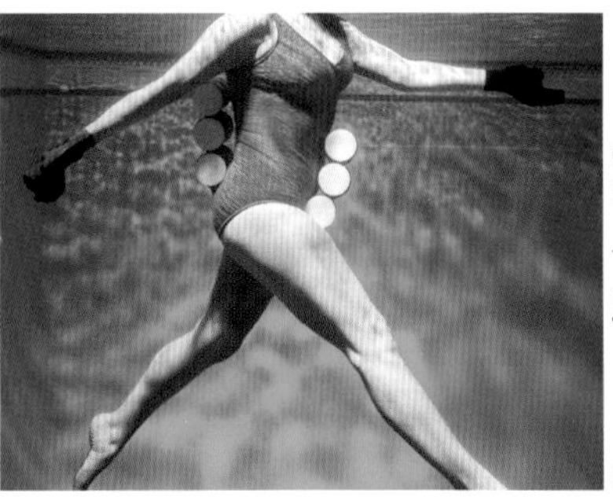

Courtesy of Hydro-Fit®

Seated flotation: This flotation option is designed for the participant to sit on, which can accommodate those who find a flotation belt too constricting or uncomfortable. Some are adjustable in the amount of flotation provided. Since this type of equipment is not attached to the body, caution should be used, especially for nonswimmers exercising in deep water.

Specialized Equipment

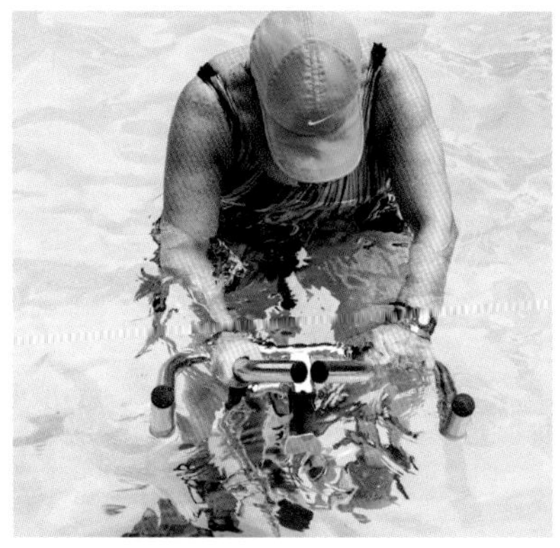

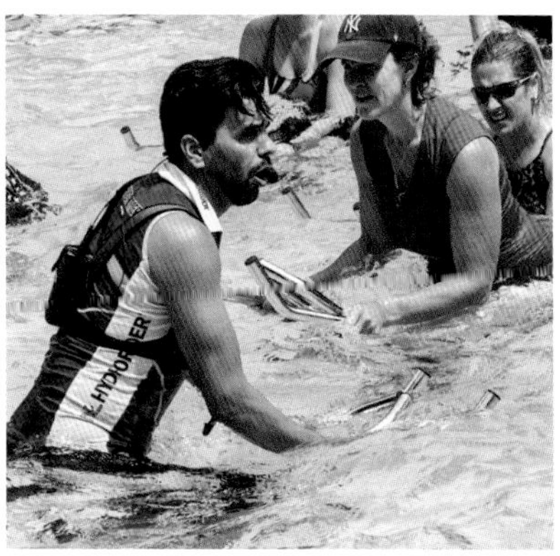

Aquatic bikes: Underwater bikes are well recognized in cardio aquatic fitness applications. They provide benefits similar to bike training on land, but with the added resistance and comfort of the aquatic environment. Generally made of high-grade, specialty-gauge steel to withstand the elements of the water, the bikes may be used for both fitness and therapy settings.

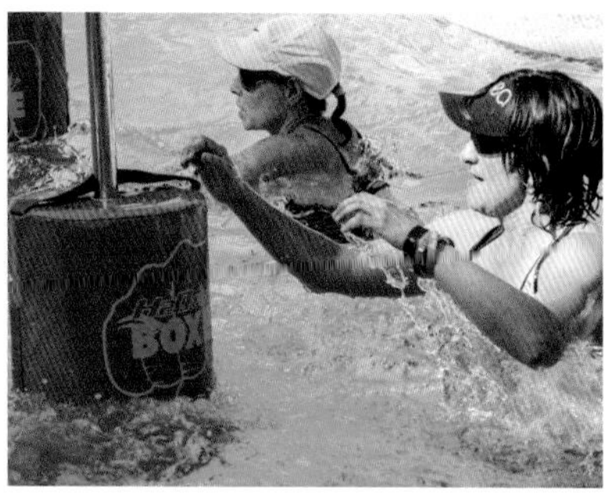

Aqua boxing bags: Weighted to anchor on the pool bottom (not permanently attached), boxing bags provide training benefits similar to land-based boxing bags. Specially designed for aquatics, the equipment provides a high-intensity training tool for martial arts programming. Offering an intense workout that simulates training on land, the equipment promotes all components of physical fitness and attracts new clientele to the pool.

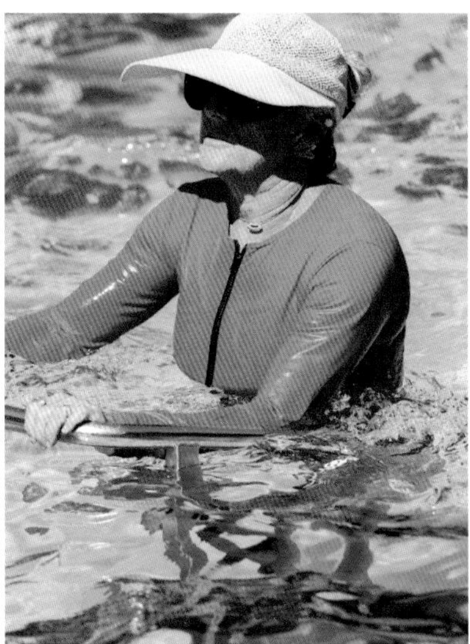

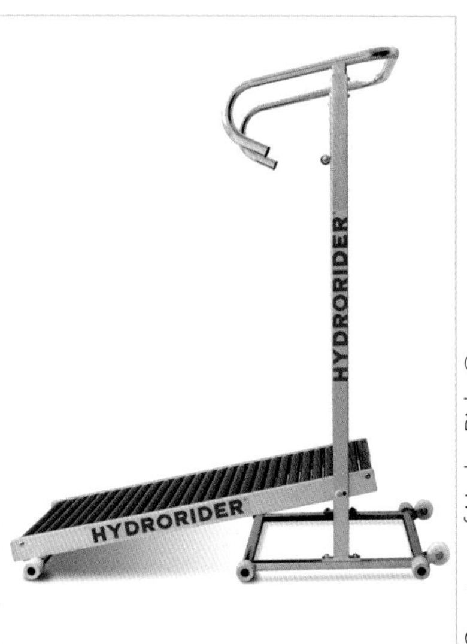

Courtesy of Hydro-Rider®

Aquatic treadmills: Like land-based treadmills, this equipment is used primarily to target cardiorespiratory endurance training, but in a reduced-gravity, low-impact setting. Designed to withstand the aquatic environment and periods of extended submersion, aquatic treadmills may be used in group settings, personal training, or therapy.

Aqua poles: This specialized type of equipment is designed specifically for pole training—dance-oriented, strength-focused, or functional fitness—in an aquatic environment. An innovative and fun approach to aquatic fitness, proper training promotes cardio and strength training of all major muscles, with a strong emphasis on the core and upper body.

(continued)

Specialized Equipment *(continued)*

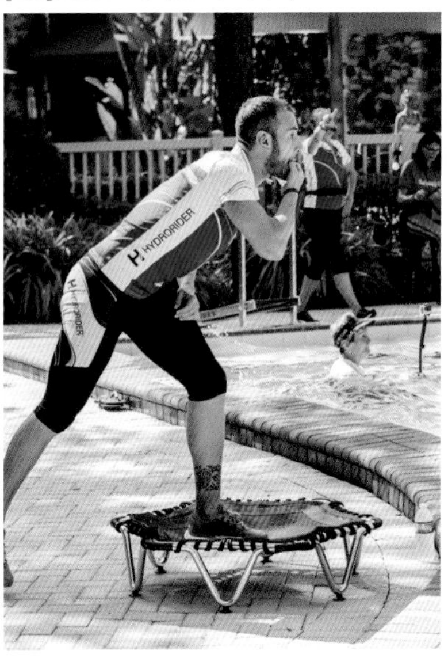

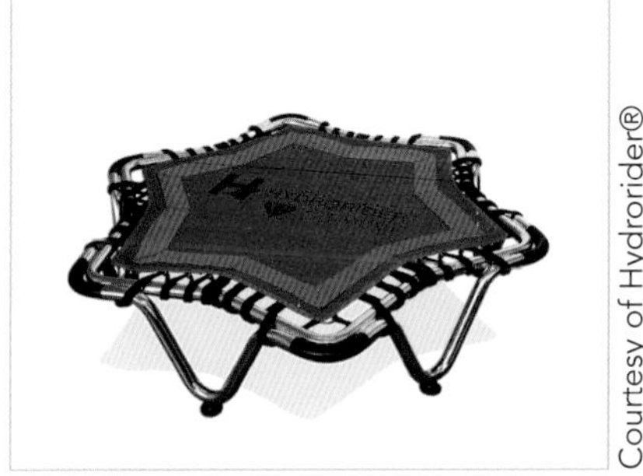

Courtesy of Hydrorider®

Aquatic trampolines: Mini trampolines are used to add variety and intensity to cardio endurance training and for lower-body and core training exercises in lessened gravity. The added benefit of the water's natural buoyancy makes trampoline training an effective advanced application.

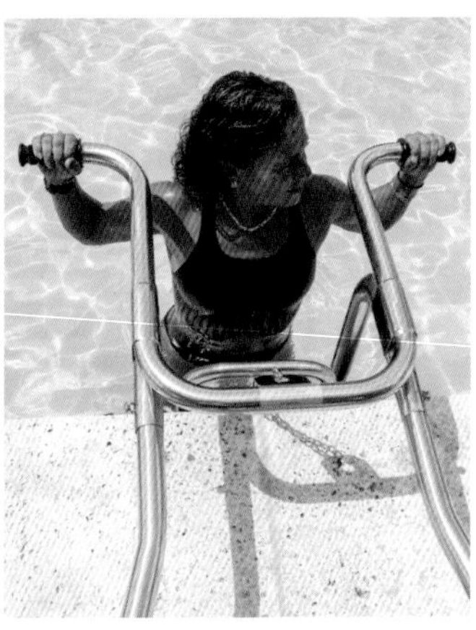

Aquatic wall stations: This stainless-steel apparatus, attached (temporarily or permanently) to the pool deck or wall, is designed as a stand-alone workout station for total-body resistance training and select cardiorespiratory endurance conditioning. The water's natural buoyancy makes this a comfortable tool for people who find similar land-based training difficult or unattainable. Some stations feature rubberized resistance tethered to the apparatus to provide total-body conditioning and increased cardio training.

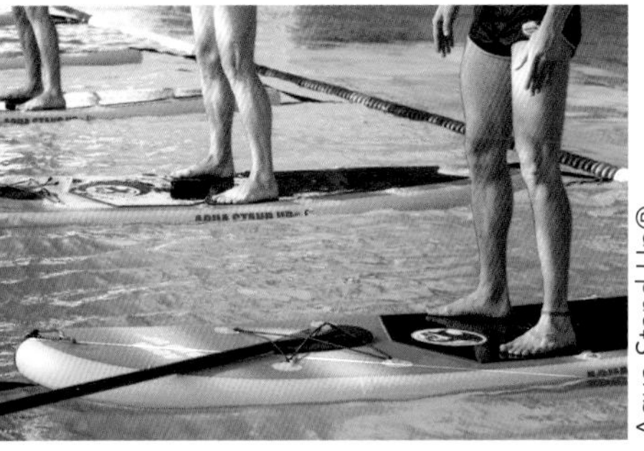

Aqua Stand Up®

Stand-up paddle boards: Stand-up paddling (SUP) is already a popular fitness trend in open water. Now, with boards designed to be anchored, SUP is also an option for the pool. Training on the boards involves paddling skills, both standing and prone, and can incorporate a variety of exercises options, such as yoga, Pilates, jump training, and stretching. This unstable surface emphasizes the core muscles, legs, and feet to maintain balance. However, programming can be designed to include exercises for all the major muscle groups.

Appendix D
Answers to Chapter Review

Chapter 1

1. Muscular strength
2. Ballistic stretching
3. Balance, coordination, speed, power, agility, and reaction time
4. Maximal heart rate is the highest heart rate a person can achieve. It is measured with a max HR test or estimated with 220 minus your age. Heart rate reserve is your maximal heart rate minus your resting heart rate.
5. The water compresses all body systems, including the vascular system, causing a smaller venous load to the heart, reducing heart rate.
6. Two to three days per week for each major muscle group.
7. The body's relative percentage of fat as compared to lean tissue (bones, muscles, and organs).
8. Improves physical appearance; increases functional capacity; heart becomes stronger; strengthens the walls of the blood vessels; improves strength and endurance; improves the efficiency of the nervous, lymph, and endocrine systems; improves psychological function.
9. b. Heart rate reserve method
10. Rating of perceived exertion

Chapter 2

1. Structure
2. Systole; diastole
3. Contractility
4. Hamstrings
5. Efferent neurons (nerve cells) that relay outgoing information from the central nervous system to the muscle cells.
6. Holding one's breath while exerting, such as during exercise, creates unequal pressure in the chest, causing blood pressure to drop and decreasing blood flow to the heart. Resuming normal breathing creates a surge in blood to the heart, causing a sharp increase in blood pressure.
7. Skeletal, muscular, nervous, respiratory and cardiovascular systems
8. Agonist
9. Visceral, cardiac, and skeletal
10. Ossification

Chapter 3

1. Specificity
2. Upper and lower
3. Oxidative system
4. During; after
5. Reduction in performance and coordination, elevated resting heart rate and blood pressure, loss of appetite, soreness, increased illness or infection, as well as issues with sleep, depression, and a reduced self-esteem.
6. Slow twitch
7. Isotonic
8. Oxygen deficit
9. Threshold of training
10. Isotonic, isometric, and isokinetic

Chapter 4

1. Abduction
2. Sagittal
3. Effort; fulcrum; resistance
4. Hinge
5. Cervical, thoracic, and lumbar
6. Buoyancy
7. Abduction and adduction; elevation and depression; protraction and retraction; pronation and supination; inversion and eversion; hyperextension; medial (internal) rotation and lateral (external) rotation; circumduction; tilt
8. The body is erect (or lying supine as if erect), arms by the side, palms facing forward, legs together, feet directed forward. Joints are neutral except for the forearms, which are supinated.
9. Assisted movement
10. Concentric

Chapter 5

1. It takes more than goals and willpower to change. There are multiple levels of influence on motivation. Finding meaning in exercise and being healthy are important.
2. Six months
3. a. True
4. b. A few days
5. Help them build an identity as an active participant and understand how being a healthier version of themselves will make a positive impact on their lives outside the water in their roles as parents, employees, or colleagues.
6. Create a task-focused, growth-oriented climate in your work. Use a motivational interviewing approach for individual encounters. Before they drop out, help participants identify and proactively address barriers to their exercise goals.
7. Their own effort and improvement
8. Autonomy (freedom of choice), competence (confidence in skills, improvement) and relatedness (meaningful connection to others)
9. a. Competence
10. Motivational interviewing

Chapter 6

1. Inertia
2. Pushing harder (applying more force) against the pool bottom to propel the body upward or through the water and pushing harder (applying more force) against the water's resistance with the arms and legs
3. Viscosity
4. An alternating wide jog traveling forward
5. Movement of the limbs (limb inertia), movement of the entire body (total-body inertia), and movement of the water (water inertia)
6. Increase (impeding arms)
7. Sink
8. The water's viscosity and drag
9. Action and reaction
10. Participant fitness and skill levels; acoustics of the pool environment

Chapter 7

1. Radiation is heat lost through vasodilation of surface vessels, and convection is the transfer of heat through the movement of a liquid or gas between areas of different temperatures.
2. Metabolic rate and heart rate decrease and the majority of the blood remains near the core of the body to keep the organs warm and functioning. When circulation is reduced to the extremities, these muscles become cold and inflexible, increasing risk of injury. Reduced circulation related to immersion in cold water also limits available oxygen for the muscles in the extremities, which may lead to muscle cramping.
3. 83 to 86 degrees F (28 to 30 degrees C)
4. A depth of 3.5 to 4.5 feet (1–1.4 m) is considered ideal for most shallow-water programs, but a slightly larger ranger (3 to 5 feet, or .9 to 1.5 meters) will accom-

modate most adult exercisers comfortably at the recommended water depth of mid–rib cage to mid-chest depth.

5. c. Slightly larger than
6. b. False
7. 75 to 85 degrees F (24–29.5 degrees C)
8. Shoes protect the skin on the soles of the feet. Traction provided by the shoes makes it easier to change direction or elevate movements. Shoes provide extra shock absorption, cushioning, and support. They also provide additional weight and resistance as well as added safety when entering and exiting the pool.
9. Instructors can experiment with different teaching locations around the pool, learn how to use hand and arm signals and other nonverbal cueing techniques effectively, and use a microphone system.
10. This depth reduces impact while still maintaining proper alignment and control of movement and allows for activities that sufficiently train all the major muscle groups against the water's resistance.

Chapter 8

1. c. Moves that land on alternating feet
2. b. False
3. Water tempo
4. b. Low impact
5. b. False
6. a. Double time
7. c. Neutral arm position
8. Float the arms on the surface of the water
9. b. Level I
10. c. Propelled movements

Chapter 9

1. a. True
2. b. False
3. Caloric expenditure
4. a. True
5. a. Dynamic stabilization
6. a. True
7. In a relaxed, motionless vertical position
8. b. Moguls
9. b. False
10. c. With all participants

Chapter 10

1. a. A cue
2. b. Feedback cues
3. Footwork
4. d. Audible
5. Advanced
6. a. True
7. d. Freestyle
8. Education and knowledge, experience, energy and enthusiasm, motivation, good interpersonal skills, adaptability, responsibility and consistency, sincerity.
9. c. Deep-water transitional move
10. e. A and B only

Chapter 11

1. a. True
2. c. Promotes more rapid removal of lactic acid.
3. b. Thermal warm-up
4. a. True
5. c. Muscular fitness training
6. b. False
7. c. The cardiorespiratory cool-down and the poststretch
8. d. Circuit training
9. b. False
10. d. A, B, and C

Chapter 12

1. 1. Decreased visual sharpness and perception, smaller visual field, and impaired judgment of the speed of moving objects. 2. Decreased hearing sharpness and reduced ability to discriminate between different sounds. 3. Reduced sensitivity to touch. 4. Decreased communication between muscles and nerves and decreased reaction time leading to altered mobility, response time, spatial awareness, and balance.

2. a. True
3. c. Hip flexion
4. b. 3-10%
5. Some muscle soreness is a normal response to exercise; if you develop joint pain that lasts for 2 hours or more after exercising, reduce exercise intensity or duration of the next class.
6. d. Fibromyalgia syndrome
7. b. False
8. c. Start in waist-deep water and gradually transition to chest-deep water.
9. a. True
10. b. Participants with multiple sclerosis

Chapter 13

1. c. Emergency action plan
2. c. Both A and B
3. a. True
4. a. True
5. d. A heart attack
6. List any three of the following: keep your throat most and your vocal chords lubricated; drink plenty of water throughout the day; avoid overuse by limiting the number of classes you teach and the use of lout vocal uses; include more body language and nonverbal cues; maintain proper breathing; use a microphone; if using music, keep it at a moderate level; consider speaker placement and the location from which you project your voice' check ventilation and chemical fume levels in the pool area; Project your voice with proper posture and body alignment; maintain the neck in neutral alignment; minimize background noise as much as possible; Limit talking when you have an upper respiratory infection; the vocal folds are already swollen and inflamed; substitute a swallow for excessive throat clearing; try to cough quietly to bring the vocal folds together gently.
7. a. True
8. b. False
9. Face. Ask the person to smile. Does one side of the face droop? Arms. Ask the person to raise both arms. Does one arm drift downward? Speech. Ask the person to repeat a simple phrase. Is their speech blurred? Time. If you observe any of these signs, call EMS immediately.
10. b. Hypoglycemia

Chapter 14

1. e. B and C only
2. a. Carbohydrates
3. c. Soluble fiber
4. d. Essential amino acids
5. a. True
6. d. Trans fats
7. a. Triglycerides
8. c. 2,000 calories
9. a. True
10. d. All of these

Chapter 15

1. c. Employee
2. b. Professional liability insurance
3. b. False
4. *AEA's Certified Aquatic Fitness Professional Code of Ethics and Conduct* and *AEA's Standards and Guidelines for Aquatic Fitness Programming*
5. a. True
6. b. Duty of care
7. Liability release or waiver of liability
8. d. Immediately after an incident
9. a. True
10. Americans with Disabilities Act (ADA)

Appendix E
Instructor Worksheets

Goal Setting

Chapter 5 explains how advanced planning may help you prepare participants for a successful exercise experience. A few simple questions can help participants recognize their reasons for participating in exercise, expectations they hold about the program, personal goals and possible barriers. Figure E.1 is a sample worksheet that you can utilize as is or modify for your specific needs, and then share with your class participants and personal training clients.

Figure E.1 Participant Assessment.

Name: ______________________________

Date: ____________________

When answering the questions below, please be as specific as possible.

1. What is the main reason you are joining this exercise program?

____
____
____

2. What are your personal fitness goals? What do you hope to get out of the program?

____
____
____

3. How might your fitness goals (if achieved) positively affect other important areas of your life (e.g., at home as a parent, at work, in your personal and social relationships)?

____
____
____

4. Has anything held you back from trying to achieve these goals in the past?

____
____
____

5. What is your plan for keeping track of your progress in this program (e.g., monitoring your exercise with a journal or smartphone app)?

____
____
____

From Aquatic Exercise Association, 2018, *Aquatic Fitness Professional Manual, Seventh Edition* (Champaign, IL: Human Kinetics).

Protocol for Kruel Aquatic Heart Deduction to Determine Target Heart Rates

The Kruel Aquatic Heart Rate Deduction is explained in chapter 1 under the section Monitoring Intensity. This protocol summarizes the formula, and can be combined with the additional worksheet provided in this appendix (figure E.2) to determine specific heart-rate training zones.

The deduction is determined by subtracting the heart rate standing in the water (water heart rate) from the heart rate standing out of the water (deck heart rate).

Step 1: Determine deck heart rate.

- Person stands out of the water for three minutes.
- After the three minutes of standing, the heart rate is taken for one full minute (with the person standing).

Step 2: Determine water heart rate.

- Person enters the water with as little movement as possible and stands in armpit-depth water.
- Person stands in armpit-depth water with as little movement as possible for three minutes.
- After three minutes of standing, the heart rate is taken for one full minute.
- Remember that environmental conditions, medication, caffeine, and excessive movement when entering the pool can affect heart rate response. Care should be taken to minimize these factors.

Step 3: Calculate aquatic heart rate deduction.

- Water heart rate is subtracted from deck heart rate.

Deck heart rate – water heart rate = aquatic heart rate deduction

Applying Kruel Aquatic HR Deduction with the Karvonen Formula

The following example applies the Kruel Aquatic HR Deduction to the Karvonen Formula to calculate a target aquatic heart rate.

[(220 – Age – RHR – Aquatic HR Deduction) × Desired Intensity Percentage] + RHR

Example:

A 50-year-old woman with a resting heart rate of 70, who wants to exercise in the water at 65% of her heart rate reserve and who has found her aquatic deduction to be 8, would calculate in the following manner.

[(220 – 50 – 70 – 8) × 0.65] + 70 = 130

Step 1: 220 – 50 (age) – 70 (RHR)
– 8 (Aquatic Deduction) = 92

Step 2: 92 × 0.65 (desired intensity) = 59.8

Step 3: 59.8 + 70 (RHR) = 129.8

Step 4: 129.8 is rounded to the nearest whole number = 130

Step 5: This woman's target heart rate is 130 beats per minute

Figure E.2 Worksheet for Determining Target Heart Rates With the Kruel Aquatic Heart Rate Deduction.

Read the protocol for Kruel Aquatic Heart Deduction to determine target heart rate found in this appendix to assist you with completing this worksheet. Additional information can be found in chapter 1.

Heart Rate Reserve:

220 – ________ – ________ = __________

AGE RHR X

Kruel Heart Rate Deduction

Participant stands out of pool for 3 minutes. Take HR for 1 minute.

HR_{Land}: ___________bpm

Participant stands in the water at armpit depth for 3 minutes. Take HR for 1 minute.

$HR_{Aquatic}$: _______________bpm

_________________ – ____________________ = ______________________

HR_{Land} $HR_{Aquatic}$ HR Deduction

Karvonen Formula with Kruel Deduction

Calculate the desired heart rate percentage (%) for the lower and upper training heart rate, and record below in Heart Rate Zone.

(_________) x (_______) + _________ – ____________ = __________

X % RHR HR Deduction

(_________) x (_______) + _________ – ____________ = __________

X % RHR HR Deduction

Heart Rate Zone

HR Zone: ___________ - ___________ BPM

From Aquatic Exercise Association, 2018, *Aquatic Fitness Professional Manual, Seventh Edition* (Champaign, IL: Human Kinetics).

Lesson Plan

A lesson plan can help you prepare for your class, develop a balanced workout, and offer reminders for important teaching tips. Lesson plans can also assist in organizing the verbal, nonverbal, and tactile cues associated with each movement or combination and keep you on track with your class schedule. The complexity and detail will depend upon your experience level and teaching style.

Refer to Chapter 11 for details on class components, including recommended durations and other considerations for each segment (summarized in Table 11. AEA Recommendations for Program Design on page 212). Figure E.3 is a simple format to follow, which you can modify to meet your personal needs.

Figure E.3 Simple Lesson Plan Format.

Class Structure: ____

Equipment: ____

Class Component	Topics and Exercises	Progressions and Cues
Warm-Up ______ minutes		
Conditioning ______ minutes		
Cool-down and stretching ______ minutes		

From Aquatic Exercise Association, 2018, *Aquatic Fitness Professional Manual, Seventh Edition* (Champaign, IL: Human Kinetics).

Example 1

Here is a simple version of a Lesson Plan that only includes key instructional reminders rather than listing every exercise (figure E.4). This option works well for experienced instructors who only want teaching tips and important concepts for discussion. This may also be sufficient when the choreography is simple.

Figure E.4 Class Structure: Shallow-Water Interval Training.

Class structure: Shallow-water interval training

Equipment: None

Class component	Topics and exercises	Progressions and cues
Warm-Up 10 minutes	• Discuss new format • Water walking alternating with practice of new exercises • Spend extra time warming up ankles for jumps	• Ankle warm up: heel-toe rocks, progress to "jump and landing" at level II, progress to low level jumps focusing on safe landing • Teach hand signals for "propulsion", "power tuck", "level III" and "speed drill" • Explain music signals for intervals
Conditioning 40 minutes total	8 Intervals 3 min : 2 min 1 = Level III exercises 2 = Propelled and tuck Jumps 3 = Speed drills 4 = Level III exercises 5 = Propelled and tuck jumps 6 = Speed drills 7 = Level III exercises 8 = Propelled and tuck Jumps	Options • Level II with tuck instead of level III • Option for level I instead of Propelled • Speed drills are self-paced Recovery • Water walking forward, backward and lateral Important cue • Jumps: Soft landing, knees bend, roll through feet
Cool-down and Stretching 10 minutes	Intersperse active stretch with static stretch Include one minute deep breathing if water warm enough	Active stretch is gentle movement, full ROM Options for cool water – practice breathing with the active stretches

Example 2

Here is a detailed lesson plan that includes all of the selected exercises plus teaching tips, progressions and cues (figure E.5). This lesson plan option works well for novice instructors and for classes with more complicated choreography. Note: This example is based upon the sample shallow water striding class found in Appendix F to demonstrate how to transfer choreography notes into a detailed lesson plan.

Figure E.5 Class Structure: Shallow-Water Striding Class.

Class structure: Shallow-water striding class
Equipment: None

Class component	Topics and exercises	Progressions and cues
Warm-Up 10 minutes	Forward walk with arms swinging at sides	• Focus on posture, alignment, and proper foot strike • Gradually increase the length of the stride without compromising form • Gradually transition to gentle jog with breaststroke arms
Conditioning 20-40 minutes	1. F Jog with knees up 4x + heels up 4x	1. Knee pointed down on heels up jog
	2. B Front kicks	2. Low kicks with assisting arms
	3. F and B tightrope walk	3. Tandem walking, gradually increase stride length
	4. L Side steps	4. Neutral arms
	5. L Side jacks	5. Jumping jack traveling laterally
	6. F and B sprint 8 counts + down run 8 counts	6. Down run = level II run with tiny steps and floating arms
	7. F Cross-country ski	7. Include level I, II, and III
	8. B Jumping Jacks	8. Include level I, II, and III
	9. L ½ WT cross-country ski with center bounce	9. Travel on center bounce, stabilize on the ski
	10. L lateral leap	10. Body facing front
	11. F and B lunge walk	11. Spine aligned and tall, core engaged; progress ROM
	12. F and B level II moguls	12. Travel forward as legs move side to side
	13. L step and cross	13. Begin grounded, progress to rebound
	14. L slide	14. Level I
	15. L glide	15. Level II

F = forward
B = backward
L = lateral
OTS = on the spot

Figure E.5 *(continued)*

Class component	Topics and exercises	Progressions and cues
Cool-Down and Stretching 10 minutes	F Walk (neutral arms) OTS Gastrocnemius stretch (stride position) with dynamic latissimus dorsi stretch (alternating reach up 3 times and pause with the arm lifted) B Walk and pause (walk back three steps and pause with leg lifted to challenge balance, progress to closing eyes on the pause) OTS Quadriceps and iliopsoas stretch (stride position) with dynamic triceps and posterior deltoid stretch (alternately reach across the body three times and pause, pulling into the stretch with the other arm) L Side steps with dynamic pectoralis and anterior deltoid stretch (arms cross front and open back four times, pausing at end position with arms back) OTS Upper trapezius and neck stretch + deep breathing	Alternating travel for warmth with static stretches to lengthen muscles Focus on proper posture throughout Add deep breathing with the stretches

Appendix F
Sample Class Formats

This appendix should be used together with chapter 11 to help you develop safe and successful aquatic programming for both group fitness and personal training. Using the general recommendations for class components, numerous formats can be designed to keep aquatic classes engaging, provide variety, and motivate a wide range of participants.

You will find six sample workouts that can be used as is or modified for your classes and training sessions. Many of the exercises and stretches included in these workouts are found in appendixes A and B. For exercises not already detailed in those two appendixes, there are movement descriptions to assist you with learning and teaching them to your classes and clients.

Sample Shallow-Water Circuit Class

Read more about this class format on page 222 in chapter 11.

Circuit training is often referred to as station training, and the activities can focus on cardiorespiratory fitness, muscular fitness, flexibility, neuromotor fitness, or any combination of these. This training format is very versatile and can be adapted for various water depths, participant ability levels, and available equipment. This specific example is designed for shallow water and combines cardio (3-minute segments) with resistance training (90-second segments).

Equipment: The resistance exercises can be done with buoyancy equipment, with drag equipment, or without equipment. However, keep in mind that the muscle actions may vary based on the equipment used.

Warm-up: 10 minutes

Heel-high jog forward, knee-high jog backward, wide jog in place. Repeat several times, adding different arm patterns; begin with short levers and progress to long levers.

Kick front (straight leg) forward and backward, pendulum in place. Repeat several times, adding different arm patterns; use long levers.

Level I jumping jacks, level I cross-country ski. Repeat several times, adding different arm patterns; use long levers.

Circuit one: 3 minutes cardio, 90 seconds resistance

Cardio: Knee-high jog traveling forward for 8 counts, knee-high jog traveling backward for 8 counts, jumping jacks for 8 counts, wide jog traveling forward for 8 counts, wide jog traveling backward for 8 counts, cross-country ski for 8 counts. Repeat for 3 minutes.

Resistance: Transverse shoulder abduction and adduction. Do 30 seconds bilateral (both arms), 30 seconds right arm, and 30 seconds left arm.

Circuit two: 3 minutes cardio, 90 seconds resistance

Cardio: Kick front (straight leg) traveling forward for 8 counts, kick front (straight leg) traveling backward for 8 counts, jumping jacks, pendulum traveling forward 8 counts, pendulum traveling backward for 8 counts, cross-country ski for 8 counts. Repeat for 3 minutes.

Resistance: Shoulder abduction and adduction. Do 30 seconds bilateral, 30 seconds right arm, and 30 seconds left arm.

Circuit three: 3 minutes cardio, 90 seconds resistance

Cardio: Knee-high jog traveling forward for 8 counts, knee-high jog traveling backward for 8 counts, level II or III jumping jack, wide jog traveling forward for 8 counts, wide job traveling backward for 8 counts, level II or III cross-country ski. Repeat for 3 minutes.

Resistance: Shoulder flexion and extension. Do 30 seconds bilateral, 30 seconds right arm, and 30 seconds left arm.

Circuit four: 3 minutes cardio, 90 seconds resistance

Cardio: Kick front (straight leg) traveling forward for 8 counts, kick front (straight leg) traveling backward for 8 counts, level II or III jumping jacks, pendulum traveling forward 8 counts, pendulum traveling backward for 8 counts, level II or III cross-country ski for 8 counts. Repeat for 3 minutes.

Resistance: Chest press transverse shoulder abduction with elbow flexion and transverse shoulder adduction with elbow extension. Do 30 seconds bilateral, 30 seconds right arm, and 30 seconds left arm.

Circuit five: 3 minutes cardio, 90 seconds resistance

Cardio: Knee-high jog with power for 8 counts, jumping jacks for 8 counts, wide jog with power, cross-country ski for 8 counts. Repeat for 3 minutes.

Resistance: Elbow flexion and extension. Do 30 seconds bilateral, 30 seconds right arm, and 30 seconds left arm.

Circuit six: 3 minutes cardio, 90 seconds resistance

Cardio: Kick front (straight leg) with power for 8 counts, jumping jacks, wide jog with power for 8 counts, cross-country ski for 8 counts. Repeat for 3 minutes.

Resistance: Internal and external shoulder rotation (keeping elbows at sides and bent so forearms are parallel to pool bottom; bring arms in across stomach and out to side). Do 30 seconds bilateral, 30 seconds right arm, and 30 seconds left arm.

Circuit seven: 3 minutes cardio, 90 seconds resistance

Cardio: Knee-high jog with power for 8 counts, level II or III jumping jacks for 8 counts, kick front (straight leg) kicks with power, level II or III cross-country ski for 8 counts. Repeat for 3 minutes.

Resistance: Spinal rotation, hold your arms straight out in front for 30 seconds. Spinal rotation, holding arms straight out in front, standing heel to toe, with right foot in front for 30 seconds. Spinal rotation, holding arms straight out in front, standing heel to toe, with left foot in front for 30 seconds.

Circuit eight: 3 minutes cardio, 90 seconds resistance

Cardio: Knee-high jog with power for 8 counts, tuck jump side to side for 8 counts, kick front (straight leg) kicks with power, tuck jump front to back for 8 counts.

Resistance: Stirring the pot: Holding the arms out in front, circle the arms as if stirring a pot. Circle to the right for 30 seconds, to the left for 30 seconds, and alternate circles for 30 seconds.

Cool-down: 10 minutes

Heel-high jog, transverse abduction and adduction with arms for 24 counts

Wide jog, abduction and adduction with arms crossing in front and behind for 24 counts

With a wide stance, stretch the following muscles:

- Gastrocnemius
- Quadriceps
- Hamstrings
- Latissimus dorsi
- Pectoralis major
- Triceps

Deep-Water High-Intensity Interval Training Sample Class

Read more about this class format on page 222-223 in chapter 11.

Interval training contains a series of training cycles that include high-intensity and low-intensity segments; both work and rest are planned and functional. HIIT, or high-intensity interval training, is designed for participants to exercise at or above their maximal capacity; rest periods vary depending on the goals of the class. This sample class is designed for deep water, but HIIT works equally well with shallow water or even with combination depths.

Table F.1 Interval Training Cycle Examples

Component	Drills	Duration
Warm-up	Jog easy and build gradually into a more challenging pace	5 minutes
	3 x 15 second hard + 45 seconds easy	3 minutes
Level 4: hard (8 on the Aquatic Exercise Intensity Scale)	Frog jog Cue quick transitions and big ROM	1 minute
	Recovery jog	5-15 seconds
	Cross country ski Cue long legs and powerful movements with both hip flexion & extension	1 minute
	Recovery jog	5-15 seconds
	5 regular jogs + 5 short and quick jogs Cue high knees for 5 and "flash-dance"; reduced ROM for 5 (faster than land tempo)	1 Minute
	Recovery Jog	5-15 seconds
	4 toe touches + 4 heel-high jogs Cue straight-leg toe touch with alternating arm and leg action with a forceful hip flexion and extension and a quick transition to a heel-high jog	1 Minute
	Recovery jog	30 seconds

(continued)

Table F.1 *(continued)*

Component	Drills	Duration
Level 5: maximal effort (10 on the Aquatic Exercise Intensity Scale)	Run hard Cue maintaining ROM, increasing power and acceleration	10 seconds
	Recovery jog	5 seconds
	Flutter kick Cue kicking hard to push shoulders out of the water	5 seconds
	Recovery jog	5 seconds
	Cross country skis popping Cue powerful hip flexion and extension to promote upward thrust out of the water	15 seconds
	Recovery jog	5 seconds
	Flutter kick Cue kicking hard to push shoulders out of the water	5 seconds
	Recovery jog	5 seconds
	Run hard Cue maintaining ROM, increasing power and acceleration	10 seconds
	Recovery jog	5 seconds
	Flutter kick Cue kicking hard to push shoulders out of the water	5 seconds
	Recovery jog	5 seconds
	Cross-country ski, popping Cue powerful hip flexion and extension to promote upward thrust out of the water	15 Seconds
	Recovery jog	5 seconds
	Flutter kick Cue kicking hard to push shoulders out of the water	5 seconds
	Recovery jog Cue breathing and slow jog with large ROM	30 sec-1 minute

Table F.1 *(continued)*

Component	Drills	Duration
Level 4: hard (8 on the Aquatic Exercise Intensity Scale)	5 jogs forward + 5 jogs backward with assistive breaststroke, arms forward and back Cue tall body and hard pulls with the arms: "Squeeze when you pull." With reverse jogs, cue leading with their toes, like digging in the sand	1 Minute
	Recovery jog	5-15 seconds
	High-knee flexed-feet run Cue big ROM with toes pulling towards the ceiling: "Pull the water up and push the water down"	30 seconds
	Recovery jog	5-15 seconds
	Cross country ski, popping every third ski Cue powerful hip flexion and extension to promote upward thrust out of the water	1 minute
	Recovery jog	5-15 seconds
	5 regular jogs + 5 wide jogs Cue big ROM, like jogging through monster truck tires	30 seconds
	5 regular jogs + 5 wide jogs Cue small ROM, like jogging through bicycle tires, short and quick	30 seconds
	Recovery jog	5-15 seconds
	Cross-body toe touches Cue maintaining shoulder abduction and rotating at the waist to bring the foot to meet the hand (should feel this in their obliques)	1 minute
	Recovery jog Cue breathing and slow jog with large ROM	30 seconds
Level 5: maximal effort (10 on the Aquatic Exercise Intensity Scale, except for the recovery jog)	Double frog jog Cue propelling the body up by bringing both legs together in a modified breaststroke kick	15 seconds
	Recovery jog	15 seconds
	Short and quick toe touches Cue half the ROM, beginning at 90 degrees, and powerful kicks upward and pull-downs Alternate arm action; cue good posture	20 seconds
	Recovery jog	15 seconds
	Flutter kick Cue kicking hard to push shoulders out of the water	15 seconds
	Recovery jog	15 seconds
	High-knee flexed-feet run Cue big ROM with toes pulling toward the ceiling: "Pull the water up and push the water down" Accelerate	30 seconds
	Recovery jog Cue breathing and slow jog with large ROM	30 sec-1 minute

(continued)

Table F.1 *(continued)*

Component	Drills	Duration
Level 4: hard (8 on the Aquatic Exercise Intensity Scale)	2 regular jog s+ 2 log (hurdler) jogs Cue tall regular jogs with big ROM + leg extension and flexion (at hip and knee), like they are jumping over a hurdle	1 Minute
	Recovery jog	5-15 seconds
	5 jogs + 5 jumping jacks Cue tall regular jogs with powerful jumping jacks	30 seconds
	Recovery jog	5-15 seconds
	5 regular jogs + 5 flutter kicks Cue tall regular jogs with flutter kicks, propelling their bodies up and out of the water	1 minute
	Recovery jog	5-15 seconds
	4 regular frog jogs + 4 double frog jogs Cue big ROM for regular frog jogs, and for double frog jogs, propelling up and out of the water	1 minute
	Recovery jog	5-15 seconds
	Elliptical (floorless jog) Cue slight body lean forward with extended ROM through the hips and knees; keep flexed feet with this motion	1 Minute
	Recovery jog	5-15 seconds
	Recovery jog Cue breathing and slow jog large ROM	30 seconds
Level 5: maximal effort (10 on the Aquatic Exercise Intensity Scale, except for the recovery jog)	Hard and fast run! Cue all-out effort, maintaining ROM and form	15 seconds
	Recovery jog They may need more recovery than this	30 seconds
	Hard and fast run! Cue all-out effort, maintaining ROM and form	15 seconds
	Recovery jog They may need more recovery than this	30 seconds
	Hard and fast run! Cue all-out effort, maintaining ROM and form	15 seconds
	Recovery jog They may need more recovery than this	30 seconds
	Hard and fast run! Cue all-out effort, maintaining ROM and form	15 seconds
	Recovery jog Cue breathing and slow jog with large ROM	30 sec-1 minute

Table F.1 *(continued)*

Component	Drills	Duration
Level 4: hard (8 on the Aquatic Exercise Intensity Scale)	4 cross-country skis + 4 x jumping jacks Jacks pop Cue Long and strong skis with powerful jumping jacks to propel the body up and out of the water	30 seconds
	4 cross-country skis + 4 x jumping jacks Skis pop Cue strong jacks with powerful cross-country skis to propel the body up and out of the water	30 seconds
	Recovery jog	5-15 seconds
	Regular jog with varied arm patterns: front punch, side punch, downward punch, criss-cross arms up and down in front	1 minute Change arm pattern every 15 seconds
	Recovery jog	5-15 seconds
	4 wide jogs + 4 wide flutter kicks Cue big ROM with wide jogs (externally rotated at the hip) and wide flutter kicks with legs abducted—powerful to push the body up and out of the water	1 Minute
	Recovery jog	5-15 seconds
	5 long cross-country skis + 5 short and quick cross-country skis (half the motion in half the time) Cue long legs, accentuating the forward and backward motion of the legs at the hip, and then shortening the movement to go faster than land tempo	1 minute
	Recovery jog	30 sec-1 minute
Level 5: maximal effort (10 on the Aquatic Exercise Intensity Scale, except for recovery jog)	Anything goes! Mix and match different exercises at maximum effort for 1 minute Example: Long cross-country skis → flutter kick up → high-knee flexed-foot jog → jumping jacks → short and quick wide jogs → wide flutter kick → short and quick cross-country skis → cross-country pop → sprint to the finish	1 minute, no rest between exercises
Cool-down with 15-second "surprises"	Slow bicycle	1.5 minutes
	Maximal effort run	15 seconds
	Slow frog jog with corresponding arms	1 minute
	Maximal effort run	15 seconds
	Tuck and row or straight body and row	1 minute forward and 1 minute back
	Maximal effort run	15 seconds
	Easy jog with emphasis on range of motion (regular, wide, and long)	5 minutes

Sample Shallow-Water Striding Class

Read more about this class format on pages 223-224 in chapter 11.

Designed around various striding patterns (e.g., walking, jogging, or other traveling exercises), this format easily adapts to various pool shapes and sizes, as well as most fitness levels. Although this specific example applies to shallow water, striding classes can be performed at any water depth with appropriate exercise choices.

Travel directions: Remain within mid-rib-cage to mid-chest water depth while traveling in the following directions:

F = forward

B = backward

L = lateral

OTS = on the spot (remain in place, not traveling)

Impact level: All exercises are at level I unless otherwise noted.

Warm-up: 10 minutes

Forward walk with arms swinging at sides:

- Focus on posture, alignment, and proper foot strike
- Gradually increase the length of the stride without compromising form
- Gradually transition to gentle jog with breaststroke arms

Conditioning: 20-40 minutes

F Jog with knees up 4× + heels up 4×

B Front kicks (low kicks with assisting arms)

F and B Tightrope walk (tandem walking, gradually increase stride length)

L Side steps (neutral arms)

L Side jacks (jumping jacks traveling laterally)

F and B Sprint for 8 counts + down run for 8 counts (drop to level II and run backward with tiny steps and floating arms)

F Cross-country ski (levels I, II, and III)

B Jumping jacks (levels I, II, and III)

L Half-WT cross-country ski with center bounce (travel on the center bounce, stabilize body on the ski)

L Lateral leap

F and B Lunge walk (keep the spine aligned and tall and the core engaged, progressive ROM)

F and B Level II moguls

L Step and cross (begin grounded, progress to rebounding)

L Slide

L Glide

Cool-down and stretching: 10 minutes

F Walk (neutral arms)

OTS Gastrocnemius stretch (stride position) with dynamic latissimus dorsi stretch (alternating reach up 3 times and pausing with the arm lifted)

B Walk and pause (walk back 3 steps and pause with leg lifted to challenge balance, progress to closing eyes on the pause)

OTS Quadriceps and iliopsoas stretch (stride position) with dynamic triceps and posterior deltoid stretch (alternately reach across the body 3 times and pause, pulling into the stretch with the other arm)

L Side steps with dynamic pectoralis and anterior deltoid stretch (the arms cross in front and open back 4 times, pausing at the end position with the arms back)

OTS Upper trapezius and neck stretch + deep breathing

Sample Shallow-Water Kickboxing Class

Read more about this class format on page 226-227 in chapter 11.

Transferring fitness kickboxing techniques and movement patterns to the water creates a high-intensity, highly resistive, yet lower-impact exercise option that can be performed by most participant levels. Attention to proper form and technique is important. If you are unfamiliar with kickboxing techniques, AEA offers a 3-hour aquatic kickboxing workshop that teaches proper stances, ring movements, punches, and kicks.

Warm-up: 10-15 minutes

Heel-high jog forward + knee-high jog backward + wide jog in place. Repeat several times, adding different arms patterns; begin with short levers and progress to long levers.

Review of punches and kicks

- Jab
- Cross
- Hook
- Upper cut
- Front kick
- Side kick
- Back kick

Conditioning: 30-40 minutes

Grounded kick drills: 8 reps of each on the right side, then repeat each series on the left side

Reverse lunge + knee lift

Reverse lunge + front kick

Squat and side kick

Double side kick and chamber (pause in knee-lift position)

Half-tempo back kick

Double-back kick and chamber

Repeat series 1-3 sets.

Punch drills: 8 reps of each on the right side, then repeat each series on the left side

Double jab + cross

Speed drill jab

Hook + upper cut + hook

Flurry (fast alternating upper cut)

Jab + cross + hook + upper cut

Repeat series 1-3 sets.

Cardio combinations: Teach each of the 3 combinations using pyramid or add-on choreography and repeat as needed to master the skills. Then, put all three combinations together.

Combination 1:

Lead-leg front kick

Jab, cross, hook 2×

Rear-leg front kick 3×

Jump turn (switch lead leg)

Combination 2:

Turning half-WT kick (front-side-front) and jack 2×, alternating lead (Note: all kicks front of pool, same leg)

Jack-ski and jab 4×, alternating lead

Combination 3:

Knee smash* right and side kick left 3×

Double-knee smash right

Repeat opposite lead

Speed drill alternating front punch (from center stance)

Speed drill upper cut (from center stance)

Repeat all three combinations together in sequence.

*Knee smash = front knee lift with arms pulling powerfully toward the knee

Cool-down and stretching: 10-15 minutes

Water walk forward across pool with exaggerated stride; arms open to stretch the chest

Pause at the wall and perform the first wall stretch listed (lower back)

Repeat, walking to the opposite side of the pool for the second stretch (hamstrings)

Continue with all seven stretches, performing on both sides of the body as needed

Wall Stretches (see deep-water wall stretches in appendix B)

- Lower back
- Hamstrings

- Inner thigh
- Outer thigh
- Iliopsoas
- Gastrocnemius
- Latissimus

Sample Deep-Water Boot Camp Workout

Read more about this class format on page 227 in chapter 11.

Boot camp classes use a combination of muscular strengthening exercises, cardiovascular exercises, power or plyometric movements, and ROM activities to challenge overall strength and conditioning. This example is a deep-water program, but classes can be created for shallow water or combination depths with appropriate exercise choices.

Warm-up: 7 minutes

Easy high-knee jog for 2 minutes

Easy wide jog for 1 minute

Easy jumping jacks for 1 minute

Easy cross-country ski for 1 minute

Repeat all exercises for 30 seconds each at a higher intensity for ample warm-up.

Conditioning

Cue: Perform each round at your individual maximum. Work hard and do your best!

Round 1: Upper body + lower body

Tuck and shoot forward and back (moguls) for 30 seconds

Boxing bag or flurry arms (legs used for balance only—wide jog) for 30 seconds

Tuck and shoot forward and back for 45 seconds

Boxing bag or flurry arms (legs used for balance only—wide jog) for 45 seconds

Tuck and shoot forward and back for 60 seconds

Boxing bag or flurry arms (legs used for balance only—wide jog) for 60 seconds

Easy jog for 1 minute

Round 2: Upper body + lower body

Jumping jacks with hard push-out and easy pull-in for 30 seconds

Internal and external shoulder rotation (flasher arms) emphasizing the open or external rotation (legs used for balance only—wide jog) for 30 seconds

Jumping jacks with hard pull-in and easy push-out for 30 seconds

Internal and external shoulder rotation (flasher arms) emphasizing the closed or internal rotation (legs used for balance only—wide jog) for 30 seconds

Jumping jacks with hard push-out and easy pull-in for 45 seconds

Internal and external shoulder rotation (flasher arms) emphasizing the open or external rotation (legs used for balance only—wide jog) for 45 seconds

Jumping jacks with hard pull-in and easy push-out for 45 seconds

Internal and external shoulder rotation (flasher arms) emphasizing the closed or internal rotation (legs used for balance only—wide jog) for 45 seconds

Easy wide jog for 1 minute

Round 3: Upper body + lower body

Cross-country ski with hard push-out and easy pull-in for 30 seconds

Palm-up scoop (legs used for balance only—wide jog) for 30 seconds

Cross-country ski with hard pull-in and easy push-out for 30 seconds

Palm-up scoop (legs used for balance only—wide jog) for 30 seconds

Cross-country ski with hard push-out and easy pull-in for 60 seconds

Palm-up scoop (legs used for balance only—wide jog) for 30 seconds

Cross-country ski with hard pull-in and easy push-out for 60 seconds

Palm-up scoop (legs used for balance only—wide jog) for 30 seconds

Easy long jog (hurdle jog) for 1 minute

Divide Class Into Teams of 3

Post a list of 5 exercises so that the class can see them.

Cue: When doing this team activity, work as hard as you can to get the exercises done as quickly as you can while still maintaining perfect form! As a *team* you will complete 100 repetitions of *each* exercise. That means that if you go slower than your teammates, they will be picking up your slack, so work to your potential! Get through as many exercises as you can in 8 minutes. If you finish, start again from the top! Don't stop moving until the time is up.

Set your timer for 8 minutes and give updates as time passes.

Exercises to be completed:

1. Hurdle jumps (right + left = 1 repetition)
2. Wall push-ups (vertically pushing up) or push-pulls (pushing and pulling to and from the wall)
3. X-jump (jump to the 4 points of an imaginary X on the bottom of the pool; knees drive up high and press down forcefully; arms used for balance) (1 X = 1 repetition)
4. Arm curls in a T (arms out to sides, bend elbow and touch fingers to shoulder, then extend elbow) (bend + extend = 1 repetition)
5. Tire run (feet in, in, out, out = 1 repetition)

Easy jog back to your spot

Back to Individual Work

Cue: Work *hard* for this last part of class! We are going to keep it simple and just run, holding our pace for 5 minutes. Start out running so it feels challenging but not too hard, so that you can maintain your pace and effort through the entire 5 minutes.

Set your timer for 5 minutes and give updates as time passes; continue to cue good form and body mechanics throughout the running piece.

Regular run for 5 minutes; work hard and maintain the effort!

Cool-down and stretching: 7 minutes

High-knee jog, gradually getting easier for 2 minutes

Easy jumping jacks emphasizing range of motion for 1 minute

Continue jumping jacks, and pause at the end range of motion for 1 minute

Easy cross-country ski emphasizing range of motion for 1 minute

Continue cross-country ski, and pause at the end range of motion, then switch legs for 1 minute

Single-leg quadriceps stretch for 30 seconds for each leg

Sample Aquatic Functional Training Class

Read more about this class format on page 228 in chapter 11.

Functional training helps give participants the strength, flexibility, power, and endurance to move effectively and efficiently throughout the day by including exercises to gain the mobility, stability, and balance needed to improve or maintain functional independence. This sample class is designed using an interval format (3 minutes of cardio and 1 minute of functional exercises), but functional training could be designed for continuous or circuit formats as well.

Equipment: Functional exercises can be completed with drag equipment or without equipment

Warm-up: 10 minutes

Heel-high jog forward, knee-high jog backward, wide jog in place. Repeat several times, adding different arm patterns; begin with short levers and progress to long levers.

Kick front (straight leg) forward and backward, pendulum in place. Repeat several times, adding different arm patterns; use long levers.

Interval one: 3 minutes cardio, 1 minute functional exercise

Cardio: Knee-high jog traveling forward across pool, knee-high jog traveling backward across pool, wide jog traveling forward across pool, wide jog traveling backward across pool, jog sideways across pool and back. Repeat for 3 minutes.

Functional exercise: Diagonal chest press: right arm with spinal rotation to the left for 30 seconds, left arm with spinal rotation to the right for 30 seconds.

Interval two: 3 minutes cardio, 1 minute functional exercise

Cardio: Alternate: 30-second knee-high jog traveling forward anywhere in the pool, 30-second knee-high jog progressively lifting knees higher and traveling forward anywhere in the pool. Repeat for 3 minutes.

Functional exercise: Squats with bilateral chest press for 30 seconds, squats with unilateral chest press (alternate right and left arms) for 30 seconds.

Interval three: 3 minutes cardio, 1 minute functional exercise

Cardio: Alternate: 30-second wide jog traveling anywhere in the pool, 30-second wide jog sideways progressively lifting knees higher and traveling anywhere in the pool. Repeat for 3 minutes.

Functional exercise: Lunge position: left leg forward, right arm, shoulder flexion or extension (as if pushing a vacuum cleaner) for 30 seconds; right leg forward, left arm, shoulder flexion or extension (as if pushing a vacuum cleaner) for 30 seconds.

Interval four: 3 minutes cardio, 1 minute functional exercise

Cardio: Alternate: 30-second knee-high jog traveling forward anywhere in the pool, 30-second knee-high jog with a longer stride traveling forward anywhere in the pool. Repeat for 3 minutes.

Functional exercise: Spinal rotation: hold your arms straight out in front for 30 seconds, hold arms down as if swinging a golf club for 30 seconds.

Interval five: 3 minutes cardio, 1 minute functional exercise

Cardio: Alternate every 15 seconds: knee-high jog traveling forward anywhere in the pool, knee-high jog with a longer stride traveling forward anywhere in the pool, knee-high jog progressively lifting knees higher. Repeat for 3 minutes.

Functional exercise: Start with shoulders abducted; bring right hand down toward right hip and back to abducted position for 30 seconds, left hand toward left hip for 30 seconds.

Interval six: 3 minutes cardio, 1 minute functional exercise

Cardio: Alternate every 15 seconds: wide jog traveling forward anywhere in the pool, wide jog with a longer stride traveling sideways to the right, wide jog with a longer stride traveling sideways to the left, wide jog traveling forward anywhere in the pool and progressively lifting knees higher. Repeat for 3 minutes.

Functional exercise: Lunge forward, alternating legs, for 30 seconds; lunge diagonally forward, alternating right and left legs, for 30 seconds.

Interval seven: 3 minutes cardio, 1 minute functional exercise

Cardio: Holding drag equipment in front of your body or holding arms out in front with wrists neutral, alternate every 15 seconds: knee-high jog forward anywhere in the pool, knee-high jog sideways to the right, knee-high jog sideways to the left, knee-high with longer stride forward, knee-high jog progressively lifting knees higher and traveling forward anywhere in the pool. Repeat for 3 minutes.

Functional exercise: Spinal rotation, holding your arms straight out in front for 30 seconds. Spinal rotation, holding arms straight out in front, standing heel to toe, with right foot in front for 30 seconds. Spinal rotation, holding arms straight out in front, standing heel to toe, with left foot in front for 30 seconds.

Interval eight: 3 minutes cardio, 1 minute functional exercise

Cardio: Alternate every 15 seconds: knee-high jog traveling forward anywhere in the pool, walk on heels, knee-high jog traveling forward with longer stride anywhere in the pool, walk on toes, knee-high jog traveling forward anywhere in the pool and progressively lifting knees higher, walk heel to toe. Repeat for 3 minutes.

Functional exercise: Squat with arms down to side, straighten legs and bring arms up to chest (as if lifting a box) for 30 seconds, straighten legs (going up on your toes) and bring arms to chest for 30 seconds.

Cool-down: 10 minutes

Heel-high jog, transverse abduction and adduction with arms for 24 counts

Wide jog, abduction and adduction with arms crossing in front and behind for 24 counts

Stretch the following muscles:

Gastrocnemius

Quadriceps

Hamstrings

Latissimus dorsi

Pectoralis major

Triceps

Glossary

abduction—Movement away from the midline (center) of the body.

acceleration—The reaction of a body is proportional to the force applied, in the same direction as the applied force, and inversely proportional to its mass.

action and reaction—For every action, there is an equal and opposite reaction.

activities of daily living (ADLs)—Activities performed in daily living, including self-care, work, and leisure; basic self-care tasks such as feeding and getting dressed.

acute injury—An injury with a sudden onset and short duration.

ADA—See **Americans with Disabilities Act**.

adaptation—The ability of a body part, system, or organ to adjust to additional stress, or overload, over time by increasing in strength or function.

additional insured—A business added to your liability insurance policy for purposes of protecting them against your negligence.

add-on choreography—A style of choreography that builds patterns gradually while providing positive reinforcement through repetition as the sequence is learned; sometimes called the *memory* or *building block method*.

adduction—Movement toward the midline (center) of the body.

adenosine triphosphate (ATP)—A chemical compound that is the most immediate source of energy for a cell.

adhesion—The tendency of molecules of one substance to stick to the molecules of another substance whose surfaces are in direct contact. For example, water adheres to the body when it is immersed.

advanced transition—A shallow-water transition that changes between a one-footed move and a two-footed move with a change in impact, or any transition that involves a change in plane *and* a change in impact level.

AEA's Certified Aquatic Fitness Professional Code of Ethics and Conduct—The definition of baseline standards that AEA-certified fitness professionals are expected to follow.

AEA's Standards and Guidelines for Aquatic Fitness Programming—Important information for professional leadership and application, environmental concerns, facility recommendations, and instructional issues for the overall safety of the participants serviced.

aerobic fitness—See **cardiorespiratory fitness**.

afferent nervous system—The part of the peripheral nervous system that conveys information via neurons, or nerve cells, from sensors in the periphery of the body to the central nervous system.

agility—The ability to rapidly and accurately change body positioning in space.

agonist—The muscle in a muscle pair that actively contracts to move the bone, also known as the prime mover.

alcohol—Although not considered a nutrient, alcohol does contain calories, but these calories provide no benefit as an energy substrate. Alcohol directly interferes with the body's absorption, storage, and use of other nutrients.

alveoli—Small balloon-like air sacs in the lungs.

American College of Sports Medicine (ACSM)—Recognized as the largest, most respected sports medicine and exercise science organization in the world. The guidelines developed by the ACSM are the primary guidelines used by the exercise profession.

Americans with Disabilities Act (ADA)—Initiated and approved in 1990, the purpose of this federal civil rights law is "to establish a clear and comprehensive prohibition of discrimination on the basis of disability." The ADA is a federal civil rights law that prohibits the exclusion of people with disabilities from everyday activities.

amino acids—Organic compounds that combine to form proteins.

anaerobic glycolysis—See **glycolytic system**.

anatomical position—The body is erect (or lying supine as if erect) with the arms by the sides, palms facing forward, legs together, and feet directed forward.

angina—Chest pain caused by lack of oxygen to the heart muscle. Angina is a symptom of heart disease.

anorexia—A condition in which a person is obsessed with being thin. It is an eating disorder characterized by an abnormally low body weight, intense fear of gaining weight, and a distorted perception of body weight.

anorexia athletica—An eating disorder, most commonly seen in competitive athletes, characterized by a preoccupation with diet, weight loss, and excessive, obsessive exercise.

antagonist—The muscle in a muscle pair that relaxes or stretches as the opposite muscle contracts.

anterior—Anatomical term describing one body part in relation to another that means "in front of."

anterior shin splint— A chronic injury causing pain in the front of the lower leg; associated with the soft tissue that connects to the tibia, or sometimes the fibula.

anterior tilt—Movement of top part of the pelvis forward.

antioxidant—A substance that protects the body from damage caused by harmful molecules known as free radicals. Found in many foods, including fruits and vegetables.

aorta—A large artery stemming from the left ventricle of the heart that transports oxygenated blood to the body.

appendicular skeleton—Refers to the bones associated with the appendages and includes the bones in the arms, shoulders, legs, and hips.

Aquatic Heart Rate Deduction—See **Kruel Aquatic Heart Rate Deduction**.

Archimedes' principle—The loss of weight of a submerged body equals the weight of the fluid displaced by the body. Thus, the amount of buoyancy a body will experience is reflected by the amount of water that is displaced.

arrhythmia—An abnormal or irregular rhythm of the heart resulting in an irregular heartbeat.

arteriole—The smallest branch of an artery.

artery—Blood vessel that carries blood away from the heart. With the exception of the pulmonary artery, blood carried by arteries is oxygenated.

arthritis—Inflammation of a joint. A broad term that covers more than 100 diseases.

articulation—The point of contact between bones or between cartilage and bone. Also known as a joint.

assisted movement—Any part in the range of motion of an exercise movement that is facilitated by gravity or buoyancy or by the properties of the equipment. The movement is an eccentric muscle action.

asthma—A chronic lung disease that inflames and narrows the airways, resulting in wheezing, chest tightness, shortness of breath, and coughing.

atherosclerosis—An abnormal collection of fat and other materials on the walls of arteries that narrow the openings and increase the risk of blockages.

ATP-PC system—An anaerobic metabolic system providing immediate fuel from stored phosphocreatine.

atrophy—The loss or wasting of muscle tissue through lack of use or disease.

audible cue—Any cue received through hearing, including spoken words (verbal) and sounds, whistles, claps, musical changes, and bells.

automated external defibrillator (AED)—A portable electronic device that automatically diagnoses heart rhythm and treats irregular rhythm through electrical therapy (defibrillation).

autonomic nervous system—The part of the efferent nervous system that transmits impulses to involuntary muscles and glands, such as the heart and the muscles involved in respiration.

autonomy—The freedom of choice; an individual's right to self-determination.

axial skeleton—Consists of the bones found around the axis (the imaginary midline of the body); includes the skull, vertebral column, sternum, and ribs.

back pain—Pain felt in any portion of the back, which may be related to the vertebrae, the ligaments around the spine, inflamation, associated nerves, and other medical conditions.

balance—The maintenance of equilibrium while stationary (static balance) or moving (dynamic balance).

ball-and-socket joint—Synovial joint where a ball-shaped surface articulates with a cup-shaped surface. Movements of this type of joint can occur in all three planes of movement and include flexion and extension, abduction and adduction, rotation, and circumduction.

basal metabolic rate—See **resting metabolic rate**.

base move—The smallest part or segment in choreography that can be modified or changed to create intensity and variety.

basic transition—A shallow- or deep-water transition in which the next move begins where the previous move ended or passes through neutral alignment.

beats per minute (BPM) — Music tempo is measured by the number of beats that occur in 60 seconds. Beats per minute may also refer to the number of contractions of the heart muscle that occur in 60 seconds (the pulse rate).

binge eating disorder—An eating disorder characterized by consuming unusually large amounts of food and, often, feeling guilty or secretive; also referred to as compulsive overeating.

biomechanics—The area of kinesiology that deals specifically with the analysis of movement.

blood pressure—The force the blood exerts against the blood vessel walls.

body composition—The body's relative percentage of fat as compared to lean tissue (bones, muscles, and organs).

body dysmorphic disorder (BDD)—A mental disorder where the individual cannot stop thinking about one or more perceived defects or flaws in their appearance, also called **dysmorphophobia**.

body mass index (BMI)—A measure of body fat based on height and weight that applies to adult men and women, commonly used as the criterion to determine the conditions of overweight and obesity.

bone resorption—The breakdown and absorption of old bone.

bradycardia—An abnormally slow or low heart rate.

bronchi—The two main branches of the trachea.

bronchial tube—Smaller branch of the bronchi.

bulimia—An eating disorder characterized by recurrent binge eating followed by compensatory behaviors (called purging) such as self-induced vomiting, fasting, exercising excessively, or using laxatives, enemas, or diuretics.

buoyancy—The upward force exerted by water on an immersed object. The tendency or ability of an object or body to float.

buoyancy assisted—Movement of a buoyant object toward the surface of the water.

buoyancy resisted—Movement of a buoyant object toward the bottom of the pool.

buoyancy supported—Movement floating on the surface of the water or movements parallel to the pool bottom while suspended below the surface.

bursitis—Inflammation of the bursa, a small fluid-filled sac near a joint that cushions bones, tendons, and muscles.

cadence training—A movement option that begins with a set movement speed (cadence) and then increases or decreases the rate of that cadence to adjust the exercise intensity.

calorie—The amount of heat energy required to raise the temperature of 1 gram of water 1 degree Celsius. Often interchanged with the word *kilocalorie*.

cancer—A collection of related diseases where some of the body's cells begin to divide without stopping and spread into surrounding tissue.

capillary—The smallest of blood vessels with very thin membranes to allow the exchange of oxygen and nutrients for carbon dioxide and waste products.

carbohydrate—An essential macronutrient that is the primary source of energy for the skeletal muscles and the exclusive source of energy for the brain and nervous system.

cardiac arrest—The abrupt loss of heart function caused when the heart's electrical system malfunctions.

cardiac cycle—The simultaneous contraction of the atria followed by simultaneous contraction of the ventricles. This sequence of events is one heartbeat.

cardiac muscle—The muscle found in the heart.

cardiac output—The volume of blood pumped by the heart in 1 minute; stroke volume times heart rate.

cardiopulmonary resuscitation (CPR)—An emergency procedure that combines chest compressions and artificial ventilation.

cardiorespiratory cool-down—The first part of the cool-down; follows the conditioning segment and consists of 5 to 10 minutes of slow, lower-intensity, controlled movement to help the body recover to pre-exercise values.

cardiorespiratory endurance—The capacity of the cardiovascular and respiratory systems to deliver oxygen to the working muscles for sustained periods of energy production.

cardiorespiratory fitness—The body's physical capacity to supply fuel and eliminate wastes in order to perform large muscle movement over a prolonged period of time. Often referred to as *aerobic fitness*.

cardiorespiratory warm-up—The third part of the warm-up where the primary purpose is to gradually elevate heart rate and respiration rate in preparation for more strenuous exercise.

cardiovascular disease (CVD)—A complex disease involving the heart and blood vessels. It may be genetic, and it includes congenital heart defects, but improper diet and lifestyle management are major contributing factors.

cardiovascular system—System composed of the heart, the blood vessels, and the blood.

carpel tunnel syndrome— A chronic injury that results in numbness and tingling in the hand and lower arm caused by a compressed nerve.

cartilage—A dense connective tissue that provides a smooth surface between two bones and acts as a shock absorber for movements in the joint.

cellular level—The second level of structural organization of the human body consisting of the basic structural and functional unit of the body called the *cell*. The body is composed of various types of cells, including muscle cells, blood cells, and adipose cells.

center of buoyancy—The center of the volume of the body displacing the water or the center of a floating object. Usually located in the chest region near the lungs; however, it will vary based on the body composition of the individual.

center of gravity—The center of mass, typically located in an object's geometric center. In the human body, the position of the body parts determines where the center of gravity is at a given time.

central nervous system (CNS)—The brain and spinal cord.

cerebral palsy (CP)—A general term referring to abnormalities of motor control caused by damage to a child's brain early in the course of development.

cervical spine—The section of the vertebral column found in the neck consisting of seven small vertebrae.

chemical level—The first level of structural organization of the human body consisting of all the chemical substances essential to maintaining life.

choreography—The arrangement or written notation of a series of movements.

choreography style—Different methods of linking together moves to create combinations.

chronic bronchitis—A type of chronic obstructive pulmonary disease (COPD) in which airways have become inflamed and thickened. An increase in mucus production contributes to excessive coughing and difficulty getting air in and out of the lungs.

chronic injury—An injury that has a long onset and long duration.

chronic obstructive pulmonary disease (COPD)—A lung disease where the lung is damaged, making it hard to breathe.

circuit training—A type of training that typically combines muscular conditioning with cardiorespiratory training. Often set up in stations, a series of exercises are performed in rotation with minimal rest, often using different types of equipment.

circumduction—Movement at a joint in a circular direction that is a combination of flexion, extension, abduction, and adduction.

coccyx—The section of the spine, also known as the tailbone, consisting of four vertebrae fused into one or two bones.

cohesion—The tendency of molecules of a substance (e.g., water) to stick together.

combination—Two or more moves linked together in sequence. Same as **pattern**.

combination circuit—A circuit training format that combines elements of instructor-guided and self-guided. For example, the instructor leads the class in a cardiorespiratory segment and then the participants move individually or in small groups to various stations.

competence—Confidence in one's skills and improvement.

complete protein—A protein-rich food that contains all nine essential amino acids in the ratio required by the body; usually comes from animal food products.

complex carbohydrate—Carbohydrate that requires a more complicated digestive process and provides a steady stream of glucose in the blood. Complex carbohydrate includes vegetables and whole-grain products that contain dietary fiber and glucose.

component—The smallest part or segment in choreography. Same as **move**.

concentric—The shortening phase of an isotonic muscle action; occurs when the muscle is creating tension while shortening or contracting.

conduction—The transfer of heat to a substance (e.g., water in the pool) or an object in contact with the body.

condyloid joint—A synovial joint formed by a convex surface and a concave surface that provides movement in two planes (flexion and extension, abduction and adduction, limited circumduction).

continuous training—After warming up, a relatively constant level of training is maintained within the targeted training zone for a designated length of time, followed by a cool-down.

contractility—The characteristic of muscle that allows it to shorten or contract when stimulated.

convection—The transfer of heat by the movement of a liquid or gas between areas of different temperatures, for example, cooler water moving by the skin when exercising in the pool.

coordination—Integrating the senses (such as hearing and vision) with movements of the body to smoothly and accurately perform motor tasks.

coronary artery—Blood vessel found in the heart.

coronary artery disease (CAD)—Develops when atherosclerosis affects the arteries of the heart muscle.

corporation—A business structure organized for the purpose of providing professional services as defined by the specific state laws.

cross training—See **variability.**

cue—A specialized form of communication used to initiate action. Used in an exercise class for many reasons, e.g., indicate a transition, provide information on safety or form, offer motivation, share feedback, or encourage relaxation.

cueing—The act of communicating information to instigate action.

deep-water basic transition—Changing from one move to another in deep water where the new movement begins where the previous movement ended.

deep-water exercise—Exercise performed suspended in water at a depth that allows the participant to remain vertical and yet not touch the bottom of the pool, providing a non-impact workout.

deep-water tempo transition—The use of half water tempo to facilitate smooth transitions in deep water exercise by using a pause in neutral alignment.

deep-water transitional move—A movement that allows more time to prepare or stabilize the body in deep water in order to perform the next movement; typically a jog or vertical flutter kick.

density—The ratio between mass and volume (density = mass/volume). The degree of compactness of an object.

depression—Movement of the shoulder girdle or scapulae down toward the hips.

diabetes mellitus—A disease characterized by abnormalities in insulin production by the pancreas, insulin action, or both that causes problems with metabolism and results in glucose intolerance.

diaphragm—The muscle that separate the chest (thoracic) cavity from the abdomen. The main muscle of respiration.

diastole (diastolic pressure)—Relaxation of the heart muscle during the cardiac cycle.

dietary fiber—The part of a plant that the human body typically cannot digest.

Dietary Guidelines for Americans—Published every 5 years by the U.S. Department of Health and Human Services and the U.S. Department of Agriculture, these guidelines offer science-based advice to promote health and reduce risk for major chronic diseases through diet and physical activity. They serve as the foundation for vital nutrition policies and programs across the United States.

digestive system—System composed of the digestive tract—a series of organs joined in a long tube—and other organs involved in digestion, including the liver, gallbladder, and pancreas.

directional cue—A type of transitional cue that communicates to exercise participants the desired direction of travel or the direction to move their bodies.

distress—In an aquatic setting, a person in distress can swim or float, is still breathing, but is having difficulty remaining on the surface to breathe.

dorsal—The back surface of the body; also refers to the top part of the foot or the instep.

dorsiflexion—Moving the dorsal surface of the foot (instep) toward the shin (anterior tibia bone).

drag—The resistance you feel to movement in the water. A function of the water's viscosity, the body's frontal shape and size, and the relative velocity between the body and the water.

drowning—A process that begins when the mouth and nose are covered with water, preventing the person from taking a breath. The process continues until the person gets a breath, either spontaneously, or through rescue breathing.

duration—The length of time an individual exercises. See **time**.

duty of care—The level of responsibility that one has to protect another from harm under the circumstances.

dynamic stabilization—The body's ability to maintain neutral, or near neutral, postural alignment (a stable position) while moving.

dynamic stretching—See **rhythmic stretching**.

eccentric—The lengthening phase of an isotonic muscle action; occurs when the muscle retains tension while lengthening.

eddy—A current moving contrary to the direction of the main current, especially in a circular motion.

efferent nervous system—The part of the peripheral nervous system that relays outgoing information from the central nervous system to the muscle cells.

effort—The amount of force needed to create the movement, such as the muscle contractions necessary to lift a weight or move through the water.

elasticity—The characteristic of muscle that allows it to return to its original shape.

elevation—Movement of the shoulder girdle or scapulae upward, as if shrugging your shoulders.

emergency action plan (EAP)—A preconceived plan of action for emergency situations intended to prepare staff to deal with emergencies in a coordinated effort.

emergency medical services (EMS)—A system of coordinated response and emergency medical care, involving multiple people and agencies.

emphysema—A type of chronic obstructive pulmonary disease (COPD) in which the walls between many of the air sacs (alveoli) in the lungs are damaged. The ability to exchange oxygen and carbon dioxide is impaired, causing shortness of breath.

employee—A person hired to provide services to a company on a regular basis in exchange for wages.

endocrine system—System composed of the glands that produce hormones. The endocrine system and the hormones it produces play an important role in regulating many exercise processes.

endosteum—The layer of old bone cells that line the medullary cavity. These cells are reabsorbed as part of the growth process to prevent the bones from becoming too thick.

energy metabolism—Chemical reactions that release or provide energy needed by the body.

epiphyseal plates—The cartilaginous growth plates located at the ends of bone, particularly in long bones.

essential amino acids—The amino acids that must be consumed in the diet because the body cannot make them.

evaporation—Loss of body heat through the sweating mechanism. The evaporation of sweat from the skin cools the body.

eversion—Turning the sole of the foot outward or laterally.

excess post-exercise oxygen consumption (EPOC)—See **oxygen debt**.

excitability—The characteristic of muscle that allows it to receive and respond to stimuli.

exercise—A type of physical activity consisting of repetitive movement that is planned and structured to maintain or improve one or more fitness components.

exercise behavior—Behaviors that motivate an individual to initiate and maintain regular exercise and influence how the person chooses to exercise.

extensibility—The characteristic of muscle that allows it to stretch.

extension—Returning to anatomical position; an increase in the angle at a joint.

external rotation—See **lateral rotation**.

fascia—A connective tissue covering found on the muscles.

fast-twitch (Type I) muscle fiber—Specialized muscle fibers characterized by their fast speed of contraction; they fatigue more quickly. Referred to as "white muscle."

fat—An energy-rich essential macronutrient that provides energy, protects vital organs, insulates, and transports fat-soluble vitamins.

fat-soluble vitamins—Vitamins that follow the same absorption pathway as fats, and are stored in the body's fatty tissues. Excess amounts can lead to toxic concentrations.

feedback cue—A type of exercise cue that is used to maintain an open line of communication between the instructor and participants.

fibromyalgia syndrome—A chronic condition characterized by fatigue and widespread pain in the muscles, ligaments, and tendons.

flexibility—The ability of limbs to move at the joints through a complete range of motion.

flexion—Moving out of anatomical position; a decrease in the angle at a joint.

footwork cue—A type of transitional cue that describes specifically how the lower body should be used; typically expressed as "right" and "left."

form and safety cue—A cue that address proper posture, safe joint action, appropriate levels of force and intensity, breathing techniques, and muscle focus.

format—The way that an exercise class is arranged.

freely movable (synovial) joints—Bones are held together by synovial membranes and the joint cavity is filled with synovial fluid that allows movement to occur with minimal friction.

freestyle—A style of choreography in which a series of moves are performed without a predictable pattern.

frequency—How often you exercise or train.

frontal plane—Plane of movement that is vertical and extends from side to side, dividing the body into anterior and posterior, or front and back segments.

frontal resistance—Resistance that results from the horizontal forces of the water as the body or body part moves through the water. A direct result of the horizontal forces of water; noticeably increases effort of movement in the water.

frontal surface area—The total area of the surface of an object moving against the resistance of the water.

fulcrum—An axis or pivot point of a lever.

functional fitness training—See **neuromotor exercise**.

general liability—A type of insurance that protects you or your company in the event that a participant is injured on your premises, or if you or one of your employees injures someone or damages property at a participant's location.

gliding joint—Also known as a plane joint, this synovial joint is formed by the proximity of two relatively flat surfaces; allows gliding movements to occur.

glucose—The simple sugar made by the body from carbohydrates.

glycogen—The principal storage form of glucose in animal and human cells.

glycolytic system (anaerobic glycolysis)—An anaerobic metabolic system that results in the incomplete breakdown of carbohydrates into lactic acid.

grounded movement—Movements performed in an upright position, similar to a level I movement, but one foot remains in contact with the pool bottom at all times.

gross negligence—reckless behavior with disregard for risks to others' safety characterized by a failure to exercise even minimal care to protect them; associated with willful indifference toward or disregard for other's rights.

growth mind-set—The understanding that one's own abilities and intelligence can be developed.

half water tempo (1/2 WT)—Movement in the pool that is performed with a bounce every other water beat; in other words, a movement (including the bounce) requires 4 beats of the music. Allows for more focused muscular force in all directions of movement and encourages a greater range of motion.

heart attack—When the blood flow in the coronary arteries becomes blocked by plaque or blood clots, a section of the heart muscle dies. Also called a *myocardial infarction*.

heart murmur—An abnormal or extra heart sound caused by the malfunctioning of a heart valve.

heart rate—The number of times the heart beats or completes a cardiac cycle in 1 minute.

heart rate reserve (HRR)—Maximal heart rate minus resting heart rate.

heart valve dysfunction—Impairment to the heart's ability to pump effectively due to the major valves of the heart being compromised. It can result in inadequate blood flow or heart failure.

heat cramps—Caused by exposure to high heat and humidity along with the loss of fluids and electrolytes, this is the least severe stage of heat-related illness, resulting in muscle pains and spasms.

heat exhaustion—Usually a consequence of losing body fluids through heavy sweating without proper rehydration, this is a more severe type of heat-related illness than heat cramps, resulting in cool, moist, pale, ashen, or flushed skin; headache; nausea; dizziness; weakness or exhaustion; and heavy sweating.

heat stroke—A potentially life-threatening heat-related illness where the individual loses the ability to sweat and cool the body because the temperature control system stops functioning. Signs include red skin that may either be dry or moist; changes in consciousness; rapid, weak pulse; and rapid, shallow breathing.

hemoglobin—A protein found in red blood cells where oxygen is carried.

high-density lipoproteins (HDL)—Known as the healthy cholesterol, HDL helps the body get rid of LDL cholesterol in the blood. Low levels of HDL increase risk of heart disease.

high-intensity interval training (HIIT)—An interval format that includes short periods of very intense anaerobic training.

hinge joint—A synovial joint where two articular surfaces restrict movement largely to the sagittal plane, typically with strong collateral ligaments to provide reinforcement to the joint. Flexion and extension are its primary movements.

homeostasis—A state of equilibrium in an organism or cell maintained by self-regulating processes.

hydrostatic pressure—The pressure exerted by molecules of a fluid on an immersed body.

hyperextension—Moving beyond anatomical position or neutral position; typically occurs in the sagittal plane.

hyperglycemia—Elevated blood sugar (glucose) levels.

hypertension—High blood pressure.

hyperthermia—An elevated body temperature that occurs when a body produces or absorbs more heat than it dissipates.

hypertrophy—An increase in the size or girth of muscle tissue.

hypoglycemia—Abnormally low blood sugar (glucose) levels.

hypothermia—A reduced body temperature that occurs when heat loss exceeds heat production; signs include shivering, numbness, glassy stare, impaired judgment, and loss of consciousness.

imagery cue—A type of exercise cue that uses vivid descriptions that appeal to one or more of the senses (sight, hearing, touch, smell, and taste) to help participants achieve a desired goal in exercise.

immovable joint—Bones are held together by fibrous connective tissue that forms an interosseous (i.e., connecting or lying between bones) ligament or membrane. These joints generally hold two parts of the body together, such as the bones in the skull.

incomplete protein—A protein food that is lacking in one or more essential amino acids. Most plant proteins are incomplete proteins.

independent contractor—An employment category where the individual is typically self-employed, and follows guidelines specified in a contract or agreement but provides services based on their schedule, expertise, and preferences. Also referred to as a subcontractor.

inertia—An object will remain at rest or in motion with constant velocity (speed and direction) unless acted on by a net external (unbalanced) force.

inferior—Anatomical term describing one body part in relation to another that means "below."

inferior vena cava—Large vein that carries deoxygenated blood from the lower half of the body into the right atrium.

informed consent—A form that explains the risks of participating in physical activity, shows that the participant or client understands these risks and voluntarily assumes responsibility for taking the risks.

injury reports—A form used to document all accidents or injuries sustained by any exercise participant or guest at a fitness facility, pool, group exercise class, or personal training session.

insertion—Most muscles have at least two tendons, each one attaching to a different bone. The attachment that is mobile is referred to as the muscle's insertion.

insoluble fiber—A type of dietary fiber that does not dissolve in water and provides roughage. It serves to soften stools, regulate bowel movements, and speed transit of fecal matter through the colon; improve the body's handling of glucose; and reduce the risk of diverticulosis, cancer, and appendicitis.

instructor-guided circuit—A circuit training format where the instructor leads everyone in the class as a group through each station at the same time.

Instrumental activities of daily living (IADLs)—More complex skills necessary for living independently, such as shopping, preparing meals and housework.

insulin—A hormone produced in the pancreas that regulates the amount of glucose in the blood.

integumentary system—System composed of the skin and all the structures derived from the skin (e.g., hair, nails).

intensity—How hard you exercise.

intermediate transition—A shallow-water transition that changes planes, changes between a one-footed and two-footed move without a center bounce, or changes between different two-footed moves without a center bounce. Requires more coordination and core strength to maintain safe alignment than a basic transition.

internal rotation—See **medial rotation**.

interval training—Harder bouts of exercise interspersed with easier bouts; these are also called *work and recovery cycles*.

intervertebral disc—A fibrocartilaginous tissue found between each vertebra of the spine.

inversion—Turning the sole (bottom) of the foot inward or medially.

irregular heart rhythms—A disturbance to the heart's electrical system causes the heart to beat too fast or too slow; extra or abnormal beats may also occur.

isokinetic—A dynamic muscle action performed at a constant velocity.

isometric—Muscle action in which tension is developed in the muscle without movement at the joint or a change in the muscle length.

isotonic—Muscle action in which the muscle shortens and lengthens; movement occurs at the joint.

joint—See **articulation**.

kilocalorie—See **calorie**.

kinesiology—The study of human motion.

kinesthetic awareness—The body's abilities to coordinate motion and its awareness of where it is in time and space.

Kruel Aquatic Heart Rate Deduction—A formula used to determine the difference in heart rate when an individual is standing immersed to chest depth in water as compared to standing on land. This deduction is then included when determining target heart rate.

kyphosis—Refers to an exaggerated curve in the thoracic spine. The head is often too far forward, with rounded shoulders and sunken chest.

lactic acid—The by-product of producing ATP through the glycolytic system (anaerobic glycolysis) that leads to muscle fatigue. Lactic acid can be converted back to glycogen in the liver.

land tempo (LT)—Movement in the pool at the same speed as used on land; sometimes cued as "double time."

lateral—Anatomical term describing one body part in relation to another that means "away from the midline."

lateral tilt—Movement of top part of the pelvis toward the right or left.

lateral (external) rotation—Rotational movement away from the midline of the body.

layer technique—A style of choreography that begins with a pattern that can be repeated. Modifications are gradually superimposed or new moves replace existing moves one at a time in the pattern.

left atrium—A receiving chamber of the heart where oxygenated blood arrives from the alveoli in the lungs.

left ventricle—A sending chamber of the heart that pumps oxygenated blood out of the heart via the aorta.

level I—Movements performed in an upright position that involve impacting movements where both feet are off the pool bottom for a brief period of time and then land or rebound.

level II—Movements performed by flexing at the hips and knees to submerge the body to shoulder depth while executing the move.

level III—Movements performed without touching the pool bottom. The body is submerged to the shoulders, as in level II, while the movement is performed suspended.

levers—A rigid bar that turns around an axis. In the body, the bones represent the rigid bars, called lever arms, and the joints represent the axes or fulcrum.

liability—An obligation, debt, or responsibility owed to someone. As an aquatic fitness instructor, you have the legal obligation and responsibility to ensure the safety of all participants.

liability release (**waiver of liability**)—A form commonly used in the fitness industry to protect the facility or fitness professional from damages and potential lawsuits. Participants agree that they are willingly using the facility and participating in the activity and waive all rights to assign damage or negligence.

ligaments—Dense connective tissue that attaches bone to bone at movable joints, helping to make the joint more stable and protect it from dislocation.

limited liability company (LLC)—A business structure common in the fitness industry where owners are called members; the IRS may treat the LLC like a partnership or a corporation, depending on how many members are involved.

lordosis—An increased curve in the lumbar spine often accompanied by an increased anterior pelvic tilt. The abdomen and the buttocks protrude and the arms hang further back.

low-density lipoproteins (LDL)—Referred to as *unhealthy cholesterol*, LDL can cause buildup of plaque on the walls of arteries. The more LDL in the blood, the greater the risk of heart disease.

lumbar spine—The lower-back area of the vertebral column consisting of five large vertebrae.

lymphatic system—System composed of the lymph, lymph nodes, lymph vessels, and lymph glands that works to protect the body against diseases.

lymphedema—Swelling that occurs in the arms or legs, most commonly caused by removal of or damage to the lymph nodes as part of cancer treatment, either through surgery or from radiation.

macronutrients—Four of the six essential nutrients required by the body for normal growth and function that are needed in large amounts every day—carbohydrate, protein, fat, and water.

maximal heart rate (HRmax)—The highest heart rate a person can achieve during exercise. A commonly accepted estimate of maximal heart rate is 220 minus age.

maximal oxygen uptake ($\dot{V}O_2max$)—The amount of oxygen a person can use during maximal exercise.

medial—Anatomical term describing one body part in relation to another that means "toward the midline."

medial (internal) rotation—Rotational movement toward the midline of the body.

medullary cavity—The space in the center of the bone filled with the bone marrow, which is where blood cells are produced.

micronutrients—Two of the six essential nutrients required by the body for normal growth and function that are needed in small amounts every day—vitamins and minerals.

minerals—Non-caloric, inorganic micronutrients that work as regulators of body processes; are components of various body cells (e.g., iron in red blood cells) or of various structures (e.g., bone).

mirror imaging—A teaching skill where the instructor faces the class while leading the exercises. The instructor is moving in opposition to what the participants should be doing (e.g., when cueing "left," the instructor is physically demonstrating with their right side).

mode—See **type**.

monounsaturated fat—Fat molecules that have one unsaturated carbon bond in the molecule.

motivational cue—A cue that encourages exercise participants to act in a positive manner, mentally or physically.

motivational interviewing—A set of counseling questions and techniques that help participants who are unmotivated or ambivalent to change.

motor neuron—Specialized cells within the efferent nervous system that innervate muscle fibers.

motor unit—One motor neuron and all of the myofibrils it stimulates.

move—The smallest part or segment in choreography. Same as **component**.

movement (step) cue—A type of transitional cue that tells exercise participants the basic movement to be performed.

Multiplane movement—Movements that occur in more than one plane.

multiple sclerosis (MS)—A chronic, potentially debilitating disease that affects the central nervous system (brain and spinal cord). Damage to the myelin sheaths surrounding the nerves causes scarring (sclerosis) that slows or blocks muscle coordination, visual sensation, and other nerve signals.

muscle balance—Balance in strength and flexibility in muscle pairs surrounding any given joint needed to promote optimal mobility and function.

muscular endurance—The capacity of a muscle to exert force repeatedly or to hold a fixed or static contraction over time.

muscular strength—The maximum force that can be exerted by a muscle or muscle group against a resistance in a single effort.

muscular system—System composed of all the skeletal muscles, visceral muscles, cardiac muscle, tendons, and ligaments.

musculoskeletal considerations—A wide range of illnesses or conditions related to the muscles, bones, joints, cartilage, tendons, ligaments, or nerves.

music beat—The steady pulse of a song. Beats can be found in music, created by a metronome or other device, or created by the instructor.

music tempo—The rate of speed at which the beats occur in music; designated as beats per minute (bpm).

MyPlate—Introduced by the USDA in 2011 to replace the previous food pyramid, a diagram designed to provide a more individualized approach to an overall food guidance system for improving diet and lifestyle. Represents the recommended portions of foods from each food group and focuses on the importance of daily making smart food choices in every food group.

negligence—The failure to use the care that a reasonably prudent person would use in a similar situation, resulting in injury or damages.

nervous system—System composed of the brain, spinal cord, nerves, and sensory organs (eyes and ears).

neuromotor exercise—*neuro* (relating to the nervous system) + *motor* (movement or motion). Includes activities to target skill-related components of agility, balance, and coordination; gait training; proprioceptive exercises; and multifaceted activities such as tai chi. Also referred to as *functional fitness training.*

neuron—Highly specialized cell of the nervous system.

neutral body alignment—The ankles, knees, hips, and shoulders are even and parallel with the floor. A vertical line should pass just anterior to the ankles, through the center of the knee, hip, and shoulder joints, and through the center of the ear.

neutral spinal alignment—A specific component of neutral body alignment. From a lateral view, the spine has three natural curves—cervical, thoracic, and lumbar. From a posterior or anterior view, the vertebrae are aligned vertically.

nonessential amino acids—The amino acids that are synthesized in the body.

numerical cue—A type of transitional cue that communicates the desired repetitions of each movement or the number of repetitions remaining before a change.

nutrient—Components of food that help to nourish the body by performing any of the following functions: provide energy, serve as building material, help maintain or repair body parts, promote or sustain growth, and regulate or assist body processes.

nutritionist—A person who advises people on dietary matters relating to health, well-being, and optimal nutrition. There is no legal definition for nutritionists, so educational levels vary.

obesity—A multifaceted health issue that results from various contributing factors, including behaviors, genetics, the community environment, as well as disease and medications. The ACSM defines obesity as a body mass index (BMI) ≥ 30.

omega-3 fatty acid—A type of fat found in certain cold-water fish, omega-3 fatty acids are associated with a decreased risk of cardiovascular disease and with other health benefits.

one-repetition maximum (one-rep max or **1RM)**—The maximum force that can be exerted by a muscle or muscle group against a resistance in a single effort.

organ level—The fourth level of structural organization of the human body, consisting of organs (various types of tissues combined based on function). Examples of organs include the heart, liver, stomach, and brain.

origin—Most muscles have at least two tendons, each one attaching to a different bone. The attachment that is immobile is referred to as the muscle's origin.

ossification—The process of new bone formation. Osteoblasts (bone formation cells) manufacture proteins or collagen molecules in response to mechanical loading or a stress on the bone.

osteoarthritis (OA)—The most common form of arthritis; referred to as *degenerative joint disease* because the cartilage in the joint breaks down, causing the bones to rub together.

osteoporosis—A systemic skeletal disease characterized by low bone mass and deterioration of bone strength, leading to bone fragility and an increased risk of fracture.

Other Specified Feeding and Eating Disorder—Formerly categorized as Eating Disorder Not Otherwise Specified (EDNOS), this diagnosis is applied when an individual's symptoms cause significant distress but do not fit neatly within the strict criteria for other eating disorders (e.g., anorexia, bulimia, or binge eating disorder).

overload—A greater-than-normal stress or demand placed on a physiological system or organ, typically resulting in an increase in strength or function.

overtraining—Long-term reductions in performance and overall ability to exercise due to an imbalance in the amount of exercise and amount of recovery. Occurs when someone trains too hard, too often, or too long.

overweight—A condition in which the individual's weight exceeds the population norm or average. The ACSM defines overweight as a BMI ≥ 25.

oxidative system—An aerobic metabolic system that yields large amounts of ATP in addition to the by-products of carbon dioxide, water, and heat, which is activated to produce energy for long-duration exercise.

oxygen debt—A time of excess oxygen supply at the cessation of exercise where oxygen supply exceeds oxygen demand. Extra oxygen is needed to help the body return to homeostasis by removing waste products, such as lactic acid. Also referred to as **excess post-exercise oxygen consumption (EPOC)**.

oxygen deficit—The period of time when beginning exercise where there is an inadequate oxygen supply.

Parkinson's disease (PD)—A disorder that affects nerve cells in the part of the brain controlling muscle movement. The four fundamental signs are resting tremors, muscle rigidity, slowness of movement, and postural instability.

partnership—A business composed of two or more people who control the business and are personally liable for the partnership's debts.

Pascal's law—Fluid exerts equal pressure on all surfaces of an immersed object when at rest at a given depth.

pattern—Two or more moves linked together in sequence. Same as **combination**.

patterned choreography—A style of choreography, a set pattern of moves is initially taught in its final form. Participants learn by repeating the total combination over and over.

periodization—A way to structure a series of workouts to help ensure that fitness gains are created and overtraining is avoided. It involves cycling of various training aspects during a specific time period.

periosteum—A dense, white fibrous sheath that covers the surface of the bone where muscles and tendons attach.

peripheral nervous system (PNS)—The various nerve processes that branch off from the spinal cord and brain, connecting with receptors, muscles, and glands.

personal training—Individualized and customized fitness programs that meet the needs and goals of a specific client.

physical activity—Movements of the body created by skeletal muscle contractions that result in a substantial increase of energy expenditure compared to resting levels.

physical fitness—A specific set of health-related and skill-related traits that are associated with an individual's ability to perform physical activity.

physiological—Relating to the mechanical, physical, and biochemical functions of a living organism.

pivot joint—A synovial joint consisting of a central bony pivot, a ring of bone and ligament that permits only rotatory movement.

plane joint—Also known as a gliding joint, this synovial joint is formed by the proximity of two relatively flat surfaces, which allows gliding movements to occur.

plantar—The bottom surface or the sole of the foot.

plantar fasciitis—A chronic injury resulting from the inflammation of the plantar fascia that runs from the heel bone to the base of the toes.

plantar flexion—Moving the plantar surface (sole) of the foot away from the body, often referred to as pointing the toes.

platelets—Blood cells that function to clot blood to prevent blood loss during an injury.

plyometrics—A technique to improve jumping ability and power by using the stretch reflex to facilitate recruitment of additional muscle motor units, also referred to as jump training. See also **propelled movements**.

polyunsaturated fat—Fat molecules that have more than one unsaturated carbon bond in the molecule.

posterior—Anatomical term describing one body part in relation to another that means "behind."

posterior tilt—Movement of top part of the pelvis backward.

poststretch—The second part of the cool-down that consists of 5 to 10 minutes of stretching exercises to return muscles to a pre-exercise length.

power—A function of strength and speed; refers to the ability to transfer energy into force at a quick rate.

power tucks—Acceleration is used to emphasize movement under the water to increase the muscular effort. The knees pull forcefully toward the chest (tucking the knees toward the body) and then the legs push forcefully away and toward the pool bottom.

prestretch—The second part of the warm-up, which is optional. Depending on the temperature of the water and the purpose of your class, you might choose not to include the prestretch or to modify it by using dynamic stretching instead of static stretching.

professional liability—A type of insurance that provides protection when you are held legally liable for how you rendered or failed to render professional services.

progression—The rate of advancement of exercise; depends on the individual's health, fitness level, training responses, and exercise goals.

progressive overload—A gradual, systematic increase in the stress or demand placed on a physiological system or organ to promote fitness gains, while avoiding the risk of chronic fatigue or injury.

pronation—Medial rotation of the forearm; turning the palm down or back.

prone—Refers to the body lying in a face-down position.

propelled movements—Refers to plyometrics performed in the water. The reduced gravity provides for reduced motor unit recruitment through the stretch reflex, but increased motor unit recruitment through the water's drag, surface tension, viscosity, and resistance properties.

property insurance—A type of insurance that protects business property and inventory (assets) against physical loss or damage by theft, accident, or other means, even if that property is removed from your place of business when it is lost or damaged.

proprioception—The body's ability to sense internal and external changes and to initiate appropriate responses.

protein—An essential macronutrient composed of long chains of amino acids that play a role in the growth, repair, and maintenance of all bodily tissues which is considered to be the building block of the human body.

protraction—Movement of the shoulder blades forward away from the spine (abduction of scapulae).

psychological—Relating to the mind, especially as a function of awareness, feeling, or motivation.

pulmonary artery—The blood vessel that carries deoxygenated blood from the right ventricle of the heart to the lungs.

pulmonary vein—A vein that carries oxygenated blood from the lungs to the left atrium of the heart.

pure movement—Muscle action void of gravity, water, or equipment.

pyramid choreography—A style of choreography where number of repetitions for each move in a combination is gradually decreased or increased.

radiation—Heat lost through dilation of the blood vessels at the surface of the body. Heat radiates from the body into the surrounding atmosphere.

range of motion (ROM)—The full movement potential of a joint.

rating of perceived exertion (RPE)—A subjective method of assessing effort, strain, discomfort, or fatigue experienced during exercise.

reaching assist—A non-swimming assist to a person in distress where the rescuer extends their arm or an object, such as a rescue tube.

reaction time—The amount of time elapsed between stimulation and acting on the stimulus.

recovery—The body's return to homeostasis.

recreational water illness (RWI)—Illness caused by germs and chemicals found in recreational bodies of water that are spread by swallowing, breathing in, or having contact with contaminated water.

registered dietitian (RD)—A food and nutrition expert who has met the minimum academic and professional requirements to qualify for the credentials.

relatedness—A meaningful connection to others.

relaxation cue—A type of exercise cue to bring awareness to muscle tension versus muscle relaxation; can be used at any point during the class to initiate proper body mechanics or alignment.

reproductive system—System composed of the organs that produce, store, and transport reproductive cells.

resistance—A force to overcome, such as a weight in your hand or the resistance of the water when exercising in a pool.

resisted movement—Any part in the range of motion of an exercise movement that is impeded by the forces of gravity or buoyancy or by the properties of the equipment. The movement is a concentric muscle action.

respiratory system—System composed of the lungs and the various passageways that lead into and out of the lungs.

resting heart rate (HRrest)—Heart rate determined from an average of three 60-second heart rate measurements; each taken prior to rising from bed on three separate days.

resting metabolic rate (RMR)—The calories needed to maintain the processes of life, such as heartbeat, respiration, and thermal regulation. In a clinical setting, RMR is referred to as **basal metabolic rate**.

retraction—Movement of the shoulder blades back toward the spine (adduction of scapulae).

reversibility—The body will gradually revert to pretraining status when exercise is discontinued.

rheumatoid arthritis (RA)—An autoimmune disease where the body's immune system mistakenly attacks the joints, which creates inflammation.

rhythmic cue—A type of transitional cue that expresses the musical counts used during movement.

rhythmic (dynamic) stretch—Type of stretch that involves moving body parts through the full range of motion in a slow, controlled manner.

right atrium—A receiving chamber of the heart where blood first arrives from the body.

right ventricle—A sending chamber of the heart that pumps blood into the pulmonary artery.

risk management—The process of measuring or assessing potential risk and developing strategies to manage the risk.

rotation—Movement around the longitudinal axis of the limb or spine; occurs in the transverse plane.

sacrum—The section of the spine located below the lumbar spine consisting of one bone made up of five fused sacral vertebrae.

saddle joint—A synovial joint, found in the thumb, with saddle-shaped articular surfaces allowing all movements except rotation.

sagittal plane—Plane of movement that is vertical and extends from front to back, dividing the body into right and left parts.

saturated fat—Fat derived mostly from animal sources that is solid at room temperature. Excess saturated fat in the diet has been associated with cardiovascular disease.

scoliosis—A lateral curvature and rotation of the spine. The shoulders and pelvis appear uneven, and the rib cage might be twisted.

seizure—A sudden surge of electrical activity in the brain that usually affects how a person appears or acts for a short time.

self-guided circuit—A circuit training format where participants or small groups rotate independently from station to station.

septum—A wall between the right and left sides of the heart.

service interruption (business interruption)—A type of insurance that covers indirect losses that occur when a direct loss (that results from a covered peril, such as a fire) forces a temporary interruption of business.

sexual abuse liability—A type of insurance that provides coverage in the event you are accused or sued for sexual harassment by a class participant or client.

shallow-water exercise—Exercise typically performed in a vertical position in a water depth from mid rib cage to mid chest, providing a reduced impact workout.

simple carbohydrate—Carbohydrate that is digested and absorbed into the blood stream from the digestive tract, providing a rapid source of energy for the muscles, brain, and nervous system. Simple carbohydrates are sugars.

skeletal muscle—The striated voluntary muscle that attaches to the bones and works with the skeletal system to create movement.

skeletal system—System composed of the bones of the body, the cartilage associated with the bones, and the joints.

skill-related components of fitness—Components of fitness that target enhanced performance in sports and improved motor skills: agility, balance, coordination, power, reaction time, and speed.

slightly movable joint—Bones are held together by strong fibrocartilaginous membranes; examples include the sacroiliac joint and symphysis pubis.

slow-twitch (Type II) muscle fibers—Specialized muscle fibers that are slow to fatigue and are designed for submaximal prolonged exercise, also referred to as "red muscle."

small-group fitness—Two to five people working under the guidance of a fitness professional to achieve health and fitness benefits through a more intimate and personal setting than group exercise classes.

sole proprietorship—A business structure in which an individual and the company are considered a single entity for tax and liability purposes.

soluble fiber—A type of dietary fiber that dissolves in water to form a gel that assists in lowering blood cholesterol levels and slows the process of digestion, allowing for greater absorption of nutrients.

somatic nervous system—The part of the efferent nervous system that transmits impulses to voluntary skeletal muscles which represents the link between the mind and the muscles to control movements.

special population—A group of people with similar characteristics, health conditions, or common age range.

specificity—Only that part of the system or body that is overloaded will adapt and achieve training results.

speed—The rate at which a movement or activity can be performed.

stabilize—A simultaneous contraction in both muscles of a muscle pair that prevents movement at that joint.

standard of care—The degree of care a reasonable person would take to prevent an injury to another.

static stretch—A slow stretch to the point of tightness or mild discomfort that is maintained in the elongated position for a period of time.

steady-state exercise—An exercise state in which the body is able to supply the oxygen needed for exercise; oxygen supply meets oxygen demand.

streamlined flow—A continuous, steady movement of a fluid past a solid object where the rate of movement at any fixed point remains constant.

stretch reflex—A muscle contraction in response to stretching within the muscle.

stroke—A disruption of the blood supply to the brain; cells in the affected area cannot function properly and might be permanently damaged. It is also known as a cerebrovascular accident (CVA).

stroke volume—The amount of blood pumped by the heart in one beat.

superior—Anatomical term describing one body part in relation to another that means "above."

superior vena cava—Large vein that carries deoxygenated blood from the upper half of the body into the right atrium.

supination—Lateral rotation of the forearm; turning the palm up or forward.

supine—Refers to the body lying in a face-up position.

surface tension—The force exerted between the surface molecules of a fluid. This creates a skin on top of the water that makes it more difficult to break through.

synergists—The muscles that contract to stabilize (or fixate) a joint or bone so that another body part can exert force against a fixed point.

synovial joint—See **freely movable joints**.

system level—The fifth level of structural organization of the human body, consisting of systems (several organs grouped together to perform a particular function). All of the systems of the body (e.g., digestion, hormone secretion, and respiration) work together to make up a functional living human.

systole (systolic pressure)—The active contraction of the heart muscle during the cardiac cycle. Ventricular contraction forces blood into the arteries.

tachycardia—An abnormally rapid or high heart rate.

tactile cue—A cue that is received by touch, such as placing a hand on the target muscle group or moving a limb only to the point of contact with an object.

talk test—A subjective measurement of exercise intensity where one's ability to talk during a workout can determine how hard they are exercising.

tempo transition—A deep-water transition that involves using a half-tempo movement (by means of a one-count return to the center position or a center tuck) to create a smooth change from one move to another.

tendon—Strong, fibrous tissue that connects the fascia of the muscles to the bones.

tendonitis—Inflammation or irritation of a tendon.

thermal warm-up—The first part of the warm-up that includes rhythmic movements to generate body heat while allowing for acclimation to the aquatic environment.

thermic effect of food (TEF)—The number of calories that are burned during digestion.

thermic effect of physical activity (TEPA)—The number of calories that are burned during physical activity or exercise.

thoracic spine—The section of the vertebral column found behind the rib cage consisting of 12 midsized vertebrae.

threshold of training—A given overload that must be exceeded in order to see improvements in fitness.

throwing assist—A non-swimming assist to a person in distress where the rescuer throws an object, such as a ring buoy.

tilt—Movements of the pelvis (anterior, posterior, and lateral).

time—The **duration**, or how long a person exercises.

tissue level—The third level of structural organization of the human body consisting of tissues, or groups of cells with similar function and structure. The body is composed of various types of tissues, including muscle tissue, nervous tissue, and connective tissue.

trachea—The tube in the respiratory tract that connects the nasal passages to the lungs.

trans fats—Hydrogenated unsaturated fats with physical properties similar to saturated fats that are typically man-made food products. Trans fats raise LDL (unhealthy cholesterol) levels while also lowering HDL (healthy cholesterol) levels.

transition—A change from one move to another move.

transitional cue—A cue that informs exercise participants that a change is about to take place and explains how to safely and effectively make that change.

transitional depth training—Aquatic exercise performed in pools with water depths between 4 and 6 feet (1–1.8 m), known as a *transitional water depth*. The water is too deep for rebounding exercises; however, the participant touches the bottom of the pool during some movements.

transitional move—Returning to a simple move (typically a bounce in shallow water) before transitioning to another move, allowing more time for the instructor and participants to prepare for the next move. See also **deep-water transitional move.**

transitional water depth—A water depth that is too deep for typical shallow-water vertical exercise, yet too shallow for conventional deep-water vertical exercise.

transverse plane—Plane of movement that is horizontal and divides the body into upper and lower portions.

triglycerides—A type of fat carried in the blood that represents the major form of fat stored and produced by the body and derived from the food we eat. High triglyceride levels increase the risk of heart disease.

turbulent flow—An irregular movement of a fluid past a solid object, with the rate of movement varying at any fixed point.

type—The mode of exercise being performed.

umbrella liability—A type of insurance sometimes referred to as a bridge or additional coverage to your professional liability coverage. It can supply additional coverage if your professional liability isn't enough to cover all expenses for damages resulting from litigation.

unsaturated fat—Fat that is liquid at room temperature. Any fat that is not completely hydrogenated (monounsaturated and polyunsaturated). It may help raise the level of healthy HDL cholesterol in the body.

urinary system—System composed of the organs that produce, collect, and eliminate urine.

U.S. 1976 Copyright Act—A law that spells out the basic rights of copyright holders. In the fitness industry, this directly affects the legal use of music. This law states that "the copyright owner has the right to charge a fee for the use of his or her music in public performance."

Valsalva maneuver—Exhalation against a closed airway, i.e., holding one's breath during the exertion phase of an exercise, which creates unequal pressure in the chest cavity.

valve—A membranous fold within the heart that opens to allow blood to flow into the chambers and then closes to prevent the backflow of blood.

variability (cross-training)—The varying of intensity, duration, or mode (cross-training) of exercise sessions to obtain better overall fitness.

vein—Blood vessel that carries blood toward the heart. With the exception of the pulmonary vein, blood carried by veins is deoxygenated.

velocity—The rate at which an object changes its position; involves speed and also direction. In movements that involve only one direction, speed and velocity are similar.

ventral—The front surface of the body.

venule—The smallest branch of a vein.

vertebrae—The individual bones that make up the vertebral column or spine.

vertebral column—The spine or spinal column of the human body is made up of 26 bones called vertebrae and is divided into five sections.

visceral muscle—The smooth involuntary muscle found in the walls of organs, such as the intestines and esophagus.

viscosity—The friction between molecules of a liquid or gas. The thickness of a fluid that determines its resistance to flow.

visual cue—A cue that is received by seeing; includes hand signals, eye contact, facial expressions, posture, physical demonstration, and body language.

vitamins—Non-caloric organic micronutrients known as the body's regulators, performing every internal action necessary to maintain life. They are classified as water soluble or fat soluble.

vocal cords—Pair of membrane-covered muscles and ligaments located in the mid throat that vibrate to produce sound.

vocal injury—Any alteration in your normal manner of speaking caused by overuse or improper voice projection.

volume—The total amount of exercise achieved during one week.

wading assist—A non-swimming assist to a person in distress where the rescuer wades into the water and typically extends an object, such as a rescue tube.

waiver of liability—See **liability release**.

water—The only non-caloric macronutrient, water is the major element for all of the workings of the human body and the single most important nutrient during exercise.

water-soluble vitamins—Vitamins that are generally absorbed directly into the bloodstream. Because they are not stored in the tissues to any great degree, excesses of these are excreted in the urine, which reduces the potential for toxicity.

water tempo (WT)—Movement in the pool that allows for full range of motion, balanced muscular conditioning, and additional time for safe transitions needed in the aquatic environment. It involves movement on every other beat of the music at the recommended 125 to 150 beats per minute (bpm).

worker's compensation insurance—A type of insurance that provides wage replacement and medical coverage for employees who sustain job-related injuries.

Index

S

T

U

V

W

Y

About the AEA

The Aquatic Exercise Association (AEA) is a nonprofit organization committed to the advancement of aquatic fitness, health, and wellness worldwide. AEA is committed to increasing awareness, education, and networking opportunities to benefit professionals as well as the general public. With AEA, achieving healthy lifestyles through aquatic fitness is a global team effort. AEA embraces cultural diversity in the industry to ensure that individuals worldwide can enjoy and employ the benefits of aquatic fitness programs regardless of age, ability, goals, or interests.

About the Editors, Contributing Authors, and Credits

Editors

Kimberly Huff, MS, CSCS, has an undergraduate degree in physical education and a master's degree in health education. She has experience in clinical and non-clinical settings, as well as in providing continuing education programs for fitness professionals. She is a certified AEA Aquatic Fitness Professional, ACE Group Fitness Instructor, and ACSM Exercise Physiologist and Personal Trainer. She is also a certified NSCA Strength and Conditioning Specialist and NCHEC Health Education Specialist. She was an Associate Editor of the AEA Arthritis Foundation Program Leader manual. A recipient of the 2015 AEA Contribution to the Aquatic Industry Global Award, she currently serves as a member of AEA's Advisory Council and contributes to *Akwa* magazine. She is an AEA Training Specialist, a presenter of certification review courses for ACSM, and an AEA Arthritis Foundation Program Leader Trainer.

Angie Proctor is the Executive Director of the Aquatic Exercise Association (AEA) and has been actively involved in the fitness industry for over 30 years. Her certifications include AEA, ACE, AFAA and IAR. She has had a long and dedicated career with experiences ranging from club management, fitness instruction, personal training and international presenting and training in over 40 countries, to producing over 100 industry videos while managing the AEA and the International Aquatic Fitness Conference (IAFC). Recognized as a pillar in the aquatic health and wellness community, she spends most of her days planning, preparing, and administrating to keep professionals and consumers safe and educated in aquatics.

Julie See serves as the Director of Education for the Aquatic Exercise Association (AEA) and as the Editor of *Akwa* magazine, AEA's member publication. With over 30 years of experience in the fitness industry, her goal has always been to share knowledge, whether through teaching classes, presenting workshops, creating programs, or writing and editing articles. She was the editor of the American Parkinson's Disease Association's 2008 publication, *Aquatic Exercise – An Exercise Program for People with Parkinson's Disease,* a contributing author to the 2013 Multiple Sclerosis Association of America manual, *Aquatic Exercise & Multiple Sclerosis: A Healthcare Professional's Guide,* and project manager for the AEA's 2015 *AEA Arthritis Foundation Program Leader – A Training Guide for Exercise and Aquatic Programming, First Edition.*

Lori Sherlock, EdD, CSCS, is a long-time supporter and educator in the field of aquatics. Dr. Sherlock has been involved with various elements of the aquatic industry since the late 1990s, including therapy and rehabilitation, exercise and personal training, and management and pool operation. As an Associate Professor in the School of Medicine within the Division of Exercise Physiology at West Virginia University, Dr. Sherlock educates and trains students through the Aquatic Therapy Emphasis. Her extensive training in the field, along with her ample certifications, allows the Aquatic Therapy Emphasis to cover the continuum of care within both the exercise and rehabilitation settings while including pool operator certification and managerial guidelines. She is certified through ATRI and serves as an AEA Training Specialist.

Contributing Authors

Deborah Ashlie-Lampl, RN, BA, is known for her special populations work, including the Aqua Hearts Fitness Program for Cardiac Rehabilitation. She has been a registered nurse for over 35 years, and she has a comprehensive background in cardiac nursing. She is a yoga instructor, a certified AEA Aquatic Fitness Professional, and a certified Ayurveda Practitioner. She has published numerous fitness articles and has presented at workshops nationwide. She has a passion for mind-body awareness for disease prevention and is currently writing a book as an in-depth study in this field.

Anne Pringle Burnell created and developed the Peyow™ Aqua Pilates program, and the Stronger Seniors™ Workout Program for older adults and people with disabilities, injuries, or chronic conditions. She has been a featured presenter at international conferences, and authored several articles for *Akwa* magazine. She is a certified faculty member and education provider for AEA, AF, AFAA, NASM, ACE, ATRI, and AquaStretch™, as well as a Stott Pilates® Instructor Trainer. She is also a professional singer in Chicago.

Laurie Denomme, BKin, FAFS, is recognized for her innovative approach to exercise. She is the founder of WECOACH, a unique water and land exercise program. Unlike most other exercise programs, WECOACH uses six directional movements targeting total body functionality. Top consumer magazines, including *Self* and *Weight Watchers,* have called upon her expertise. She has collaborated with industry experts to develop new education programs for exercise professionals, including Aquatic Options, AquaStretch™, and BioExercise. Laurie is the recipient of the 2013 AEA Global Aquatic Fitness Professional Award and 2014 ATRI Tsunami Spirit Award.

Mushi Harush, MA, has been an AEA International Aquatic Training Specialist since 1994. She holds a master's degree from Idaho State University in athletic management and a master's degree from Haifa and Wingate College, Israel, in education and physical education. She works in many areas of aquatics, including fitness programming and hydrotherapy. Her areas of expertise include special populations (overweight, older adults, and bone density concerns) as well as recreation and sport. She is the founder of the Israeli Aquatic Exercise Center which certifies hundreds of instructors throughout Israel. She is also an international presenter and a frequent contributing author for *Akwa* magazine.

Spencer Ingels, MA, is a Provost Fellow in the sport and exercise psychology doctoral program, and in the community counseling master's degree program at West Virginia University. He completed his master's degree in sport and exercise psychology from John F. Kennedy University in California. His experience includes work as a health coach, as a personal trainer, and as a sport and exercise psychology consultant. His research focuses on managing chronic illness through behavior change with a focus on how to empower and train peers to deliver coaching and support to improve health.

Melissa Layne, MEd, is a faculty member in the Kinesiology Department of the University of North Georgia. She began her career 30 years ago after earning a master's degree in exercise physiology from Auburn University. She has been teaching kinesiology students sports nutrition, exercise physiology, and public health for the past 13 years. Melissa is the author of *Water Exercise*, a national fitness presenter, and DVD featured presenter. She is known for her ability to take complicated subject material and break it down into easily understood examples and pieces.

Donna Lewen, BA, owns and operates a mobile post-rehab company in Phoenix, AZ. Her company works with geriatrics, pediatrics, and clients with a variety of health challenges, with a specialization in chronic pain. She has been recognized with the Arthritis Foundation Regional Public Health Partnership Award, the University of Pittsburgh Community Service Award, the Aquatic Therapy Professional of the Year Award (2016), and the Tsunami Spirit Award (2012). She is a co-author of the *Aquatic Solutions for Chronic Conditions Manual*, and is a consultant at Ability360. Certified with AEA and ATRI, she is an international presenter and continuing education provider.

Mick Nelson, BS, MS, is the Club Facilities Development Director for USA Swimming. Mick and his wife, Sue, built their first indoor facility in Danville, Illinois, in 1973, One year later, they opened Nelson's Swim Supply. Through the years, they have formed NSS Inc., WaterWay Therapy Inc., and Poolside Health & Wellness Center. Since joining USA Swimming in 2004, he and Sue have presented at over 70 aquatic conferences, conducted more than 60 Build and Program a Pool Conferences, and been involved in the design and programming of 144 new facilities. Mick's specialty areas include business development, water treatment, and aquatic facility design.

Sue Nelson, BS, is the Aquatic Programs Specialist for USA Swimming. Sue and her husband, Mick, built their first indoor facility in Danville, Illinois, in 1973. One year later, they opened Nelson's Swim Supply. Through the years, they have formed NSS Inc., WaterWay Therapy Inc., and Poolside Health and Wellness Center. Since joining USA Swimming in 2004, she and Mick have presented at over 70 aquatic conferences, conducted more than 60 Build and Program a Pool Conferences, and been involved in design and programming of 144 new facilities. With a degree in exercise science, Sue specializes in aquatic programming for all populations.

Eduardo Netto, MS, graduated from the University of Rio de Janeiro in physical education. He holds a master's degree in human movement and is the Fitness Director of the Body Tech Health Club, with 103 facilities in Brazil. He is responsible for training approximately 3,000 instructors as well as for creating and implementing fitness programs. He is an international presenter, a well-respected fitness professional, and a consultant in Brazil. He holds certifications with ACSM, AEA, AFAA, and ACE, and he has written four books on fitness programs. He is a contributing author for *Akwa* magazine and serves as a continuing education provider in the fitness industry.

Charlotte O. Norton, DPT, MS, ATC, CSCS practices physical therapy in Sacramento, California. She specializes in orthopedics, sports medicine, home health, and aquatic physical therapy. Her company, Building Bridges, is committed to facilitating relationships to provide a holistic continuum of care for her clients. She is the current President for the APTA Aquatic Section. Dr. Norton co-authored *The Aquatic Continuum of Care* and the *Aquatic Tool Box*. She received the 2007 Judy Cirullo Award for Leadership in Aquatic Physical Therapy and the 2016 UC Davis Health Mentoring Award.

Jill E. White, BSE, is an internationally recognized safety, risk management, and training specialist in the field of aquatics. She is the co-founder of the Starfish Aquatics Institute (certification agency for lifeguards, swimming instructors and pool operators) and the managing partner of StarGuard

Elite (provider of training, aquatic risk prevention, and operational support services to waterparks, the cruise industry, and public aquatic venues). She was recognized by *Aquatics International* magazine as one of the "Power 25 of the last 25 years." She was inducted into the World Waterpark Association Hall of Fame. She has received the National Drowning Prevention Alliance Lighthouse Award and the USA Swimming Adolph Kiefer Safety Award.

Flávia Giovanetti Yázigi, PhD, MS, is an assistant professor in the Faculty of Human Kinetics at the University of Lisbon. She received her PhD in physical activity and health and holds a master's degree in exercise and health. She has also completed two post-graduate programs, Exercise Physiology (FMU-SP, Brazil) and Aging and Quality of Life (FMH-UL, Lisbon). She is a member of the Exercise Physiology and Biochemistry Lab, and has 28 years of experience related to exercise and health, especially in designing and developing exercise programs for special populations. She has been actively involved with the Aquatic Exercise Association (AEA) in many projects.

Marjorie P. Zimmerman, BS, received her degree from Douglass College at Rutgers University. She has multiple fitness certifications, including ACE Medical Exercise Specialist, ACSM Cancer Exercise Trainer, Cancer Exercise Specialist, ATRI Ai Chi Trainer, AEA Aquatic Fitness Professional, and AEA Arthritis Foundation Aquatic and Exercise Program Leader. She was on the Arthritis Foundation's national review and revision committee, which revised and updated the AF Aquatic program. In 2006, she developed one of the first exercise programs devoted solely to cancer survivors of all ages and types for a large medically accredited fitness facility in New Jersey.

Sam Zizzi, EdD, CC-AASP, is the Dr. Pat Fehl Endowed Professor of Sport and Exercise Psychology in the College of Physical Activity and Sport Sciences at West Virginia University. He is a certified consultant and Research Fellow in the Association for Applied Sport Psychology. Since 2008, he has served as the principal investigator on a contract with West Virginia's public employees' insurance agency to coordinate the states' largest weight loss program. In addition to publishing more than 60 journal articles and book chapters, he serves on the editorial board of the *Journal of Applied Sport Psychology*. His recent work focuses on health behavior change primarily related to physical activity promotion and obesity prevention.

Photo Contributors

Jeroen Brockweg
Sheryl Ewart
Carolyn MacMillan
Troy Nelson
Debra Zimmerman
AQUA STAND UP®
HYDRO-FIT®
H2O Wear®
HYDRORIDER®
WaterGym®

Models

Monique Acton
Miff Hendriksen
Julia Sullivan
Danielle Yeats
Declan Yeats
Ella Yeats
Matthew Yeats
Heather Zipperer

Apparel, Shoes, and Equipment

H2O Wear®
WaterGym®